HEMATOLOGY, ONCOLOGY SECRETS

Second Edition

MARIE E. WOOD, M.D.
Assistant Professor of Medicine
Division of Hematology and Oncology
University of Vermont College of Medicine
Burlington, Vermont

HANLEY & BELFUS, INC./ Philadelphia

Publisher: HANLEY & BELFUS, INC.
              Medical Publishers
              210 South 13th Street
              Philadelphia, PA 19107
              (215) 546-7293; 800-962-1892
              FAX (215) 790-9330
              Web site: http://www.hanleyandbelfus.com

Note to the reader: Although the information in this book has been carefully reviewed for correctness of dosage and indications, neither the authors nor the editor nor the publisher can accept any legal responsibility for any errors or omissions that may be made. Neither the publisher nor the editor makes any warranty, expressed or implied, with respect to the material contained herein. Before prescribing any drug, the reader must review the manufacturer's current product information (package inserts) for accepted indications, absolute dosage recommendations, and other information pertinent to the safe and effective use of the product described.

Library of Congress Cataloging-in-Publication Data

Hematology/Oncology Secrets / edited by Marie E. Wood.
        p.   cm. — (The Secrets Series®)
    Includes bibliographical references and index.
    ISBN 1-56053-313-7 (alk. paper)
        1. Hematology—Examinations, questions, etc.. 2. Oncology—
    Examinations, questions, etc. I. Wood, Marie E. II. Series.
        [DNLM: 1. Hematologic Diseases examination questions.
    2. Neoplasms examination questions.   WH 18.2 H487 1999]
    RB145.H429726 1999
    616.1'5'0076—dc21
    DNLM/DLC
    for Library of Congress   99-11380
                                                        CIP

HEMATOLOGY/ONCOLOGY SECRETS, 2nd edition   ISBN 1-56053-313-7

Last digit is the print number: 9 8 7 6 5 4 3 2

CONTENTS

iii

IV. GENERAL CARE OF THE CANCER PATIENT

VI. PEDIATRIC ONCOLOGY

VII. HIV-RELATED DISEASES

VIII. CANCER GENETICS

CONTRIBUTORS

Dorothy M. Adcock, M.D.
Assistant Professor of Pathology, University of Colorado Health Sciences Center, Denver; Staff Pathologist, Kaiser Permanente, Aurora, Colorado

Dennis J. Ahnen, M.D.
Professor of Medicine, Department of Medicine, University of Colorado School of Medicine and Denver Veterans Affairs Medical Center, Denver, Colorado

Edythe A. Albano, M.D.
Assistant Professor of Pediatrics, University of Colorado Health Sciences Center, Denver; Pediatric Oncologist, Children's Hospital, Denver, Colorado

Clay M. Anderson, M.D.
Assistant Professor of Medicine, Department of Medicine, Division of Hematology/Oncology, University of Missouri Health Sciences Center, and Attending Physician, Ellis Fischel Cancer Center, Columbia, Missouri

Elizabeth L. Aronsen, M.D.
Clinical Assistant Professor, Department of Medicine, Division of Pulmonary Diseases and Critical Care Medicine, University of Colorado School of Medicine, Denver; Vice-Chairman, Department of Medicine, Rose Medical Center, Denver, Colorado

Louis Bair, D.O.
Department of Family Practice, Presbyterian–St. Luke's Hospital, Denver, Colorado

Mona Bernaiche Bedell, R.N., B.S.N., M.S.P.H., O.C.N.
Nurse Epidemiologist, Denver Public Health Department, and Denver Health Medical Center, Denver, Colorado

S. Mark Bettag, M.D.
Private Practice, Sheboygan, Wisconsin

Samer E. Bibawi, M.D.
Senior Fellow, Hematology-Oncology Unit, and Clinical Instructor of Medicine, Department of Medicine, Hematology-Oncology Unit, University of Vermont College of Medicine, Fletcher Allen Health Care, Burlington, Vermont

Mitchell A. Bitter, M.D.
Clinical Professor, Department of Pathology, University of Colorado Health Sciences Center, Denver, Colorado

Richard F. Branda, M.D.
Professor, Departments of Medicine and Pharmacology, University of Vermont School of Medicine, Burlington, Vermont

Kerry E. Brega, M.D.
Director of Neurosurgery, Denver Health Medical Center, and Assistant Professor of Neurosurgery, University of Colorado Health Sciences Center, Denver, Colorado

Tim Byers, M.D., M.P.H.
Professor, Department of Preventive Medicine, University of Colorado School of Medicine, Denver, Colorado

Allen L. Cohn, M.D.
Associate Professor, Department of Medicine, University of Colorado Health Sciences Center, Denver, Colorado

Michael R. Cooper, M.D.
Director, Experimental Therapeutics Program; Associate Professor of Medicine, Department of Medicine, Division of Medical Oncology, Duke University School of Medicine, Durham, North Carolina

Jeffrey W. Cronk, M.D.
Fellow in Hematology Oncology, Department of Hematology/Oncology, University of Virginia Health Sciences Center, Charlottesville, Virginia

Todd M. De Boom, M.D.
Chief Resident, Department of Pathology, University of Colorado Health Sciences Center, Denver, Colorado

Robert E. Donohue, M.D.
Professor of Surgery, Department of Surgery, Division of Urology, University of Colorado Health Sciences Center, Denver; Chief, Urology Section, Denver Veterans Affairs Medical Center, Denver, Colorado

Lyndah K. Dreiling, M.D.
Instructor, Department of Internal Medicine, Division of Hematology/Oncology, University of Colorado Health Sciences Center, Denver, Colorado

Timothy Egbert, B.S
University of Colorado Health Sciences Center, Denver, Colorado

Brad A. Factor, M.D.
Formerly Fourth-Year Medical Student, University of Colorado School of Medicine, Denver, Colorado

Kyle M. Fink, M.D.
Rocky Mountain Cancer Centers, Columbia Presbyterian–St. Luke's Medical Center, Denver, Colorado

Christina A. Finlayson, M.D.
Assistant Professor, Department of Surgery, Division of Gastrointestinal, Tumor, and Endocrine Surgery, University of Colorado Health Sciences Center, Denver, Colorado

Kerry Scott Fisher, M.D.
Saint Joseph Hospital, Denver, Colorado

Nicholas K. Foreman, M.B., B. Chir.
Associate Professor, Department of Pediatric Surgery, University of Colorado School of Medicine, Denver; Director, Neuro-Oncology, The Children's Hospital, Denver, Colorado

Helen L. Frederickson, M.D.
Gynecologic Oncologist, Saint Joseph Hospital, Denver, Colorado

Ann D. Futterman-Collier, Ph.D.
Senior Lecturer, Department of Psychological Medicine; Co-Director, National Centre for Treatment Development (Alcohol, Drugs, and Addiction), Christchurch School of Medicine, University of Otago, Christchurch, New Zealand

David H. Garfield, M.D.
Associate Clinical Professor of Medicine, University of Colorado Health Sciences Center, Denver, Colorado

William J. Georgitis, M.D., FACP
Associate Clinical Professor, Division of Endocrinology, University of Colorado Health Sciences Center, Denver; Staff Physician, Kaiser Permanente, Denver, Colorado

Barbara W. Grant, M.D.
Associate Professor of Medicine, Department of Medicine, Hematology-Oncology Unit, University of Vermont School of Medicine, Fletcher Allen Health Care, Burlington, Vermont

Marc S. Greenblatt, M.D.
Assistant Professor, Department of Medicine, University of Vermont School of Medicine, Burlington, Vermont

Brian S. Greffe, M.D., C.M.
Staff Oncologist and Assistant Professor of Pediatrics, Department of Pediatrics, University of Colorado Health Sciences Center, and The Children's Hospital, Denver, Colorado

David S. Hanson, M.D.
Clinical Assistant Professor of Medicine, Louisiana State University Earl K. Long Hospital, Baton Rouge; Chief of Medical Oncology, Mary Bird Perkins Cancer Center, Baton Rouge, Louisiana

Kathryn L. Hassell, M.D.
Assistant Professor of Medicine, Division of Hematology, University of Colorado Health Sciences Center, Denver, Colorado

Bryan R. Haugen, M.D.
Assistant Professor, Department of Medicine, University of Colorado Health Sciences Center, Denver, Colorado

Julie Heimbach, M.D.
Third-year Resident, Department of General Surgery, University of Colorado Health Sciences Center, Denver, Colorado

Richard B. Hesky, M.D.
Assistant Clinical Professor, Department of Oncology, University of Colorado Health Sciences Center, Denver, Colorado

Fred D. Hofeldt, M.D., FACP
Professor of Medicine, Department of Medicine, Denver Health Medical Center, University of Colorado Health Sciences Center, Denver, Colorado

Stephen J. Hoffman, M.D., Ph.D.
Formerly Fellow, Department of Dermatology, University of Colorado School of Medicine, Denver, Colorado

Christine M. Holm, M.D.
Adjunct Professor, Department of Hematology/Oncology, University of Osteopathic Medicine and Health Sciences, Des Moines; Staff, The Cancer Center, Des Moines, Iowa

Kathryn T. Howell, M.D.
Private Practice, Englewood, Colorado

Madeleine A. Kane, M.D., Ph.D.
Professor, Department of Medicine, Division of Medical Oncology, University of Colorado Health Sciences Center and Denver Veterans Affairs Medical Center, Denver, Colorado

Robert S. Kantor, M.D.
Private Practice, Lakewood, Colorado

James P. Kelly, M.D.
Associate Professor of Rehabilitation Medicine and Neurology, Northwestern University Medical School, and Director, Brain Injury Program, Rehabilitation Institute of Chicago, Chicago, Illinois

Karen Kelly, M.D.
Associate Professor, Division of Medical Oncology, University of Colorado Health Sciences Center, Denver, Colorado

Douglas Jerome Kemme, M.D.
North Colorado Medical Center, Greeley, Colorado

Catherine E. Klein, M.D.
Associate Professor of Medicine, University of Colorado School of Medicine, Denver, Colorado

J. Frederick Kolhouse, M.D.
Professor of Medicine, Division of Hematology, University of Colorado Health Sciences Center, Denver, Colorado

Robin J. Kovachy, M.D.
Director of Medical Oncology Services, Rocky Mountain Cancer Centers–South Swedish Medical Center, Englewood, Colorado

Jill Lacy, M.D.
Associate Professor of Medicine, Department of Medicine, Yale University School of Medicine, New Haven, Connecticut

Steven P. Lawrence, M.D
Assistant Professor of Medicine, Department of Medicine, University of Colorado Health Sciences Center; Denver Veterans Affairs Medical Center, Denver, Colorado

William E. Lee, M.D.
Clinical Assistant Professor, Department of Medicine, Division of Oncology, University of Colorado Health Sciences Center, Denver; Staff Physician, Centura Health–St. Anthony's Hospitals, Denver, Colorado

Jerry B. Lefkowitz, M.D.
Assistant Professor, Department of Pathology, University of Colorado Health Sciences Center, and Director, University Hospital Coagulation Laboratory, Denver, Colorado

Charles E. Leonard, B.A., M.D.
Clinical Assistant Professor, Department of Radiation Oncology, University of Colorado Health Sciences Center, Denver, Colorado

Bertrand C. Liang, M.D.
Associate Professor, Departments of Medicine and Neurology, University of Vermont School of Medicine, Burlington, Vermont

Alice M. Luknic, M.D.
Instructor, Department of Medicine, Division of Medical Oncology, University of Colorado School of Medicine, Denver, Colorado

Henry T. Lynch, M.D.
Professor and Chairman, Department of Preventive Medicine, Creighton University School of Medicine, Omaha, Nebraska

Jane F. Lynch, R.N., B.S.N.
Instructor, Department of Preventive Medicine, Creighton University School of Medicine, Omaha, Nebraska

Kelly C. Mack, R.N., M.S.N., A.O.C.N.
Oncology Clinical Nurse Specialist, Rocky Mountain Cancer Centers, Denver, Colorado

Richard A. Marlar, PhD.
Director, Coagulation Laboratories, Denver Veterans Affairs Medical Center; Associate Professor of Pathology, Department of Pathology, University of Colorado Health Sciences Center, Denver, Colorado

George Mathai, M.D.
Senior Consultant Physician and Medical Oncologist, Department of Medicine, Christian Medical College, Ludmiana Punjab, India

Jeffrey V. Matous, M.D.
Assistant Clinical Professor, Department of Medicine, University of Colorado School of Medicine, Denver, Colorado

Lori A. McBride, M.D.
Chief Resident, Department of Neurosurgery, University of Colorado Health Sciences Center, Denver, Colorado

Jane M. McCabe, R.N., B.S.N., O.C.N.
Oncology Nurse Clinician, Department of Medicine, Division of Hematology/Oncology, Denver Health Medical Center, Denver, Colorado

Michael T. McDermott, M.D.
Professor of Medicine, Division of Endocrinology, Diabetes, and Metabolism, University of Colorado Health Sciences Center, Denver, Colorado

Wendy C. McKinnon, M.S.
Clinical Assistant Professor, Department of Pediatrics, University of Vermont School of Medicine, Burlington, Vermont

Laura Boehnke Michaud, Pharm.D.
Adjunct Professor of Pharmacy Practice, Department of Clinical Sciences and Administration, University of Texas—Houston Medical School; M.D. Anderson Cancer Center, Houston, Texas

Jeanette Mladenovic, M.D.
Professor and Vice Chair (Education), Department of Medicine, University of Colorado Health Sciences Center, Denver; Director, Medicine and Education, HealthONE Affiliated Hospitals, Denver, Colorado

Bradley J. Monk, M.D.
Assistant Professor, Division of Gynecologic Oncology, University of California, Irvine, College of Medicine, Orange, California

George E. Moore, M.D., Ph.D.
Professor Emeritus of Surgery, Department of Surgery, Denver Health and Hospitals, University of Colorado Health Sciences Center, Denver, Colorado

Patrick L. Moran, M.D.
Assistant Clinical Professor, Department of Medicine, University of Colorado Health Sciences Center, Denver, Colorado

Lisa G. Mullineaux, M.S., C.G.C.
Genetic Counselor, University of Colorado Cancer Center, University of Colorado Health Sciences Center, Denver, Colorado

Nathan A. Munn, M.D.
Staff Psychiatrist, Behavioral Health Services, St. Peter's Hospital, Helena, Montana

Bronagh P. Murphy, M.D
Assistant Professor of Medicine, Division of Hematology/Oncology, University of Vermont College of Medicine, Burlington, Vermont

Adam M. Myers, M.D., FACP
Professor of Medicine, Department of Medicine, Division of Medical Oncology, University of Colorado Health Sciences Center and Denver Health Medical Center, Denver, Colorado

Lorrie F. Odom, M.D.
Professor of Pediatrics, Department of Pediatrics, Division of Pediatric Hematology/Oncology, University of Colorado School of Medicine, and The Children's Hospital, Denver, Colorado

David Ospina, M.D.
Clinical Instructor, Department of Medicine, Division of Hematology-Oncology, University of Vermont College of Medicine, Burlington, Vermont

Eduardo R. Pajon Jr., M.D.
Associate Professor of Medicine, Department of Medicine, Division of Hematology/Oncology, University of Colorado Health Sciences Center, Denver, Colorado

Polly E. Parsons, M.D.
Associate Professor of Pulmonary and Critical Care Medicine, University of Colorado School of Medicine; Director, Medical Intensive Care Unit, Denver Health Medical Center, Denver, Colorado

Daniel G. Petereit, M.D.
Assistant Professor, Department of Radiation Oncology, University of Wisconsin, Madison, Wisconsin

George K. Philips, M.D.
Formerly Clinical Fellow in Hematology/Oncology, University of Colorado School of Medicine, Denver, Colorado

Mark K. Plante, M.D., FRCS
Assistant Professor of Surgery, Department of Surgery, Division of Urology, University of Vermont School of Medicine, Burlington, Vermont

Sheila A. Prindiville, M.D., M.P.H.
Assistant Professor of Medicine, Division of Medical Oncology, University of Colorado Health Sciences Center, Denver, Colorado

Malcolm Purdy, M.D.
Formerly Instructor, Bone Marrow Transplant Program, Department of Medicine, University of Colorado School of Medicine, Denver, Colorado

Julie Pysklo, M.D.
Associate Program Director at Presbyterian-St. Luke's Medical Center, Department of Internal Medicine, University of Colorado Health Sciences Center, Denver, Colorado

Rachel Rabinovitch, M.D.
Assistant Professor and Clinical Director, Department of Radiation Oncology, University of Colorado Health Sciences Center, Denver, Colorado

Peter C. Raich, M.D., FACP
Clinical Associate Professor, Department of Medicine, University of Colorado Health Sciences Center, Denver; Senior Scientist, AMC Cancer Research Center, Denver, Colorado

Haleem J. Rasool, M.D.
Postdoctoral Fellow, Department of Internal Medicine, Division of Hematology/Oncology, University of Missouri—Columbia School of Medicine, and Ellis Fischel Cancer Center, Columbia, Missouri

William A. Robinson, M.D., Ph.D.
Formerly Professor of Medicine, Division of Medical Oncology, University of Colorado School of Medicine, Denver, Colorado

Maureen Ross, M.D., Ph.D.
Professor of Medicine and Pathology, University of Virginia School of Medicine; Director, Bone Marrow Transplant Program, University of Virginia Health Sciences Center, Charlottesville, Virginia

Dennis A. Sanders, M.D.
Assistant Professor of Medicine, Department of Medicine, University of Vermont School of Medicine, Burlington, Vermont

David M. Schrier, M.D.
Physician, Rocky Mountain Cancer Centers–South Swedish Medical Center, Englewood, Colorado

Miho Toi Scott, M.D.
Clinical Assistant Professor, Department of Medicine, Division of Medical Oncology, University of Colorado Health Sciences Center, Denver; Private Practice, Fort Collins, Colorado

Scot M. Sedlacek, M.D.
Clinical Associate Professor of Medicine, Division of Medical Oncology, University of Colorado Health Sciences Center, Denver, Colorado

Paul A. Seligman, M.D.
Professor of Medicine, Department of Medicine, Division of Hematology, University of Colorado Health Sciences Center, Denver, Colorado

Victor Shada, D.O.
Formerly Third-Year Resident, Presbyterian–St. Luke's Hospital, Denver, Colorado

George R. Simon, M.D.
Assistant Professor of Medicine, Division of Medical Oncology, University of Colorado Health Sciences Center and Denver Health Medical Center, Denver, Colorado

Sharon L. Space, M.D.
Fellow, Department of Pediatric Oncology and Bone Marrow Transplant, University of Colorado School of Medicine, Denver, Colorado

Austin L. Spitzer, B.A.
Third-Year Medical Student, University of Colorado School of Medicine, University of Colorado Health Sciences Center, Denver, Colorado

Alka Srivastava, M.D.
Fellow, Hematology-Oncology, Division of Hematology-Oncology, University of Vermont School of Medicine, Fletcher Allen Health Care, Burlington, Vermont

Sally P. Stabler, M.D.
Associate Professor of Medicine, Department of Medicine, Division of Hematology, University of Colorado Health Sciences Center, Denver, Colorado

Andrew W. Steele, M.D., M.P.H.
Assistant Professor, Department of Medicine, University of Colorado Health Sciences Center, Denver, Colorado

Linda C. Stork, M.D.
Associate Professor, Department of Pediatrics, University of Colorado Health Sciences Center, and The Children's Hospital, Denver, Colorado

Douglas Y. Tamura, M.D.
Surgical Resident, Department of Surgery, University of Colorado Health Sciences Center, Denver, Colorado

Russell C. Tolley, M.D.
Physician, Rocky Mountain Cancer Centers, Denver, Colorado

Amy Strauss Tranin, R.N., M.S., O.C.N.
Genetic Cancer Risk Counselor, and Manager, Cancer Prevention Program, The Cancer Institute of HealthMidwest, Kansas City, Missouri

Paul S. Unger, M.D.
Clinical Assistant Professor of Medicine, and Clinical Director of Stem Cell Transplantation, University of Vermont, Fletcher Allen Health Care, Burlington, Vermont

Amy W. Valley, Pharm.D., BCPS
Clinical Assistant Professor of Pharmacy, Clinical Pharmacy Programs, Department of Pharmacology, University of Texas Health Science Center at San Antonio, San Antonio, Texas

Patrick Walsh, M.D.
Assistant Professor, Department of Dermatology, University of Colorado Health Sciences Center, Denver, Colorado

Lari B. Wenzel, Ph.D.
Associate Scientist, Department of Behavioral Science, AMC Cancer Prevention Research Center, Denver, Colorado

Madeline J. White, M.D.
Clinical Associate Professor, Department of Medicine, University of Colorado Health Sciences Center, Denver, Colorado

Ross M. Wilkins, M.D., M.S.
Assistant Clinical Professor, Department of Orthopedics, University of Colorado Health Sciences Center, Denver; Medical Director, Institute for Limb Preservation, Denver, Colorado

Marie E. Wood, M.D.
Assistant Professor of Medicine, Department of Medicine, University of Vermont College of Medicine, Burlington, Vermont

David W. Yandell, Sc.D.
Director, Vermont Cancer Center, Burlington; Professor of Pathology and Medicine, University of Vermont College of Medicine, Burlington, Vermont

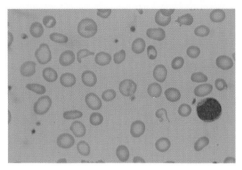

Figure 1. Peripheral blood film showing iron deficiency anemia. The red blood cells are small (compared to a lymphocyte nucleus) and hypochromatic. Notice the rare targets and absence of polychromatophilia. (See p. 23.)

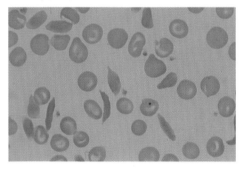

Figure 2. Bone marrow aspirate from a patient with megaloblastic anemia. Megaloblastic erythroid precursors may be mistaken for blasts by the inexperienced morphologist. (See p. 38.)

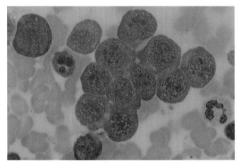

Figure 3. Peripheral blood film showing sickle cell anemia. Sickled erythrocytes are prominent. Polychromatophilia suggests a reticulocytosis and functional hyposplenia is indicated by the presence of a Howell-Jolly body (nuclear remnant in erythrocyte [center]). (See p. 50.)

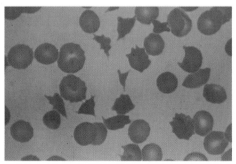

Figure 4. Peripheral blood film from a patient with thrombotic thrombocytopenic purpura. Fragmented cells are prominent. Platelets are decreased. This smear could also be seen in patients with disseminated intravascular coagulation, hemolytic uremic syndrome, malignant hypertension, prosthetic or pathologic heart valves, or large hemangiomas. (See pp. 22, 46, 65, 68.)

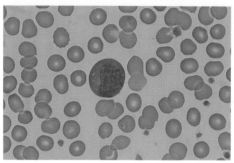

Figure 5. Peripheral blood film showing a reactive lymphocyte. Notice the large size, basophilic cytoplasm, and clumped chromatin (See p. 116.)

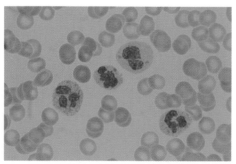

Figure 6. Peripheral blood film from a patient with a leukemoid reaction. Notice the toxic granulation (prominent cytoplasmic granules), and Döhle bodies (blue structures in cytoplasm) within neutrophils. The above findings, in addition to vacuolated polys (not seen in this field), are common in reactive neutrophilias (See p. 31.)

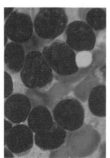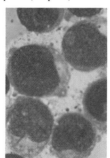

Figure 7. Bone marrow aspirate showing acute myelogenous leukemia (AML) *(left)* and acute lymphoblastic leukemia *(right)*. The myeloblasts are large with fine chromatin and moderate amounts of cytoplasm. An Auer rod *(bottom, center)* is virtually diagnostic of AML. Lymphoblasts are generally smaller with coarse chromatin and scant cytoplasm. (See p. 116.)

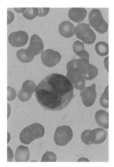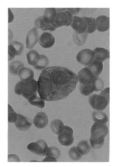

Figure 8. Peripheral blood film showing acute promyelocytic leukemia (APL) (FAB M3) usual form *(left)* and microgranular variant *(right)*. The typical APL cell on the left has a bilobed nucleus and prominent cytoplasmic granules. The microgranular variant (M3v) *(right)* shows cells with the same bilobed nucleus as is seen in the hypergranular form. However, the granules are below the resolution of the microscope and are therefore not visualized. (See p. 120.)

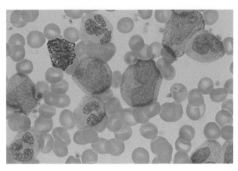

Figure 9. Peripheral blood film from a patient with chronic myelogenous leukemia. Neutrophils at various stages of maturation are seen. Thrombocytosis is common and basophilia is invariably seen. Basophilia can be very helpful in distinguishing this disorder from the leukemoid reaction. (See p. 130.)

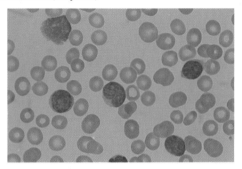

Figure 10. Peripheral blood film from a patient with chronic lymphocytic leukemia (CLL). A lymphocytosis is comprised of small, mature-appearing lymphocytes. Note the smudge cell (degenerated cell) in the lower right corner. Smudge cells are characteristic but not diagnostic of CLL. (See p. 126.)

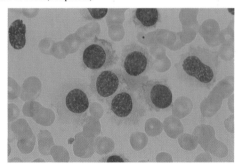

Figure 11. Peripheral blood film from a patient with hairy cell luekemia (HCL). The malignant cells show characteristic nuclear morphology and "hairy" cytoplasmic projections. This illustration is not typical of HCL because it is extremely unusual to find such large numbers of hairy cells circulating in the peripheral blood. (See p. 133.)

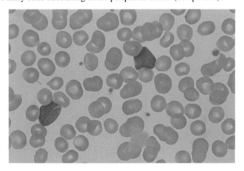

Figure 12. Peripheral blood film showing leukemic involvement by small-cleaved lymphoma. It is not uncommon to see small numbers of circulating lymphoma cells; however, overt leukemia is unusual.

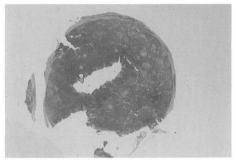

Figure 13. Lymph node showing follicular lymphoma. The neoplastic follicles are numerous and assume a back-to-back arrangement. (See p. 144).

Figure 14. Lymph node from a patient with small, noncleaved (Burkitt's) lymphoma. Notice the prominent "starry sky" appearance. This finding is not limited to small noncleaved lymphoma, but is common in any high-grade lymphoma. (See p. 149.)

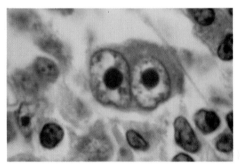

Figure 15. Lymph node from a patient with Hodgkin's disease. A Reed-Sternberg cell shows the typical "owl eye" nuclear appearance. (See p. 159.)

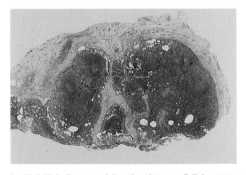

Figure 16. Lymph node showing Hodgkin's disease, nodular sclerosing type. Cellular areas are surrounded by dense fibrous bands. (See p. 160.)

PREFACE TO THE FIRST EDITION

Hematology/Oncology Secrets is intended to provide useful information to medical students, housestaff, and primary care practitioners. The book contains 89 individual chapters under these five broad section headings: General Concepts, General Hematology, Malignant Hematology, General Care of the Cancer Patient, and Solid Tumors. The table of contents will not be reiterated here. Instead, a few areas of possible interest are highlighted.

The first section, General Concepts, addresses the evaluation of eight common problems, with the goal of presenting questions and answers to guide the practitioner before the patient even sees a specialist.

The section on General Care of the Cancer Patient covers management of pain, various complications of chemotherapy, and newer treatment modalities (bone marrow transplantation, growth factors, and monoclonal antibodies), to name a few. Chapters on carcinogenesis, molecular diagnostics, and cancer prevention are meant to introduce the reader to interesting and rapidly developing areas of oncology.

In a section of color plates in the front of the book, 16 illustrations are presented in full color, depicting different types of anemias, leukemias, and lymphomas.

As with other volumes in The Secrets Series®, this book is not meant to be a comprehensive textbook, but rather is meant to provide a general overview of the field. We trust the reader will find the material in these pages readable as well as informative.

Marie E. Wood, M.D.
Paul A. Bunn, Jr., M.D.

PREFACE TO THE SECOND EDITION

The rapidly changing nature of hematology and oncology is reflected in the new information presented in this second edition. Two new timely sections also are included: HIV-related Diseases, which covers malignancies and hematologic abnormalities, and Cancer Genetics, which includes counseling, cancer prevention strategies, hereditary malignancies, and the genetic components of breast and colon cancer.

Several new chapters have been introduced to enhance the section on General Care of the Cancer Patient: Cancer in the Elderly is relevant to all facets of medicine due to the rates of cancer and comorbid diseases in this population, and the chapters that discuss Psychosocial Aspects of Cancer Care and Palliative Care and End-of-Life Decision Making describe effective and empathic clinician-patient communication and ways to alleviate psychological and physical pain.

Again, this book is not meant to be a comprehensive review but rather a general overview, often reflecting the biases and clinical opinions of the authors. I appreciate the input of the authors in this edition who have taken time from very busy schedules to assist in this effort.

Marie E. Wood, M.D.

I. General Concepts

1. EVALUATION AND MANAGEMENT OF THE PALPABLE BREAST MASS

Julie Heimbach, M.D., and Christina A. Finlayson, M.D.

1. What are the characteristics of a dominant breast mass?

Identification of a dominant mass, especially in premenopausal women, can be very challenging. Typically, a dominant mass can be palpated in three dimensions and its density is distinct from surrounding breast tissue. Synonyms of equal importance are nodule, lump, thickening, and asymmetry. Breast cancer cannot be excluded by physical examination alone. "Failure to be impressed by physical exam findings" was the most common reason cited for a delay in the diagnosis of breast cancer.

2. What are the four most common palpable breast masses?

Most dominant masses are benign. These include cysts, fibroadenomas, and fibrocystic masses. Carcinoma, although not the most common type of mass, is the reason that all persistent, dominant masses require a tissue diagnosis. Other less common causes of palpable breast masses are lipomas, granulomas, fat necrosis, epidermal inclusion cysts, and lactational adenomas.

3. What are the differential characteristics of the most common palpable masses?

Although physical examination has only a 75% accuracy in distinguishing benign from malignant abnormalities, certain characteristics may be appreciated on examination of the breast that can be used to generate a differential diagnosis for a specific abnormality. Typically, a **cyst** is a regular, mobile mass that may be tender. It also may be quite firm or fluctuant. A **fibroadenoma** is usually smooth, firm, elongated (longer than it is wide), and mobile, with discreet borders. **Fibrocystic changes** are often described as "lumpy-bumpy" breast tissue. There may be a discrete focal area of fibrosis that is more dominant than the background irregular tissues. **Carcinoma** is traditionally described as an irregular, hard, painless mass. In advanced stages it may become fixed to the chest wall or be associated with overlying skin changes. Although this is the classic presentation, it may present in a form similar to the description for the benign lesions. Lobular carcinoma often appears as a soft mass or area of thickening. Because physical examination alone is unreliable in definitively excluding breast cancer, a biopsy must be obtained for all persistent, dominant masses.

4. A 32-year-old woman presents to the clinic with the complaint of a breast lump. Which questions regarding a patient's history are important in the evaluation of the mass?

Specific questions regarding the size of the mass, whether it has changed in size, how long it has been present, and whether or not it is painful provide clues to the differential diagnosis of this lesion. Other questions regarding skin changes, nipple discharge, or changes in relation to the menstrual cycle may provide helpful information. Evaluation of any breast condition should include an assessment of risk factors for breast cancer, which include personal or family history of breast or other cancers, age of menarche, age at first full-term pregnancy, age of menopause (if applicable), birth control or hormone replacement use, and history of previous breast biopsy.

1

5. The mass identified in question 4 is discrete, not tender, easily palpable, and has been gradually increasing in size. What is the most appropriate next step?

Breast imaging can be useful in further defining the characteristics of a breast mass. Ultrasound of a discrete mass can determine if it is cyst or solid. There are specific ultrasound criteria for defining a simple cyst. A simple cyst may be aspirated or observed. A complex cyst must be further evaluated, which may be done by aspiration to see if it completely resolves or by excisional biopsy. With a complex cyst, fine-needle aspiration (FNA) or core biopsy have a higher risk of sampling error of the solid component. A solid mass requires a tissue diagnosis.

6. How is a cyst aspiration performed?

An 18–22 gauge needle is inserted into the cyst and fluid is withdrawn. Generally, a 10-cc syringe is adequate, although occasionally cysts may contain larger amounts of fluid. If the cyst is quite deep and difficult to fix between your fingers, the aspiration may be performed under ultrasound guidance. Aspiration of a cyst is both diagnostic and therapeutic. After aspiration, the mass should completely resolve. If a mass persists or recurs after two aspirations, the lesion should be excised. Cyst fluid may be clear or cloudy yellow, green, gray, or brown. A purely bloody aspirate or an aspirate of what appears to be old blood should be sent for cytology; consideration should be given to excising the lesion.

7. What techniques are available for diagnosis of a solid breast mass?

Fine-needle aspiration (FNA), core biopsy, incisional biopsy, and excisional biopsy are different techniques that have a role in diagnosing palpable breast masses. Which technique is used depends on the nature of the lesion and available technical support. **FNA** recovers cells from the mass and requires a skilled cytopathologist for accurate interpretation. Several benign and malignant lesions can be accurately characterized by FNA, but it cannot discriminate between invasive and in situ carcinoma. To be used effectively, it must be correlated with physical examination and breast imaging.

Core biopsy is a sampling technique that removes 14–18 gauge pieces of tissue for histologic evaluation by the pathologist. Because it is a sampling, it is possible to "miss" the lesion and obtain a false-negative result. Again, correlation with physical examination and imaging is important to avoid failing to diagnose a breast cancer.

Incisional biopsy is rarely used today. However, it does have a role when a highly suspicious lesion that is also a candidate for neoadjuvant treatment fails to be definitively diagnosed on core biopsy.

Excisional biopsy completely removes the target lesion. It provides the most tissue for pathologic evaluation and, in benign disease, is both diagnostic and therapeutic.

8. What is the role for breast imaging in the evaluation of a palpable breast mass?

Mammography has its greatest success in identifying early breast cancer before it becomes palpable. Annual mammography in women > 40 years of age decreases the risk of dying from breast cancer by approximately 30%. When a woman presents with a palpable abnormality, breast imaging can help to define the lesion as well as screen the remainder of the breast for secondary lesions. In general, breast imaging is done before biopsy because the artifact from the biopsy can interfere with the interpretation of the study. In women < 30 years, when the risk of malignancy is low, mammography should be reserved for only the most suspicious lesions. For women > 30 years, evaluation of a mass suspicious for malignancy includes mammography to characterize the mass as well as evaluate the remainder of the breast. For masses with a low suspicion for malignancy, ultrasound can reliably differentiate between cystic and solid masses. A cyst aspiration or biopsy can be performed accordingly. A negative mammogram does not exclude malignancy: mammography has a false-negative rate of at least 15%. Every solid mass requires a tissue diagnosis.

9. What is meant by the "triple negative test" or "diagnostic triad"?

The three components to diagnosing a palpable breast abnormality are: physical examination, breast imaging, and biopsy. Benign lesions do not have to be removed, but the difficulty is in differentiating between a benign and a malignant lesion. When the characteristics of a mass on physical examination are of low suspicion for malignancy, the mammogram is benign, and FNA recovers benign cells, the chance that the lesion is benign is 98%. Treatment options include excision for definitive diagnosis or observation. If observation is elected, the abnormality should be reexamined within 3 months to confirm that it is stable. If any component of the diagnostic triad is questionable, then definitive diagnosis, usually with excisional biopsy, is necessary.

10. Describe three pitfalls that may occur in the management of palpable breast masses.
   1. **"Your mammogram is fine, there's no problem."**

Mammography is but one tool in the diagnosis of breast cancer and cannot be relied on exclusively. The false-negative rate for mammography is at least 15%. Each persistent, palpable breast mass requires a tissue diagnosis.

   2. **"You have an abnormality on mammography, and I can feel it on examination."**

Occasionally, the palpable abnormality on examination is **not** the same lesion as that seen on mammography. Careful correlation with the mammographic location is necessary to confirm the presence of one lesion and not two that require investigation. Usually the breast imaging center will mark the palpable abnormality with a BB or marker to help prevent this type of error.

   3. **"I don't feel anything, you are fine."**

Often a patient can feel an abnormality that the physician does not appreciate. If you do not appreciate a lesion at the site of the patient's clinical concern and breast imaging does not demonstrate an abnormality, a repeat examination within 8 weeks is appropriate. The physician needs to work with the patient until both are satisfied that the lesion has either been evaluated or has resolved.

BIBLIOGRAPHY

1. Cady B, Steele GD, Morrow M, et al: Evaluation of common breast problems: Guidance for primary care providers. Cancer 48:49–63, 1998.
2. Foster RS: Limitations of physical examination in the early diagnosis of breast cancer. Surg Oncol Clin North Am 3:55–65, 1994.
3. Harris JR, Lippman ME, Morrow M, et al (eds): Diseases of the Breast. Philadelphia, Lippincott-Raven, 1996.
4. Morris A, Pommier RF, Schmidt WA, et al: Accurate evaluation of palpable breast masses by the triple test score. Arch Surg 133:930–934, 1998.
5. Singletary SE, Bevers T, Dempsey P, et al: Screening for and evaluation of suspicious breast lesions: NCCN practice guidelines. Oncology 12:89–138, 1998.

2. EVALUATION OF A LUNG MASS

Elizabeth L. Aronsen, M.D., and Polly E. Parsons, M.D.

1. What are the causes of a lung mass?

Lung masses may have benign and malignant causes. Although many other causes exist, benign masses are often granulomas or hamartomas. The frequency of benign disease depends on the patient population studied but may represent 75% of lung masses in some series of solitary pulmonary nodules. Young age, nonsmoking status, stable (small) size of the mass over 2 years, and a benign pattern of calcification in the mass all favor a nonmalignant cause. Metastases from a nonpulmonary site, especially breast, head and neck, or colon, constitute up to 30% of malignant lung masses. The remainder are due to primary bronchogenic cancer or to malignant transformation of other tissues (such as thymus or lymph nodes) within the thorax.

2. How do patients with malignant lung masses present?

Patients with primary bronchogenic cancer generally present in one of four ways:

Asymptomatic. Fifteen percent of all patients with lung cancer are asymptomatic at the time of their diagnosis. Their disease is discovered by routine chest roentgenograph (CXR).

Local disease. Patients with local disease present with symptoms referable to the primary tumor itself or to local invasion of adjacent structures such as bronchi, vessels, or mediastinal structures. Symptoms include cough, dyspnea, chest pain, hemoptysis, wheezing, hoarseness, recurrent pneumonia, pleural effusion, dysrhythmias, dysphagia, Horner's syndrome, and superior vena cava (Hunter's) syndrome.

Metastatic disease. Some patients with metastatic lung cancer present with complaints dependent on the site of the extrapulmonary metastasis. Examples of this may be cerebrovascular accident, hepatomegaly, bone pain, and anemia. Fatigue, anorexia, and malaise, which occur in 20% of patients with lung cancer, are nonspecific systemic symptoms that are not necessarily associated with metastatic disease.

Paraneoplastic syndromes. A large number of paraneoplastic syndromes are associated with lung cancer, particularly squamous cell lung cancer (hypercalcemia) and small cell lung cancer (syndrome of inappropriate secretion of antidiuretic hormone and hypercortisolemia). The importance of correctly diagnosing a patient's symptoms as a part of a paraneoplastic syndrome lies in the fact that the syndrome does not represent metastatic disease and, unlike metastatic disease, does not prevent the patient from pursuing a curative surgical therapy.

3. What other paraneoplastic syndromes are associated with lung cancer?

Endocrine and metabolic. Gene deregulation results in polypeptide release by the tumor and many endocrinologic and metabolic manifestations of paraneoplastic syndromes, including:

Hypercalcemia	Hypercortisolemia	Hyperthyroidism
Hyponatremia	Hypophosphatemia	Hypercalcitonemia
Acromegaly		

Neurologic. A number of neurologic paraneoplastic syndromes associated with small cell lung cancer have autoimmune mechanisms, including:

Eaton-Lambert myasthenia
Limbic encephalitis
Necrotizing myelopathy
Subacute peripheral sensory neuropathy
Chronic intestinal pseudo-obstruction

Hematologic
Anemia
Polycythemia
Coagulopathy

Cutaneous
Clubbing
Acanthosis nigricans
Hypertrophic pulmonary osteoarthropathy
Tylosis

Renal
Membranous glomerulonephritis
Nephrotic syndrome

4. What are the risk factors for lung cancer?

By far the biggest risk for lung cancer is tobacco use. Smoking causes approximately 85% of the 170,000 lung cancers diagnosed in Americans each year. According to the Surgeon General, 5000 of the 145,000 deaths due to lung cancer each year occur in patients exposed to passive smoke. Other risk factors that increase the incidence of lung cancer include occupational exposures to asbestos, arsenic, radon, ionizing radiation, chloromethyl methyl ether, and chromium. Tobacco abuse is synergistic to these other exposures. An increased incidence of lung cancer in males and in African-Americans independent of smoking history also may be observed.

5. Is there a noninvasive means of distinguishing benign vs. malignant causes of a lung mass?

There is a great deal of interest in the use of single-photon emission computed tomography (SPECT) to measure 18F-fluorodeoxyglucose (FDG) uptake in pulmonary masses. SPECT imaging is generally positive in malignant masses > 2 cm and negative in benign masses, making this a potentially useful imaging modality in patients who may be poor surgical risks. However, ultimately one needs a histologic diagnosis requiring tissue sampling.

6. Why is the histology of a lung cancer important?

The major histologic types of primary bronchogenic cancer are small cell lung cancer (SCLC), which accounts for 20% of all lung cancers, and non-small cell lung cancer (NSCLC). NSCLC may be further divided into squamous cell (30%), adenocarcinoma (30%), large cell undifferentiated (15%), and bronchoalveolar (< 5%) carcinomas. Knowing the histology of a lung mass is important for several reasons:

To direct further work-up. For example, adenocarcinoma and SCLC metastasize to the central nervous system more frequently than other cell types. Some physicians argue that all patients with lung cancer due to one of these two cell types should undergo head CT scan as part of their work-up.

To direct therapy. Chemotherapy is considered primary therapy for SCLC, whereas early stages of NSCLC require surgical resection for definitive cure. Metastatic lesions from other primary sites carry a different prognosis and require different therapy than primary bronchogenic lung carcinoma.

Paraneoplastic syndromes. Specific cell types often are associated with specific paraneoplastic syndromes. Therefore, knowing the histology of the lung mass alerts the physician to be especially vigilant for such symptoms.

7. Discuss specific procedures that can be used to determine the histology of a lung mass.

Lung mass tissue may be obtained in several ways:

Sputum cytology is most helpful in central lesions, which are often due to squamous cell carcinoma. Sensitivity and specificity are affected by the method of obtaining the specimen (spontaneous vs. induced), the care taken in preserving the specimen, primary tumor size and location, and skill of the pathologist in interpreting the results. Both false-negative and false-positive specimens are obtained. A negative sputum cytology from a patient with a lung mass on CXR does **not** rule out malignancy, and further work-up must be done.

Fiberoptic bronchoscopy (FOB). The success of FOB in establishing the cause of a lung mass ranges from 50–85% in most studies and depends on the size and location of the lesion, the sharpness of its borders, and whether or not multiple sampling techniques (bronchial wash, bronchial brush, transbronchial needle aspiration, transbronchial biopsy) were used during the procedure. This approach offers the additional advantage of visualization of the airways to look for endobronchial involvement and to determine proximity of the mass to the carina, which is important in staging the tumor. Central tumors often have squamous cell or small cell histologies.

Percutaneous transthoracic fine-needle aspiration (PTFNA). Peripheral lesions, especially those abutting the chest wall, are amenable to computed tomography (CT) or fluoroscopy-guided PTFNA. Diagnostic sensitivity may be as high as 90% in an experienced operator's hands. The histology of such tumors is most frequently adenocarcinoma or large cell carcinoma.

Open lung biopsy (OLBx). Small peripheral lung masses without evidence of nodal involvement or metastatic disease, termed solitary pulmonary nodules (SPN), are often removed entirely during OLBx through thoracotomy or thoracoscopy. The advantage of this approach is that the surgery is not only diagnostic (in greater than 95% of patients) but frequently curative.

Biopsy of a peripheral metastatic lesion. Lung cancer can metastasize to sites such as the supraclavicular lymph nodes or skin where the tissue becomes readily accessible to biopsy.

Thoracentesis. A pleural effusion can be associated with lung masses of multiple causes. Thoracentesis may be diagnostic as well as therapeutic for those patients presenting with shortness of breath. Two-thirds of malignant pleural effusions result from lymphoma or breast cancer.

8. Who is a candidate for surgical resection of a lung mass?

Simply put, a patient with NSCLC at clinical stage IIIa or less is a surgical candidate. (For further classification and staging information on primary bronchogenic carcinomas, see chapter

63, Lung Cancer.) Other candidates may include patients in whom the diagnosis is still in doubt, or patients in whom the lung mass represents a single metastatic lesion from a nonlung primary. However, further work-up must be done before recommending surgery, which includes assessing the patient's general ability to undergo surgery, evaluating the patient for pulmonary reserve sufficient to withstand resection of lung parenchyma, and determining the resectability of the tumor. Controversy exists about whether a patient with SCLC is ever a surgical candidate (see question 13.)

9. What general and pulmonary-specific preoperative assessments should be done for a patient before recommending thoracotomy for a lung mass?

Preoperative assessment of a patient about to undergo thoracotomy for resection of a malignancy includes determining the general risks of surgery as well as predicting the pulmonary-specific morbidity associated with the planned operation. Obviously, someone who has medical conditions prohibiting him or her from undergoing the risks of surgery does not need extensive work-up to assess the resectability of his or her disease.

General assessment. Any patient undergoing anesthesia for surgery requires a thorough history and physical as part of the preoperative assessment. The patient with lung cancer often has a history of tobacco use associated with a higher risk of other diseases such as hypertension and cardiovascular disease, which may increase the risk of the operation. Comorbid diseases need to be assessed and optimal medical therapy instituted before operation. Routine laboratory analysis includes complete blood count, creatinine and electrolyte analyses, coagulation studies, and liver function tests. All patients with risk factors for cardiovascular disease require electrocardiograms. Nutritional assessment should be done and every effort made to optimize the patient's performance status.

Pulmonary-specific assessment. Patients who will undergo parenchymal resection for a lung mass also need specific assessment of their pulmonary reserve. Spirometry is often the first pulmonary function test ordered. In general, a reasonable **post**operative goal is a forced expiratory volume in 1 second (FEV_1) of 0.8 liters (L). Patients with a preoperative $FEV_1 > 2$ L ordinarily may undergo resection, including pneumonectomy, without further testing. An FEV_1 of 0.8 L or less excludes virtually all patients from consideration of surgical therapy. For the majority of patients, additional work-up includes differential ventilation or perfusion lung scanning to determine the contribution of the parenchyma planned for resection to the overall FEV_1. For example, a patient in whom 60% of lung function is contributed by the right lung would likely be able to undergo total **left** pneumonectomy with a preoperative FEV_1 of approximately 1.3 L. However, the same patient would need a preoperative FEV_1 of at least 2 L to undergo total **right** pneumonectomy. Similar calculations may be made for smaller resections such as lobectomies or wedge resections. For indeterminate cases, many physicians would recommend further testing, including maximal voluntary ventilation (MVV), exercise testing, or ventilation-perfusion (V/Q) lung scanning. Finally, hypercarbia is associated with a higher surgical risk (although many such patients also will be excluded for insufficient pulmonary reserve), and most patients should have a preoperative arterial blood gas analysis.

10. What work-up is necessary to assess the resectability of a chest malignancy?

Once it has been established that surgery is not contraindicated in a patient, then the resectability of the lung mass must be established within the limits of a clinical assessment. This is done in several ways:

Chest computed tomography (CT). Virtually all patients will have a chest CT. This procedure establishes the boundaries of the primary tumor and suggests the minimal extent of parenchymal resection required. Multiple nodules not visible on plain film are sometimes found this way. It also can suggest invasion of adjacent structures, lymph node involvement, and liver or adrenal metastasis.

Bronchoscopy. Patients who have not undergone bronchoscopy as part of their initial work-up of a lung mass should probably have it done as part of the staging. Bronchoscopy is necessary to evaluate the endobronchium for metastatic lesions and to assess the extent of proximal bronchial involvement that may exclude the patient from consideration of surgical therapy.

Mediastinoscopy. In patients with lymph nodes > 1 cm in diameter by chest CT, mediastinoscopy with lymph node biopsy is often recommended to stage the disease; enlarged lymph nodes are not specific for locally metastatic disease and do not necessarily exclude the patient from surgical resection. In contrast, for the patient with borderline function, mediastinoscopy as an intermediate step to surgery may prove nonresectable disease and avoid the larger, more morbid procedure.

Thoracentesis. All patients with pleural effusions and lung cancer should have thoracentesis to rule out metastatic disease. The characteristic effusion associated with lung cancer is hemorrhagic and exudative. Sensitivity of diagnosis is increased with repeat thoracenteses.

Brain CT is often recommended for all patients with lung cancer, especially those with adenocarcinoma or SCLC, but probably should be reserved for patients with neurologic signs or symptoms. Frontal lobe metastases may result only in behavioral changes.

Bone marrow aspirate and biopsy. This is often done in patients with SCLC as part of the routine staging procedure and should be strongly considered for all patients with SCLC being considered for surgical resection (see also Controversies) to rule out extensive disease.

11. Which modalities besides surgery are available for treating lung cancer?

No therapy of lung cancer should be considered exclusive of combination modalities.

Chemotherapy remains the primary therapy for most, if not all, cases of SCLC. Most regimens include cyclophosphamide and/or platinum combination chemotherapy. Chemotherapy is less successful for the most resistant NSCLC. Tumor susceptibility testing is often done on resected tissue.

External beam radiation therapy (XRT) is often used as palliative treatment, but long-term survival is reported with this therapy for both NSCLC and SCLC.

Photodynamic therapy (PDT) is used with success most often for carcinomas in situ. Photosensitizing agents given intravenously are concentrated in the cancer cells. The bronchoscope directs an argon laser light (wavelength 630 nm) to the lesion where toxic oxygen radicals are formed, causing cell death.

Laser therapy. The neodymium-yttrium-aluminum-garnet (Nd-YAG) laser (wavelength 1064 nm) induces photocoagulation and thermal necrosis in endobronchial lesions. Its primary use has been in palliative therapy of metastatic disease.

Brachytherapy is endobronchial radiation therapy used in cases of carcinoma in situ as well as for endobronchial metastatic lesions.

Immunotherapy is likely to be used in the future as tumor-specific cell surface markers are identified.

CONTROVERSIES

12. Why not screen all high-risk patients for lung cancer with routine CXR and/or sputum cytology?

For:

1. The most curable lung cancer, i.e., stage I disease, usually presents asymptomatically. Therefore, screening is the only method available for detection.

2. Although periodic CXR screening has not been shown to reduce mortality, it does appear to improve stage distribution and resectability of lung cancer. CXR and sputum cytology represent complementary, noninvasive methods of screening for a disease with high morbidity and mortality.

3. Prolonging even one life through early detection of lung cancer is worth whatever the cost.

Against:

1. The prevalence of lung cancer was less than 0.7% for all ages in a large multicenter study of high-risk patients screened by these methods. Screening these patients alone would represent

an enormous economic burden on the health care system. Even in patients with a lung mass on CXR, the cost of sputum examination per correct diagnosis is over $63,000.

2. The vast majority of resectable lung masses have a benign cause. The finding of an incidental lung mass on screening CXR will impel such patients to undergo further unnecessary, expensive, and potentially morbid diagnostic procedures in order to reassure both patient and physician that the mass is not malignant.

3. Most lung cancer is associated with tobacco use. The money would be better spent in education to prevent smoking.

13. Should patients with limited SCLC be offered surgical therapy?

For:

1. About 4% of SPNs are SCLC histologically. In such patients, surgical resection is potentially curative.

2. After chemotherapy and/or radiotherapy, the incidence of local recurrence is high, suggesting a role for adjuvant surgical therapy.

3. The primary tumor may be mixed NSCLC and SCLC cell type, suggesting a role for combining surgical therapy with standard SCLC chemotherapy and/or radiotherapy. Others have suggested that a carcinoid SCLC subtype may be more favorable for surgical resection.

Against:

1. No controlled studies demonstrate that patients with SCLC treated surgically have any survival advantage over those treated with chemotherapy and/or radiotherapy alone.

2. Most patients with SCLC, including those with SPN, have micrometastases at the time of diagnosis, suggesting that they also must receive adjuvant chemotherapy.

3. There is no evidence that partial resection of a primary SCLC tumor has any advantage for subsequent conventional chemotherapy or radiotherapy.

BIBLIOGRAPHY

1. Beckett WS: Epidemiology and etiology of lung cancer. Clin Chest Med 14:1–15, 1993.
2. Cortese DA, Edell ES: Role of phototherapy, laser therapy, brachytherapy, and prosthetic stents in the management of lung cancer. Clin Chest Med 14:149–159, 1993.
3. Faber LP: Issues in the management of chest malignancies. Clin Chest Med 13:113–135, 1992.
4. Midthun DE, Swensen SJ, Jet JR: Clinical strategies for solitary pulmonary nodule. Annu Rev Med 43:195–208, 1992.
5. Patel AM, Davila DG, Peters SG: Paraneoplastic syndromes associated with lung cancer. Mayo Clin Proc 68:278–287, 1993.
6. Reilly JJ Jr: Preoperative and postoperative care of standard and high risk surgical patients. Hematol Oncol Clin North Am 11:449–459, 1997.
7. Rubins JB, Rubin HB: Temporal trends in the prevalence of malignancy in resected solitary pulmonary lesions. Chest 109:100–103, 1996.
8. Worsley DF, Celler A, Adam MJ, et al: Pulmonary nodules: Differential diagnosis using 18F-fluorodeoxyglucose single-photon emission computed tomography. Am J Roentgenol 168:771–774, 1997.
9. Goldberg-Kahn B, Healy JC, Bishop JW: The cost of diagnosis: A comparison of four different strategies in the workup of solitary radiographic lung lesions. Chest 111:870–876, 1997.
10. Lillington GA, Caskey CI: Evaluation and management of solitary and multiple pulmonary nodules. Clin Chest Med 14:111–119, 1993.
11. Strauss GM: Prognostic markers in resectable non-small cell lung cancer. Hematol Oncol Clin North Am 11:409–434, 1997.
12. Schaffer K: Imaging and medical staging of lung cancer. Hematol Oncol Clin North Am 11:197–213, 1997.
13. Strauss GM, Gleason RE, Sugarbaker DJ: Screening for lung cancer. Another look: A different view. Chest 111:754–768, 1997.

3. EVALUATION OF A TESTICULAR MASS

Robert E. Donohue, M.D.

1. Name the structures normally palpated during the routine scrotal examination and the most common abnormality involving each structure.

The structures to be palpated are the testis, epididymis, the space between the testis and epididymis to allow localization of a mass, the vas deferens, the veins of the pampiniform plexus, if present, and the contents of the tunica vaginalis. The most common abnormality of each structure is listed below:

Testis: germ cell tumor, 7,000 new cases per year (diagram 2 below)

Epididymis: epididymitis, lower pole (diagram 3)

Space between the testis and epididymis: to distinguish a testicular from an epididymal mass (diagrams 1, 2, and 3)

Vas deferens: sperm granuloma from previous vasectomy (diagram 3)

Spermatic veins: varicocele

Tunica vaginalis: hydrocele (diagram 4)

Examine the patient supine first and then upright. The normal scrotal side should be examined first. The examination should be completed with adequate exposure and without gloves. If an abnormality is detected, it should be diagrammed, and the diagram should be labeled as to the side of the scrotum. The diagram is completed as if the patient were standing and turned 90° (see below).

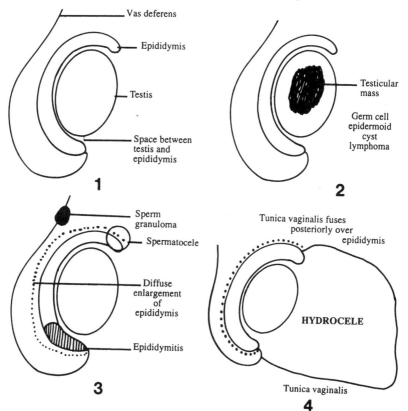

2. What are the significant events in the past history of a patient with a testicular mass thought to be a germ cell tumor?

The three significant events in the past history of a patient with a germ cell tumor are (1) cryptorchidism, either corrected or uncorrected (the age at correction is irrelevant); (2) testicular atrophy (most commonly from postpubertal mumps orchitis); and (3) recent trauma.

3. What percentage of intratesticular masses are germ cell tumors? Of these, what percentage are a single histologic type and what percentage are mixed tumors?

Ninety-seven percent of all intratesticular masses are germ cell tumors. Sixty percent of all germ cell tumors are a single histologic type, whereas 40% are mixed tumors.

4. Name the germ cell tumors and give their clinical incidence.

Seminoma: 40%   Teratocarcinoma: 25–30%
Embryonal cell carcinoma: 20–25%   Choriocarcinoma: 1%
Teratoma: 5–10%

5. What are the non-germ cell tumors of the testis?

The interstitial tumors of the testis are the Leydig cell and the Sertoli cell tumors. They account for about 2% of testis tumors. Lymphoma occurs in older men (50 plus years), whereas metastatic disease from any primary extragonadal lesion may occur. Lung tumors are the most common metastatic tumors to the testis; prostatic tumors are the most common genitourinary tumors metastatic to the testis.

6. Which structures should be examined in a directed physical examination in a patient with suspected testis tumor?

- The supraclavicular lymph nodes—metastatic spread of tumor filtered from the thoracic duct lymph
- Breasts for gynecomastia—elevated human chorionic gonadotropin (hCG) from tumor leads to symmetric or asymmetric breast enlargement
- Upper abdomen, subxiphoid—first site of nodal metastases, the perirenal hilar area
- Lower abdomen for inguinal scars from previous surgery and masses—scars suggest a previous orchidopexy, hernia, or varicocele and possible altered lymphatic drainage to the inguinal nodes; a mass suggests inguinal adenopathy or tumor in an undescended testis
- Testis with the mass in it
- Opposite testis—the contralateral testis may be the site of the tumor when the ipsilateral testis was cryptorchid. The patient also may have simultaneous bilateral tumors. Lymphomas are the most common tumors to present simultaneously bilaterally.

7. If a testis tumor is suspected, what serum markers should be drawn preoperatively? What are the half-lives of these markers? Can their value after orchiectomy be of use?

The serum markers to be drawn are the alpha-fetoprotein (AFP), beta-chain human chorionic gonadotropin (β-hCG), and lactic dehydrogenase. The AFP half-life is 5–7 days; the β-hCG half-life is 24–36 hours. If the values of the markers decline with respect to their half-lives, it suggests that no other tumor is present in the patient.

8. Is age significant in the final histology of the patient with a testis tumor?

The three peak periods for testis tumors are the 20–40 age group, infancy, and late adulthood (> 60 years). The testis tumor is the most common solid tumor in men between 20 and 35 years of age. Infants have benign teratomas, whereas preteens suffer from yolk sac tumors. Young adult men, aged 25–35, have embryonal cell carcinomas and teratocarcinomas (embryonal cell carcinomas with teratomas). Men aged 35 and older have a higher percentage of seminomas, whereas the most common testicular tumor in men over age 60 is lymphoma.

9. What is the initial treatment for a suspected testis tumor?

Radical inguinal orchiectomy is the treatment of choice. An inguinal incision is made; the testis is delivered into the inguinal canal, and after high ligation of the spermatic cord at the internal inguinal ring, orchiectomy is completed. If doubt exists as to the diagnosis, the tunica vaginalis can be opened in the inguinal area and the testis examined directly.

10. How do you stage a testis tumor?

Staging of the diagnosed testis tumor consists of determining the extent of the tumor in the testis and surrounding structures, chest PA and lateral films, serum markers preoperatively and postoperatively, CT scan of the abdomen and possibly of the chest, and possibly a brain scan. The venous and lymphatic channels of the testis also should be carefully examined for tumor cells or tumor thrombus within them. Tumor stage is as follows:

Stage A: confined to scrotum
Stage B1:   < 6 retroperitoneal lymph nodes: none larger than 2 cm
Stage B2:   > 6 retroperitoneal lymph nodes: none larger than 5 cm
Stage B3:   palpable retroperitoneal nodes: nodes larger than 5 cm
Stage C: metastatic disease anywhere beyond the retroperitoneal lymph nodes—supra-
clavicular nodes, mediastinum, lung, liver, or brain metastases

11. If a testicular tumor is diagnosed and orchiectomy does not show the intratesticular mass to be a malignancy, what is the lesion, how common is it, and could it have been correctly diagnosed preoperatively?

The mass is an epidermoid cyst and its incidence is 1% of intratesticular masses. Fifty percent occur in the third decade of life. No diagnostic study at the present time short of orchiectomy allows the diagnosis to be made with certainty. The lesion may represent a monolayer teratoma and is benign.

12. Acute unilateral painful scrotal swellings associated with nausea and vomiting in a teenager or adult are most likely caused by what entity? What is the natural history of this entity?

The most likely entity is torsion of the spermatic cord. In any acute unilateral scrotal swelling, testicular torsion, testicular appendage torsion, epididymitis, epididymo-orchitis, and trauma must be considered.

The natural history of torsion of the spermatic cord is sudden onset of pain, often awakening the patient from sleep, with the pain peaking immediately, and associated with nausea and vomiting. Scrotal swelling occurs almost immediately. If asked, the patient often relates a history of multiple previous episodes. The spermatic cord torsion is produced by the heightened cremasteric reflex activity of puberty with a congenital abnormality of testicular fixation to the spermatic fascia of the scrotum.

Remember, the majority of patients with mumps orchitis have a preexisting parotid inflammation. Recall that mumps orchitis is a postpubertal infection of the testis.

13. What is the treatment of choice for acute spermatic cord torsion?

Manual untwisting of the spermatic cord torsion should be attempted if the event has occurred within 6 hours. This procedure allows an elective bilateral orchidopexy. If the attempt at untwisting is unsuccessful or if the acute torsion has persisted for more than 6 hours, immediate scrotal exploration and ipsilateral orchiectomy or orchidopexy (testicular fixation to the internal spermatic fascia) and contralateral orchidopexy must be accomplished.

14. How many hours of ischemia may elapse before the testis suffers irreversible ischemic damage and atrophies?

In our study, if the torsion of the spermatic cord was corrected by surgical untwisting and fixation within 6 hours, none of our patients had any atrophy when examined from 6 months to 10 years after the acute episode. The opposite testis, also fixed at the original surgery, was used as the normal testis size for each patient.

15. What time period must elapse after torsion of the spermatic cord and testicular fixation before the physician can state that the testis will undergo no atrophy or undergo no further atrophy?

Testis atrophy from the ischemic episode that results from torsion of the spermatic cord will usually occur within 6 months.

16. Name the three most common organisms that cause bacterial epididymitis.

Bacterial epididymitis is the most common type of epididymitis. The most common organisms causing this condition are *Chlamydia trachomatis* and *Neisseria gonorrhoeae* in males under 35 years of age and *Escherichia coli* in men over 35 years of age.

17. How does bacterial epididymitis present?

Bacterial epididymitis presents as gradually increasing scrotal pain, peaking over many hours; possible inguinal discomfort; and urethral discharge or urinary frequency, urgency, and burning, without anorexia, nausea, or vomiting. The patient may be febrile. Physical examination reveals a lower pole mass of the epididymis. The urinalysis is abnormal. Prehn's sign, improvement in the pain with ipsilateral elevation of the swollen scrotal content, is suggestive of epididymitis and may be positive.

18. Name the most common lesion of the head of the epididymis.

A spermatocele is the most common lesion (diagram 3, page 9).

19. Is unilateral absence of the vas deferens a significant physical finding? What other scrotal abnormalities are associated with its absence?

Yes. Unilateral absence of the vas deferens is associated in 70–90% of cases with ipsilateral absence or agenesis of the kidney. The contralateral solitary kidney has a significant abnormality in 33% of patients. Associated scrotal and pelvic abnormalities include absence of the ipsilateral epididymis and seminal vesicle and an ipsilateral spermatocele. The testis is normal.

20. How should a varicocele be examined?

A varicocele is varicosities of the pampiniform plexus of the internal spermatic vein. The variocele should collapse with elevation: the ipsilateral testis may be smaller in up to 25% of adult men with a varicocele because of failure of the testis to grow during puberty.

There are three periods of significance to the patient with a varicocele:

1. Preteens and teenagers because of impaired growth of the developing testis on the side of the varicocele

2. Adult men because of impaired fertility

3. Sudden onset in the adult man suggesting increased pressure in or on a large venous vessel, the renal vein or inferior vena cava

21. Is the sudden appearance of a varicocele in an adult a significant finding?

The sudden appearance of a varicocele suggests either intrinsic or extrinsic compression of the renal vein or inferior vena cava by a mass, which is most commonly malignant. The most common lesions are metastatic testicular carcinoma, lymphoma, renal cell carcinoma, and primary retroperitoneal malignancies. Abdominal ultrasonography should be performed to evaluate the patient initially. A CT scan of the abdomen may be required.

22. List the three most common entities that involve the tunica vaginalis.

1. Clear fluid within the tunica vaginalis from an inflammatory, ischemic, or traumatic testicular or epididymal event is a **hydrocele**.

2. Bloody fluid, usually after trauma, is a **hematocele**.

3. Omentum or small or large intestine entering into the scrotum via a patent processus vaginalis is an **incarcerated, indirect inguinal hernia**. An impulse may not be detected on examination.

BIBLIOGRAPHY

1. Berger R, et al: Etiology, manifestations and therapy of acute epididymitis, a prospective study of 50 cases. J Urol 121:750–757, 1979.
2. Coolsaet B: The varicocele syndrome: Venography determining the optimum level for surgical management. J Urol 124:833–839, 1980.
3. Donohue R, et al: Torsion of the spermatic cord. Urology 11:33–37, 1978.
4. Donohue R, et al: Unilateral absence of the vas deferens—A useful clinical sign. JAMA 261:1180–1181, 1989.
5. Meacham RB: Testicular metastases as the first sign of colon cancer. J Urol 140:621, 1988.
6. Prehn DT: A new sign in the differential diagnosis between torsion of the spermatic cord and epididymis. J Urol 32:191, 1934.
7. Richie J: Neoplasms of the testis. In Walsh PC, et al (eds): Campbell's Urology, 6th ed. Philadelphia, W.B. Saunders, 1992, pp 1222–1266.
8. Vordermark J, et al: Epidermoid cysts of the testes and the role of sonography. Urology 41:75–78, 1993.
9. Whitmore WF: Testicular cancer in cryptorchids. Cancer 49:1023–1030, 1982.

4. INTRACRANIAL MASSES

Lori A. McBride, M.D., and Kerry E. Brega, M.D.

1. How do intracranial masses commonly present?

1. **Focal deficits** secondary to local mass effects of the tumor in the brain are the presenting signs in 68% of intracranial tumors and may have significant localizing value. For example, a patient with aphasia and right-sided hemiparesis most likely has a left posterior frontal mass.

2. **Seizures** secondary to irritation of cerebral cortex are the presenting symptoms in 26% of tumors. All patients with a first-time seizure should be evaluated by computed tomography (CT) or magnetic resonance imaging (MRI) with and without IV contrast.

3. **Increased intracranial pressure** (ICP) secondary to large tumor size or multiple small tumors is often seen with lesions localizing to the "silent" areas of the brain.

4. **Hydrocephalus** may result from mechanical obstruction of cerebrospinal fluid (CSF) flow. Mechanical obstruction and resulting hydrocephalus also may produce signs and symptoms of increased ICP.

2. What are the signs and symptoms of increased ICP?

Headache, vomiting with (or especially without) nausea, papilledema, and decreased level of consciousness.

3. What other entities may present as intracranial masses? How are they differentiated from tumors?

1. **Abscess**—Abscesses are ring-enhancing on contrast CT and MRI. Patients may have other infections, especially of the lungs or sinuses, or a history of facial/head trauma or surgery.

2. **Stroke**—CT and MRI appearance may mimic tumor. Strokes tend to have mass effect only in younger patients. Strokes may be clinically distinguished from tumors by the abrupt onset of symptoms and by the presence of specific risk factors.

3. **Hemorrhage**—Acutely, hemorrhages are uniformly bright on noncontrast CT scans. They also ring-enhance after the first few days.

4. **Aneurysm**—Aneurysms appear bright on noncontrast CT, roundly shaped, and usually located at the circle of Willis.

PRIMARY CENTRAL NERVOUS SYSTEM TUMORS

4. What are the most common primary brain tumors in adults? How can they be recognized radiographically?

Primary brain tumors make up one-half to two-thirds of all adult brain tumors.

1. **Gliomas** account for 40–67% of primary CNS tumors in adults. There are several types. Grade IV astrocytomas, also known as *glioblastomas*, are the most common and most aggressive type. They account for 50% of all supratentorial gliomas and 15% of all intracranial tumors. They are unencapsulated and heterogeneously enhancing with areas of central necrosis and significant surrounding edema on CT and MRI scans. Less aggressive forms of gliomas are *astrocytomas* (grades I–III), which make up 25–30% of all supratentorial gliomas. Peak incidence is between 20 and 50 years of age. On imaging studies, they may be cystic. Lower-grade astrocytomas are homogeneous and show minimal enhancement, whereas higher-grade forms are more heterogeneous and contrast enhancement is the rule. The more aggressive forms also tend to create more edema. *Oligodendroglioma*, a less common type of glioma, is seen most often in patients in the 4th and 5th decades of life. These tumors make up 5–7% of all intracranial tumors. Radiographic appearance is similar to the lower-grade astrocytomas, but calcification is common.

2. **Meningiomas** represent 15–18% of intracranial tumors and are usually seen in patients aged 40–60 years. On CT they are homogeneous, hyperdense tumors with homogeneous enhancement. Generally, there is a clear dural attachment (50% parasagittal, 20% sphenoid wing, and 5–10% in the posterior fossa). The dural attachment is often better seen on MRI. Hyperostosis of the adjacent bone is common. Meningiomas are usually solitary but may be multiple, especially in the setting of neurofibromatosis.

3. **Pituitary adenomas** are also common tumors in adults (10–15% of all intracranial tumors). Secreting tumors usually are diagnosed by their endocrine symptoms (prolactin-secreting tumors are most common). Prior to the onset of mass effects, tumors tend to present at a smaller size when endocrinopathies are present, prior to the onset of mass effects. Nonsecreting tumors become symptomatic secondary to their mass effects, usually on the optic chiasm.

5. Identify the more frequent pediatric brain tumors and their characteristics.

Supratentorial tumors (50% of pediatric brain tumors)
- **Astrocytomas.** Low-grade gliomas of the cerebral hemispheres make up 50% of astrocytic tumors in pediatrics. Optic chiasm and hypothalamic gliomas are usually low-grade gliomas as well (10–20% of these patients have neurofibromatosis).
- **Craniopharyngiomas.** These sellar region tumors account for 6–8% of pediatric brain tumors. They may present with hormonal derangements, visual problems, or signs and symptoms of increased ICP. Calcification is common on CT scans.

Infratentorial tumors (make up the remaining 50% of pediatric brain tumors, along with spinal cord tumors, and are much less common in adults)
- **Primitive neuroectodermal tumors (PNET)** are a group of highly malignant tumors including medulloblastoma, pineoblastoma, retinoblastoma, and others. **Medulloblastomas** alone account for one-third of posterior fossa tumors in pediatric patients. They are thought to arise from the superior medullary velum and are therefore usually midline tumors involving the vermis. They often contain cysts or blood on imaging scans, are enhancing, and frequently are associated with obstructive hydrocephalus. Such patients should be evaluated with total spine MRI to rule out CSF seeding of tumors, or "drop mets" in the spinal canal.
- **Cerebellar astrocytomas** are generally low-grade tumors, but the most common subtype (juvenile pilocytic astrocytoma) often has a heterogeneous, cystic, contrast-enhancing appearance on CT and MRI scans. Most often located in the cerebellar hemispheres, they account for 30–40% of posterior fossa tumors in children.
- **Ependymomas** arise from the floor of the fourth ventricle and generally enhance on contrasted scans. Of infratentorial tumors in this age group, 10–20% are ependymomas.

Because of their intraventricular location, they may seed in the CSF pathway and present with obstructive hydrocephalus or cranial nerve palsies due to brainstem compression.

• **Brainstem gliomas.** Ten to 20% of pediatric posterior fossa tumors are gliomas intrinsic to the brainstem. They appear as a low-density enlargement of the brainstem without enhancement. Presenting symptoms reflect their slowing progressive brainstem compression or infiltration, which result in cranial nerve palsies, motor or gait difficulties, or signs of hydrocephalus.

METASTATIC LESIONS OF THE CENTRAL NERVOUS SYSTEM

6. What is the incidence of metastatic tumors to the brain?

Metastases make up one-third to one-half of all adult brain tumors. Metastases are seen in 20–40% of adult and 10–15% of pediatric cancer patients. Two-thirds of these metastases become symptomatic. One-third of patients with brain metastases have no primary diagnosis.

7. Name the most common sources of metastatic disease to the brain.

Bronchogenic carcinoma remains the most common source of brain metastases. In adults, the most frequent sources of brain metastases are, in descending order, lung (44–57%) > breast (10–19%) > GI (primarily colon) > GU (primarily kidney) > melanoma. In patients under age 21, metastases usually result from neuroblastoma, sarcoma (osteogenic sarcoma, rhabdomyosarcoma, Ewing's sarcoma), and germ cell tumors. Conversely, certain tumors (which may themselves occur infrequently) have a strong tendency to metastasize to the brain. At autopsy, 46% of patients with testicular cancer are found to have brain metastases. Similarly, 40% of melanoma, 21% of lung, 20% of renal cell, and 9% of breast cancer patients have brain lesions at the time of death.

8. What are the radiographic characteristics of brain metastases?

Brain metastases have several classic features on imaging studies. Generally, they appear well-circumscribed and enhance on contrasted scans. A significant ring of peritumoral edema is the norm. Their expected location is at the gray-white junction. The most common site is near the junction of the temporal, parietal, and occipital lobes, posterior to the sylvian fissure. A probable mechanism is embolic spread to the narrow terminal branches of the middle cerebral artery found in this region. Tumors known for metastasizing to the meninges are adenocarcinomas (of the lung, breast, stomach, and colon), lymphomas, and leukemias.

Approximately 50% of metastases are single on CT scan. Colon, breast, and renal cell cancer typically produce single metastases, whereas melanoma (and occasionally lung malignancies) leads to multiple metastases. Eighty percent of solitary metastases are found in the cerebrum and 16% in the cerebellum, corresponding roughly to the relative volumes of brain in each compartment. Metastases from GI and pelvic sources may spread more frequently via the spinal epidural venous plexus or patent foramen ovale (rather than the usual hematogenous route), because these tumors have three times the rate of posterior fossa metastases compared with other malignancies.

INTRACRANIAL MASSES IN HIV/AIDS

9. What is the differential diagnosis of an intracranial mass in a patient with HIV or AIDS?

Forty percent to 50% of AIDS patients experience CNS dysfunction secondary to direct HIV infection, primary CNS lymphoma, or opportunistic infection. The features of a few of these are reviewed below:

Toxoplasmosis. Infection with *Toxoplasma gondii* is responsible for 70–80% of mass lesions in AIDS patients. The incidence seems to be decreasing, possibly because of the widespread use of pentamidine prophylaxis in AIDS patients. It is usually believed to be a reactivation of prior exposure, and 30% of seropositive AIDS patients will develop active infection.

Abscesses are most commonly located in the basal ganglia or cortex. A ring-enhancing appearance is classic, but inflammation (and therefore enhancement) in the lesions decreases as the immunosuppression worsens.

Primary CNS lymphoma. This rare tumor (2% of primary brain tumors) is usually seen in older or immunocompromised patients—especially those on immunosuppressive therapy (after transplant) or those with AIDS. Lymphomas may have a thick-walled ring of enhancement on CT and MRI scans and often are located in the frontal lobes, deep nuclei, cerebellum, or in a periventricular arrangement. CSF cytology is diagnostic in only 10% of patients; most lumbar punctures reveal only increased protein and cell count. Surgery should be used for biopsy only, because operative removal (even gross total resection) does not change outcome.

Progressive multifocal leukoencephalopathy (PML). PML usually may be diagnosed by its classic radiographic appearance: focal myelin loss causes ill-defined areas of low density in the white matter on CT scans, without contrast enhancement. There is no edema or evidence of mass effect.

10. What is an effective protocol for evaluating patients with AIDS who have unidentified intracranial masses?

Because toxoplasmosis and CNS lymphoma are not readily distinguishable radiographically and must be differentiated to provide appropriate therapy, some method of determining which patients should have a biopsy is needed. No absolute algorithm has been established to determine which patients should be empirically treated and which should be biopsied, but a reasonable protocol is as follows:

1. For patients with possible toxoplasmosis, begin trial of pyrimethamine/sulfadiazine/folic acid. Substitute clindamycin for sulfa-allergic patients.

2. Clinical (radiographic) improvement should be visible in 2–3 weeks. If so, treatment should be continued **for life** to keep toxoplasmosis under control (recurrences are the rule). Doses may be halved after 6–12 weeks.

3. If no response is seen after 2–3 weeks of antibiotics (7–10 day minimum), consider a biopsy (usually stereotactic).

4. Proceed to biopsy without antibiotic trial if:
   (a) The patient's toxoplasmosis titers are negative
   (b) The patient has a rapidly progressive neurologic deficit, and a two-week trial of therapy (if not effective) could potentially significantly alter outcome
   (c) The patient has other known infections or malignancies suggestive of an atypical diagnosis

ANATOMIC SUMMARY

11. What are the most likely diagnoses by region for intracranial masses?
  A. **Cerebellopontine angle tumors**
   1. Schwannoma (usually eighth nerve, i.e., acoustic neuroma)
   2. Meningioma
   3. Epidermoid
  B. **Sellar region tumors**
   1. Pituitary adenoma
   2. Craniopharyngioma—especially in children
   3. Aneurysm
   4. Meningioma
   5. Optic chiasm/hypothalamic glioma—especially in children
  C. **Pineal region tumors**
   1. Germ cell tumors
   2. Pineocytoma/pineoblastoma
   3. Glioma

D. **Deep white matter or periventricular region**
  1. Glioma
  2. Lymphoma
E. **Cortical lesions** (think hematogenous spread)
  1. Metastasis
  2. Abscess
  3. Infarct
F. **Deep cerebellar (adult)**
  1. Metastasis
  2. Glioma
  3. Hemorrhage/infarct
  4. Hemangioblastoma
G. **Posterior fossa (pediatric)**
  1. Medulloblastoma (one-fourth to one-third of tumors)
  2. Juvenile pilocytic astrocytoma (one-fourth to one-third)
  3. Ependymoma (one-sixth)
  4. Brainstem glioma (one-sixth)

MANAGEMENT OF METASTASES

12. What are the management options for metastatic tumors to the CNS?

Radiotherapy. Should be considered standard therapy for brain metastasis.

Chemotherapy. Reserved for malignancies most likely to respond (i.e., lymphoma, small-cell lung cancer). Treatment, however, should include consolidation with radiotherapy.

Surgical resection. Once thought too radical a treatment for patients with metastatic disease, this modality is being increasingly used. Decreased perioperative risk and shorter recuperation times now make surgery a more attractive option. Sawaya et al. reviewed outcomes in patients with newly diagnosed and recurrent brain metastases after surgical removal, whole-brain radiation therapy, or stereotactic radiosurgery. Their results show that surgical tumor resection leads to longer survival and improved quality of life for such patients.

Stereotactic radiosurgery. Recently considered as a treatment option, even for tumors that have proved resistant to conventional radiation therapy. Early results are promising. Kida et al. report a series of 26 metastatic lesions from various primary tumors treated with gamma knife stereotactic radiosurgery. Tumor control rates (cessation in growth or regression in tumor size) averaged 85.7% at 9 months. Eighteen of the 26 patients were neurologically stabilized or improved at follow-up. The advantage to this treatment is that there is only one treatment session, not a series as with conventional radiotherapy. It should be noted that it is fairly new; longer follow-up is needed as well as other studies to confirm the early data.

13. When is surgical therapy considered for patients with solitary or multiple brain metastases?

  1. When the lesion is located in an area that is surgically accessible.
  2. When the lesion has become symptomatic or life-threatening due to compression of nearby structures or overall increased ICP. The surgeon must weigh the quality of life in making this decision, not just overall survival.
  3. When the primary disease is reasonably well controlled (i.e., a life expectancy of more than 4 months).
  4. When a diagnostic biopsy is needed (i.e., the primary tumor is unknown).

BIBLIOGRAPHY

1. Galicich JH, Arbit E: Metastatic brain tumors. In Youmans (ed): Neurological Surgery. Philadelphia, W.B. Saunders, 1990, pp 3204–3222.
2. Greenberg MS: Handbook of Neurosugery. Lakeland, FL, Green Graphics, 1994.

3. Kida Y, et al: Gamma-radiosurgery of metastatic tumors. No Shinkei Geka 21(11):991–997, 1993.
4. Morantz RA, Walsh JW: Brain Tumors: A Comprehensive Text. New York, Marcel Dekker, 1994.
5. Osborn AG: Diagnostic Neuroradiology—A Text/Atlas. St. Louis, Mosby, 1993.
6. Sawaya R, et al: Surgical treatment of metastatic brain tumors. J Neurooncol 27(3):269–277, 1996.
7. Smirniotopoulos JG: Correlation of neuroradiology and neuropathology. In Mena H, et al: 35th Annual Armed Forces Institute of Pathology Neuropathology Review. Washington, DC, Armed Forces Institute of Pathology, 1997.

5. EVALUATION OF ANEMIA

Samer E. Bibawi, M.D., and Richard F. Branda, M.D.

1. What are the first steps in evaluating a patient with anemia?

The first steps should include the evaluation of a peripheral smear, a reticulocyte count, and red cell indices. The smear can yield useful information about the cause of anemia, e.g., the association of hypersegmented neutrophils with B_{12} or folate deficiency, spherocytes with autoimmune hemolysis or hereditary spherocytosis, schistocytes with microangiopathy (e.g., thrombotic thrombocytopenic purpura [TTP] or disseminated intavascular coagulopathy [DIC]) and changes such as basophilic stippling commonly seen with lead toxicity. The reticulocyte count is significant because if elevated, it indicates blood loss due to hemolysis or bleeding. On the other hand, a low or normal reticulocyte count indicates a marrow underproduction process, such as iron deficiency, anemia of chronic disease, or myelodysplasia. Further work-up of the anemia will depend on the findings of a peripheral smear and reticulocyte count.

Similarly, evaluating red cell indices can yield helpful information. The mean corpuscular volume (MCV) refers to the mean (or average), red blood cell (RBC) volume and should be interpreted with the RDW (RBC distribution width), which is a measure of the homogeneity of size of the red cell population. A high MCV with a normal RDW indicates a homogenous state of macrocytosis, making megaloblastic anemia a likely cause. On the other hand, a normal MCV with a high RDW indicates a potential coexistence of mixed etiologies, e.g., iron and folate/B_{12} deficiency. The RDW is also useful when evaluating microcytosis with mild or no anemia; in cases of iron deficiency it will be elevated, whereas in certain thalassemia traits it will be normal.

Red Cell Morphologies and Commonly Associated Anemic Processes

RED CELL	DESCRIPTION	ASSOCIATED DISEASE(S)
Basophilic stippling	Basophilic inclusions, fine or course	Fine: various anemias Coarse: lead toxicity, thalassemia
Howell-Jolly bodies	Small, single, basophilic inclusion	Postsplenectomy
Hypochromic cells	Central pallor > $\frac{1}{3}$ RBC diameter	Iron deficiency, thalassemia
Polychromatophilia	Grayish-blue hue	Reticulocytosis
Schistocyte (helmet cell)	Red cell fragment	TTP, DIC
Spherocyte	Spherical cell with absent central pallor	HS, AIHA
Target cell	Target-like appearance	Liver disease, thalassemia
Tear drop cell	Drop-shaped cell	Myelofibrosis, myelopthisic process

AIHA = autoimmune hemolytic anemia; DIC = disseminated intravascular coagulopathy; HS = hereditary spherocytosis; TTP = thrombotic thrombocytopenic purpura.

Evaluation of Anemia Based on Red Cell Indices

MCV LOW RDW NORMAL	MCV LOW RDW HIGH	MCV NORMAL RDW NORMAL	MCV NORMAL RDW HIGH	MCV HIGH RDW HIGH
Thalassemia trait	Thalassemia major	Chronic disease	Combined deficiency	Folate or B_{12} deficiency
Chronic disease	Iron deficiency	Hereditary spherocytosis	Early iron, folate or B_{12} deficiency	Autoimmune hemolysis

MCV = mean corpuscular volume; RDW = RBC distribution width.

2. Discuss how to correct the reticulocyte count; is this process necessary?

The reticulocyte count is reported as a percentage of circulating red cells; hence, it will vary with the degree of anemia. Correction can be done in one of two ways: the first is to multiply the observed reticulocyte percent by the absolute RBC count, which yields the absolute reticulocyte count (normal range: 24,000–84,000/mm^3). Another way to correct for the level of anemia is to multiply the observed reticulocyte percent by the observed hematocrit and divide by the normal hematocrit (45). Note that correction for anemia always lowers the reticulocyte percent; thus, if the observed percent is already low, correction will not add any useful information. Correct the reticulocyte percentage only if it seems elevated.

3. In the evaluation of iron deficiency, should a ferritin level be obtained, or will serum iron and iron-binding capacity (IBC) suffice?

Classically, iron deficiency anemia is associated with a low serum iron and an elevated IBC. The transferrin saturation (obtained by dividing iron by IBC) should be less than 10%. However, serum iron is a negative acute phase reactant, meaning that iron levels will be low in cases of acute stress. Also, a normal serum iron may reflect the patient's intake of a single high-iron meal or a multivitamin and minerals pill (such pills are frequently given to hospitalized patients). If a patient has a coexistent chronic inflammatory process, his or her IBC may be decreased. Therefore, it is important to routinely integrate ferritin, which reflects body stores of iron, into the work-up of iron deficiency anemia. Despite being an acute phase reactant, if the body stores of iron are low, it is unlikely that ferritin levels will increase substantially. Similarly, a markedly elevated ferritin, even in the face of acute stress, rules out iron deficiency.

4. What are the hallmarks of anemia of chronic disease and what are the mechanisms involved in its pathogenesis?

First, a chronic inflammatory disease underlies this type of anemia. Malignancy leads to anemia by a similar mechanism and hence is frequently included in this category. The hallmarks are a normochromic/normocytic anemia (sometimes hypochromic/microcytic), normal or low reticulocyte count, low serum iron and IBC, and an elevated ferritin. Such findings reflect impaired iron utilization in spite of abundant iron stores. Chronic inflammation or malignancy is associated with inflammation-associated cytokines, namely interleukins (IL-1 and IL-6), tumor necrosis factor (TNF-α) and interferon (IFN-γ), and underproduction of erythropoietin by the kidneys. These abnormalities lead to the development of anemia of chronic disease.

5. Is checking serum erythropoietin levels of any value?

This depends on the disorder associated with anemia. After other possible causes of end-stage renal disease have been ruled out, patients may be given erythropoietin (EPO) without checking its level. Similarly, anemic patients with advanced malignancy or patients undergoing active chemotherapy do not need their levels checked. On the other hand, some patients with myelodysplastic syndrome may benefit from EPO replacement, provided their levels are less than 500 mIU/ml. Because EPO replacement is expensive, first check levels in this group of patients to identify the subset that might benefit from this approach.

6. How long does it take to deplete the body stores of folate and vitamin B$_{12}$?

The folic acid storage pool in the body is relatively small, which leads to deficiency in a matter of weeks if intake is decreased (folate deficiency is rampant among alcoholics) or if demands are increased (e.g. during pregnancy or in chronic hemolytic states). On the other hand, B$_{12}$ stores are much larger and daily requirements are small; deficiency takes years to develop and occurs mainly in patients with impaired absorption (e.g., patients with pernicious anemia or postgastrectomy states) or in strict vegetarians.

7. Are serum folate and B$_{12}$ levels diagnostic of their tissue status?

Not always. Extremely low serum levels are indicative of deficiency and very high levels probably rule it out, especially with B$_{12}$. Serum folate levels fluctuate widely with intake, and one folate-rich meal can temporarily normalize blood levels. If in doubt, RBC folate is a better reflection of body stores. B$_{12}$ levels that are in the low-normal or upper-low range are best described as indeterminate. A confirmatory test is the serum methylmalonic acid (MMA) test, the levels of which will be increased in B$_{12}$ deficiency. MMA is a co-enzyme for mitochondrial methylmalonyl-CoA mutase and responsible for converting potentially toxic methylmalonyl-CoA to succinyl-CoA, which is readily metabolized. Note that the kidneys clear MMA, and elevated levels should be interpreted in the presence of normal renal function only.

8. Is bone marrow examination a necessary step in evaluating anemia?

Although a bone marrow biopsy is considered the gold standard for diagnosing most cases of anemia, it is usually not a necessary step. The investigative methods descibed previously usually reveal the cause of anemia. Although it is a low-risk procedure, bone marrow biopsy is an uncomfortable procedure and should be done only when indicated. Older patients with unexplained anemia usually require this procedure to evaluate for myelodysplastic syndrome, which is not infrequent in the elderly. Needless to say, if a neoplastic process such as lymphoma or leukemia is suspected as the cause of anemia, bone marrow examination becomes mandatory.

9. Explain how to evaluate a case of suspected hemolytic anemia.

The first step is to establish hemolysis. First, evaluate the reticulocyte count, which should be elevated, and examine the peripheral smear for nucleated red cells, reticulocytes, schistocytes or microspherocytes. In hemolytic states, bilirubin (mainly of the unconjugated portion) is frequently elevated. Serum lactate dehydrogenase (LDH) should be elevated as well. Once hemolysis is established, you should search for the cause (see question 10).

10. How is intravascular hemolysis distinguished from extravascular hemolysis?

After hemolysis is established, it is important to distinguish intravascular from extravascular hemolysis. The prototype for intravascular hemolysis is incompatible blood transfusion; other causes are microangiopathic processes such as TTP or DIC. Serum haptoglobin is universally decreased in intravascular hemolysis because it binds free hemoglobin and is rapidly eliminated. Urine hemosiderin is an evidence of recent (up to 3 months) intravascular hemolysis, because it is slowly released with the normal sloughing of aging renal papillae. Characteristic red cell fragments, called helmet cells or schistocytes, are seen with microangiopathy due to the sheering of red cells on fibrin strands. (See Figure 4, Color Plates.) Extravascular hemolysis occurs in the reticuloendothelial system, mainly the spleen. The prototype for this process is autoimmune hemolytic anemia. Microspherocytes are abundant on the peripheral smear but the serum haptoglobin is normal (unless hemolysis is so severe with spillover into the intravascular space where it may be lowered) and the direct Coomb's test is positive.

11. Is it possible to have a hemolytic anemia with a normal reticulocyte count?

Yes. This may happen due to one of five causes. The first is the presence of a coexistent marrow hypoproduction process, such as iron deficiency or an underlying myelodysplastic syndrome. The second possibility is antibody-mediated destruction of erythroid precursors. The third possibility, which is sometimes overlooked, is folate deficiency due to chronic hemolysis and folate loss. Other possibilities are cases associated with renal failure and decreased erythropoietin and infection with parvovirus B19.

12. How is thalassemia diagnosed?

Thalassemia is a disorder of hemoglobin synthesis and can present with a wide range of clinical pictures, from asymptomatic trait to severe thalassemia major. In considering the diagnosis, one should look at ethnic background; these disorders are more common in patients of Mediterranean descent, patients from Southeast Asia, and to a lesser extent, African-Americans.

In thalassemia trait the cells are microcytic but, unlike iron deficiency, they are uniformly small and the RDW is usually normal. Occasionally, basophilic stippling and target cells will be seen. Hemoglobin electrophoresis and quantification of A_2 hemoglobin (Hg-A_2) and fetal hemoglobin (Hg-F) are usually diagnostic, although they may be normal in α-trait. Typically, Hg-A_2 is elevated and Hg-F is normal. (See Figure 1, Color Plates.)

Full-blown thalassemia major is more easily diagnosed. Untreated, these patients exhibit thalassemic facies (with frontal bossing) and hepatosplenomegaly, both related to extramedullary hematopoiesis. The smear is more abnormal with microcytosis, poikilocytosis, anisocytosis, target cells, basophilic stippling, and nucleated red cells. Hemoglobin electrophoresis and quantification of Hg-A_2 and Hg-F are usually diagnostic, showing normal Hg-A_2 and elevated Hg-F.

13. How are sickling disorders diagnosed?

The individual with sickle cell disorder is usually African-American, anemic (except patients with sickle cell trait), and may present with a sickling crisis. The smear reveals microcytosis and sickle cells, and a sickle preparation is usually positive. Diagnosis is confirmed by hemoglobin electrophoresis.

Note that depending on the pattern of the hemoglobinopathy, sickling disorders present with a wide range of severity. Patients with sickle cell trait (Hg A > Hg S) are asymptomatic with near-normal hemoglobin levels. Patients with sickle cell disease are moderately symptomatic with a hemoglobin level in the range of 10–12 gm/dl and few sickle cell crises. Severely symptomatic patients with hemoglobin in the range of 6–9 gm/dl and frequent painful crises usually suffer from sickle cell anemia (Hg S, no Hg A).

14. Can impaired hemoglobin affinity for oxygen lead to anemia? How is this entity diagnosed?

Abnormal hemoglobin affinity resulting from the presence of certain mutations in the hemoglobin molecules may lead either to anemia or polycythemia, depending on the type of impairment. Patients with unstable hemoglobin and low affinity for oxygen suffer an underproduction anemia due to shifting of the oxygen dissociation curve to the right. This rare type of anemia should be suspected after all other causes have been eliminated. Diagnosis may be difficult and requires sensitive assays of hemoglobin stability.

BIBLIOGRAPHY

1. Bertero MT, Caligaris-Cappio F: Anemia of chronic disease in systemic autoimmune diseases. Haematologica 82:375–381, 1997.
2. Bessman JD, Gilmer PR, Gardner FH: Improved classification of anemias by MCV and RDW. Am J Clin Pathol 80:322–326, 1983.
3. Chang CC, Kass L: Clinical significance of immature reticulocyte fraction determined by automated reticulocyte counting. Am J Clin Pathol 108:69–73, 1997.
4. Hyun BH: Bone marrow examination. Hematol Oncol Clin North Am 2:(4), 1988.
5. Lichtman MA, Murphy MS, Adamson JW: Detection of mutant hemoglobins with altered affinity for oxygen, a simplified technique. Ann Intern Med 84:517–520, 1976.
6. Saba HI: Myelodyplastic syndromes in the elderly: The role of growth factors in management. Leuk Res 20:203–219, 1996.
7. Savage DG, Lindenbaum J, Stabler SP, Allen RH: Sensitivity of serum methylmalonic acid and total homocysteine determination for diagnosing cobalamin and folate deficiencies. Am J Med 96:239–246, 1994.
8. Tabbara IA: Hemolytic anemias. Diagnosis and management. Med Clin North Am 76:649–668, 1992.
9. Weatherall DJ: The thalassemias. BMJ 314:1675–1678, 1997.

6. EVALUATION OF THE PATIENT WITH A BLEEDING DIATHESIS

Kathryn L. Hassell, M.D.

1. What are the considerations in a patient who seems to bleed "too much"?

Excessive bleeding occurs when one or more components of the hemostatic mechanism are dysfunctional. The first step in the evaluation of a patient is to look carefully for areas of trauma or postoperative bleeding that may require mechanical repair. In the absence of obvious reasons for bleeding, function of the hemostatic system should be measured by assessing platelets, blood coagulation proteins, and breakdown products.

2. Are there any helpful questions to ask when taking a history to determine a bleeding risk?

The best predictors of bleeding risk can be found in taking a history. A patient should be asked about a personal history of bleeding. A lifelong history of easy bruising, nose bleeds, gum bleeding, or heavy menses may indicate a quantitative or qualitative platelet problem. Tonsillectomy and wisdom tooth extraction are two common surgeries that greatly stress the entire hemostatic system. If a patient has tolerated these procedures or other surgery/trauma in the past, it is unlikely that he or she has a severe inherited bleeding disorder.

A careful family history should be taken for bleeding symptoms because mild hemophilia and von Willebrand's disease are relatively common inherited mild bleeding disorders.

A careful medication history, including use of over-the-counter drugs, should be taken because medications can significantly alter hemostasis. Aspirin, nonsteroidal antiinflammatory drugs, and some "cold" remedies (pseudoephedrine) can affect platelet function, as can many prescription medications. Heparin and coumadin (including prophylactic "low" doses) can also change test results and cause bleeding.

3. Are there any useful signs on physical examination to determine a bleeding disorder?

Petechiae (small purplish subcutaneous "spots" found especially on the dependent parts of the body) may indicate a quantitative or qualitative platelet disorder. Ecchymoses (bruises), especially in different stages of healing, can indicate either a platelet or blood coagulation protein disorder. Oozing or bleeding from old puncture sites or wounds may indicate inadequate platelets, inadequate blood coagulation factors, or an increase in fibrinolytic activity associated with disseminated intravascular coagulation (DIC).

4. Which tests assess platelets?

Both quantitative and qualitative abnormalities in platelets may cause excessive bleeding.

Quantitative testing is done using a platelet count. A normal platelet count is approximately 150,000–400,000/mm^3; spontaneous bleeding in the absence of trauma is uncommon with a platelet count above 20,000/mm^3, but a platelet count of 50,000–60,000/mm^3 is necessary to maintain hemostasis postoperative or with injury. Occasionally, patients with a very low platelet count (< 20,000/mm^3) may have immune-mediated thrombocytopenia (ITP). These patients produce young platelets with increased function, resulting in less bleeding than would be expected in a patient with a very low platelet count. In contrast, some patients with myeloproliferative disorders (where the bone marrow is producing excessive blood cells) may have platelet counts of up to 1,000,000/mm^3, but the platelets function poorly, resulting in bleeding. When assessing the platelet count, a final consideration is pseudothrombocytopenia, which occurs because platelets from some patients will clump with EDTA (the anticoagulant used for the CBC "purple-top" tube): the peripheral blood smear will show this clumping, and a repeat platelet count should be done using a heparinized ("green top" Vacutainer tube) blood sample.

Qualitative platelet function can be assessed by the bleeding time. In this test, a nick is made in the skin using a standardized template under standardized conditions, and the time to first formation of a blood clot is measured. The bleeding time can be prolonged by a number of factors other than qualitative platelet function, including platelet count, skin integrity, and blood vessel integrity, and needs to be interpreted with caution (see Controversies below). Platelet aggregation studies are done to assess responses to various agents that cause platelets to adhere and aggregate. These studies can be used to detect inherited or acquired platelet function disorders.

5. Which tests assess the blood coagulation proteins?

Screening tests for abnormalities in the coagulation proteins include the prothrombin time (PT) and activated partial thromboplastin time (aPTT). Prolongation of these tests indicates either deficiencies of blood coagulation factors or interference with the function of these factors by an inhibitor. To determine whether an inhibitor or deficiency state exists, the prolonged test (PT or aPTT) is repeated by mixing the patient's plasma with normal plasma (1:1 mixing study). If the prolonged test corrects to normal, this indicates the patient is missing some factor that can be corrected by adding normal plasma. If it does not correct, the patient may have an inhibitor that blocks the function of factors when normal plasma is added. This mixing study is the first step to evaluate an abnormal PT or aPTT.

6. What does a prolonged PT mean?

The PT assesses the function of the extrinsic pathway (tissue factor, factor VII) and common pathway (factors X, V, II, fibrinogen) of coagulation. If any of these factors are low (< 30–40% of normal), the PT will be prolonged. Although inherited deficiencies and inhibitors of these factors are rare, acquired deficiencies occur. Factors II, VII, and X require vitamin K and adequate liver function for production, so a patient with moderate-to-severe liver disease or poor vitamin K intake (from malabsorption, malnutrition, antibiotic therapy impairing gut production of vitamin K) will have a prolonged PT. Coumadin and rat poison, by inhibiting vitamin K metabolism, will also prolong the PT by inhibiting production of these factors. In very severe liver disease, all factors measured by the PT (including fibrinogen) will be decreased. Bleeding can occur in patients with only mild prolongation of the PT (1–2 seconds above the normal range) but is more common with more prolonged values (> 3 seconds above normal).

7. What does a prolonged aPTT mean?

The aPTT assesses the function of the intrinsic pathway (factors XII, XI, IX, VIII) and common pathway (factors X, V, II, and fibrinogen) of coagulation. If any of these factors are low (< 30–40% of normal), the aPTT will be prolonged. Inherited deficiencies of factor VIII (hemophilia A) and factor IX (hemophilia B) may be seen. In patients with mild hemophilia (factor levels of 10–30%), bleeding may occur only with trauma or surgery. Inherited deficiencies or other factors are rare.

Acquired deficiencies of these factors can be seen in severe liver disease (the site of production of the factors) and in long-term coumadin therapy (because factors II, IX, and X require vitamin K for production).

Von Willebrand's disease, an inherited disease that is characterized by low levels of factor VIII, and von Willebrand's factor with prolonged bleeding time due to platelet dysfunction also can prolong the aPTT because von Willebrand's factor carries factor VIII.

Specific inhibitors against factors VIII and IX are uncommon but result in severe bleeding disorders. *Nonspecific* inhibitors (e.g., lupus anticoagulant) can prolong the aPTT but are not associated with a bleeding diathesis. Bleeding can occur in patients with only mild prolongation of the aPTT (3–4 seconds above normal range) but is more common with more prolonged values (> 5 seconds above normal).

8. Are there other tests that help to evaluate the bleeding patient?

Measurement of the actual factor levels, including von Willebrand's factor, will confirm a deficiency or the activity of an inhibitor detected by the screening tests (PT, aPTT) or the 1:1 mixing study. Knowing that a specific factor is low may guide the choice of therapy; for example, the use of factor VIII concentrate in a hemophiliac, cryoprecipitate in a patient with an abnormal fibrinogen or 1-deamino-8-D-arginine vasopressin (DDAVP) in a patient with von Willebrand's disease. Screening for von Willebrand's disease should be considered in a patient with a chronic bleeding disorder even if the aPTT or bleeding time is normal.

Measurement of fibrin split products (FSPs), which accumulate when a large amount of clot has been formed and then broken down, can be useful. Increased FSPs develop in disseminated intravascular coagulation (DIC), and in conjunction with an elevated PT or aPTT, low fibrinogen levels and falling platelets help to make the diagnosis of DIC. In addition, elevated FSP can interfere with the measurement of the PT and aPTT, causing prolonged test results without necessarily increasing the risk of bleeding.

Assessment of hepatic and renal function is important. Because the liver makes all coagulation factors, liver enzymes (aspartate aminotransferase [AST], alanine aminotransferase [ALT], alkaline phosphatase) and liver function tests (total/direct bilirubin, albumin) should be measured. Blood urea nitrogen (BUN) and creatinine should be measured because uremia affects platelet function.

9. In patients with a chronic bleeding problem, which diseases or conditions are likely?

A lifelong history of bleeding problems, especially if they began in childhood or at puberty, make an inherited condition more likely. Von Willebrand's disease, mild hemophilia, and qualitative platelet function disorders need to be considered, along with rare isolated factor deficiencies. If the problem is longstanding but has developed over time, an acquired disorder is more likely. Chronic liver disease, chronic renal disease, vasculitis with vascular damage, and chronic use of medications may affect hemostasis.

10. In patients with an acute bleeding problem, which diseases or conditions should be considered?

In the absence of a significant past history of bleeding, acquired disorders need to be considered. Consumption of platelets and coagulation factors can occur in instances of massive trauma, severe bleeding, overwhelming infection, severe liver disease, or because of DIC associated with any of these conditions. An isolated fall in platelets can be seen in ITP, thrombotic thrombocytopenia purpura/hemolytic uremic syndrome (TTP/HUS), or because of ingestion of a toxic drug. Finally, it is possible that a previously mild inherited disorder (e.g., von Willebrand's disease) has become apparent in the setting of a hemostatic stress (e.g., surgery, trauma).

CONTROVERSIES

11. Is the bleeding time of any value?

The bleeding time is affected by several hemostatic factors, including the qualitative function of platelets, the number of platelets, and the integrity of capillary vessels and of the skin itself. It is not specific to platelet function and may not correlate with the risk of bleeding from nonskin surfaces such as the mucosa, visceral organs, or other tissues that may sustain injury or surgical trauma. Several studies have shown it has no value in predicting the risk of bleeding in patients undergoing cardiac bypass surgery, gastrointestinal biopsy, percutaneous renal biopsy, or general surgery. Because it is nonspecific, it is unclear if an elevated bleeding time performed on a hospitalized patient who is acutely ill and on multiple medications indicates a bleeding diathesis. The main use for a bleeding time would be to screen for von Willebrand's disease or an inherited platelet defect; even in these diseases, the bleeding time is variable.

BIBLIOGRAPHY

1. Bick RL: Acquired platelet function defects. Hematol Oncol Clin North Am 6:1203, 1992.
2. Bloom AL: Von Willebrand factor: Clinical features of inherited and acquired disorders. Mayo Clin Proc 66:743, 1991.
3. Fareed J, et al: Drug-induced alterations of hemostasis and fibrinolysis. Hematol Oncol Clin North Am 6:1229, 1992.
4. Galanakis DK: Fibrinogen anomalies and disease. A clinical update. Hematol Oncol Clin North Am 6:1171, 1992.
5. Kitchen CS: Approach to the bleeding patient. Hematol Oncol Clin North Am 6:983, 1992.
6. Lusher JM: Screening and diagnosis of coagulation disorders. Am J Obstet Gynecol 175:778–783, 1996.
7. Mammen EF: Coagulation abnormalities in liver disease. Hematol Oncol Clin North Am 6:1247, 1992.
8. Peterson P, Hayes TE, Arkin CF, et al: The preoperative bleeding time test lacks clinical benefit: College of American Pathologists' and American Society of Clinical Pathologists' position article. Arch Surg 133:134–139, 1998.
9. Scott-Timperly LJ, Haire WD: Autoimmune coagulation disorders. Rheum Dis Clin North Am 23:411–423, 1997.
10. Wu KK: Endothelial cells in hemostasis, thrombosis, and inflammation. Hosp Pract 27(4):145, 1992.

7. EVALUATION OF ADENOPATHY

*George K. Philips, M.D., Catherine E. Klein, M.D.,
and Lyndah K. Dreiling, M.D.*

1. What is adenopathy?

The term *adenopathy* refers to enlargement of the lymph nodes. In general, lymph nodes are discrete, soft, ovoid structures that vary from a few millimeters to 2 cm in length. They are connected to both afferent and efferent lymphatics. Their internal structure is both complex and highly organized with aggregates of lymphoid tissue containing specific regions of B-cells, T-cells, plasma cells, and some lymphocytes. These structures are never static; their size and morphology are modified by stress, thyroid and adrenal function, and immune responses.

2. What method of physical examination best allows detection of adenopathy?

Place the patient in a relaxed position (e.g., in examining the axilla, the arm should be flaccid and to the side; in examining the neck, the head should be flexed slightly forward). Use the pads of the index and middle fingers, moving the skin over the underlying tissues rather than moving the fingers over the skin. The examiner should be able to roll a node in two directions, side to side, and up and down. Muscles and arteries cannot be similarly manipulated. Small, mobile, nontender nodes can be easily found in normal people. Tender or enlarged lymph nodes require careful assessment of the regions that they drain and evaluation of lymph nodes elsewhere to distinguish between regional and generalized lymphadenopathy.

3. What is the differential diagnosis of a swelling in the neck?

Not all lumps in the neck are lymph nodes. Abscesses (particularly periodontal), infections in salivary glands, thyroid cysts, or thyroglossal duct cysts may present as masses in the neck. Many of these entities are midline, whereas nodes are usually lateral or may move in conjunction with the thyroid during swallowing. Such observations may help to differentiate the mass from true adenopathy.

4. When should a posterior cervical lymph node raise concern?

Careful examination of the patient with isolated cervical adenopathy usually reveals an infection as the cause. The most common infections are viral or bacterial and involve the face or oropharynx. Infectious mononucleosis may present with posterior cervical adenopathy, but a careful search usually reveals mild splenomegaly and other swollen nodes as well as the typical pharyngitis. With the recent increase in mycobacterial disease, related in part to its associations with infection by the human immunodeficiency virus (HIV) and with the immigrant Asian population, more patients present with tuberculous cervical adenopathy. Other less common infections include cat-scratch fever, toxoplasmosis, histoplasmosis, and cytomegalovirus (CMV). Hodgkin's disease and other lymphomas present only rarely as isolated cervical adenopathy. Another common cause of posterior cervical adenopathy is scalp lesions of any type, including scabies.

5. What entities cause swelling in the groin?

Enlarged lymph nodes in the groin are common, often resulting from minor infections in the feet. Bilateral tender groin adenopathy may signal a venereal disease; herpes usually causes unilateral swelling. Inguinal hernias and vascular aneurysms occasionally may be mistaken for adenopathy.

6. Can drugs cause adenopathy?

Phenytoin is associated with a hypersensitivity reaction that gives the picture of pseudolymphoma. A small portion of patients develop true lymphoma. Antithyroid agents and isoniazid are also associated with occasional adenopathy.

7. What benign conditions cause generalized adenopathy?

Conditions associated with widespread adenopathy are systemic in nature. Many are infectious (Epstein-Barr virus [EBV], CMV, and HIV infection, tuberculosis, histoplasmosis, syphilis, brucellosis, leptospirosis). Rheumatologic diseases such as lupus, and widespread skin diseases, such as eczema, drug eruptions, and psoriasis, also may present with diffuse adenopathy. Occasionally patients with thyrotoxicosis, lipidoses, or sarcoidosis have generalized adenopathy.

8. What are the causes of adenopathy in the patient with acquired immunodeficiency syndrome (AIDS)?

Patients with AIDS frequently have generalized adenopathy of unclear etiology; for this condition, no therapy is needed. However, fungi and mycobacterial infections must be carefully excluded. The most common malignancies in patients with AIDS are Kaposi's sarcoma and lymphoma, both of which are associated with enlarged lymph nodes.

9. What are the common malignancies that cause adenopathy?

Cancerous lymph nodes may be either single or multiple, localized or widespread. The causes of widespread cancerous lymph nodes are usually systemic in nature—lymphoproliferative or, less commonly, myeloproliferative disorders. When the malignancy is solitary or localized to one or two lymph node groups, one should consider not only lymphomas and Hodgkin's disease but also metastatic carcinomas. Primary tumors of the head and neck often present with an abnormal node in the neck. Women with breast cancer may have detectable nodes in the axilla before the primary tumor has been diagnosed.

10. How does age affect the likelihood of finding tumor in an isolated enlarged node?

On average, 20% of patients under the age 25 years who have a node biopsied are found to harbor a malignancy, whereas patients over age 50 years have an 80% probability of cancer at biopsy.

11. Are there characteristics of the node that should raise the suspicion of cancer?

Generally, the larger the node, the greater the concern. Location is important: supraclavicular nodes are almost always malignant, whereas posterior cervical nodes are rarely malignant. Rock-hard nodules are highly worrisome for metastatic carcinoma. Painful nodes are less likely to be cancerous. Matted nodes, fixed to underlying structures and growing steadily over weeks to months, are suggestive of cancer. Of importance, none of these characteristics is diagnostic, and tissue for microscopic examination is required.

12. Which tests may be done to help establish a diagnosis before the patient undergoes a lymph node biopsy?

Although not specific for any disease, the complete blood count (CBC) is frequently abnormal in patients with infections, malignancies, or rheumatologic disorders associated with adenopathy. A Venereal Disease Research Laboratory (VDRL) or rapid plasmin reagin (RPR) test may help to rule out syphilis and should be considered in any sexually active patient. HIV antibody testing in persons at risk is essential. In addition to liver function tests, serologic studies to detect the hepatitis virus (both B and C), EBV for infectious mononucleosis, antinuclear antibodies (ANA) for rheumatologic disease, and thyroid-stimulating hormone (TSH) for thyroid disease are probably warranted. A chest radiograph may be helpful in identifying mediastinal adenopathy in patients with sarcoidosis or lymphoma.

13. What is scrofula?

Scrofula is an old term referring to the presentation of mycobacterial disease as cervical adenopathy. Because of its worldwide prevalence, it is associated most commonly with *Mycobacterium tuberculosis*, even though *Mycobacterium scrofulaceum* is the organism most prone to present in this manner.

14. What is the best approach to diagnosing a patient with adenopathy?

Not all patients with enlarged lymph nodes need histologic examination of tissue to establish a diagnosis. Many infectious diseases or rheumatologic disorders are better diagnosed from history, serologic examination, or cultures. In fact, the microscopic appearance of lymph nodes from these patients is often nonspecific. When suspicion of infection is high, a trial of antibiotics may be warranted, with reexamination in 2–3 weeks. For patients in whom the adenopathy does not regress as expected or in whom the likelihood of cancer is significant at presentation, tissue should be obtained for biopsy. The best specimen for histopathologic study is the excisional biopsy, in which the entire lymph node, fresh and in saline, is submitted to the pathologist for sectioning, staining, and culture. Sections are necessary to assess the architecture of the node, a fundamental part of the diagnosis of any lymphoma.

15. When should fine-needle aspiration (FNA) be used?

FNA of a node provides small samples for culture and cytologic examination. It can be useful when the patient is known to have cancer and is now suspected of having recurrent or metastatic disease. FNA is also useful in the documentation of suspected new malignancy, although histologic specimens are generally preferred in this setting. When the aspiration is unrevealing, the next step is to biopsy the node.

16. What are the potential risks of FNA?

With proper sterile technique, the risk of infection is extremely low. Obviously there is a small risk of bleeding, particularly if a vascular structure is biopsied by mistake, but serious bleeding in patients with normal hemostatic function is rare. Of concern has been the possibility of seeding tumor cells along the tract of the needle, which may reduce the curability of some malignancies. This risk seems to be more theoretic than actual.

17. In the patient with multiple enlarged nodes, which one(s) should be biopsied?

In general, one diagnostic specimen is adequate, although more specimens may be required to document the exact stage of lymphoma. Biopsies of groin nodes are usually avoided because these nodes are commonly enlarged from other dermatopathic causes and are of low yield. Otherwise we look for large, readily accessible nodes. Nodes in the axilla, which often require more extensive dissection, are avoided if more superficial cervical nodes appear pathologically enlarged.

BIBLIOGRAPHY

1. Fijten GH, et al: Unexplained adenopathy in family practice: An evaluation of the probability of malignant causes and the effectiveness of the physician's work-up. J Fam Pract 27:373, 1988.
2. Greenfield S, et al: The clinical investigation of lymphadenopathy in primary care practice. JAMA 240:1388, 1978.
3. Kline TS, et al: Lymphadenopathy and aspiration biopsy cytology. A review of 376 superficial nodes. Cancer 54:1076, 1984.
4. Kunitz A: An approach to peripheral lymphadenopathy in adult patients. West J Med 143:393, 1985.
5. Libman H: Generalized adenopathy: Clinical reviews. J Gen Intern Med 2:48, 1987.
6. Slap GB, et al: When to perform biopsies of enlarged peripheral lymph nodes in young patients. JAMA 252:1321, 1984.
7. Tschammler A, Wirkner H, Ott G, Hahn D: Vascular patterns in reactive and malignant lymphadenopathy. Eur J Radiol 6:473–480, 1996.

8. EVALUATION OF LEUKOCYTOSIS

David S. Hanson, M.D., George Mathai, M.D.,
and William A. Robinson, M.D., Ph.D.

1. Define leukocytosis.

An elevation in the total white blood cell (WBC) count greater than two standard deviations above the mean (usually 20,000 cells/mm^3) constitutes leukocytosis. This elevation may involve one or more subsets of the circulating WBCs, including neutrophils, monocytes, eosinophils, basophils, and lymphocytes (when the primary cause of leukocytosis is an elevation of lymphocytes, the term lymphocytosis is often used). Neutrophilia is a specific elevation of the absolute neutrophil count and is the most common cause for leukocytosis.

2. What is a leukemoid reaction?

Elevation of the WBC (50,000 cells/mm^3) constitutes a leukemoid reaction. This increase is generally characterized by increased numbers of both mature neutrophils and band forms, although immature cells (including blast forms) may be seen. (See Figure 6, Color Plates.) A leukemoid reaction must be distinguished from acute leukemia, chronic myelogenous leukemia, and leukoerythroblastic reaction.

3. What are the different types of leukemoid reactions?

Myeloid, lymphoid, and monocytoid are the three different types of leukemoid reactions. Myeloid leukemoid reactions are the most common and consist primarily of an elevation of mature neutrophils and band forms. Bacterial infections are the most common cause of a myeloid leukemoid reaction. Lymphoid leukemoid reactions are characterized by a lymphocytosis that may appear atypical and are usually seen with viral infections, such as mononucleosis or hepatitis. Monocytic leukemoid reactions have been identitifed, although they are uncommon. These reactions are generally associated with parasitic infections.

4. Review a step-by-step approach to evaluating a patient with leukocytosis.

- Evaluate the patient for signs and symptoms suggestive of acute or chronic inflammatory illness. Relevant tests may include blood cultures (bacterial, fungal, and/or viral), smears, tissue biopsies, and radiologic studies.
- Examine the peripheral smear to confirm the nature of the leukocytosis and determine the type and maturation of the WBCs. Also evaluate for concomitant abnormalities of the red blood cells (RBCs) and platelets.

- Obtain a leukocyte alkaline phosphatase (LAP) score. The LAP score will be high in a leukemoid reaction but low in CML.
- Examine parents' or siblings' blood to detect genetic or familial causes of leukocytosis.
- Bone marrow biopsy, aspiration, and cytogenetic studies may confirm the diagnosis of CML or other myeloproliferative disorders. A bone marrow exam also confirms leukoerythroblastosis and detects infiltrative marrow disease by cancer, inflammatory disorders, or fungal infections.

5. When should a marrow examination be performed early in a patient's evaluation?

If the diagnosis of acute leukemia or a myeloproliferative disorder is suspected on the basis of the appearance of the peripheral smear, prominent splenomegaly, or other findings, a bone marrow biopsy should be performed early. In an individual infected with the human immunodeficiency virus (HIV), the bone marrow may be done early to evaluate for lymphoma or to provide culture material.

6. What is a leukoerythroblastic reaction?

It is a reaction of the bone marrow to an infiltrating process such as metastatic carcinoma (e.g., breast, prostate, or lung cancer) or infection (e.g., tuberculosis, fungus). A leukoerythroblastic blood smear is characterized by the presence of nucleated RBCs, tear drop-shaped red cells, and early myeloid cells (i.e., promyelocytes and metamyelocytes).

7. Distinguish a leukemoid reaction from chronic or acute leukemia.

In **chronic myelogenous leukemia**, the LAP score is low and generally the spleen is palpable. The blood smear often contains increased numbers of eosinophils and basophils. Cytogenetic or fluorescence in-situ hybridization (FISH) techniques should reveal the presence of the characteristic Philadelphia translocation t(9,22).

In **acute leukemia**, a higher percentage of blast forms should be evident on the peripheral smear. The marrow examination should reveal an excess of clonal blasts effacing the marrow.

8. What causes a leukemoid reaction?

Although the exact cause is not clear, it is postulated that certain malignancies or inflammatory processes result in the elaboration of certain growth factors or growth factor-like substances. In addition, release of endogenous epinephrine, cortisol, or histamine may contribute to elevation of the WBC count.

9. Do any drugs cause an elevated WBC count?

Yes. Epinephrine and steroids may cause a doubling of the WBC count due to demargination. Lithium also contributes to elevated WBC counts by increasing white cell numbers. Growth factors developed with recombinant deoxyribonucleic acid (DNA) technology that are administered in pharmacologic doses may cause significant elevation of the WBC count, marrow expansion, and subsequent bone pain.

10. Can the WBC count be falsely elevated?

Yes. False elevation of the automated determination of the WBC count may be caused by clotting, cryoglobulins, or platelet aggregation. In addition, nucleated RBCs may be inappropriately counted as WBCs.

11. What are the most common causes of a leukemoid reaction?

The two most common causes are bacterial infection or underlying malignancy.

12. Should leukocytosis be treated?

Treatment of leukocytosis depends on the underlying cause. In cases of congenital idiopathic neutrophilia, treatment is unnecessary.

13. How can congenital or idiopathic neutrophilia be identified?

Idiopathic neutrophilia, a cause of chronic neutrophilia, occurs in healthy people. Usually the WBC is 20,000 cells/mm^3. All other causes of leukocytosis should be excluded before this diagnosis is made, because congenital neutrophilia is rare. Personal and family histories can be useful in making this diagnosis. Acute and chronic leukemoid reactions also may be seen in Down syndrome.

14. Does smoking cause leukocytosis?

Yes. Nicotine can induce leukocytosis. One study identified the degree of leukocytosis in smokers as a risk factor for myocardial infarction.

15. Does a past leukemoid reaction or history of neutrophilia predict the subsequent development of acute leukemia or CML?

No. Patients with idiopathic leukopenia have not been found to be at increased risk for subsequent disease, specifically CML.

16. Is the level of leukocytosis useful in distinguishing the diagnosis?

No. There are no studies correlating the level of leukocytosis with specific diagnoses. Even idiopathic neutrophilia, commonly associated with modest WBC counts, may be associated with counts of 40,000 cells/m^3.

BIBLIOGRAPHY

1. Brodeur GM, Dahl GV, Williams DL, et al: Transient leukemoid reaction and trisomy 21 mosaicism in a phenotypically normal newborn. Blood 55:691–693, 1980.
2. Dale DC, Fauci AS, Guerry D, Wolff SM: Comparison of agents producing a neutrophilic leukocytosis in man. J Clin Invest 56:808–813, 1975.
3. Herring WB, Smith LG, Walker R, Herion JC: Hereditary neutrophilia. Am J Med 56:729–734, 1974.
4. Reding MT, Hibbs JR, Morrison VA, et al: Diagnosis and outcome of 100 consecutive patients with extreme granulocyte leukocytosis. Am J Med 104:12–16, 1998.
5. Walker RI, Willemze R: Neutrophil kinetics and the regulation of granulopoiesis. Rev Infect Dis 2:282, 1980.
6. Ward HN, Reinhard EM: Chronic idiopathic leukocytosis. Ann Intern Med 75:193–198, 1971.
7. Zalokar JB, Richard JL, Claude JR: Leukocyte count, smoking and myocardial infarction. N Engl J Med 304:465–468, 1981.

II. General Hematology

9. IRON DEFICIENCY ANEMIA

Richard F. Branda, M.D.

1. Does the intake of iron in a typical American diet meet body requirements?

The daily dietary intake of iron in the United States averages 10–20 mg, of which approximately 10% is absorbed. Adult males and nonmenstruating females lose about 1 mg/day and therefore are in iron balance. Menstruating women lose the equivalent of another 0.5–1 mg/day, and pregnant women require 4–6 mg/day of iron for the use of mother and fetus and to replace blood loss at parturition. Consequently, most menstruating women and all pregnant women are in negative iron balance. Infants at special risk for iron deficiency live in low socioeconomic conditions, are started on cow's milk before six months of age, consume formula not fortified with iron, or are of low birth weight. Rapid growth during infancy and adolescence increases the demand for iron.

2. Which segments of the population in the United States are most susceptible to iron deficiency?

Toddlers, adolescent girls, and women of childbearing age have the highest prevalence of iron deficiency and iron deficiency anemia.

3. Does a vegetarian diet predispose to iron deficiency?

Heme iron from meat is much better absorbed than nonheme iron because of specific heme-binding sites in the intestine. Therefore, the nonheme iron in dairy products, eggs, and all plant foods is not as well absorbed. In addition, some compounds such as phytates and polyphenolics in plant foods and tannins in teas and coffee interfere with iron absorption. Vitamin C counteracts these inhibitory effects. It is important that vegetarian diets contain substantial amounts of plants rich in iron and vitamin C, such as whole-grain cereals, legumes, brown rice, nuts, seeds, and fruits.

4. Who should be screened for iron deficiency anemia or supplemented with iron?

The hemoglobin or hematocrit should be measured once during the following periods: infancy (between 6 and 9 months of age); early childhood (between 1 and 5 years of age); late childhood (between 5 and 12 years of age); and adolescence (between 14 and 20 years of age). Dietary iron intake should be evaluated; if inadequate, iron supplementation should be considered. All pregnant women should be supplemented routinely with iron. Adequate iron intake during pregnancy is provided by 30 mg of elemental iron (150 mg ferrous sulfate or 250 mg ferrous gluconate).

5. What is the distribution of iron in the body?

Each 1 ml of whole blood contains approximately 0.5 mg of iron, or a total of 2,000 mg of iron in the blood. Storage iron (500 mg in women and 1000 mg in men) and about 500 mg in iron-containing proteins account for the rest of body iron.

6. What are the most common causes of iron deficiency anemia?

Iron deficiency anemia occurs when iron loss exceeds iron intake. The most common causes are blood loss from the gastrointestinal (GI) tract in males and postmenopausal females and from the GI tract or from menstruation in premenopausal females. As little as 1–2 ml of chronic blood loss eventually will result in iron deficiency because of the low iron intake in most diets.

7. Loss of a unit of blood would be expected to produce what change in the hematocrit of a normal person?

The hematocrit decreases approximately three points and the hemoglobin decreases approximately 1 gm/dl for each unit of blood lost. Therefore, for each unit of blood loss and drop in the hematocrit of three points, approximately 250 mg of iron is required to regenerate a normal hematocrit and hemoglobin in a normal person.

8. How sensitive is the stool Hemoccult test as an indication of excessive blood loss?

The stool Hemoccult test is useful only if it is positive. False-negative tests occur because of insensitivity of the test and because bleeding from the GI tract is frequently intermittent. False-positive tests may occur with the ingestion of certain heme-containing foods.

9. How is iron deficiency evaluated in men and postmenopausal women?

Such individuals have a high probability of GI disease whether or not occult blood is found in their stool. The combination of a positive Hemoccult test and site-specific symptoms may increase the likelihood of identifying a lesion, but a negative test should not preclude further evaluation. Esophagogastroduodenoscopy and colonoscopy should be performed. A majority of patients have an upper GI source, usually peptic ulcer disease, and 20–30% have a colonic source such as a polyp, cancer, or angiodysplasia. Concurrent upper and lower bleeding sources are rare. However, in patients aged 50 or older, colonoscopy should be strongly considered even if an upper GI source of blood loss was found. If bidirectional endoscopy is negative, small-bowel biopsy should be performed, since occult celiac disease is a common cause of iron deficiency in this age group. If all the tests are negative and the patient is asymptomatic, no further evaluation is necessary. Iron supplementation usually corrects the deficiency, and 90% remain hematologically normal 5 years later. Patients who fail to respond to iron or who become progressively anemic should be evaluated further.

10. What other causes of blood loss should be considered?

Sports anemia, particularly in long-distance runners, may increase blood loss in the stool. Excessive blood donation or frequent phlebotomies in hospitalized patients can cause iron depletion. Intravascular hemolysis due to prosthetic heart valves or paroxysmal nocturnal hemoglobinuria results in the loss of iron in the urine that may be detected by the presence of urinary hemosiderin.

11. What is sports anemia?

Sports anemia is a cause of iron deficiency anemia in endurance athletes, particularly marathon runners. Following a marathon race, runners frequently have blood in their stools for several days. Blood loss is thought to be due to ischemia of the GI tract because blood is diverted to muscles. Use of nonsteroidal antiinflammatory drugs (NSAIDs) may aggravate this blood loss. In addition, some runners have chronic intravascular hemolysis (footstrike hemolysis) and urinary loss of iron. The degree of anemia may be exaggerated by an expanded plasma volume. Elite distance runners have an increase of both plasma and red cell volumes, but the gain in plasma volume exceeds the gain in red cell volume. Non-elite runners and joggers seem to have an increase of plasma volume alone.

12. What are the clinical features of iron deficiency?

If the anemia developed slowly, many patients are asymptomatic. Others may complain of fatigue, decreased exercise tolerance, weakness, sore tongue, or brittle nails. Pica, the unusual craving for a single food item or ingestion of nonfood items such as clay or laundry starch, is common in some population groups. Physical findings include glossitis, angular cheilitis, and spoon nails (koilonychia).

13. Which laboratory tests should be used to diagnose iron deficiency?

The peripheral smear should be examined for hypochromia and microcytosis. With more severe anemia, poikilocytosis is common. The reticulocyte count is low, and the leukocyte count and differential are normal. Thrombocytosis may be present. The serum ferritin is probably the most useful test in otherwise normal individuals, because it correlates well with total body iron stores. However, ferritin is an acute phase reactant. Chronic infection, chronic inflammation, liver disease, and malignant disease may raise the ferritin level and obscure the presence of iron deficiency. Thus, healthy individuals may be screened for iron deficiency with a serum ferritin and hemoglobin; if both are normal, iron deficiency is excluded. Low serum ferritin and normal hemoglobin indicates storage depletion. If anemia is present with normal or elevated ferritin levels, a search for other causes should be initiated. In typical iron deficiency anemia, the serum iron and transferrin saturation are low and the iron-binding capacity is high, but these tests are relatively insensitive. They may be normal even though iron stores are depleted as would be detected by the serum ferritin.

14. What is the role of bone marrow examination in the evaluation of iron deficiency?

The presence of any storage iron in the bone marrow essentially excludes the diagnosis of iron deficiency anemia. For this reason, bone marrow examination is considered the gold standard for diagnosis. However, it is painful and expensive. Most cases of iron deficiency can be diagnosed without resorting to this test.

15. What other conditions should be considered in the differential diagnosis of microcytic anemia?

The anemia of chronic disease, thalassemia, and sideroblastic anemia may be confused with iron deficiency anemia. In all of these conditions, the serum ferritin is normal or elevated. However, if the serum ferritin falls in the low normal range (20–100 ng/ml), it may be difficult to distinguish the anemia of chronic disease from iron deficiency. Moreover, in some patients the two conditions coexist.

16. Describe the characteristic test abnormalities in the anemia of chronic disease.

In this disorder, certain conditions impair iron use by the body. The characteristic finding is iron in the reticuloendothelial system of the bone marrow but not in red cell precursors. Oral iron therapy is of questionable or no benefit. This disorder is characterized by a reduced serum iron, a reduced total iron-binding capacity, and frequently an elevated ferritin and sedimentation rate. Usually the etiology of these abnormalities is clear (active rheumatoid arthritis, osteomyelitis, pulmonary tuberculosis, neoplastic disease), but on occasion the patient may have to be followed and retested at intervals to establish the reason for having anemia of chronic disease.

17. What is emerging as the single best test to discriminate between iron deficiency anemia, the anemia of chronic disease, and combined anemia?

An elevated level of serum transferrin receptor is a sensitive indicator of iron deficiency. Transferrin receptors are upregulated on red cell precursors and shed into the serum in increased amounts when the iron supply is inadequate. Serum transferrin receptor levels are normal in the anemia of chronic disease. Measuring the combination of serum transferrin receptor levels and ferritin provides very high sensitivity and specificity to detect iron depletion and will probably replace conventional indices of iron status, such as serum iron, transferrin, and ferritin alone.

Comparison of Laboratory Tests for Iron Status

	IRON DEFICIENCY	CHRONIC DISEASE	IRON DEFICIENCY AND CHRONIC DISEASE
Serum iron	↓	↓	↓
TIBC or transferrin	↑	↓	↓ Normal ↑
Ferritin	↓	↑	Normal ↓
Serum transferrin receptor	↑	Normal	Normal ↑

TIBC = total iron-binding capacity.

18. What pitfalls may be expected from a therapeutic trial of iron sulfate?

The hematocrit may fail to rise during a therapeutic trial of iron for presumed iron deficiency anemia because (1) the patient is noncompliant with the iron supplementation; (2) blood loss exceeds the ability to absorb increased iron from supplementation; (3) the iron preparation is ineffective (enteric coated iron is not well absorbed); (4) antacid administration may inhibit iron absorption because of an increased gastric pH; (5) the patient has a malabsorption syndrome; or (6) the diagnosis of iron deficiency is in error. Regardless of whether a therapeutic trial of iron successfully increases the hematocrit, presumed iron deficiency requires further documentation and subsequent gastrointestinal tract evaluation for a source of blood loss.

19. How long should a patient with iron deficiency take replacement iron?

Replacement of iron stores takes at least 4–6 months.

20. What are the side effects of oral iron?

Ten to 20% of patients have side effects that lead to noncompliance, including diarrhea, constipation, nausea, and abdominal pain. If such symptoms occur, the dosage should be decreased to 1–2 tablets per day with meals.

21. What is the role of parenteral iron treatment?

Indications include severe intolerance of oral preparations, malabsorption, and iron losses exceeding maximal oral replacement. Intravenous iron dextran is effective but is accompanied by an approximate 10% incidence of serious side effects, such as anaphylaxis, wheezing, fever, seizures, hypotension, hives, or pain in the chest, abdomen, or back. A test dose should be given with the infusion administered over 4–6 hours.

22. Does iron deficiency occur in the setting of renal failure?

Patients with renal disease are predisposed to iron deficiency because of blood loss during dialysis and an increased bleeding tendency accompanying uremia. Patients at risk for iron deficiency should be supplemented with oral iron. This is particularly important in renal patients treated with erythropoietin; the increase in the hematocrit during erythropoietin therapy requires a massive transfer of iron from the storage pools to red cell precursors. If storage pools are depleted, iron deficiency results and limits the hematopoietic response.

23. Are there other clinical uses of erythropoietin that require iron supplementation?

In addition to chronic renal failure patients, erythropoietin is approved for use in anemic HIV-infected patients and cancer patients. It also is used to reduce allogeneic blood transfusion in elective surgery patients (with the exception of cardiac and vascular surgery). In some European countries, erythropoietin is approved to enhance preoperative autologous blood donation. Iron supplementation routinely should be given during the first 4–6 weeks of erythropoietin treatment to all such patients except those with increased serum iron and transferrin saturation. Iron status should be monitored, and iron should be supplemented more aggressively if the transferrin saturation drops below 20% or if the serum ferritin is less than 100 μg/L. Erythropoietin therapy has been reported to be of benefit in some patients with rheumatoid arthritis and inflammatory bowel disease. Many such patients may be resistant to oral iron but respond to IV iron. The presence of a serum ferritin below 70 μg/L or an increased serum transferrin receptor level suggests coexistent iron depletion and inflammation. Patients should be treated with IV iron before erythropoietin therapy.

BIBLIOGRAPHY

1. Allen LH: Nutritional supplementation for the pregnant woman. Clin Obstet Gynecol 37:587–595, 1994.
2. Cook JD, Skikne BS: Iron deficiency: Definition and diagnosis. J Intern Med 226:349–355, 1989.
3. Craig WJ: Iron status of vegetarians. Am J Clin Nutr 59(Suppl):1233S–1237S, 1994.
4. Farley PC, Foland J: Iron deficiency anemia: How to diagnose and correct. Postgrad Med 87:89–101, 1990.

5. Lipschitz DA: The anemia of chronic disease. J Am Geriatr Soc 38:1258–1264, 1990.
6. Looker AC, Dallman PR, Carroll MD, et al: Prevalence of iron deficiency in the United States. JAMA 277:973–976, 1997.
7. Moses PL, Smith RE: Endoscopic evaluation of iron deficiency anemia. Postgrad Med 98:213–226, 1995.
8. Punnonen K, Irjala K, Rajamäki A: Serum transferrin receptor and its ratio to serum ferritin in the diagnosis of iron deficiency. Blood 89:1052–1057, 1997.
9. Massey AC: Microcytic anemia: Differential diagnosis and management of iron deficiency anemia. Med Clin North Am 76:549–566, 1992.
10. Swain RA, Kaplan B, Montgomery E: Iron deficiency anemia: When is parenteral therapy warranted? Postgrad Med 100:181–193, 1996.
11. US Public Health Service: Anemia in children. Am Fam Physician 51:1121–1123, 1995.
12. Van Wyck DB: Iron deficiency in patients with dialysis-associated anemia during erythropoietin replacement therapy: Strategies for assessment and management. Semin Nephrol 9 (Suppl 2):21–24, 1989.

10. MEGALOBLASTIC ANEMIA

Sally P. Stabler, M.D.

1. Define megaloblastic anemia.

Megaloblastosis refers to a pathologic process characterized by delay in maturation of the nucleus of blood cell precursors and continuing development of the cytoplasm. The result of this nuclear-cytoplasmic dissociation is production of cells that are larger than normal. Therefore, the red blood cells have an elevated mean cell volume (MCV > 100 fl or higher than the patient's baseline MCV). A bone marrow sample reveals giant bands, and the mature granulocytes are often hypersegmented. Other causes of large red blood cells, termed macrocytosis, are technically not megaloblastic, but in practice it is difficult to differentiate them. (See Figure 2, Color Plates.)

2. How are megaloblastic anemia and macrocytic anemia different?

Megaloblastic anemia is thought to be due to problems with DNA synthesis. Therefore, generally all cells in the bone marrow are affected to some degree. Other rapidly dividing cells, such as the epithelial surface of the tongue and the lining of the gastrointestinal tract, also may show megaloblastic changes. In contrast, macrocytic anemia simply refers to large red blood cells, which may be caused by problems unrelated to DNA synthesis.

3. Name the causes of megaloblastic anemia and macrocytic anemia.

Vitamin B_{12} (cobalamin) and folate deficiency are common causes of megaloblastic anemia. These common vitamin deficiencies must be differentiated from bone marrow failure syndromes such as aplastic anemia, refractory anemia, and/or preleukemia (myelodysplastic syndromes). Both hypo- and hyperthyroidism cause macrocytic anemia with pancytopenia, which is difficult to distinguish from cobalamin deficiency in some cases. Alcoholism, chronic liver disease, chronic renal failure, and cigarette smoking also may cause macrocytosis. A high reticulocyte count can increase the MCV (less than 110 fl) because reticulocytes are large. Thus, hemolytic anemia may be misdiagnosed as a macrocytic process. The MCV may be falsely high in patients with hypergammaglobulinemia or paraproteinemias due to clumping of red blood cells in the blood cell counter.

4. Do any drugs cause megaloblastic or macrocytic anemia?

Many medications that interfere with folate metabolism have been shown to cause megaloblastic anemia, such as methotrexate, carbamazepine, diphenylhydantoin, triamterene, trimethoprim, and pyrimethamine. Any drugs that interfere with DNA synthesis may cause megaloblastic anemia and pancytopenia, such as azidothymidine, hydroxyurea, and many common chemotherapy agents. Alcohol abuse may cause megaloblastic anemia or macrocytic anemia in several ways: (1) alcohol interferes with folate metabolism, (2) chronic alcoholics rarely have enough folate intake to counteract the effect of alcohol, and (3) alcohol is a common cause of chronic liver disease, which causes macrocytosis because of red cell membrane abnormalities.

5. What is ineffective erythropoiesis?

In severe megaloblastic anemia and refractory anemia many developing red blood cells are destroyed in the bone marrow before they are released into the circulation. This intramedullary destruction of the red blood cells increases the serum levels of indirect bilirubin and lactate dehydrogenase. In addition, the bone marrow is hypercellular. On occasion, the hypercellular bone marrow of megaloblastic anemia has been confused with acute leukemia. Generally the cytology of the bone marrow aspirate differentiates severe megaloblastic changes from acute leukemia.

6. How do you distinguish cobalamin and folate deficiency?

Cobalamin and folate deficiencies cause identical hematologic abnormalities of megaloblastic anemia. Both vitamins are cofactors for the enzyme methionine synthase. In this reaction, methyltetrahydrofolate is converted to tetrahydrofolate, which is necessary for some enzymes of DNA synthesis. Homocysteine, a sulfhydral-containing amino acid, is converted to methionine in this reaction also. Therefore, both cobalamin and folate deficiencies cause elevated levels of serum total homocysteine. Cobalamin is also required for the pathway in which L-methylmalonyl-CoA is converted to succinyl-CoA. When the cobalamin cofactor is decreased, increased levels of methylmalonyl-CoA are hydrolyzed to methylmalonic acid, which can be detected in both serum and urine.

7. What other organ system is affected by cobalamin deficiency?

The nervous system requires cobalamin for normal growth and functioning. People with cobalamin deficiency may develop a demyelinating disorder (formerly termed combined systems disease) that affects the brain, the dorsal columns of the spinal cord, and occasionally the peripheral nerves. The most frequent symptoms are painful paresthesias and gait ataxia. Untreated lesions progress over months to years to complete sensory loss and motor weakness and eventually to frank paralysis. The optic nerves and autonomic nervous system also may be involved. Disorders of vibration sense and proprioception can be detected on physical examination. An occasional patient has a neuropsychiatric presentation with depression, paranoia, emotional lability, memory problems, and a predominantly organic psychosis.

8. Is the presence of megaloblastic anemia a good screening test for cobalamin deficiency of the nervous system?

No. There is a marked inverse relationship between the severity of neurologic abnormalities and megaloblastic anemia. At least 25% of patients with cobalamin deficiency present mainly with neurologic abnormalities and normal or nearly normal hematologic indices.

9. What are the causes of cobalamin deficiency?

Most patients with severe cobalamin deficiency have an autoimmune illness called pernicious anemia. Patients with pernicious anemia have gastric achlorhydria and atrophy of the gastric parietal cells, which normally produce intrinsic factor. Intrinsic factor is necessary for the normal absorption of cobalamin. Occasionally this autoimmune disease is accompanied by other autoimmune diseases, especially of the thyroid. Pernicious anemia is usually found in middle-aged or older persons, but it is overlooked in a significant number of young patients because of lack of suspicion on the part of health care providers. Pernicious anemia is equally common in blacks and whites in the United States, but it is somewhat more common in women than men. Recently it also has been shown that up to 20% of elderly persons are cobalamin-deficient, probably because of varying degrees of malabsorption of cobalamin (so-called food cobalamin malabsorption). Dietary insufficiency is rare in the United States because cobalamin is available in all foods of animal origin and the requirement (1 μg) is small. Surgical causes of cobalamin deficiency include ileal resection, total gastrectomy (inevitable), partial gastrectomy, and jejunal or other intestinal bypass procedures. Pancreatic insufficiency and bacterial overgrowth of the small intestines also may cause malabsorption of cobalamin.

10. When is a Schilling test useful?

The Schilling test measures the absorption of ingested radioactive crystalline cobalamin. Usually a dual label test is performed in which the uptake with added intrinsic factor is also measured. The Schilling test detects classic pernicious anemia. It is not useful in conditions of mild malabsorption of cobalamin, which are common in the elderly. Modifications of the test, termed the food cobalamin Schilling test, have not been widely validated clinically. The Schilling test is infrequently performed at present because of newer methods of diagnosis.

11. What are the causes of folate deficiency?

Folate deficiency frequently results from a diet deficient in folic acid or chronic alcoholism. Organ meats, leafy green vegetables, and enriched breakfast cereals are the main sources of folic acid in the American diet. Since January 1998 all enriched grain products also have contained folic acid, and it seems likely that dietary folate deficiency will decrease in prevalence. People with rapid growth, pregnancy, or hemolytic anemia require more folate and may become deficient even on an adequate diet. Sprue and other disorders of the upper gastrointestinal tract may result in folate malabsorption and deficiency. Medications and alcohol, as described earlier, also may result in an increased need for folate.

12. Describe the problems with serum vitamin levels.

Both serum cobalamin and serum and red-cell folate levels have major problems with sensitivity and specificity in diagnosing the deficiency syndromes. Generally if the serum cobalamin or serum folate levels are extremely low, the patient has clinically important cobalamin or folate deficiency. Such patients are rare, however. The common clinical situation is a patient with mild megaloblastic anemia and serum cobalamin or folate level in the low normal range. An improper clinical practice is to repeat the vitamin level with the hope that it will become frankly normal or frankly abnormal. There is no scientific reason, however, to value the second result over the first. It is not surprising that serum levels of vitamins do not always accurately reflect the intracellular biochemical processes. Assessment of folate in red blood cells, as commonly performed, is not clinically validated, not reproducible and, therefore, not recommended. When a low normal serum vitamin level is detected, the clinician can either treat with the suspected vitamin and watch carefully for clinical response or follow-up with the assays for methylmalonic acid and total homocysteine.

13. What are the causes of elevated methylmalonic acid?

The only known causes for elevated serum methylmalonic acid are cobalamin deficiency, congenital disorders of cobalamin metabolism, and renal insufficiency. Renal insufficiency causes modest increases in serum methylmalonic acid (usually < 500–1000 nmol/L). If renal disease is excluded, elevated methylmalonic acid is diagnostic of a tissue deficiency of cobalamin. The elevated levels decrease readily after adequate cobalamin treatment. Ninety-nine percent of patients with clinical abnormalities due to cobalamin deficiency, such as megaloblastic anemia, have elevated methylmalonic acid.

14. What does an elevated total homocysteine level mean?

Total homocysteine may be elevated not only in cobalamin or folate deficiency but also in homocystinuria, renal failure, and rarer inborn errors of metabolism involving folate and cobalamin metabolism. If both methylmalonic acid and total homocysteine are elevated, *at least* cobalamin deficiency is present; folate deficiency also may exist. Elevated total homocysteine levels due to cobalamin deficiency do not respond to folate therapy and vice versa; thus, a clinical trial of specific vitamin therapy sometimes differentiates the two disorders.

15. Can serum cobalamin and folate levels be falsely low?
The serum cobalamin and folate levels can be quite nonspecific; many normal people have levels in the frankly low or low normal range. Such people do not have elevated methylmalonic acid or total homocysteine and will not benefit clinically from vitamin therapy. The lack of specificity of the serum cobalamin level may be problematic in evaluating older patients with refractory anemia or a patient with neurologic problems compatible with cobalamin or folate deficiency but due to another cause. Megaloblastic anemia that does not respond to specific vitamin therapy is *not* caused by vitamin deficiency. A further diagnostic work-up is required. Obtaining methylmalonic acid or, in the case of suspected folate deficiency, homocysteine levels before treatment confirms the deficient state and prevents delay in diagnosis of other conditions such as preleukemia or multiple sclerosis.

16. How do you treat cobalamin deficiency?
For many years the standard of care has been to administer cyanocobalamin only by parenteral methods, because deficiency is caused by malabsorption in almost every case. However, 1% of an oral dose is absorbed by an unknown mechanism in the stomach. Therefore, oral regimens using high doses (1 mg) of cyanocobalamin may be effective. A daily supplement may be less convenient to the patient, however, than a self-administered injection once a month. The choice of therapy at this point is 1 mg cyanocobalamin intramuscularly every 30 days (in some patients every 2 weeks) or 1 mg cyanocobalamin orally every day. Standard multivitamin pills usually contain only 6 µg of cobalamin and are not effective in the malabsorption syndrome.

17. What is the treatment for folate deficiency?
In most patients folate deficiency can be treated with 1 mg of oral folate per day.

18. What if you choose the wrong vitamin?
If a cobalamin-deficient patient is treated with folic acid, hematologic abnormalities may respond partially, leading the clinician to believe that the patient is improving. Unfortunately, neurologic lesions may progress because cobalamin is not being replaced. Therefore, it is extremely important to treat cobalamin-deficient patients with cobalamin. Patients with elevated methylmalonic acid should not be treated with folic acid alone.

19. Administration of folate in the periconceptual period may reduce the incidence of which group of congenital anomalies?
In numerous studies, the periconceptual administration of folate has been shown to reduce the incidence of neural tube defects in offspring by approximately 50%. As a result, the Food and Drug Administration (FDA) recently advised women who are contemplating pregnancy and who are of childbearing age to increase intake of folate in their diet. The Folate Food Fortification Program begun in January 1998 should decrease the incidence of neural tube abnormalities. It will also increase folate intake in cobalamin-deficient persons and thus possibly mask hematologic abnormalities. Clinicians need to be aware of this phenomenon and to pursue diagnosis aggressively in patients with neurologic abnormalities.

20. What is the newest indication for vitamin B_{12} and folate treatment?
Many reports show that elevated total homocysteine levels are associated with cardiovascular and thrombotic disease. No intervention studies show that lowering homocysteine levels in patients with mild hyperhomocysteinemia will benefit cardiovascular disease, however. The hyperhomocysteinemia in such patients is related to vitamin status as well as renal status. Many patients with hyperhomocysteinemia also have elevated methylmalonic acid and require combination vitamin therapy, including cobalamin and folic acid. Because vitamin therapy is inexpensive, safe, and convenient, many health experts recommend a "shotgun approach" with vitamins in the hope that lower homocysteine levels will prevent cardiovascular disease.

BIBLIOGRAPHY

1. Allen RH: Megaloblastic anemias. In Wyngaarden JB, Smith LH Jr, Bennett JC (eds): Cecil Textbook of Medicine, 19th ed. Philadelphia, W.B. Saunders, 1992, pp 846–854.
2. Allen RH, Stabler SP, Savage DG, Lindenbaum J: Metabolic abnormalities in cobalamin (vitamin B12) and folate deficiency. FASEB J 7:1344–1353, 1993.
3. Boushey CJ, Beresford SAA, Omenn GS, Motulsky AG: A quantitative assessment of plasma homocysteine as a risk factor for vascular disease. Probable benefits of increasing folic acid intakes. JAMA 274:1049–1057, 1995.
4. Centers for Disease Control: Recommendations for the use of folic acid to reduce the number of cases of spina bifida and other neural tube defects. MMWR 41(RR-14):1–7, 1992.
5. Stabler SP, Allen RH, Savage DG, Lindenbaum J: Clinical spectrum and diagnosis of cobalamin deficiency. Blood 76:871–881, 1990.
6. Toh BH, van Driel IR, Gleeson PA: Pernicious anemia. Ne Engl J Med 337:1441–1448, 1997.

11. HEMOLYTIC ANEMIAS

Richard F. Branda, M.D., and J. Frederick Kolhouse, M.D.

1. Which test best indicates a compensatory increase in erythrocyte production in hemolytic anemia?

The reticulocyte count, a measure of new red blood cell production, is the most sensitive test to measure adequacy of bone marrow response to hemolysis or blood loss. Erythroid hyperplasia is noted in the bone marrow, but bone marrow examination is generally not required to evaluate hemolytic anemia.

2. What chemistry laboratory tests are useful for the diagnosis of hemolytic anemias?

Numerous tests have been developed to help in the diagnosis of hemolytic anemia, but no single test is definitive. The **serum haptoglobin**, when saturated with hemoglobin from hemolysis, does not bind radioactive hemoglobin and thus is reported as absent. Approximately 2% of the population has congenitally absent haptoglobin, and liver disease can interfere with its synthesis. Because haptoglobin is an acute-phase reactant, it is most interpretable when it is absent. Low levels are seen regularly with intravascular hemolysis but also occur in extravascular hemolysis, particularly if it is chronic.

Hemopexin, a beta globulin that binds heme, is often reduced in patients with intravascular hemolysis. Once the binding capacity of haptoglobin and hemopexin are saturated, **methemalbumin** is formed, the **plasma hemoglobin** level rises, and free hemoglobin is filtered by the renal glomeruli and excreted as **hemoglobinuria**. Chronic hemoglobinuria is detected by staining for **urinary hemosiderin** in the sediment. An elevation of plasma or urine hemoglobin indicates brisk intravascular hemolysis.

The **erythrocyte lactate dehydrogenase** (LDH) and **indirect reacting bilirubin tests** also are indicators of hemolysis. However, both tests may be elevated in megaloblastic anemias because of hemolysis within the bone marrow (ineffective erythropoiesis). LDH can be elevated by numerous other problems in ill patients. The bilirubin level depends on liver function as well as red cell mass. For example, the indirect bilirubin is elevated in the 2% of the population who have Gilbert's disease. Increased hemoglobin breakdown results in delivery of additional bilirubin to the intestine and increased excretion of **urinary and fecal urobilinogen**.

3. What are the most important historical facts to obtain about a patient with a presumptive hemolytic anemia?

Documentation that the patient once had a normal hematocrit (particularly with a normal reticulocyte count) establishes that the anemia is most likely acquired as opposed to inherited. It is important to ask about a family history of anemia. Gallstones at an early age suggest chronic hemolysis. A careful drug history is essential.

4. What clues observed in the peripheral blood smear help to evaluate hemolytic anemias?

Patients with spherocytes or microspherocytes in the peripheral smear have hemolytic anemia that is usually due to either hereditary spherocytosis or autoimmune hemolytic anemia. Schistocytes, helmet cells, and red cell fragments indicate a microangiopathic process. Spur cells are seen in patients with liver failure. Target cells are associated with thalassemia, hemoglobin C disease, and liver disease. Sickle cells are characteristic of sickle cell anemia, and blister forms suggest glucose-6-phosphate dehydrogenase (G-6-PD) deficiency. Identifying intraerythrocytic parasites helps to diagnose hemolytic anemia due to malaria, babesiosis, and bartonellosis.

5. Which test is used to determine the presence of autoimmune hemolytic anemia?

The direct antiglobulin test (Coombs test) is used to determine the presence of autoimmune hemolytic anemia. Positivity of an indirect antiglobulin test or antibody screen with a negative direct antiglobulin test is meaningless with regard to autoimmune hemolytic anemia. This situation occurs in people who have been previously transfused and multiparous women. A positive antibody screen causes difficulties with cross-match in the blood bank but has no other pathophysiologic significance. A positive direct antiglobulin test is meaningful with regard to hemolytic anemia, although all patients with a positive direct antiglobulin test do not necessarily have hemolytic anemia. Conversely, some patients with a negative direct antiglobulin test may have autoimmune hemolytic anemia. Commercial reagents cannot detect fewer than 100–500 antibody molecules per cell, but fewer than 100 molecules per cell may shorten red cell survival in vivo. In addition, these reagents detect IgG and C3; therefore IgA antibodies are not detected.

6. What classes of antibodies are usually involved in autoimmune hemolytic anemias?

The two most common classes of antibodies involved in autoimmune hemolytic anemia are IgG and IgM. Certainly IgA has been associated with autoimmune hemolytic anemia, but this association appears to be rare. Approximately 30–40% of patients with autoimmune hemolytic anemia have only IgG on the red cells, a slightly larger number have both IgG and C3, and about 10% have C3 alone. Complement-only direct antiglobulin positivity is usually related to a cold-reacting IgM antibody. In this setting, the IgM is not present on the erythrocytes at the core body temperature. However, because IgM antibodies actively fix complement and complement stays on the erythrocytes, a complement-only positive antiglobulin test is found in this disorder.

7. Which diseases are associated with cold agglutinin disease?

Infection with Epstein-Barr virus is sometimes complicated by antibody production against the I red cell antigen, and mycoplasmal pneumonia is associated with antibody directed against the I antigen. These postinfectious cold agglutinin diseases are self-limited. If not infection-related, cold agglutinin disease may indicate an underlying lymphoproliferative disorder.

8. What conditions are associated with warm-reacting autoantibodies?

About one-half of cases are idiopathic. Identifiable causes include collagen diseases, lymphoproliferative disorders, and drug reactions. The drugs most commonly implicated are α-methyldopa, levodopa, procainamide, nonsteroidal antiinflammatory drugs (NSAIDs), quinidine and quinine, and penicillins and cephalosporins.

9. Which treatment modalities are used in patients with autoimmune hemolytic anemias?

Direct antiglobulin positivity to IgG alone or with complement in **warm-mediated autoimmune hemolytic anemia** results in removal of erythrocytes mainly by the spleen. Glucocorticoids such as prednisone are the first line of treatment. Once the hemoglobin is normal, a slow taper of prednisone can be started. About one-half of patients relapse. Splenectomy helps about one-half of this group. The remainder are often treated with immunosuppressive drugs such as azathioprine or cyclophosphamide. Other therapeutic approaches include intravenous immunoglobulin and cyclosporine. Thus, immunosuppression and splenectomy are usually successful treatments for warm-mediated autoimmune hemolytic anemia, which can be severe and life-threatening. If the hemolysis is secondary to a drug, simply stopping the drug is usually effective.

In contrast, **cold antibody-mediated autoimmune hemolytic anemia** is rarely as severe with regard to the anemia as warm-mediated autoimmune hemolytic anemia. Of interest, steroids, splenectomy, and frequently immunosuppression are relatively ineffective because most of the erythrocytes are removed by the liver rather than the spleen. Immunosuppression may be of benefit if an underlying secondary malignancy, causing the cold-mediated autoimmune hemolytic anemia, is treated by this therapeutic maneuver or with chemotherapy.

10. What is the role of transfusion therapy in autoimmune hemolytic anemia?

Blood transfusion may be necessary in severe cases of anemia. Cross-matching is difficult because the autoantibody may prevent accurate identification of coexisting alloantibodies induced by prior transfusions or pregnancies. This difficulty increases the risk of an alloantibody-induced hemolytic transfusion reaction. In addition, the autoantibody may decrease the survival of transfused red cells. Compatible red cells should be administered slowly while the patient is observed closely for transfusion reactions. Because the serologic evaluation may be time-consuming, the blood bank should be notified as soon as transfusion is considered. Prior identification of alloantibodies and knowledge of recent transfusions may expedite the evaluation. In many cases the signs and symptoms of anemia can be alleviated by relatively small quantities of blood, such as 0.5–1 unit. In patients with cold-reacting anti-I or anti-i autoantibodies, blood lacking these antigens may not be available, and red cells transfused through a blood warmer may survive adequately.

11. What is the most prominent inherited abnormality of the erythrocyte membrane that results in hemolysis?

Several proteins in the submembrane surface of erythrocytes help to maintain a normal biconcave disk shape. These proteins are referred to as ankyrin, spectrin, and protein band 4.1. In hereditary spherocytosis, spectrin deficiency is present in nearly all patients, and the degree of the deficiency correlates directly with the severity of hemolysis. Some patients have a primary defect of spectrin, whereas others have defective membrane proteins such as ankyrin and band 3 that attach spectrin to the membrane. The lipid bilayer is destabilized, leading to loss of membrane lipid and surface area and resulting in spherocyte formation. These rigid cells are retained and destroyed in the spleen. In hereditary elliptocytosis, the defect involves horizontal interactions between spectrin-spectrin and spectrin protein band 4.1. This defect weakens the skeleton, decreases membrane stability, and leads to red cell fragmentation. As with hereditary spherocytosis, the elliptocytes are removed by the spleen.

12. How are hereditary spherocytosis and elliptocytosis diagnosed and treated?

The mean corpuscular hemoglobin count (MCHC) is typically elevated in hereditary spherocytosis. The most reliable diagnostic test for hereditary spherocytosis is the incubated osmotic fragility test. Hereditary elliptocytosis is diagnosed by examination of the peripheral smear and by evidence of similar red cell abnormalities in family members. Splenectomy should be considered in patients with hereditary spherocytosis who are symptomatic from the hemolytic anemia or its complications, particularly gallstones. However, splenectomy should not be performed in children younger than 3–5 years to avoid postsplenectomy infections. All patients should be immunized with polyvalent vaccine against pneumococcus, *Haemophilus influenzae*, and meningococci several weeks before splenectomy. Most patients with hereditary elliptocytosis are asymptomatic, but occasional patients with more severe disease require splenectomy. For patients with the most severe form of elliptocytosis, hereditary pyropoikilocytosis, splenectomy is the treatment of choice.

13. What is the most common cause of hemolytic anemia as a result of erythrocyte glycolytic enzyme abnormalities?

Pyruvate kinase deficiency accounts for 95% of the hemolytic anemias due to abnormalities of the glycolytic pathway. This pathway produces adenosine triphosphate (ATP), which is necessary to maintain red cell shape and deformability. Pyruvate kinase deficiency is observed almost entirely in children, and moderately severe hemolysis is present from birth onward. The peripheral smear shows echinocytes, spherocytes, acanthocytes, and dehydrated red cells (xerocytes). The diagnosis is made by performing enzymatic assays. Splenectomy is used in patients with failure to thrive, chronic transfusion requirements, and severe anemia.

14. What is the most common abnormality of the red cell hexose-monophosphate shunt that is associated with hemolytic anemia?

G-6-PD deficiency is the most frequent abnormality of red cell metabolism and the most important defect of the hexose-monophosphate shunt. This pathway is necessary to preserve and regenerate reduced glutathione, which protects hemoglobin and other proteins from oxidant damage. G-6-PD deficiency is seen in approximately 10% of African-American men and is associated with episodic hemolysis. G-6-PD deficiency follows a pattern of development in the malaria belt. It is a genetic polymorphism that protects individuals from death from malaria. In the rare Mediterranean form of G-6-PD deficiency, the hemolysis is persistent and chronic but may become severe and even fatal after ingestion of fava beans (favism). In the United States, the episodic form of hemolysis is most common and is frequently induced by drugs that produce an excessive oxidant stress on erythrocytes.

A classic example is the antimalarial primaquine, which produces an immediate drop in the hematocrit and a small rise in the reticulocyte count. Increasing the dose of primaquine results in a further drop in the hematocrit and further small increase in the reticulocyte count. Thus, in the anemia induced by primaquine and other oxidant drugs in a patient with episodic hemolysis from G-6-PD deficiency, the hemolysis is dose-related because only the oldest erythrocytes are hemolyzed at a given dose. The older the erythrocyte, the less G-6-PD is available and thus the more sensitive the cells. As the dose of the oxidant drug is increased, an increasingly greater proportion of younger erythrocytes with greater amounts of G-6-PD are caused to hemolyze. Other drugs that cause significant hemolysis in patients with G-6-PD deficiency include sulfa drugs, nitrofurantoin, and nalidixic acid. The oxidation of hemoglobin produces intracellular precipitates (Heinz bodies) that can be detected by special stains. The removal of Heinz bodies by the spleen leads to the appearance of "bite" cells or blister forms. The diagnosis of G-6-PD deficiency should be considered in African-American patients who develop acute hemolysis and is made by measuring erythrocyte G-6-PD content.

15. Discuss the causes of a sudden drop in the hematocrit in patients with hemolytic anemias.

When the hematocrit suddenly drops from increased hemolysis, the reticulocyte count should reveal whether the bone marrow is responding properly to a worsening hemolytic rate. If the hematocrit is dropping and the reticulocyte count is also decreasing, one must look immediately for causes of relative bone marrow failure resulting in the sudden drop of hematocrit. The drop in hematrocit in each circumstance can be rather dramatic because the patients have an ongoing hemolytic anemia and are now not producing new erythrocytes. The cause may be (1) advancing chronic renal failure with a relative reduction in erythropoietin production (usually a slower, gradual drop in hematocrit): (2) reduction in micronutrients required for normal erythrocyte production (folate and iron); (3) acute infection; (4) infection of the bone marrow with parvovirus; or (5) drug suppression of the bone marrow. In this setting, the clinician usually orders a number of tests, including bone marrow aspiration and biopsy, to determine a cause of the aplastic crisis. All patients with hemolytic anemia should receive supplemental folic acid to avoid this cause of aplastic crisis.

16. Describe the characteristic features of the hemolytic anemia of paroxysmal nocturnal hemoglobinuria (PNH).

The reticulocyte count is usually elevated, and the erythrocyte morphology on peripheral smear is normal. The features of intravascular hemolysis are present—namely, absent haptoglobin, elevated LDH, excessive iron in the urine, and absent bone marrow iron. The white cell count and platelet count are often reduced, probably as a result of decreased production. PNH should be suspected in patients with a history of unexplained hemolysis, pancytopenia, marrow aplasia, and thrombotic events.

17. How is the diagnosis of PNH established?

PNH is a clonal stem cell disorder. The erythrocytes, leukocytes, and platelets of patients with PNH have an abnormally increased sensitivity to normal complement activation. The defect involves the cell membranes: proteins that carry a glycosylphosphatidylinositol anchor and normally inactivate activated complement are missing. Thus, the PNH erythrocyte is far more sensitive than normal red cells to hemolysis after activation of normal complement in serum. Activation of serum complement may be produced by a mild acidification of the serum (Ham acid hemolysis test) or reduction of the ionic strength of serum using sucrose to maintain tonicity (sucrose hemolysis test). The second test is more sensitive and less specific than the Ham test.

18. Describe the clinical course and treatment of PNH.

The degree of anemia varies but can be severe. Spontaneous long-term remissions may occur. Some patients have recurrent bacterial infections, and 10% of deaths are attributable to infection. Patients with PNH are prone to thrombosis of veins in unusual sites. Most patients die from clotting abnormalities in unusual places, such as the mesenteric veins, hepatic veins, and venous sinuses in the brain. Arterial occlusions are rare. Other patients die of hemorrhage. In addition, patients with PNH ultimately may develop a myelodysplastic picture that can evolve into frank leukemia. Treatment includes corticosteroids, androgens, iron therapy to replace losses in the urine, and transfusion as necessary. Thrombotic complications must be treated aggressively. Many patients require chronic anticoagulation. Bone marrow transplantation has been used in some patients with PNH.

19. What is a possible explanation for the clonal expansion of the PNH stem cells?

Mutations in the X-linked gene that codes for the enzyme required for the first step in the biosynthesis of glycosylphosphatidylinositol anchors confer a survival advantage by making the cells relatively resistant to apoptotic death. This abnormality may contribute to the tendency of PNH to transform to acute leukemia.

20. What is footstrike hemolysis?

Intravascular hemolysis with hemoglobinemia and hemoglobinuria has been described in runners and after prolonged marching. Footstrike hemolysis is probably due to trauma to the red cells and may lead to iron deficiency anemia.

21. What conditions are associated with a microangiopathic hemolytic anemia?

Microangiopathy occurs in conjunction with intravascular hemolysis secondary to vasculitis; for example, certain infections causing disseminated intravascular coagulation, thrombotic thrombocytopenic purpura, hemolytic-uremic syndrome, malignant hypertension, or collagen vascular diseases. The pathophysiology is endothelial damage and fibrin deposition leading to shearing of red cells. Pathologic heart valves may cause mechanical fragmentation of red cells. Microangiopathic disease may be a sign of disseminated malignancy. Abnormal tumor vessels and tumor-released thromboplastins contribute to the process. (See Figure 4, Color Plates.)

BIBLIOGRAPHY

1. Arese P, De Flora A: Pathophysiology of hemolysis in glucose-6-phosphate dehydrogenase deficiency. Semin Hematol 27:1–40, 1990.
2. Brodsky RA, Vala MS, Barber JP, et al: Resistance to apoptosis caused by PIG-A gene mutations in paroxysmal nocturnal hemoglobinuria. Proc Natl Acad Sci USA 94:8756–8760, 1997.
3. Collins PW, Newland AC: Treatment modalities of autoimmune blood disorders. Semin Hematol 29:64–74, 1992.

4. Cynober T, Mohandas N, Tchernia G: Red cell abnormalities in hereditary spherocytosis: Relevance to diagnosis and understanding of the variable expression of clinical severity. J Lab Clin Med 128:259–269, 1996.
5. Hillmen P, Lewis SM, Bessler M, et al: Natural history of paroxysmal nocturnal hemoglobinuria. N Engl J Med 333:1253–1258, 1995.
6. Jefferies LC: Transfusion therapy in autoimmune hemolytic anemia. Hematol Oncol Clin North Am 8:1087–1104, 1994.
7. Lubran MM: Hematologic side effects of drugs. Ann Clin Lab Sci 19:114–121, 1989.
8. Petz LD: Drug-induced autoimmune hemolytic anemia. Transfus Med Rev 7:242–254, 1993.
9. Rosse WF: Paroxysmal nocturnal hemoglobinuria. Curr Top Microbiol Immunol 178:163–173, 1992.
10. Tabbara IA: Hemolytic anemias: Diagnosis and management. Med Clin North Am 76:649–668, 1992.

12. APLASTIC ANEMIA

Eduardo R. Pajon Jr., M.D.

1. Discuss the differential diagnosis of pancytopenia.

Pancytopenia may be caused by two basic mechanisms: (1) relative bone marrow failure and (2) excessive peripheral destruction of cells. Relative bone marrow failure may be caused by folate or vitamin B_{12} deficiency, which leads to ineffective erythropoiesis with a hypercellular marrow. The marrow may be replaced with destruction of the normal architecture by myelofibrosis, metastatic carcinoma, acute leukemia, or even disseminated infection, such as tuberculosis or fungal infections. Clonal or premalignant disorders leading to depletion of the common stem cell compartment, such as paroxysmal nocturnal hemoglobinuria or hypocellular myelodysplastic syndromes, also may lead to relative bone marrow failure. Finally, the marrow may be hypocellular, as in aplastic anemia. The most frequent type of disorder associated with increased peripheral destruction is seen in hypersplenism, although autoimmune destruction of progenitor cells also may be a cause.

2. Are splenomegaly and lymphadenopathy usually found in patients with aplastic anemia at presentation?

No. Splenomegaly may develop after several blood transfusions, but in general the presence of splenomegaly and/or lymphadenopathy should raise a question as to the correct diagnosis.

3. Give the general categories of causes of aplastic anemia.

The causes of aplastic anemia may be divided into several categories, some of which may overlap in pathophysiology. In the first category is the idiopathic form of constitutional Fanconi's anemia, as well as the less frequent Estren-Dameshek anemia. A more frequent cause is exposure to **environmental toxins** such as benzene, cleaning solvents, or glues, **drugs,** such as chloramphenicol, quinine derivatives, gold salts, and antiepileptic drugs. **Ionizing radiation** that leads to a dose-dependent bone marrow aplasia is in contrast to the usual bone marrow aplasia seen with **chemotherapeutic drugs**, which, although dose-dependent, rarely lead to irreversible aplasia. Infections, particularly non-A, non-B, and non-C hepatitis, are notoriously associated with aplastic anemia. **Infections** seen with the Epstein-Barr virus, human immunodeficiency virus (HIV), and parvovirus also have been associated with varying degrees of bone marrow depression and aplastic anemia. In addition, other seemingly physiologic disorders such as pregnancy may be associated with aplastic anemia. In the last few years, it has been increasingly recognized that a significant number of cases of aplastic anemia are due to **aberration of the immune system** (e.g., T-gamma lymphocytosis or cases associated with abnormal CD-8 suppressor activity), resulting in agranulocytosis and pure red cell aplasia, or due to a **basic stem cell** disorder, such as paroxysmal nocturnal hemoglobinuria. Additional evidence for the autoimmune basis for the development of aplastic anemia is indirectly found in the association of aplastic anemia with various immune disorders, such as graft-versus-host disease, diffuse fasciitis, and systemic lupus erythematosus.

4. What is the appearance of the bone marrow in aplastic anemia?

The bone marrow is markedly hypocellular in aplastic anemia and the bone marrow space is occupied by fat. However, all degrees of aplastic anemia may be observed. In fact, a single blood cell line may be reduced in the beginning of aplastic anemia, which if followed long enough will frequently develop into full pancytopenia. Some physicians recommend bone marrow biopsy (the only way to accurately assess marrow cellularity) in at least two sites before establishing the diagnosis of aplastic anemia. More recent studies also have shown the value of magnetic resonance imaging (MRI) scans in evaluating bone marrow cellularity in patients with aplastic anemia.

5. How is the severe form of aplastic anemia distinguished from the highly severe form?

Although this may seem like a trivial distinction, it is an important one. Persons with early, highly severe aplastic anemia that is not treated have a median survival of only a few months (3 to 6 months), whereas those with severe aplastic anemia may have a much more prolonged survival with some hope of spontaneous recovery or at least a partial response to less aggressive treatment. Highly severe aplastic anemia is categorized as a granulocyte count of < 500, a platelet count of < 20,000, and a reticulocyte count of < 10,000/μl (< 0.1%). Patients with severe aplastic anemia who develop highly severe aplastic anemia over the ensuing months have an equally grim prognosis. It is important to distinguish individuals with highly severe aplastic anemia, because such patients should be treated as soon as possible with aggressive forms of therapy (see question 6).

6. Discuss the treatment of aplastic anemia.

All patients should be carefully questioned about exposure to drugs known to induce aplastic anemia (note: withdraw all drugs that are not absolutely necessary), and conditions in the workplace or home that may have caused aplastic anemia. Precautions with regard to gum damage (such as with toothbrushing) and good perirectal care (stool softeners, cleansing) help minimize infectious and bleeding complications. Patients with moderate-to-severe aplastic anemia may be observed or placed on androgen therapy unless their counts begin to deteriorate.

Patients with very severe aplastic anemia should be immediately considered for bone marrow transplantation (BMT) if they are under 45 years of age. In patients > 45 years difficulty with graft-versus-host reactions and other complications make BMT an especially risky procedure. In older patients therapy with a combination of antilymphocytic globulin (ALG), methylprednisolone (Solumedrol), and cyclosporine gives the best chance for a hematologic response. Caution should be taken in administering ALG because of the frequent development of serum sickness or even anaphylactic reaction; virtually all patients should receive the drug while under observation in the hospital. Although the remission rate to the above three drug protocols is approximately 70%, it must be remembered that many patients may relapse following such remissions. Retreatment with antithymocyte globulin (ATG) or ALG has been successful in many cases. The incidence of ultimate conversion of chronic aplastic anemia to acute leukemia or a myelodysplastic syndrome may be high. If a patient with aplastic anemia is considered for BMT, a major bone marrow transplant center should be contacted immediately to receive instructions as to how to maximize the chances of a successful transplant with regards to transfusions and other medical management issues.

7. What precautions should be taken when transfusing patients with aplastic anemia, particularly if they are candidates for BMT?

Because the success of BMT and the incidence of graft-versus-host reactions have been correlated with leukocyte alloimmunization, every effort should be made to minimize the use of blood products. When ordering blood products specifying leukodepleted, remember that irradiated products help to minimize alloimmunization.

8. Which blood abnormalities suggest pure red blood cell aplasia?

As the name implies, pure red blood cell aplasia involves only the red blood cell progenitors, sparing granulopoiesis and megakaryopoiesis. Therefore, the leukocyte count, differential, and platelet count are normal. The diagnosis can be established by bone marrow biopsy where few, if any, erythroid precursors are observed in the marrow and the white cell precursors and megakaryocytes are found in normal numbers.

9. Explain the causes of idiopathic pure red cell aplasia.

Idiopathic pure red cell aplasia may represent an extreme example in the spectrum of auto-antibody-mediated autoimmune hemolytic anemia. In the case of pure red cell aplasia, the difficulty may be that the antibody is directed against an antigen on the very early erythroid precursors. Based on elegant studies performed by Krantz, clearly the disease is mediated by antibody. The primary treatment of pure red cell aplasia involves immunosupression with steroids and occasionally immunosupressive agents. The majority of patients will respond dramatically to steroid therapy, but it is difficult to taper off steroids completely. Secondary causes of pure red cell aplasia have been associated with thymomas as well as other lymphoid malignancies. Removal of thymomas in some cases has led to remission of the anemia.

10. What is the typical mean corpuscular volume (MCV) in patients with aplastic anemia or pure red cell aplasia?

The MCV is typically elevated above 100 in patients with either aplastic anemia or pure red cell aplasia, which may sometimes cause initial confusion and suggest that the cause of the anemia may be folate or B_{12} deficiency. The question can be resolved by measuring levels of folate and B_{12} and performing a bone marrow biopsy. In folate or B_{12} deficiency, the bone marrow is characteristically highly cellular and sometimes confused with acute leukemia. The high MCV is presumably caused by early release of cells, because the few erythoid cells that are produced are intensely stimulated by erythropoietin.

11. What is the cause of secondary pure red cell aplasia in patients with a chronic hemolytic anemia?

Patients with a chronic hemolytic anemia may develop aplastic crisis resulting from micronutrient deficiency. In such a case significant numbers of erythroid precursors will be present, some of which may be megaloblastic. However, the culprit also may be a parvovirus that causes a severe depletion of erythroid precursors in the marrow with giant pronormoblasts. The diagnosis of parvovirus can be established by examination of the bone marrow and serologies for parvovirus B-19 antibodies.

BIBLIOGRAPHY

1. Brodsky RA: Biology and management of acquired severe aplastic anemia. Curr Opin Oncol 10:95–99, 1998.
2. Brown KE, Young NS: Parvovirus B19 in human disease. Annu Rev Med 48:59–67,1997.
3. Brown KE, Tisdale J, Barrett AJ, et al: Hepatitis-associated aplastic anemia. N Engl J Med 336: 1059–1064, 1997.
4. Camitta BM, O'Reilly RJ, Sensenbrenner L, et al: Antithoracic duct lymphocyte globulin therapy of severe aplastic anemia. Blood 62:883–888, 1983.
5. Clark CA, Dessypris EN, Krantz SB: Studies of pure red cell aplasia. IX: Results of immunosuppressive treatment of 37 patients. Blood 63:277–286, 1984.
6. Deeg HJ, Leisenring W, Storb R, et al: Long-term outcome after marrow transplantation for severe aplastic anemia. Blood 91:3637–3645, 1998.
7. Doney K, Leisenring W, Storb R, Appelbaum FR: Primary treatment of acquired aplastic anemia outcomes with bone marrow transplantation and immunosuppressive therapy. Ann Intern Med 126:107–115, 1997.
8. Kanwar VS, Wang WC, Winer-Muran HT, et al: Magnetic resonance imaging for evaluation of childhood aplastic anemia. J Pediatr Hematol Oncol 17:284–289, 1995.
9. Krantz SB, Kao V: Studies on red cell aplasia. I. Demonstration of a plasma inhibitor to heme synthesis and an antibody to erythroblastic nuclei. Proc Natl Acad Sci USA 58:493–500, 1967.

10. Marsh JC, Gordon-Smith EC: Treatment options in severe aplastic anemia. Lancet 351:1830–1831, 1998.
11. Najean Y: For joint group for the study of aplastic and refractory anemia: Long term follow up in patients with aplastic anemia. A study of 137 androgen-treated patients surviving more than two years. Am J Med 71:543–551, 1981.
12. Rosenfeld SJ, Kimball J, Vining D, et al: Intensive immunosuppression with antithymocyte globulin and cyclosporine as treatment of severe acquired aplastic anemia. Blood 85:3058–3065, 1995.
13. Young NS, Maciejewski J: The pathophysiology of acquired aplastic anemia. N Engl J Med 336: 1365–1372, 1997.

13. SICKLE CELL DISEASE AND THALASSEMIAS

Kathryn L. Hassell, M.D.

SICKLE CELL DISEASE

1. What is the genetic basis of sickle cell disease?

Sickle cell disease is caused by an inherited mutation of adult hemoglobin in which glutamic acid is replaced by valine as the sixth amino acid of the beta-globin chain. Sickle disorders are inherited in an autosomal manner because the gene for beta-globin is located on chromosome 11. Persons heterozygous for sickle hemoglobin are asymptomatic carriers of sickle cell disease and are said to have sickle trait. Homozygosity for the sickle gene causes sickle cell anemia, which is the most common form of sickle cell disease. Other common forms of sickle cell disease occur in individuals who are compound heterozygotes for the sickle cell gene and a second beta-globin abnormality such as hemoglobin C or β-thalassemia.

2. Who is affected by sickle cell disease?

In the United States, sickle disorders are encountered most frequently in African-Americans. The sickle gene also occurs in high frequency in India, Saudi Arabia, Turkey, Greece, Southern Italy, and Sicily. Thus, sickle cell trait and sickle cell disease occur in both African-Americans and Caucasians.

3. What two pathophysiologic processes are responsible for the clinical manifestations of sickle cell disease?

The signs and symptoms of sickle cell disease result from decreased red blood cell survival (hemolysis) and from the tendency of sickle cells to cause vasoocclusion, especially in the microvasculature. Hemolysis causes varying degrees of anemia, jaundice, increased cardiac output (heart murmur and cardiomegaly), and delayed growth; it also predisposes patients to cholelithiasis and to anemic crises (aplastic and sequestration). (See Figure 3, Color Plates.) Vasoocclusion causes tissue ischemia and organ dysfunction and frequently manifests as intermittent episodes of pain. Other important vasoocclusive complications include pulmonary infarction, stroke, hepatic and renal dysfunction, aseptic necrosis of the femoral head, priapism, leg ulcers, and proliferative retinopathy.

4. Do all patients with sickle disease have anemia?

No. The severity of hemolysis varies among the different forms of sickle cell disease, and for each syndrome there is much individual heterogeneity. Some persons with sickle hemoglobin C disease and sickle β⁺-thalassemia have mild hemolysis, and compensatory reticulocytosis prevents development of anemia (see table with question 6). Thus absence of anemia does not exclude sickle cell disease.

5. Describe the solubility test for sickle hemoglobin (Sickle Screen, Sickledex, or Sickle-quick). What does a positive result indicate?

The solubility test screens for the presence of sickle hemoglobin and is positive in persons with sickle cell trait as well as sickle cell diseases. Thus, a positive result does not differentiate persons with symptomatic disease from asymptomatic carriers. False negatives also occur, and the test does not identify carriers of β-thalassemia or hemoglobin C. Thus, hemoglobin electrophoresis is always necessary to evaluate the possibility of sickle cell disease or, in the context of genetic counseling, to identify persons at risk for having children with sickle cell disease.

6. How is sickle cell disease diagnosed?

The diagnosis of sickle syndrome requires quantitative hemoglobin electrophoresis. Typical results for the common sickle cell diseases and for sickle cell trait are shown in the table below.

Common Sickle Syndromes: Estimates of Clinical Severity and Typical Hemoglobin Electrophoresis Results

SYNDROME	β-GLOBIN GENOTYPE	HEMOLYSIS	VASOOCCLUSIVE COMPLICATIONS	HEMOGLOBINS (%)				
				A	A₂	F	S	C
Sickle cell diseases								
Sickle cell anemia	S-S	+ + + +	+ + + +	0	3	7	90	0
Sickle Hgb C disease	S-C	+	+ +	0	*	1	50	49
Sickle β⁰-thalassemia	S-β⁰†	+ + +	+ + +	0	7	8	85	0
Sickle β⁺-thalassemia	S-β⁺‡	+	+	20	6	7	67	0
Sickle trait	A-S	0	0	56	3	1	40	0

* High A_2 cannot be quantitated in presence of Hgb C.
† β^0 denotes β-thalassemia mutation that causes absent production of beta-globin.
‡ β^+ denotes β-thalassemia mutation that causes decreased production of beta-globin.

7. Are persons with sickle cell disease at increased risk for bacterial infections?

Yes. Numerous immunologic defects have been described in patients with sickle cell disease. The most important of these is the development (often early in life) of functional asplenia. Fulminant sepsis with pneumococcal and other encapsulated bacteria is the leading cause of death in childhood and remains a significant risk in adults.

8. What is the rationale for neonatal screening for sickle cell disease?

Sickle cell anemia is frequently asymptomatic during the first 1–2 years of life. The first manifestation of the disease is often pneumococcal sepsis or splenic sequestration, both of which are potentially fatal complications. Identification of sickle cell anemia at birth provides an opportunity to educate families and health care providers about the nature of sickle cell disease and to institute prophylactic penicillin and comprehensive care. These interventions have been shown definitively to reduce morbidity and mortality in early childhood.

9. How can pneumonia and pulmonary infarction be reliably differentiated in patients with acute respiratory symptoms?

They cannot be differentiated reliably. Patients with sickle cell disease are at increased risk for pneumonia as well as pulmonary infarction. Both complications typically present with fever, cough, chest pain, tachypnea, hypoxemia, and the presence of a new infiltrate on the chest radiograph. The term "acute chest syndrome" is used to describe such illness. Medical treatment generally includes antibiotics for infection as well as hydration, analgesia, oxygen, and sometimes exchange transfusions for vasoocclusion.

10. What is the most commonly performed surgical procedure in persons with sickle cell disease?

Cholecystectomy. Most patients with sickle cell anemia develop cholelithiasis during childhood and adolescence. Many patients subsequently become symptomatic. Elective cholecystectomy for asymptomatic gallstones is often recommended.

11. Describe important therapeutic considerations in the management of patients with sickle cell disease who require general anesthesia.

General anesthesia for surgical procedures is associated with a significant risk of intraoperative and postoperative complications. These complications include acute chest syndrome, pain episodes, infection, stroke, renal failure, and death. Thus, the intraoperative and postoperative management of patients with sickle cell disease requires scrupulous efforts to prevent dehydration or overhydration, hypoxemia, acidosis, and pulmonary atelectasis. To prevent sickling complications, many institutions routinely perform exchange transfusion before surgery to obtain a hemoglobin level of ≥ 10 gm/dl and a percentage of sickle hemoglobin $< 30\%$. Other institutions recommend simple transfusion with packed red blood cells before general anesthesia. A multicenter study of preoperative transfusion therapy has demonstrated that conservative therapy with simple transfusion to attain $< 60\%$ sickle hemoglobin is as effective as aggressive transfusion therapy in preventing perioperative complications for elective surgery.

12. What are the leading causes of death in adults with sickle cell disease?

- Cardiopulmonary disease (acute chest syndrome or chronic lung disease with cor pulmonale)
- Chronic renal failure
- Stroke
- Infection

13. What are new approaches to the treatment of sickle cell disease?

Several therapeutic approaches have been developed to attempt to ameliorate the severity of sickle cell anemia and sickle β^0-thalassemia, the most severe forms of sickle cell disease. Agents such as erythropoietin, hydroxyurea, and butyrate increase fetal hemoglobin levels and alter other RBC parameters (e.g., increased mean corpuscular volume [MCV]) in patients with sickle cell anemia. A study using hydroxyurea in adults with severe sickle cell disease demonstrated a 50% decrease in the incidence of painful events and acute chest syndrome in the group receiving the drug compared with the placebo group. This study did not include patients with milder forms of sickle cell disease or children. Bone marrow transplantation has been successfully performed in children with sickle cell anemia, and there are ongoing bone marrow transplantation trials for children and young adults with severe complications of sickle cell disease.

14. Is sickle cell trait associated with any medical complications?

Persons with sickle cell trait are generally asymptomatic, and the diagnosis of sickle cell trait is important principally for genetic counseling implications. However, red blood cells in sickle trait may sickle under hypoxemic, acidotic, or hypertonic conditions. Persons with sickle cell trait often develop mild hyposthenuria, and some may have intermittent episodes of painless microscopic or macroscopic hematuria. Exposure to environmental hypoxia (unpressurized aircraft, high mountain altitudes) may occasionally precipitate splenic infarction, but an overwhelming majority of persons with sickle cell trait can participate in mountain recreation such as hiking and skiing without adverse effects. Sickle cell trait is not a contraindication to participation in competitive athletics. Life expectancy is not altered by the presence of sickle cell trait.

THALASSEMIA

15. Define thalassemia.

Thalassemia syndromes constitute a heterogeneous group of genetic disorders whose clinical manifestations result from the decreased or absent production of normal globin chains of hemoglobin. These abnormalities result in hypochromic, microcytic anemias of varying severity. Alpha-thalassemia is caused by the decreased production of alpha-globin chains, and β-thalassemia by the decreased production of beta-globin chains.

16. Who is affected by thalassemia?

Thalassemia may be encountered in persons of all ethnic backgrounds. In the United States, the thalassemia syndromes occur with greatest frequency among persons whose ancestors originated from Africa, the Mediterranean Basin, the Middle East, Southern and Southeast Asia, Southern China, and the Pacific Islands.

17. With what disorder is thalassemia most often confused?

Iron deficiency. An almost universal manifestation of thalassemia is microcytosis (low MCV). Thalassemia is the most common inherited cause of microcytosis, and iron deficiency is the most common acquired cause of microcytosis. Thus, thalassemia should always be suspected in a person with low MCV, especially when iron deficiency has been excluded by laboratory tests or by failure to respond to therapeutic administration of iron.

18. Describe the genetic basis, clinical manifestations, and laboratory diagnosis of β-thalassemia minor.

Beta-thalassemia minor occurs in persons heterozygous for a β-thalassemia gene. Most are asymptomatic and many are not anemic, but their red blood cells are hypochromic and microcytic. The MCV is low unless the blood picture is clouded by coexistent folate or cobalamin deficiency. The diagnosis is confirmed by detecting elevated levels of hemoglobin A_2 and/or hemoglobin F by hemoglobin electrophoresis.

19. Since β-thalassemia minor is usually asymptomatic, why is it important to make this diagnosis?

Heterozygous β-thalassemia may have important genetic counseling implications. In addition, unnecessary administration of supplemental iron in a futile attempt to correct the microcytosis should be avoided. Women with β-thalassemia minor also may develop symptomatic anemia during pregnancy and rarely may require blood transfusion.

20. What is Cooley's anemia?

Cooley's anemia is homozygous β-thalassemia, or β-thalassemia major. Patients with Cooley's anemia develop a severe hydrochromic microcytic anemia during the first year of life and require chronic blood transfusions with iron chelation or bone marrow transplantation for survival.

21. Describe the genetic basis of α-thalassemia.

Most α-thalassemia syndromes are due to deletions of the alpha-globin genes. Normal persons have four alpha-globin genes, two on each chromosome 16. Thus, the severity of α-thalassemia syndromes is related to the number of gene deletions. The α-thalassemia syndromes have important genetic counseling implications because deletion of all four alpha-globin genes results in fetal hydrops, which is incompatible with life, and because such pregnancies are associated with significant maternal morbidity.

Alpha-Thalassemia Syndromes

USUAL GENOTYPES	ALPHA GENE NO.	CLINICAL FEATURES
αα/αα	4	Normal
α–/αα	3	Silent carrier
α–/α– or – –/αα	2	α-Thalassemia trait
– –/α–	1	Hemoglobin H disease
– –/– –	0	Fetal hydrops

α, presence of α gene; –, deletion of α gene.

22. What is α-thalassemia trait? How is it diagnosed?

Alpha-thalassemia trait is a mild, asymptomatic form of α-thalassemia caused by the deletion of two of four alpha-globin genes. The MCV is low, but anemia may not be present. Hemoglobin electrophoresis results are normal, so the diagnosis is often a presumptive one based on the exclusion of iron deficiency and β-thalassemia trait. DNA studies are usually required for a definitive diagnosis and should be obtained in the context of genetic counseling or prenatal diagnosis.

23. What is hemoglobin H disease?

Hemoglobin H disease is a moderately severe form of α-thalassemia that is usually caused by deletion of three of four alpha-globin genes. Affected patients typically have a moderately severe hypochromic microcytic anemia (hemoglobin 7–9 g/dl) with an elevated reticulocyte count. Clinical manifestations may include jaundice, splenomegaly, and cholelithiasis. Hemoglobin electrophoresis of fresh blood shows hemoglobin H (a tetramer composed of four beta-globin chains), and incubation of blood with brilliant cresyl blue (hemoglobin H prep) shows red blood cell inclusions.

BIBLIOGRAPHY

1. Bunn HF, Forget BG: Hemoglobin: Molecular, Genetic and Clinical Aspects. Philadelphia, W.B. Saunders, 1986.
2. Charache S, Barton FB, Moore RD, et al: Hydroxyurea and sickle cell anemia. Clinical utility of a myelosuppressive "switching" agent. The Multicenter Study of Hydroxyurea in Sickle Cell Anemia. Medicine 75:300–326, 1996.
3. Charache S, Lubin B, Reid CD (eds): Management and Therapy of Sickle Cell Disease. U.S. Department of Health and Human Services, NIH Publication No. 89-2117, revised September 1989.
4. Consensus Development Panel: Newborn screening for sickle cell disease and other hemoglobinopathies. JAMA 258:1205, 1987.
5. Gaston NH, Verter JI, Woods G, et al: Prophylaxis with oral penicillin in children with sickle cell anemia: A randomized trial. N Engl J Med 314:1593, 1986.
6. Giardina PJ, Hilgartner MW: Update on thalassemia. Pediatr Rev 13:55, 1992.
7. Koshy M, Entsuah R, Koranda A, et al: Leg ulcers in patients with sickle cell disease. Blood 74:1403, 1989.
8. Mentzer WC, Wagner GM (eds): The Hereditary Hemolytic Anemias. New York, Churchill Livingstone, 1989.
9. Milner PF, Kraus AP, Sebes JI, et al: Sickle cell disease as a cause of osteonecrosis of the femoral head. N Engl J Med 325:1476, 1991.
10. Ohene-Frempong K: Stroke in sickle cell disease: Demographic, clinical, and therapeutic considerations. Semin Hematol 28:213, 1991.
11. Platt OS, Thorington BD, Brambilla DJ, et al: Pain in sickle cell disease: Rates and risk factors. N Engl J Med 325:11, 1991.
12. Powars DR, Elliott-Mills DD, Chan L, et al: Chronic renal failure in sickle cell disease: Risk factors, clinical course and mortality. Ann Intern Med 115:614, 1991.
13. Powars D, Weidman JA, Odom-Maryon T, et al: Sickle cell chronic lung disease: Prior morbidity and the risk of pulmonary failure. Medicine 67:66, 1988.
14. Rackoff WR, Kunkel N, Silber JH, et al: Pulse oximetry and factors associated with hemoglobin oxygen desaturation in children with sickle cell disease. Blood 81:3422, 1993.
15. Serjeant GR: Sickle Cell Disease, 2nd ed. Oxford, England, Oxford University Press, 1992.
16. Vichinsky EP, Haberkern CM, Neumayr L, et al: A comparison of conservative and aggressive transfusion regimens in the perioperative management of sickle cell disease. The Prospective Transfusion in Sickle Cell Disease Study Group. N Engl J Med 333:206–213, 1995.
17. Walters MC, Patience M, Leisenring W, et al: Bone marrow transplantation for sickle cell disease. N Engl J Med 335:369–376, 1996.
18. Wayne AS, Kevy SW, Nathan DG: Transfusion management of sickle cell disease. Blood 81:1109, 1993.
19. West MS, Wethers D, Smith J, et al: Laboratory profile of sickle cell disease: A cross-section analysis. J Clin Epidemiol 45:893, 1992.
20. Zarkowsky HS, Gallagher D, Gill FM, et al: Bacteremia in sickle hemoglobinopathies. J Pediatr 109:579, 1986.

14. POLYCYTHEMIC STATES

Christine M. Holm, M.D., and Marie E. Wood, M.D.

1. What does the term *polycythemia* refer to?

Polycythemia literally means *(too) many cells.* Practically speaking, the term refers to (1) an increased hematocrit (erythrocytosis) or (2) increased hematocrit and increased platelets with or without increased leukocytes. An increase only in platelets is called thrombocythemia, whereas an increased white blood count alone is called leukocytosis.

2. What disease states should you consider in a patient with polycythemia?

In general, it is useful to think of two diagnostic categories, primary and secondary. **Primary erythrocytosis** is typified by the incessant, unregulated bone marrow production of cells, as with the myeloproliferative disorders polycythemia vera (PCV) and erythroleukemia (M6; extremely rare). **Secondary erythrocytosis** is a nonmalignant manifestation or response to another condition and, accordingly, is either relative (spurious) *or* real. The category of real polycythemia can be further divided into appropriate or inappropriate. Patients with **relative (or spurious) polycythemia** have normal red blood cell (RBC) mass and conditions that reduce the plasma volume, causing hemoconcentration. Examples include dehydration from high altitude, medications, decreased oral intake, and burns or stress (i.e., pheochromocytoma). A specific and common example of relative polycythemia is Gaisbock's syndrome, which characteristically occurs in hypertensive, obese men who smoke. Patients with real polycythemia have an elevated RBC mass (> 36 ml/kg for men or > 32 ml/kg for women). Generally, the hematocrit is > 60% without evidence of dehydration. Lower values may need to be verified by red blood cell mass measurements.

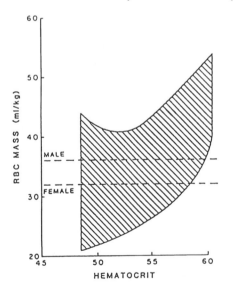

Range of red cell masses that may be seen in clinically stable patients with hematocrits in the range of 45–60 ml/dl. The interrupted horizontal lines depict the upper limits of the normal range for men and women. Patients with hematocrits in the range of 48–58 may or may not have increased red cell mass. (From Murphy S: Polycythemia vera. Dis Month 3:158–212, 1992, with permission.)

3. What is the differential diagnosis and evaluation of erythrocytosis?

The causes of erythrocytosis are quite diverse. Determining the underlying cause is essential to proper management. It is helpful to understand the normal regulation of erythropoiesis and then simply to apply Murphy's Law: Anything that can go wrong will go wrong at one time or another!

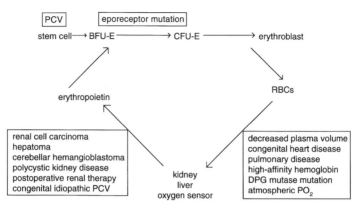

Varying causes of erythrocytosis. PCV = polycythemia vera; BFU-E = burst-forming unit, erythrocytes; CFU-E = colony-forming unit, erythrocytes; DPG = 2,3-diphosphoglycerate. (Courtesy of Mark A. Goldberg, M.D.)

4. What clinical clues may help to diagnose the cause of polycythemia?

The history and physical examination should focus on symptoms or signs of secondary erythrocytosis as mentioned above. A family history of polycythemic disorders (e.g., PCV, high-affinity hemoglobinopathies) is also important. The patient with PCV often has symptoms of vascular congestion or occlusion, central nervous system (CNS) symptoms, headache, peripheral vascular disease (PVD), gout, and/or weight loss. Pruritus, especially after a hot shower, is often reported. The physical examination in patients with polycythemia vera may reveal ruddy cyanosis, hypertension, gout, a palpable spleen or liver, and findings of PVD. Signs or symptoms of infection should not be present.

5. How common is PCV?

It is quite common. The incidence is about 1:100,000; men are affected slightly more often than women (1.2:1). The average age at diagnosis is 60 years. Less than 5% of patients with PCV are under 40 years old, and less than 0.1% are under 20. Few patients (0.4%) have a family history of PCV. Radiation exposure (e.g., atomic bomb fallout) may increase the risk for PCV.

6. Is PCV a malignancy?

Yes. It is a clonal disorder—unregulated growth of a malignant cell. Studies in heterozygote glucose-6-phosphate dehydrogenase (G-6-PD)-deficient women initially demonstrated the clonality of PCV. The malignant precursor is thought to be the pluripotent stem cell, thus accounting for involvement of all three cell lines in the bone marrow. Patients with PCV have increased numbers of CFU-GEMM (colony-forming units—granulocytes, erythroids, macrophages, megakaryocytes), a progenitor cell close to the pluripotent stem cell in the blood and bone marrow. CFU-GEMMs demonstrate unregulated proliferation in culture in the absence of erythropoietin. Increased tyrosine kinase activity also has been identified in progenitor cells; possibly influencing proliferation and/or survival of the cells.

7. What is the natural history of PCV?

Untreated controls have a median survival of about 18 months from diagnosis. Treated patients, however, may live 10–15 years.

8. How does the spent phase of PCV vary from the proliferative phase?

The **proliferative phase** is the initial phase of PCV and is typified by effective hematopoiesis. Bone marrow biopsy may reveal trilinear hyperplasia and increased cellularity. The peripheral blood smear may reflect this trilinear hyperplasia, demonstrating elevation of hemoglobin, platelets, and white blood cells. Vascular congestion, splenomegaly, bleeding, and thrombosis are also seen during the proliferative phase.

The **spent phase** or postpolycythemic myeloid metaplasia (PPMM) is seen after about 10 years in only 5–15% of patients. It is characterized by a decreased need for cytoreductive treatment, decreased red cell mass, and increasing splenomegaly. A leukoerythroblastic blood smear, pancytopenia, extensive bone marrow fibrosis, and ineffective and extramedullary hematopoiesis are common features of PPMM. Anemia in such patients is due to increased splenic sequestration, iron deficiency, and bleeding (secondary to platelet dysfunction). A decreased platelet count as well as platelet dysfunction may be observed. Among cases of PPMM, 20–50% evolve to acute leukemia. The prognosis for such patients is poor; only 30% are alive at 3 years. Patients who received 32P or alkylating agents have the highest incidence of acute leukemia.

9. Is splenomegaly seen during the proliferative phase as a result of extramedullary hematopoiesis?

No. Hematopoiesis is effective in this stage. Splenomegaly results from increased platelet and red blood cell sequestration within the spleen. The spleen can contain 2–3 times the platelet count (as estimated by a CBC), a splenectomy may result in a dramatic and dangerous increase of the platelet count.

10. What are the complications of PCV?

The most common complications are hemorrhage, thrombosis, PPMM, and leukemic transformation. Thrombosis is the most frequent cause of mortality (30–40%). Unusual sites such as the splenic vein and hepatic artery and vein are common, including portal vein thrombosis. About 10% of patients with the Budd-Chiari syndrome have underlying PCV. An elevated hematocrit with resultant viscous blood, elevated platelet count, and abnormal platelet function contribute to the thrombotic tendency. Surgery involves an especially increased risk of thrombosis or hemorrhage; 79% of patients with untreated polycythemia and 28% of treated patients risk these complications. Surgical complications in untreated patients consist of hemorrhage (52%), thrombosis (18%), or both (14%) as well as a postoperative mortality of 18%.

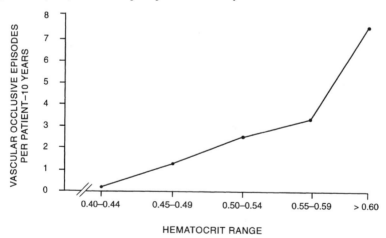

(Modified from Pearson TC, Weatherley-Mein G: Vascular occlusive episodes and venous hematocrit in primary proliferative polycythemia. Lancet 2:1219–1222, 1978, with permission.)

11. Which laboratory tests help to isolate the cause of polycythemia?

1. **Secondary erythrocytosis.** Patients have evidence of tissue hypoxia (low PO_2 or local tissue hypoxia) or conditions of elevated erythropoietin secretions. Both situations may be associated with elevated erythropoietin levels.

2. **High-affinity hemoglobinopathies.** Patients have a decreased P_{50} on the oxygen dissociation curve (see question 14).

3. **Polycythemia vera.** Patients demonstrate an increased RBC mass (> 36 ml/kg in men; > 32 ml/kg in women) and may have evidence of the following:

- Iron deficiency anemia
- Leukocytosis (66% of patients) without evidence of an infection
- Basophilia (one-third of patients)
- Elevated leukocyte alkaline phosphatase (LAP) score (if the WBC is increased and the LAP < 100, the diagnosis of chronic myelogenous leukemia [CML] should be considered)
- Increased vitamin B_{12} (due to increased binding protein, transcobalamin I, produced by white blood cells)
- Increased uric acid and increased lactate dehydrogenase (moderately increased in proliferative phase but may exceed 1000 mg/dl in PPMM)
- Increased platelet count (50% of patients have a platelet count > 500,000; 10% have a platelet count > 1,000,000)

12. Does the serum erythropoietin level help in the differential diagnosis?

Elevation of the serum erythropoietin level indicates a secondary erythrocytosis. If the laboratory is truly capable of sensitive and accurate low-level measurements, a very low level in the face of an elevated RBC mass indicates an autonomic proliferative disorder.

13. What is a "dry tap"?

A dry tap is the inability to aspirate bone marrow during a bone marrow biopsy. It is commonly seen in PCV and may be due to hypercellularity or fibrosis of the bone marrow.

14. What are the bone marrow findings in patients with PCV?

During the proliferative phase, the bone marrow is hypercellular, often demonstrating trilinear hyperplasia. One may see abnormal megakaryocytes, and > 5% of bone marrow biopsies have stainable marrow iron. A mild increase in reticulin, which is consistent with marrow fibrosis, may be seen. The spent phase of PCV is identified by an extreme clustering of megakaryocytes and an increase in reticulin, fibrosis, and disordered hematopoiesis.

15. Why would a physician order cytogenetic studies? Is PCV associated with chromosomal abnormalities?

Of patients with PCV, 15% have chromosomal abnormalities. The percentage increases with increasing years of the disease. The presence of Philadelphia chromosome (t[9,22] or BCR-ABL rearrangement) suggests CML.

16. How do I diagnose PCV?

Polycythemia Vera Study Group Criteria*

CATEGORY A: MAJOR	CATEGORY B: MINOR
A1: increased red cell mass (men: $\geq$ 36 ml/kg; women: $\geq$ 32 ml/kg)	B1: thrombocytosis (platelet count > 400,000)
A2: normal anterial saturation (> 92% on room air)	B2: leukocytosis (WBC > 12,000 without evidence of infection)
A3: splenomegaly	B3: increased LAP > 100 in absence of fever or infection
	B4: increased vitamin B_{12} (> 900 pg/ml) or unbound vitamin B_{12} (binding capacity > 2200 pg/ml)

* The diagnosis of PCV can be made if all three criteria from category A are present or with documentation of A1 + A2 + two criteria from category B.
From Berlin JJ: Diagnosis and classification of the polycythemias. Semin Hematol 12:339–351, 1975, with permission.

17. How should PCV be treated?

Control of the white blood cell count and hemoglobin and platelet counts decreases the incidence of hemorrhage and thrombosis. Treatment may include the following:

1. If phlebotomy is used to maintain the hemoglobin > 500,000/μl and/or thrombosis is clinically evident, cytoreductive drugs (i.e., hydroxyurea or interferon) should be used. This therapy may be used in addition to phlebotomy.

2. For the proliferative phase patients should be phlebotomized to a hematocrit of 43%. For patients over 70 years old or with thrombotic manifestations, hydroxyurea, interferon, or anagrelide should be used.

3. 32P and chlorambucil have been shown to be effective, but the markedly increased incidence of leukemia associated with these drugs precludes their use except as a last resort.

4. Hydrea has not been shown to cause a statistically significant increase in the incidence of leukemia, but the results were close. The question is still often raised.

5. Anagrelide and interferon are not thought to be leukemogenic.

6. Interferon may be considered in pregnant patients.

7. Pruritus may respond to myelosuppressive treatment.

8. There is no effective treatment for PPMM. Supportive care is generally offered.

9. Secondary leukemic transformation responds poorly to standard regimens, and treatment decisions should be individualized for each patient.

10. Aspirin does not decrease thrombosis but may increase bleeding events.

18. In the following case history, what is the differential diagnosis? Why?

A hematology consultation was requested for a 17-year-old white man with an elevated hemoglobin. He was admitted to the hospital with acute psychotic symptoms and a history of drug abuse. The patient denied any history of medical problems, but he had a family history of PCV (paternal aunt, paternal uncle, and father). Physical examination revealed mild rubor, no ecchymosis or petechiae, no cyanosis, no clubbing, and no adenopathy. His liver span was 14 cm, and the spleen tip was palpable. The laboratory evaluation revealed a white blood count of 5000/μl, hemoglobin of 17 gm/dl, and normal mean corpuscular volume (MCV) and mean corpuscular hemoglobin concentration (MCHC). The platelet count was normal at 184,000/μl. Electrolytes were normal, and the erythropoietin level was 6 μ/ml (normal: 0–50 μ/ml). A head CT scan was normal, and an abdominal ultrasound revealed only splenomegaly.

One may suspect PCV or a high-affinity hemoglobinopathy. Consistent with the diagnosis of PCV, the patient had an elevated hematocrit, splenomegaly, and a positive family history. The erythropoietin level was normal, as in PCV, and most secondary causes of polycythemia have been ruled out. Against the diagnosis of PCV is the fact that no other blood cell lines were elevated (WBC or platelets). There was no personal or family history of bleeding or thrombosis, and the patient is unusually young for a diagnosis of PCV.

Thus, support for the diagnosis of PCV is weak, and another diagnosis should be suspected, such as high-affinity hemoglobinopathy. High-affinity hemoglobinopathy is often an autosomal dominant disorder. The high-affinity hemoglobin releases a smaller percent of oxygen to the tissues than normal hemoglobin; thus, a higher volume of RBC is needed to achieve the same oxygen delivery stoichiometrically. At equilibrium erythropoietin is usually normal. The diagnosis is made by constructing an oxygen-hemoglobin dissociation curve. Hemoglobin electrophoresis may identify some but not all increased-affinity hemoglobins. If the abnormal-affinity hemoglobin is unstable, signs and/or symptoms of chronic hemolysis are seen. It is important to distinguish high-affinity hemoglobinopathy from PCV, thus avoiding misdiagnosis and possibly inappropriate treatment.

CONTROVERSIES

19. Should iron-deficient patients with PCV be given exogenous iron?

For:

• Iron deficiency has been implicated in pruritus and may contribute to fatigue.

• Iron deficiency can make the red blood cells less deformable. Some argue that this contributes to thrombosis.

Against:

• The resulting erythrocytosis is often uncontrollable without excessive phlebotomy or addition of myelosuppressive drugs.

• Increased hemoglobin predisposes to thrombosis.

• Finally, according to Rector et al., no nonhematologic sequelae of iron deficiency were found in patients with PCV who were studied over 25 years. Treadmill performances were similar to normal controls, patients developed no dysphagia or esophageal changes, and physical examinations failed to reveal the skin and nail changes described in other iron-deficient patients.

20. Should all patients with an elevated hemoglobin be phlebotomized, regardless of the underlying cause?

Generally not in secondary erythrocytosis. The hemoglobin is often increased in an attempt to compensate for the common denominator of tissue hypoxia. However, hematocrit over 60% may cause such sludging that oxygen delivery is impaired despite the hemoglobin increase. Acutely, phlebotomy may be indicated for patients with hematocrit > 60–65% and signs of sludging and/or tissue hypoxia. Hydration should precede and follow careful phlebotomy, and oxygen should be given. In special patients with high-affinity hemoglobin, acute difficulty due to sludging, and impaired tissue oxygenation, one should consider phlebotomy and replacement with normal blood (exchange transfusion). Anticoagulation with Coumadin may help to avoid sludging in patients with high-affinity hemoglobin and mild sludging symptoms. However, most patients with high-affinity hemoglobin do not require treatment.

On a more chronic basis, oxygen should be administered to patients with secondary polycythemia and hypoxia. Erythropoietin-secreting tumors should be resected.

Pitfalls

• Iron deficiency may mask increased RBC volume.

• Folate or B_{12} deficiency may mask polycythemia.

• RBC volume determinations in obese patients are somewhat imprecise.

• A patient with evidence of secondary polycythemia (e.g., hypoxic smokers) also may have PCV—both diseases are common. A major clue is an elevated WBC or an elevated platelet count in addition to elevated hemoglobin.

• Splenectomy during the proliferative phase of PCV may cause dangerously high thrombocytosis from release of the large volume of pooled platelets.

BIBLIOGRAPHY

1. Adamson JW, Fialkow PJ, Murphy S, et al: Polycythemia vera: Stem-cell and probable clonal origin of the disease. N Engl J Med 295:913–916, 1976.
2. Berk PD, Goldberg JD, Donovan PB, et al: Therapeutic recommendations in polycythemia vera based on polycythemia vera study. Semin Hematol 23:132–143, 1986.
3. Berlin NJ: Diagnosis and classification of polycythemias. Semin Hematol 12:339–351, 1975.
4. Fruchtman SM, Mack K, Kaplan ME, et al: From efficacy to safety: A Polycythemia Vera Study Group report on hydroxyurea in patients with polycythemia vera. Semin Hematol 34:18–23, 1997.
5. Gruppo Italiano Studio Policitemia: Polycythemia vera: The natural history of 1213 patients followed for 20 years. Ann Intern Med 123:656–664, 1995.
6. Meytes D, Katz D, Ramot B: Prognostic parameters in myeloid metaplasia: Agnogenic vs. post polycythemic myelofibrosis. Isr Med J 12:534–542, 1976.
7. Najean Y, Rain JD: The very long-term evolution of polycythemia vera: An analysis of 318 patients initially treated by phlebotomy or 32P between 1969 and 1981. Semin Hematol 34:6–16, 1997.
8. Petitt RM, Silverstein MN, Petrone ME: Anagrelide for control of thrombocythemia in polycythemia and other myeloproliferative disorders. Semin Hematol 34:51–54, 1997.
9. Rector WG, Fortuin NJ, Conley CL: Non-hematologic effects of chronic iron deficiency: A study of patients with polycythemia vera treated solely with vera sections. Medicine (Baltimore) 61:382–398, 1992.

10. Silverstein MN, Lanier AP: Polycythemia vera 1935–1969: An epidemiologic survey in Rochester, Minnesota. Mayo Clin Proc 46:751–753, 1971.
11. Silver RT: Interferon alfa: Effects of long-term treatment for polycythemia vera. Semin Hematol 34:40–50, 1997.
12. Swolin B, Weinfeld A, Wostin J: A prospective long-term cytogenic study in polycythemia vera in relation to treatment and clinical course. Blood 72:386–395, 1988.
13. Weatheral DJ: Polycythemia resulting from abnormal hemoglobins. N Engl J Med 280:604–606, 1969.
14. Weinreb NJ, Shin CF: Spurious polycythemia. Semin Hematol 12:397–406, 1975.

15. IRON OVERLOAD

S. Mark Bettag, M.D., Julie Pysklo, M.D., and Paul A. Seligman, M.D.

1. What is the definition of iron overload?

The definition of iron overload is an excess amount of total body iron. In the normal individual, two-thirds of the total body iron is found in red blood cells, making up about 2 grams (gm) of iron. The remaining one-third is almost exclusively found in storage iron that is sequestered in the iron storage protein, ferritin. Conditions that result in excess storage iron (i.e., more than 1 gm of iron sequestered in ferritin) cause iron overload. The pathologic entities responsible for iron overload are hemochromatosis and hemosiderosis. Hemochromatosis is defined as iron overload with resultant tissue damage. Hemosiderosis is iron overload not associated with tissue damage. Pathologically, hemochromatosis implies excessive iron deposition in various parenchymal cells of the body, besides deposition in cells associated with iron storage, i.e., macrophages. In hemosiderosis, the vast majority of excess iron is found in the macrophages.

2. What are the causes of iron overload?

Causes of iron overload are generally divided into genetic and acquired. The main genetic cause is hereditary hemochromatosis (see question 3). Other genetic causes include refractory anemias including thalassemia major or hereditary sideroblastic anemia. In most cases, the genetic causes of iron overload are associated with obvious hemochromatosis (deposition of excess iron in parenchymal cells). Acquired causes include refractory anemias including aplastic anemia necessitating transfusion (which also results in iron overload), or chronic ingestion of medicinal iron. This includes thalassemia or congenital hemolytic anemias with or without blood transfusions. Blood transfusions do exacerbate the hemochromatosis in these instances. The acquired cause of iron overload are at first associated with hemosiderosis. However, with increased ingestion of iron or increased transfusions, iron excess associated with hemosiderosis eventually results in "spillover" of iron so that hemochromatosis associated with tissue damage becomes evident.

3. What genetic defect has been associated with hemochromatosis?

The genetic defect associated with hemochromatosis is a mutation of the HLA-H protein, a novel MHC class 1-gene. Similar to the other MHC class 1-genes, it is located on the short arm of chromosome 6. Classically, MHC class 1-molecules are part of the immune system and act as antigen presentation molecules. The role of the HLA-H protein and the common genetic defect in normal iron metabolism or in causing the defect in hemochromatosis is not clear. However, it is known that this protein binds beta-2 microglobulin, a protein whose deficiency has been found to be associated with iron loading in mice. The identification of a single mutation (C282Y) that is present in most well-defined pedigrees with hemochromatosis has allowed for a reevaluation of various diagnostic criteria using a genotypic gold standard. Finding this mutation, however, is not a perfect genetic test for hemochromatosis because patients with clinical disease may show this defect in only one or neither of their HLA-H proteins. This suggests that other mutations in this protein may be associated with the same genotypic abnormalities as shown in hemochromatosis. So far, however, only one other genetic defect at the 63-amino acid position has been found to be associated with iron overload, and in such cases virtually all of the patients have one of these mutations and another mutation at C282Y.

4. What is the mode of inheritance of the hereditary hemochromatosis?

Primary hereditary hemochromatosis is of autosomal recessive inheritance. Heterozygotes have no clinical expression associated with iron overload, but if affected with another condition such as hemolytic anemia, this mixed heterozygous state may show evidence of clinical disease. Hereditary hemochromatosis is one of the most common hereditary diseases in North America. The gene incidence is about 10% and 1 in 200–400 individuals are homozygotes, although such patients generally have subclinical disease. A form of hemochromatosis seen in African-Americans originally called "African nutritional hemochromatosis" appears to have a genetic basis not related to the gene defect seen in hereditary hemochromatosis.

5. Since hereditary hemochromatosis is so common, why does clinical presentation have such a low incidence?

People with homozygous hemochromatosis have a defect in iron absorption that results in accumulation of excess iron over decades. Because women generally have a negative iron balance during childbearing years, they accumulate on average much less excess iron than men. It is estimated that about 20 gm of excess iron is necessary to cause clinically significant disease; therefore, individuals with homozygous hemochromatosis, particularly women, may never accumulate this much excess iron in the period of the average life span (i.e., 75 years). However, homozygous hemochromatosis is underappreciated in the clinical population because diseases such as diabetes, arthritis, impotence, and congestive heart failure are so common. Individuals with homozygous hemochromatosis, who have other reasons for organ system involvement, may have exacerbation of their disease process due to damage caused by iron. Based on such considerations, it is important to diagnose homozygous hemochromatosis.

6. What is the best screening test for homozygous hemochromatosis?

Screening tests used for the detection of homozygous hereditary hemochromatosis are the serum ferritin and the transferrin saturation. The transferrin saturation is the best screening test: a saturation value > 62% predicts the homozygous state in 92% of cases. The serum ferritin value is generally increased only with iron overload. The transferrin saturation is increased even in individuals with homozygous hemochromatosis screened during childhood or early adulthood.

7. Which genetic test is used?

In general, treatment decisions are based on the finding of a markedly increased transferrin saturation and the degree of iron overloading is revealed by the ferritin value and a liver biopsy to determine the quantity of excess iron in the body. However, genetics testing for hemochromatosis is often helpful in patients who have "borderline" values or other diseases associated with iron overload. Additionally, in most instances, family studies require the genetics test. When following pedigree studies, the prevalence of two C282Y mutations has been described in 95% or more of the homozygotes for the disease. When unrelated patients exhibit genotypic expression of this disease as indicated by high transferrin saturation, closer to 80% of the patients have homozygosity for this mutation. The test itself uses a polymerase chain reaction amplification and digestion of the DNA with a restriction enzyme.

8. If a person is diagnosed as hemochromatic, should the rest of the family be evaluated?

Once an index case of homozygous hemochromatosis is found in a family, the presence of the hemochromatosis gene can be followed. If the patient is homozygous for the C282Y mutation, it can be determined in family members, whether they are homozygous or heterozygous for the condition. Thus, family members can be screened by the genetics test and the clinical diagnosis or phenotypic expression confirmed by transferrin saturation. If the index case does not show homozygosity for the genetic defect, then genetics testing is much less useful, but these individuals can still be screened by transferrin saturation. Clinicians should make it clear to people with one mutation that they are "carriers" but not at risk for iron overload unless they have another condition that causes iron overload. Homozygotes determined by the genetics test (or those who have high saturations) and a high serum ferritin value or evidence for a liver disease should have a liver biopsy to determine the amount of iron overload by quantitating the amount of iron found in the liver (hepatic iron index) and the amount of damage to the liver, because patients with cirrhosis even after phlebotomy therapy have a poor prognosis (see question 12). The amount of iron loading allows the physician and the patient to better estimate the total number of phlebotomies necessary to deplete iron to normal levels.

9. How does iron overload cause tissue damage?

It is believed that excess iron accumulation in parenchymal cells causes enhanced lysosomal fragility associated with increased iron laden ferritin that is denatured to hemosiderosis. Perioxidation of membrane lipids mediated by free radical formation, a reaction catalyzed by iron also may occur. The parenchymal cells most damaged by excess iron correlate with the clinical signs of disease discussed below.

10. What are the early and late clinical features of iron overload?

The diagnosis of early hemochromatosis may be associated with only subtle findings. In many instances, the presenting finding may be hepatomegaly, mild diabetes mellitus, or mild arthritis, particularly of the large joints or the metacarpophalangeal (MCP) joints. In some cases, other endocrinologic findings may be evident, including impotence or hypothyroidism. Cardiomyopathy is usually not the presenting finding of hemochromatosis in older individuals. A rare young individual (i.e., 20–30 years old) with markedly excessive iron accumulation may present with congestive heart failure as an early manifestation. The clinical manifestations of the disease are due to parenchymal cell damage caused by iron overload in hepatocytes, pancreatic islet cells, or the pituitary. The arthritis associated with hemochromatosis may be similar to that seen with osteoarthritis, or in rarer instances the classic findings of chondrocalcinosis are evident. The late clinical manifestations of hemochromatosis such as the classic triad of cirrhosis, diabetes mellitus, and bronze skin (due to excessive melanin production), is rarely seen in patients who present with the disease in modern times.

11. What is the therapy for hemochromatosis?

The best therapy for homozygous hemochromatosis is phlebotomy. Because such patients have marked iron overload, the removal of 1 or even 2 units of blood per week is generally well tolerated unless the patient is severely ill. At least 10 gm of iron is associated with clinical manifestations of the disease. One unit of blood contains about 250 mg of iron. It should be anticipated, therefore, that at least 40–80 phlebotomies would be necessary to normalize the total body iron. During phlebotomy therapy the patient is monitored with blood counts to ensure that they have maintained an adequate hemoglobin level. Serial ferritin values follow the decrease in total body iron stores for individual patients receiving phlebotomy therapy. Once symptomatic patients have a normalized total body iron, a maintenance phlebotomy regimen of 2–4 phlebotomies per year may be adequate to maintain body iron stores at normal levels. In patients who have hemochromatosis due to hereditary or acquired anemic conditions associated with transfusion therapy, treatment with an iron chelator such as deferoxamine is necessary in order to remove iron. In such individuals it must be ensured that they receive adequate iron chelation therapy, particularly if transfusions are necessary to maintain their hemoglobin in an acceptable range.

12. What is the overall prognosis of patients with hemochromatosis?

Treated patients with hemochromatosis who present with mild clinical disease or subclinical disease generally have a normal lifespan if iron stores are maintained at optimal levels. Patients who already have cardiac damage or severe diabetes generally will have only partial reversal of their disease state with phlebotomy therapy and will have decreased survival based on complications. Patients with hepatic cirrhosis also have decreased survival. Although it has been suggested that in some instances phlebotomy therapy may reverse this process, patients with cirrhosis, even if treated with phlebotomy therapy, are at risk for the development of hepatoma.

13. What is the best treatment for patients with hemochromatosis acquired from transfusions?

The best therapy in this instance is not phlebotomy because the patient depends on transfusions to keep the hemoglobin in an acceptable range. So the best therapy would be chelation therapy, usually with deferoxamine.

14. Can hemochromatosis be cured?

At present, no. Hemochromatosis is similar to diabetes mellitus, in which insulin is needed to keep the glucose in check. In hemochromatosis, maintenance therapy with phlebotomy and/or chelation is required to keep the iron from accumulating. In the future, gene therapy may be available to cure patients, but at present there is no cure.

BIBLIOGRAPHY

1. Adams PC, Chakrabarti S: Genotypic/phenotypic correlations in genetic hemochromatosis: Evolution of diagnostic criteria. Gastroenterology 114:319–323, 1998.
2. Adams PC, Speechley M, Kertesz AE: Long-term survival analysis in hereditary hemochromatosis. Gastroenterology 101:368–372, 1991.
3. Edwards CQ, Griffen LM, Goldgar D, et al: Prevalence of hemochromatosis among 11,065 presumably healthy blood donors. N Engl J Med 318:1355–1362, 1988.
4. Fairbanks V, Baldus W: Iron overload. In Hoffman R, Benz EJ Jr, Shattil SJ, et al: Hematology: Basic Principles and Practice. New York, Churchill Livingstone, 1991, pp 752–758.
5. Gordeuk V, Mukiibi J, Hasstedt SJ, et al: Iron overload in Africa. Interaction between a gene and dietary iron content [see comments]. N Engl J Med 326:95–100, 1992.
6. Jazwinska EC, Cullen LM, Busfield F, et al: Haemochromatosis and HLA-H [letter; comment]. Nat Genet 14:249–251, 1996.
7. Nichols GM, Bacon BR: Hereditary hemochromatosis: Pathogenesis and clinical features of a common disease [see comments]. Am J Gastroenterol 84:851–862, 1989.
8. Powell LW, Summers RM, Board PG, et al: Expression of hemochromatosis in homozygous subjects. Implications for early diagnosis and prevention. Gastroenterology 98:1625–1632, 1990.
9. Skikne BS, Cook JD: Screening test for iron overload. Am J Clin Nutr 46:840–843, 1987.
10. Weintraub LR, Conrad ME, Crosby WH: The many faces of hemochromatosis. Hosp Pract 26:49–52, 55–59, 1991.
11. Weintraub LR, Conrad ME, Crosby WH: The treatment of hemochromatosis by phlebotomy. Med Clin North Am 50:1579–1590, 1996.

16. DISSEMINATED INTRAVASCULAR COAGULATION

Robin J. Kovachy, M.D., and David M. Schrier, M.D.

1. What is disseminated intravascular coagulation (DIC)?

It is the widespread deposition of fibrin in small blood vessels that may cause tissue or organ damage from ischemia. Depletion of clotting factors and platelets result in a bleeding diathesis. Simultaneous activation of plasmin and resulting fibrinolysis also occur. This has been reported in association with any severe illness or may be more insidious in certain chronic diseases.

2. How common is DIC?

DIC is second only to liver disease as a cause of *acquired* coagulopathy. In the hospitalized population, DIC may be as common as 1 per 1000 admissions.

3. What illnesses are associated with DIC?

Common illnesses associated with DIC include:

Obstetric complications: abruptio placentae, septic abortion, chorioamnionitis, amniotic fluid embolism, intrauterine fetal death, postpartum hemolytic-uremic syndrome, and severe eclampsia

Infections: viral, bacterial (especially meningococcemia and gram-negative sepsis, rickettsial, mycotic, protozoal)

Neoplasms: carcinoma of the prostate, pancreas, breast, lung, ovary, gastric, and others

Intravascular hemolysis (e.g., transfusion reaction)

Vascular disorders: aneurysms, giant hemangiomas, or vasculitis

Massive tissue injury and trauma

Miscellaneous: snake bite, anaphylaxis, drug reactions, hypothermia, transplant rejection, acute respiratory distress syndrome (ARDS), acidosis, acute pancreatitis

4. Describe the clinical picture of acute DIC.

The major clinical finding is generalized bleeding. Patients may ooze from venipuncture sites and have widespread ecchymoses and petechiae. Bleeding into the kidneys, lungs, gastrointestinal tract, or central nervous system (CNS) may occur as well. Evidence of thromboembolic phenomena may also be present. Acral cyanosis (gray to purple discoloration of the tips of the fingers and toes) is occasionally seen, especially in patients with shock.

5. Describe the clinical picture of chronic DIC.

Chronic DIC is usually manifested by bruising and mucosal bleeding. Thrombophlebitis is common and often occurs in unusual sites. Evidence of renal dysfunction or transient neurologic syndromes is common.

6. What laboratory tests are needed to diagnose DIC?

In acute DIC, usually the prothrombin time (PT), partial thromboplastin time (PTT), and thrombin time are prolonged. The platelet count is decreased. Fibrin degradation products (FDPs) are elevated. Multiple clotting factors, especially fibrinogen and factors V, VIII, and XIII, are usually depressed. In chronic DIC, the platelet count and clotting factor levels may be normal. However, FDPs are elevated. Review of the peripheral blood smear shows schistocytes (fragmented RBCs) in 50% of cases. (See Fig. 4, Color Plates.)

7. Name two conditions that may be confused clinically with DIC. How can they be distinguished?

1. Severe liver disease can look the same with thrombocytopenia, prolonged PT and PTT, and elevated FDPs. Usually factor VIII is normal or increased in liver disease, whereas it is more likely to be depressed in DIC.

2. Primary fibrinogenolysis is a *rare* disorder with hemorrhagic tendencies from increased breakdown of fibrinogen. The PT and PTT are prolonged. Usually the platelet count is normal. Schistocytes are not seen on the peripheral blood smear.

8. What is the most important treatment of DIC?

Treatment of the underlying illness is the cornerstone of treatment. Spontaneous reversal of DIC often occurs if the underlying illness is successfully treated. Frequently patients require transfusions of red blood cells and aggressive management of shock. Platelets should be transfused if there is severe hemorrhage and the platelet count is < 50,000.

CONTROVERSIES

9. Should clotting factor replacement be given?
For:

Cryoprecipitate, rich in fibrinogen, should be given when the fibrinogen level is < 100 mg/dl, especially in the presence of hemorrhage. In most series, infusion of fresh frozen plasma or cryoprecipitate has not been associated with adverse effects.

Against:

Infusion of fibrinogen may add "fuel to the fire" and aggravate the deposition of fibrin in small blood vessels. Thromboembolic complications have been reported with replacement of clotting factors. With large volumes of blood products, the risk of hepatitis or acquired immunodeficiency syndrome (AIDS) increases.

10. Should heparin be used to treat DIC?
For:

Heparin activates antithrombin III, which neutralizes free thrombin and inhibits its further formation. Because DIC is the abnormal activation of the clotting pathway, heparin should improve the coagulation abnormalities. Heparin is considered useful in patients with clinical signs of major thrombotic events, such as acral ischemia, or chronic DIC, as seen with malignancies.

Against:

No randomized trials have shown improved outcome in acute DIC with the use of heparin. Beneficial effects of heparin have been reported mostly in situations in which DIC is self-limited and would be expected to resolve spontaneously anyway. Heparin may increase the bleeding tendency.

11. Should antithrombin III be used in the treatment of DIC?

Giving antithrombin III in the form of antithrombin III concentrates or fresh frozen plasma should theoretically neutralize excessive thrombin and slow down the intravascular coagulation process. The main use of antithrombin III concentrates should be in patients with DIC-associated hepatic failure, because the functional antithrombin III levels can be extremely low due to decreased synthesis in the setting of increased consumption. Pregnant patients with fatty liver and DIC may also benefit from antithrombin concentrates. The role of antithrombin III in the setting of DIC due to other causes besides hepatic failure has not been established.

BIBLIOGRAPHY

1. Bick RL: Disseminated intravascular coagulation and related syndromes: A clinical review. Semin Thromb Hemost 14:299, 1988.
2. Djulbegovic B: Reasoning and Decision Making in Hematology. New York, Churchill Livingstone, 1992, pp 215–219.
3. Feinstein DI: Disseminated intravascular coagulation. J Crit Illness 4:21, 1989.
4. Feinstein DI: Treatment of disseminated intravascular coagulation. Semin Thromb Hemost 14:351, 1988.
5. Hoffman R, Benz EJ, Shattil SJ, et al (eds): Hematology: Basic Principles and Practice, 2nd ed. New York, Churchill Livingstone, 1995.
6. Lee GR, et al: Wintrobe's Clinical Hematology. Philadelphia, Lea & Febiger, 1993, pp 1480–1493.
7. Ratnoff OD: Disorders of Hemostasis, 2nd ed. Philadelphia, W.B. Saunders, 1991, pp 292–326.

17. THROMBOTIC THROMBOCYTOPENIC PURPURA AND HEMOLYTIC UREMIC SYNDROME

Kathryn L. Hassell, M.D.

1. What is thrombotic thrombocytopenic purpura (TTP)?

TTP is a clinical syndrome classically characterized by a pentad of signs and symptoms:
1. Low platelet count
2. Microangiopathic hemolytic anemia
3. Neurologic changes
4. Impaired renal function
5. Fever

In many cases, not all five of these characteristics are present, but this diagnosis should be considered in a patient with hemolytic anemia with schistocytes (broken RBCs) on the peripheral smear (see Figure 4, Color Plates), low platelet count, and a rising creatinine.

2. Are there other syndromes related to TTP?

Yes. Hemolytic uremic syndrome (HUS) is a disease characterized by renal failure, microangiopathic hemolytic anemia, and a low platelet count. It is considered to be part of a clinical spectrum of diseases, which include TTP, and has major features similar to TTP.

Hemolytic anemia with Elevated Liver enzymes and Low Platelets (HELLP syndrome) is seen in pregnant women usually in the late second or third trimester. It can occur in conjunction with signs of preeclampsia (hypertension, proteinuria, edema) and is characterized by microangiopathic hemolytic anemia, low platelet count, and marked elevation in liver enzymes. HELLP is thought to represent another disease in the spectrum of TTP.

3. What mechanisms are at work in TTP and HUS?

The precise pathophysiologic changes that occur in TTP are not clear. Based on biopsy and autopsy material, the primary pathologic change appears to be platelet microthrombi in the small arterioles and capillaries of all organs (including kidneys, liver, brain). These microthrombi consume platelets and impede blood flow, resulting in tissue damage and organ dysfunction. In addition, these microthrombi impede passage of the red blood cells, resulting in fragmentation and hemolysis (microangiopathic hemolytic anemia).

The events that promote the initial platelet aggregation and microthrombi are not known. A great deal of work has centered on the observation that patients with relapsing TTP have an increased amount of high molecular weight von Willebrand's factor in the circulation that may promote platelet aggregation. Because TTP has occurred after viral illness, in human immunodeficiency virus (HIV)-infected patients, after use of certain medications, during pregnancy, and in conjunction with autoimmune diseases, the role of endothelial cell inflammation and/or an autoimmune "trigger" to this disease has been considered. It is not known why some organs (brain, kidney, liver) are affected more than others in these syndromes. Some childhood cases of HUS have been associated with toxins produced by infections with *Shigella* species and *Escherichia coli*.

4. Are there other diseases that are often confused with TTP/HUS?

TTP and its related diseases are diagnosed clinically, so other possible diagnoses need to be eliminated. Disseminated intravascular coagulation (DIC) has many features similar to TTP, especially in a patient who is septic. Patients with DIC have a microangiopathic hemolytic anemia and a low platelet count due to the intravascular coagulation and may develop fever, mental status changes, and renal failure due to overwhelming infection. In DIC, however, the prothrombin time (PT) and activated partial thromboplastin time (aPTT) are elevated because of the consumption of coagulation factors; this does **not** occur in TTP.

Malignant hypertension may be associated with acute renal failure, mental status changes, and, when severe, with microangiopathic hemolytic anemia and thrombocytopenia, as is seen in HUS. Very high blood pressure (as seen in malignant hypertension) is not common in HUS, however, and the lowering of blood pressure should result in resolution of these changes if they are due to malignant hypertension.

Acute liver failure can complicate pregnancy characterized by marked elevations in liver enzymes and (in some cases) a fall in platelet count resembling HELLP. However, microangiopathic hemolytic anemia is not seen and must be present to consider the diagnosis of HELLP.

5. How is the diagnosis of TTP/HUS made?

Because it is a clinical diagnosis, TTP and related disorders may be diagnosed only by identifying typical features and ruling out other possible disorders. Thrombocytopenia, sometimes mild but often severe ($< 30,000$ to $40,000/mm^3$), must be present. Microangiopathic hemolytic anemia is diagnosed by the presence of anemia, elevated reticulocyte count, schistocytes on the peripheral smear, elevated indirect bilirubin, lactate dehydrogenase (LDH), and aspartate aminotransferase (AST; SGOT), indicating red blood cell destruction. Elevations in creatinine may be mild in TTP but are characteristically higher in HUS. Neurologic changes range from minor mental status changes and headaches to seizures, stroke, and coma. Fever is not always present. Coagulation tests (PT, aPTT) should be checked and should be normal to exclude the diagnosis of DIC. Gingival biopsy looking for arteriolar microthrombi can be helpful, but when it is negative, it does not exclude the diagnosis of TTP. The same is true for the value of renal biopsy in HUS.

6. What is the treatment of TTP/HUS?

Two main approaches to treatment involve (1) an attempt to decrease the formation of microthrombi and (2) the use of plasma and plasmapheresis.

Because the primary pathophysiology appears to center on the development of platelet microthrombi, antiplatelet agents, including aspirin and dipyridamole, have been used during acute episodes of TTP. Steroids, usually prednisone (1–2 mg/kg), are given to reduce any possible role of autoimmunity or other inflammatory stimuli in the development of vasculopathy. Heparin and other anticoagulants have not shown any benefit.

Fresh frozen plasma (FFP) has been used both by simple transfusion and via plasmapheresis with plasma exchange. Initially, plasmapheresis with total plasma exchange was thought to be necessary to remove unknown factors in the patient's circulation that were promoting platelet aggregation, but some patients seemed to improve with simple transfusion of FFP. It is now thought that some regulatory product, present in donor FFP but missing in the patient, can be replaced with FFP transfusion. Currently, plasmapheresis using donor FFP for replacement is used to treat acute episodes of TTP and HUS in conjunction with prednisone with or without aspirin.

In refractory cases, vincristine (a chemotherapeutic agent that alters microtubular function and may impair platelet function) has been used. Intravenous gamma globulin and splenectomy have also been tried with mixed success.

HELLP syndrome, in contrast with TTP/HUS, is treated with steroids and termination of the pregnancy. Most cases of HELLP reverse spontaneously once the baby has been delivered; in cases in which the symptoms persist, a more typical TTP-like syndrome is suspected, and the patient is treated as though she has TTP. Because TTP does not require termination of pregnancy, distinguishing it from HELLP is important but not easy. In TTP, severe liver disease is unusual and suggests the diagnosis of HELLP.

7. Is there any harm in transfusing platelets for a low platelet count?

Platelet transfusions should be avoided in TTP/HUS. Because the basic pathophysiology seems to be related to platelet aggregation, it is theoretically possible to worsen the course of

TTP/HUS markedly by platelet transfusion. Anecdotal data suggest that increased microthrombi deposition with development of stroke, worsening hemolytic anemia, and renal dysfunction has occurred with platelet transfusions.

8. How are patients monitored to determine if treatment is working?

Successful therapy of TTP/HUS will be reflected in improvement in neurologic and renal function. Daily determination of hemoglobin/hematocrit, platelet count, reticulocyte count, LDH, and creatinine should be done. Over the course of several days, a fall in reticulocyte count with a rise in hemoglobin and a reduction in LDH and schistocytes herald improvement in the microangiopathic process. Daily plasmapheresis should not be discontinued until there are signs of improvement, and some series suggest that "tapering" plasmapheresis over several days to weeks may reduce the acute relapse rate. Prednisone should be continued until the episode is clearly remitted and then tapered slowly.

9. How successful is treatment?

Acute, severe episodes of TTP can be difficult to treat, with a mortality rate of up to 30–40% despite therapy. Early recognition and appropriate treatment may reduce this mortality. Response rates of up to 90% have been reported in episodes where fresh frozen plasma is used.

10. Is there a high relapse rate if a patient is successfully treated?

A subgroup of patients appear to have a chronic, relapsing form of TTP, where episodes can be triggered by recognized stimuli (e.g., certain medications, viral illnesses) or occur without apparent cause. Some of these patients have a large amount of high molecular weight von Willebrand's factor in their circulation chronically. Patients who have had TTP or HELLP in association with pregnancy may be at risk for recurrence with another pregnancy.

CONTROVERSIES

11. Should aspirin be used in the treatment of TTP?

Because patients with TTP have low platelet counts and often have associated bleeding, there is hesitation to add aspirin, which will compromise the function of the few remaining platelets and increase the risk of bleeding. Nonetheless, because functional platelets are thought to contribute significantly to the underlying pathophysiology of the disease, aspirin should theoretically be used. More recent studies have suggested that aspirin does not alter the overall course of TTP and therefore should not be used. Some continue to advocate its use, however, especially if thrombocytopenia is mild, there is little clinical bleeding, and plasmapheresis is not immediately available.

12. Is simple transfusion with FFP enough or is plasmapheresis always necessary?

Plasma exchange has been done, in part, because the concept involves removing "negative factors" in the patient's blood that may be promoting platelet aggregation. Evidence now suggests that some regulatory factor may be missing from the patient's blood that is given back by transfusing FFP, and that this represents the main benefit of exchange. Some series do show an improvement in an episode of TTP with simple transfusion of FFP. Nonetheless, current practice still includes plasmapheresis with plasma exchange, although the patient is often treated initially with simple transfusion of FFP until plasmapheresis can be initiated.

13. Is there a relationship between TTP and human immunodeficiency virus (HIV) infection?

An unexpected number of cases of TTP have been reported in patients infected with HIV. Given the alterations in the immune system associated with HIV infection (e.g., autoimmune diseases such as idiopathic thrombocytopenic purpura, polyclonal gammopathy), some investigators have postulated a theoretical link between this abnormal immune response and TTP/HUS. Proof of this relationship, however, has not yet been found.

BIBLIOGRAPHY

1. Barton JR, Sibai BM: Care of the pregnancy complicated by HELLP syndrome. Obstet Gynecol Clin North Am 18:165, 1991.
2. Kaplan BS, Meyers KE, Schulman SL: The pathogenesis and treatment of hemolytic uremic syndrome. J Am Soc Nephrol 9:1126–1133, 1998.
3. Kelton JG, et al: The platelet aggregating factor(s) of thrombotic thrombocytopenic purpura. Prog Clin Biol Res 337:141, 1990.
4. Martin JN Jr, Stedman CM: Imitators of preeclampsia and HELLP syndrome. Obstet Gynecol Clin North Am 18:181, 1991.
5. Miller JM Jr, Pastorek JG II: Thrombotic thrombocytopenic purpura and hemolytic uremic syndrome in pregnancy. Clin Obstet Gynecol 34:64, 1991.
6. Moake JL: The role of von Willebrand factor (vWF) in thrombotic thrombocytopenic purpura (TTP) and the hemolytic-uremic syndrome (HUS). Prog Clin Biol Res 337:135, 1990.
7. Neild GH: Hemolytic uremic syndrome/thrombotic thrombocytopenic purpura: Pathophysiology and treatment. Kidney Int 64(Suppl):S45–S49, 1998.
8. Ranicle DP, et al: Should intravenous immunoglobulin G be first-line treatment for acute thrombotic thrombocytopenic purpura? Case report and review of the literature. Am J Kidney Dis 18:264, 1991.
9. Rarick MU, et al: Thrombotic thrombocytopenic purpura in patients with human immunodeficiency virus infection: A report of three cases and review of the literature. Am J Hematol 40:103, 1992.
10. Rock G, et al: Comparison of plasma exchange with plasma infusion in the treatment of thrombotic thrombocytopenic purpura. Canadian Apheresis Study Group. N Engl J Med 325:7, 1991.
11. Stricker RB, et al: Thrombotic thrombocytopenic purpura complicating systemic lupus erythematosus. Case report and literature review from the plasmapheresis era. J Rheumatol 19:1469, 1992.
12. Thompson CE, et al: Thrombotic microangiopathies in the 1980s: Clinical features, response to treatment, and the impact of the human immunodeficiency virus epidemic. Blood 80:1890, 1992.

18. IDIOPATHIC THROMBOCYTOPENIC PURPURA

Robin J. Kovachy, M.D., and David M. Schrier, M.D.

1. Define idiopathic thrombocytopenic purpura (ITP).

ITP is a condition in which low platelet counts are due to increased destruction of platelets by immunoglobulin G (IgG) platelet antibodies. Platelet production in the bone marrow is increased. It is a relatively common cause of thrombocytopenia and the most common immunologic disorder in women of childbearing age.

2. What laboratory abnormalities other than a low platelet count may be noted in the complete blood cell count (CBC)?

Unless bleeding has been severe enough to cause iron deficiency anemia, the CBC is relatively normal. Occasionally, the mean platelet volume (MPV) is increased.

3. What can cause a falsely low or elevated platelet count on an automated CBC machine?

Ethylenediamine tetraacetic acid (EDTA)-induced platelet clumping, paraproteinemias, hyperlipidemia, giant platelets counted as white blood cells, or fragmented red blood cells counted as platelets. In all patients with decreased platelet counts, the peripheral blood smear should be reviewed to confirm the automated count.

4. Name the single test that establishes the definitive diagnosis of ITP.

There is no such test. ITP is a diagnosis of exclusion. Platelet-associated antibodies are not sensitive or specific enough. There are many false positives and false negatives. Other causes of thrombocytopenia must be ruled out, particularly thrombocytopenia related to drugs, which may be indistinguishable from ITP. The diagnosis of ITP is based on the history, physical exam, CBC, and review of peripheral blood smear.

5. How can ITP be distinguished from thrombotic thrombocytopenic purpura (TTP), he-molytic uremic syndrome (HUS), and disseminated intravascular coagulation (DIC)?

Review of the peripheral smear reveals normal red blood cells and white blood cells in ITP. HUS and TTP always have fragmented red blood cells on the peripheral blood smear. With DIC, usually the protime and partial thromboplastin time (PTT) are prolonged, fibrinogen is low, and fibrin split products are elevated.

6. How can ITP be distinguished from disorders of the hematopoietic system such as aplastic anemia, acute leukemia, myelodysplastic syndromes, and myeloma?

Review the peripheral blood smear. In ITP, red blood cell morphology is usually normal. Bone marrow biopsy and aspiration show increased megakaryocytes as the only abnormality. Other primary hematologic disorders are obvious on bone marrow biopsy.

7. Is it necessary to do a bone marrow biopsy for all patients with suspected ITP?

No. Most patients do not require a bone marrow biopsy. Bone marrow biopsy and aspiration are appropriate to establish the diagnosis in patients over 60 years old and in patients contemplating splenectomy.

8. Which infectious diseases may be associated with thrombocytopenia without a presumed immune mechanism?

- Viral infections, including herpes, pertussis, rubella, infectious mononucleosis, chicken-pox, hepatitis, Colorado tick fever, and AIDS
- Rickettsial infections, such as Rocky Mountain spotted fever and typhus
- Bacterial infections, especially subacute bacterial endocarditis, meningococcemia, and gram-negative sepsis

9. What commonly used drugs have been associated with thrombocytopenia and a presumed immune mechanism?

Acetaminophen	Gold salts	Quinidine
Cephalothin	Heparin	Quinine
Diazepam	Penicillin	Sulfisoxazole

10. How do patients with ITP usually present?

Patients usually feel reasonably well and have no systemic symptoms such as fatigue, weight loss, or fever. They often have minor bleeding such as epistaxis, menorrhagia, easy bruising, and petechiae. Hematuria, melena, and hematemesis are not common but may be presenting symptoms.

11. What are the most common clinical characteristics of acute ITP?

Acute ITP occurs most often in children, with a peak incidence at 2–6 years of age. Usually the disorder starts abruptly with hemorrhagic complications and follows a viral illness by 1–3 weeks. Spontaneous remission is common. There is no gender predilection.

12. What are the most common clinical characteristics of chronic ITP?

Chronic ITP occurs primarily in adults, with a peak incidence at 20–40 years of age. Women are three times more likely to be affected than men. A recent history of infection is unusual. Spontaneous remission is rare. The onset is somewhat more insidious than in acute ITP.

13. How often is ITP associated with splenomegaly?

In 10–20% of patients, mild splenomegaly may be noted. More significant splenomegaly (i.e., more than 2–3 cm below the left costal margin) should prompt consideration of other diseases of the spleen, such as neoplastic infiltration and congestive or infectious splenomegaly.

14. What is the most serious complication of ITP? How should it be treated?

Spontaneous intracranial hemorrhage can be life-threatening but fortunately occurs in less than 1% of patients with ITP. It is unlikely to occur unless platelets are < 10,000. Once intracranial bleeding or other life-threatening hemorrhage is diagnosed, the patient should be given a large dose of gammaglobulin, intravenous steroids, and platelet transfusions. Neurosurgical consultation should be obtained, and splenectomy should be considered.

15. Name the three main therapies for ITP.

Corticosteroids (usually at an initial dose of 60 mg/day), splenectomy, and high-dose gammaglobulin. Most patients respond to steroids, although sometimes steroids need to be continued for 2 weeks before response is seen. Only 10–30% of patients maintain a long remission with steroid therapy only.

16. At what platelet count do patients with ITP need to be treated?

Patients with platelet counts > 50,000 do not require treatment. In patients who have platelet counts of 30,000–50,000 and either mucocutaneous bleeding or significant risk factors for bleeding (hypertension, peptic ulcer disease, physically active lifestyle), glucocorticosteroid therapy should be initiated. Patients with platelet counts < 20,000 and significant mucous membrane bleeding should be hospitalized.

17. What are the indications for splenectomy in ITP?

Splenectomy should be considered when patients are unable to be tapered off prednisone within 3–6 months. Complications from long-term steroids are more severe than from splenectomy. Patients who fail to respond to steroid therapy and patients with severe contraindications to steroid usage (i.e., steroid psychosis, brittle diabetes) should be offered splenectomy.

18. When is splenectomy contraindicated in ITP?

Splenectomy is contraindicated early in the first episode of ITP, because most patients respond to steroids. It is especially contraindicated in children because of frequent spontaneous remission. Children under 2 years of age have a much higher risk of overwhelming sepsis if the spleen has been removed. Splenectomy should be avoided in pregnant women and in patients with severe cardiac and pulmonary disease who are at risk from any major surgery.

19. How effective is splenectomy? What is the mortality rate? How can response to splenectomy be predicted?

Approximately 80% of patients respond initially to splenectomy, and 60% have a sustained remission. There is no way to predict who will respond to splenectomy. The mortality rate is < 1%. All patients should be treated with pneumococcal, meningococcal, and *Hemophilus influenzae* vaccines several weeks before splenectomy to minimize complications from sepsis.

20. List other treatments that are used in refractory ITP.

Cyclophosphamide	Danazol	Colchicine
Vincristine	Azathioprine	Plasmapheresis

21. List other conditions associated with ITP.

Sarcoidosis	Chronic lymphocytic leukemia
Non-Hodgkin's lymphoma	Systemic lupus erythematosus
Hodgkin's lymphoma	Thyrotoxicosis

22. What are additional concerns in pregnant patients with ITP?

Usually pregnant patients can be managed with prednisone and/or high-dose gammaglobulin. Splenectomy is to be avoided if at all possible. In mothers with a history of ITP and increased levels of platelet IgG antibodies, severe thrombocytopenia may occur in the fetus, resulting in spontaneous bleeding.

BIBLIOGRAPHY

1. Abrams RA, et al: Intravenous gammaglobulin in refractory immune thrombocytopenia purpura: Efficiency with or without concomitant steroid therapy. Am J Hematol 18:85, 1985.
2. Berchtold P, et al: Therapy of chronic thrombocytopenia purpura in adults. Blood 74:2309, 1989.
3. Cortelazza S, et al: High risk of severe bleeding in aged patients with chronic idiopathic thrombocytopenic purpura. Blood 77:31, 1991.
4. Djulbegovic B: Reasoning and Decision Making in Hematology. New York, Churchill Livingstone, 1992, pp 195–200.
5. George J, et al: Idiopathic thrombocytopenic purpura: A practice guideline developed by explicit methods for the American Society of Hematology. Blood 88(1):3–40, 1996.
6. Lee GR, et al: Wintrobe's Clinical Hematology. Philadelphia, Lea & Febiger, 1993, pp 1329–1347.
7. Ratnoff OD: Disorders of Hemostasis, 2nd ed. Philadelphia, W.B. Saunders, 1991, pp 108–130.
8. Steinberg MH, et al: An aid in the classification of thrombocytopenic disorders. N Engl J Med 317:1037, 1987.

19. THROMBOCYTOSIS

Eduardo R. Pajon, Jr., M.D., and Douglas Jerome Kemme, M.D.

1. What is a normal platelet count?

It ranges from 150–450 thousand platelets per microliter (K/μl).

2. What is thrombocytosis?

A platelet count > 400 K/μl.

3. What are the two broad categories of thrombocytosis?

Reactive thrombocytosis is due to an increased production of platelets or decreased destruction of platelets from another process. **Primary thrombocytosis** is due to a primary bone marrow disease that causes increased production of platelets.

4. List ten conditions that can cause reactive thrombocytosis.

1. Inflammatory diseases (rheumatoid arthritis, ulcerative colitis, vasculitis)
2. Acute trauma or stress
3. Iron deficiency
4. Acute and chronic infections (e.g., tuberculosis, osteomyelitis)
5. Blood loss
6. Hemolytic anemia
7. Splenectomy
8. Malignancy
9. Rebound after bone marrow suppression of platelet production (alcohol, chemotherapy, malnutrition)
10. Surgery or postoperative state

5. How do inflammatory and infectious diseases cause reactive thrombocytosis?

Chronic inflammation and infection may result in the production of increased amounts of various cytokines, such as interleukin (IL)-1, IL-6, granulocyte-macrophage colony-stimulating factor, and IL-3, that stimulate platelet production by inducing hematopoietic stem cell development and promoting megakaryocyte maturation.

6. Can alcohol cause an increase as well as a decrease in platelet count?

Yes. Alcohol may decrease the platelet count by a direct toxic effect on the megakaryocytes. Thrombocytosis is commonly observed as the patient recovers from this effect.

7. Can iron deficiency cause an increase as well as a decrease in platelet count?

Yes. Children and elderly patients may develop thrombocytopenia with iron deficiency. Severe iron deficiency in adults may cause thrombocytopenia, although most adults develop thrombocytosis.

8. When are patients with reactive thrombocytosis at risk for thrombosis?

Few patients with reactive thrombocytosis develop thrombosis when the platelet count is < 1,000 K/μl. Above that, the risk is proportional to the platelet count, with patients with platelet counts > 2,000 K/μl at highest risk. Management of such patients is difficult. After excluding essential thrombocytosis (see below), aspirin is usually sufficient prophylaxis until the platelet count returns to normal with correction of the underlying problem. Patients with proven thromboembolism should receive standard anticoagulation.

9. When are patients with reactive thrombocytosis at risk for bleeding complications?

Bleeding is rare in patients with reactive thrombocytosis and is usually related to the underlying condition or its treatment.

10. What disorders are associated with primary thrombocytosis?

Patients with myeloproliferative disorders often have thrombocytosis. Examples include polycythemia vera (PCV), chronic myelogenous leukemia (CML), and myelofibrosis with myeloid metaplasia (described elsewhere) as well as essential thrombocytosis (also known as essential thrombocythemia, or ET).

11. What is essential thrombocytosis (ET)?

ET is a chronic myeloid disorder that has been shown to be clonal, with origin in a multipotent stem cell whose predominant disease expression is thrombocytosis. The elevated platelet count is frequently associated with abnormal function of the platelets and an increased frequency of thromboembolic as well as bleeding complications.

12. What causes the increased platelet count?

The megakaryocyte precursor, known as colony-forming unit-megakaryocyte (CFU-MK), has been shown to be abnormal in ET. These cells appear to replicate in the absence of the normal growth factors (tryptophan peroxidase [TPO], thrombopoietin), demonstrating the loss of a normal feedback system. Abnormal binding of TPO to platelets of patients with ET has also been demonstrated to lead to elevated levels of circulating TPO, further evidence of a loss of normal feedback inhibition. The abnormal CFU-MK cells have been shown to be clonally derived.

13. Why do other myeloproliferative disorders demonstrate increased platelet counts?

The abnormal clone causing increased growth of white blood cells in CML or red blood cells in PCV appears to be an early progenitor cell capable of differentiation to the CFU-MK line as well. Furthermore, it has been shown that the megakaryocyte progenitors in PCV are hypersensitive to TPO and lead to increased megakaryocyte colony formation.

14. In patients with primary thrombocytosis, do the platelets function normally?

No. In addition to an increase in number, the platelets frequently have functional abnormalities. Thus one patient may have both bleeding and clotting problems.

15. What platelet functional abnormalities have been described in ET?

Functional abnormalities include prolonged bleeding time, spontaneous platelet aggregation, decreased platelet aggregation to agents such as adrenaline, and abnormal intraplatelet and serum contents of B-thromboglobulin, 5-hydroxytryptamine, and platelet factor 4.

16. How is ET diagnosed?

1. Platelet count > 600 K/μl
2. Absence of conditions associated with reactive thrombocytosis
3. Confirmation of normal iron stores
4. Normal erythrocyte mass (to rule out PCV)
5. No Philadelphia chromosome
6. Bone marrow collagen fibrosis must be absent or, in the absence of both splenomegaly and leukoerythroblastosis, it must be restricted to < ⅓ of the area of the biopsy specimen.

17. How can reactive thrombocytosis be excluded?

This may be difficult in some patients, particularly those that have two concurrent disorders. Elevated levels of IL-6 or C-reactive protein as well as fibrinogen or vWf antigen may be indicative of a reactive process. Abnormal CFU-MK growth on bone marrow aspirate samples or circulating levels of thrombopoetin have been associated with ET. Bone marrow morphology may show increased reticulin content in ET compared with reactive thrombocytosis.

18. How can the possibility of CML be eliminated?

This distinction is important, because treatment and prognosis are different for CML. Careful examination of the bone marrow by a hematopathologist and chromosome analysis for the Philadelphia chromosome are helpful. Polymerase chain reaction (PCR) amplification of DNA from marrow or peripheral blood samples to look for the *bcr/abl* gene rearrangement characterized by the Philadelphia chromosome should be performed in any patient in whom the correct diagnosis of CML is critical.

19. Who may develop ET?

This rare disorder affects women and men equally around the age of 50–60 years.

20. What are common presenting symptoms of ET?

Often the disorder is found incidentally during laboratory analysis for an unrelated reason, especially with the routine use of automated complete blood cell count (CBC) machines. Patients may present with clotting disorders or bleeding complications.

21. What types of thromboembolic events may a patient experience?

Patients may present with arterial thrombosis leading to cerebral or myocardial ischemia or infarction. Large vessel thrombosis may lead to limb ischemia or even bowel infarction. Venous thrombosis, particularly in unusual locations (as in Budd-Chiari disease) or in people with no predisposition to venous thromboembolism, may be another manifestation.

22. Define erythromyalgia.

Erythromyalgia is a painful red rash in patients with ET due to clotting of the superficial skin vessels. Response of this disorder to aspirin is diagnostic of ET.

23. Discuss the type of bleeding problems that develop in patients with ET.

Patients may develop gastrointestinal, mucosal, or skin bleeding, none of which is life-threatening. Bleeding may be aggravated by the concurrent use of antiplatelet drugs such as aspirin or ticlopidine. Problems are more prevalent when the platelet count exceeds 1,500 K/μl.

24. Can patients have both clotting and bleeding problems?

Yes. A patient with clotting problems may develop bleeding problems at any platelet level. Thus, the routine use of aspirin or ticlopidine without evaluating the clinical situation or analyzing platelet function can be risky.

25. How do you manage a patient with life-threatening thromboembolic situations due to ET?

Hydroxyurea, anagrelide, or platelet pheresis are commonly used to decrease platelet counts rapidly.

26. What is the goal in the treatment of ET?

The goal is to decrease the thromboembolic complications. Clinical studies have shown a decreased frequency of thromboembolic complications when the platelet count is maintained below 600 K/μl. Transient ischemic attacks and erythromyalgia respond well to aspirin or ticlopidine; however, caution should be used, because these medications also increase the risk of bleeding complications.

27. Are there any special recommendations for pregnant patients with ET?

Pregnancy in patients with ET is reported to be often complicated by recurrent abortion and fetal growth retardation. Use of aspirin and subcutaneous heparin appears to improve outcome.

28. Are there any long-term complications from hydroxyurea therapy?

Acute leukemia has been reported in as many as 8% of patients treated with long-term hydroxyurea.

29. Does anagrelide have a role in the treatment of ET?

Anagrelide is a new drug that promotes thrombocytopenia by an unknown mechanism. It is not leukemogenic and has minimal effect on red blood cell production and even less effect on white blood cell production. In clinical studies over 70% of treated patients responded with normalization of platelet counts. The drug, however, is very expensive.

30. Is there a role for interferon in the treatment of ET?

Yes. Interferon has been shown to decrease the platelet count in patients with myeloproliferative diseases but has more side effects than hydroxyurea. It may be useful in patients refractory to hydroxyurea or anegralide.

BIBLIOGRAPHY

1. Beressi AH, et al: Outcome analysis of 34 pregnancies in women with essential thrombocythemia. Arch Intern Med 11:1217–1222, 1995.
2. Chloe EI, et al: Thrombocytosis after major lower extremity trauma: Mechanism and possible role in free flap failure. Ann Plast Surg 5:489–494, 1996.
3. Corteazzo S, et al: Hydroxyurea for patients with essential thrombocythemia and a high risk of thrombosis. N Engl J Med 17:1132–1136, 1995.
4. Johnson M, et al: Essential thrombocytosis: Underemphasized cause of large-vessel thrombosis. J Vasc Surg 4:443–447, 1995.
5. Juvonen E, et al: Megakaryocyte and erythroid colony formation in essential thrombocythemia and reactive thrombocytosis: Diagnostic value and correlation to complications. Br J Haematol 2:192–197, 1993.
6. Kiladjian JJ, et al: Hydroxyurea-related acute leukemia in essential thrombocythemia. Long term results of a prospective study. Abstract 3552, American Society of Hematology Meeting, Orlando, Florida, December 6–10, 1996.
7. Michiels JJ, et al: Erythromelalgic, thrombotic and hemorrhagic manifestations in 50 cases of thrombocythemia. Leuk Lymphoma 22(Suppl 1):47–56, 1996.
8. Ruggeri M, et al: Is ticlopidine a safe alternative to aspirin for management of myeloproliferative disorders? Haematologica 78 (6 Suppl 2):18–21, 1993.
9. Sagripanti A, et al: Thrombotic and hemorrhagic complications in chronic myeloproliferative disorders. Biomed Pharmacother 50:376–382, 1996.
10. Schrier SL: Leukemias and the myeloproliferative disorders. Scientific American Medicine SAM-CD, Scientific American, Inc., New York, 1997.
11. Silverstein MN: Anagrelide, a therapy for thrombocythemic states: Experience in 577 patients. Anagrelide Study Group. Am J Med 92:69–76, 1992.
12. Sutor AH: Thrombocytosis in childhood. Semin Thromb Hemost 21:330–339, 1995.
13. Tefferi A, et al: Issues in the diagnosis and management of essential thrombocythemia. Mayo Clin Proc 69:651–655, 1994.
14. Torenbohm-Roche E, et al: Alpha-2a interferon therapy and antibody formation in patients with essential thrombocythemia and polycythemia vera with thrombocytosis. Am J Hematol 48(3):163–167, 1995.
15. Yohaman MD, et al: Thrombocytosis. Etiologic analysis of 663 patients. Clin Pediatr 33(6):340–343, 1994.

20. HEMOPHILIA

Sally P. Stabler, M.D.

1. Define hemophilia.

In a general sense hemophilia refers to any of a number of congenital factor deficiencies that result in a bleeding diathesis; more specifically, hemophilia A refers to factor VIII deficiency and hemophilia B to factor IX deficiency. Factor VIII deficiency, or classic hemophilia, is the most common severe congenital clotting deficiency. It cannot be distinguished from the second most common disorder, factor IX deficiency, without specific assays. Von Willebrand's disease is the most common mild disorder. In some populations (such as Ashkenazi Jews), factor XI deficiency is actually more common than either factor VIII or factor IX deficiency. Factor XI deficiency causes a much less serious bleeding diathesis than the other two. Less common but of clinical significance is factor VII deficiency, which presents usually in milder, probably heterozygous forms but occasionally as postoperative hemorrhage without a previously known coagulopathy.

2. What is the best screening test for hemophilia?

In evaluating patients with a suspected factor deficiency, the first screening tests should be the prothrombin time (PT), activated partial thromboplastin time (aPTT), thrombin time (TT), fibrinogen, and bleeding time. In the cases of mild deficiency, the aPTT may be prolonged only 1–4 seconds compared with normal controls. In general, the more prolonged the aPTT, the more severe the hemophilia. The rest of the above screening tests are usually normal in hemophilia. An isolated elevated PT is found in congenital factor VII deficiency. Factors IX and XII deficiencies cause a prolonged aPTT similar to that found in patients with factor VIII deficiency. The next step is to mix normal plasma with the patient's plasma. Correction of the aPTT suggests a factor deficiency. Specific factor assays are then performed for factors VII, VIII, IX, XI, and XII. If the factor VIII or IX level is 1% of normal or less, the patient has severe hemophilia. Levels between 1 and 3% are considered moderate hemophilia, and levels above 5% are considered mild hemophilia. Normal levels are usually 60–120%.

3. List the clinical situations in which factor VIII levels are decreased.
- Hemophilia A and the carrier state
- Acquired factor VIII inhibitor (acquired hemophilia, an uncommon but devastating autoimmune disorder)
- Disseminated intravascular coagulation (DIC)
- Von Willebrand's disease (In all patients with a low level of factor VIII, von Willebrand's factor antigen and von Willebrand's ristocetin cofactor should be assayed.)

4. Why don't women get hemophilia?

Hemophilia A and B are X-linked disorders—that is, the gene is on the X chromosome and women are carriers. Although previously carriers were thought not to manifest bleeding tendencies, this has been shown not to be true. Because of lyonization of the X chromosome, some carrier women have low levels of either factor VIII or IX—often in the 30–50% range. They may have major postoperative hemorrhage, although they do not bleed spontaneously. Each son of a carrier woman has a 50:50 chance of having hemophilia. All daughters of a hemophiliac man are obligatory carriers of hemophilia. All sons of a hemophiliac man are normal. The sisters of a hemophiliac or of a hemophiliac carrier each have a 50:50 chance of being carriers.

5. Does a negative family history preclude the diagnosis of hemophilia?

No. New molecular biology techniques have shown that approximately one-third of all patients with hemophilia are either new mutations themselves or sons of a woman with a new mutation.

Thus the population of hemophiliacs is constantly renewed, and the family history may be highly unreliable. Patients with mild hemophilia are often not diagnosed until after they experience postsurgical bleeding. In such cases, all family members should be screened because it is possible that some affected members (even elderly men) have not had a hemostatic challenge that previously led to diagnosis.

6. What are the most common manifestations of hemophiliac bleeding?

Severe and moderately severe hemophiliacs (factor levels < 3%) have frequent spontaneous hemorrhages into joints and soft tissues. Untreated, such hemarthroses result in an arthropathy, leading to total destruction of the knees, elbows, ankles, and hips. In addition, hemophiliacs have frequent spontaneous intracerebral hemorrhages, renal bleeding, and retroperitoneal hemorrhages. Gastrointestinal hemorrhaging also is frequent and usually due to underlying peptic ulcer disease, Mallory-Weiss tears, or other pathology.

7. Should transfusion of clotting factors be avoided because of the risk of transmission of viral diseases?

No. All currently available factor VIII and factor IX products have been treated so that they are not contaminated with human immunodeficiency virus (HIV), hepatitis B, or hepatitis C. They are safer than fresh frozen plasma or cryoprecipitate from the blood bank that has not been virally inactivated. The choices of factor VIII products include recombinant factor VIII, monoclonally purified factor VIII from human plasma, or a less pure preparation of factor VIII. All are virally safe, but the cost differs markedly among different preparations. A new recombinant factor IX product and monoclonally purified factor IX are available as well as prothrombin complex, which includes other vitamin K-dependent factors. Factor treatment should not be withheld because of a fear of infectious complications.

8. How and when does one decide on the amount of factor to give for a specific episode?

Always remember to transfuse immediately. There is no point in measuring aPTT before transfusion because all hemophiliacs have an elevated aPTT. Appropriate doses for different clinical situations are given below. In general, patients are transfused to approximately 40% of normal levels for soft tissue hemorrhages and mild-to-moderate joint bleeding. In life-threatening situations and after surgery, we transfuse more aggressively to maintain normal levels of factor VIII, never letting the trough level fall below 40–50%. The half-life of factor VIII is about 12 hours; thus, patients are dosed every 12 hours to maintain adequate trough levels. The half-life of factor IX is longer (about 24 hours); thus, a once-daily transfusion usually maintains adequate levels. However, twice as much factor IX is required to obtain the same levels as factor VIII.

Required Factor Doses in Bleeding Hemophiliacs

EPISODE	FACTOR VIII DEFICIENCY	FACTOR IX DEFICIENCY
Soft tissue bleed or mild joint bleed	20 μ/kg × 1	40 μ/kg × 1
Severe joint or soft tissue bleed	40 μ/kg × 1, then 20 μ/kg q 12 hr × 2	80 μ/kg × 1, then 40 μ/kg q 24 hr × 1
Compartment syndrome	40 μ/kg × 1, then 20 μ/kg q 12 hr until resolved	80 μ/kg × 1, then 40 μ/kg q 24 hr until resolved
Laceration with sutures	20 μ/kg during suturing, then q.o.d. until sutures are removed	40 μ/kg during suturing, then q.o.d. until sutures are removed
Dental cleaning and restoration	20 μ/kg × 1	40 μ/kg × 1

Table continued on following page.

Required Factor Doses in Bleeding Hemophiliacs (Continued)

EPISODE	FACTOR VIII DEFICIENCY	FACTOR IX DEFICIENCY
Oral surgery	40 μ/kg × 1, then 20 μ/kg q 24 hr × 2 Aminocaproic acid (Amicar) 6 gm q 6 hr × 4–6 days	80 μ/kg × 1, then 40 μ/kg q 24 hr × 1 Aminocaproic acid (Amicar) 6 gm q 6 hr × 4–6 days
Central nervous bleeding	40 μ/kg prior to CT scan, then 20 μ/kg q 12 hr until resolved, then q 24 hr to finish 10–14 days	80 μ/kg prior to CT scan, then 40 μ/kg q 24 hr until resolved, then q.o.d. to finish 10–14 days
Major surgery and joint synovectomy	50 μ/kg on induction of anesthesia, then 20 μ/kg q 12 hr for 14 days	100 μ/kg on induction of anesthesia, then 40 μ/kg q 24 hr for 14 days
Major orthopedic surgery, especially joint replacement	60 μ/kg on induction 20 μ/kg after 4 hr in surgery, then 2 μ/kg/hr IV drip × 72 hr, then 20 μ/kg q 12 hr 10 days, then 40 μ/kg/day × 7 days, then 20 μ/kg q.o.d. × 2 wk	120 μ/kg on induction 50 μ/kg q 24 hr × 3 days, then 40 μ/kg × 11 days, then 40 μ/kg q.o.d. × 3 wk
Bronchoscopy, lumbar puncture, bone marrow biopsy, other endoscopy	40 μ/kg × 1; treat any hematoma again	80 μ/kg × 1; treat any hematoma again

9. How long do I need to treat a patient with factor replacement?

The length of treatment depends on the lesion. One or two doses usually stop the bleeding for a mild joint bleed or soft tissue hemorrhage. In compartment syndromes and severe soft tissue hemorrhage, treatment should continue until the entire area has softened and all hematomas have resolved. After surgery, treatment should continue until the wound has completely healed, usually between 10 and 14 days for abdominal and chest surgery. In orthopedic surgery, adequate levels of factors must be maintained for 3–6 weeks. Inexperienced physicians often discontinue factor replacement after surgery on the third or fourth postoperative day, which results in hematoma formation at the edges of the wound and dehiscence. The wound then becomes infected because of the large amount of blood and requires a prolonged period of factor coverage while healing by secondary intention.

10. What is the best treatment for mild factor VIII deficiency?

For female carriers of hemophilia A with factor VIII levels < 50% and mild hemophiliacs with levels of > 10%, 1-deamino-8-D-arginine vasopressin (DDAVP) is often the treatment of choice. DDAVP, 0.3 μ/kg given intravenously over 15 minutes, usually raises factor VIII levels 3–4 times the baseline level. A new high-potency nasal spray preparation also may be used. DDAVP can only be used once daily. Because hyponatremia may be a serious side effect, patients should be fluid-restricted. This protocol is adequate for many minor procedures and in female carriers is usually adequate for major surgery. In life-threatening hemorrhage or surgery on mucosal surfaces such as nose or sinuses, tonsillectomy, transurethral resection of the prostate, or cone biopsy of the cervix, the levels obtained with DDAVP usually are not sufficient; recombinant or monoclonally purified factor VIII is a better choice. DDAVP does not increase factor IX levels.

11. What is an inhibitor of factor VIII?

The worst complication of hemophilia is the development of neutralizing IgG antibodies to factor VIII, which occurs after treatment in about 15% of patients with severe hemophilia A and rarely in patients with hemophilia B. These inhibitors are measured in an assay in which the amount of residual factor VIII is determined in normal plasma after 2 hours of incubation with the patient's plasma. The amount of inhibition is assigned a titer known as the Bethesda unit (BU). Low-titer inhibitors (< 5 BU) usually can be overwhelmed with large amounts of either human factor VIII or factor VIII purified from pig plasma (porcine factor VIII). In most patients, however, the Bethesda titers are high (> 20 BU), and it is difficult to overwhelm them with factor VIII. In such cases, factor IX concentrate or an activated factor IX complex is used. Both products have some bypassing activity and may promote hemostasis of a bleeding lesion. The activated material is cleared quickly by the patient's liver; thus, the infusion has no lasting benefit and rebleeding is common. Once patients have developed an inhibitor, they are in danger of sustaining a fatal central nervous system hemorrhage and should not undergo elective surgery. Minor surgical procedures or intramuscular injections may result in life- and limb-threatening hemorrhage and are contraindicated. New methods of suppression of the inhibitors are under development, but they are expensive and still experimental.

12. How do you choose a factor IX product?

Because multiple doses of the standard factor IX-containing concentrates can cause thrombotic complications, purified coagulation factor IX has been developed. The two forms of purified factor IX are monoclonally purified from human plasma and a new recombinant preparation. For one-dose use, patients should receive standard factor IX concentrate, which also contains other vitamin K-dependent factors. For surgery, massive trauma, or in patients with severe liver disease, purified factor IX (coagulation factor IX) should be used instead.

13. Is hemophilia always hereditary, or can it be acquired?

Acquired hemophilia is the development of an antibody to factor VIII in a person who does not have a history of hemophilia. This condition arises in patients with autoimmune diseases or lymphoproliferative illness, postpartum patients, in the very elderly population, and in patients who have had antibiotics or blood transfusions and often a complicated ICU course for an unrelated illness. The patient has a prolonged PTT and evidence of hematomas at sites of mild trauma. The 1:1 mix with normal plasma may correct immediately, but the PTT is prolonged after a 2-hour incubation. The factor VIII level will be low (usually < 20%), and the Bethesda titer may range from 5–30 BU. These inhibitors respond well to prednisone, high-dose intravenous gammaglobulin, and other forms of immunosuppression. Unfortunately, there is a 25% mortality rate from bleeding before the patient responds. The treatment of choice to treat hemorrhage is porcine factor VIII in high enough doses to overwhelm the inhibitor. Patients should not undergo surgical procedures until hemostasis can be guaranteed. The response to immunosuppression may be as prompt as 2 weeks. Even if there is no response to immunosuppression, the inhibitors usually remit spontaneously within several years. A hemophilia center or hematologist experienced in coagulation should care for such patients.

14. Although factor products are now virally safe, is it not true that previously most hemophiliacs were infected with transfusion-related viruses?

Approximately 80–90% of adults with severe hemophilia were infected with HIV during the years 1979–1984. In addition to HIV, most hemophiliacs have evidence of past infection with hepatitis C. Because this cohort of hemophiliacs became HIV-positive at approximately the same time, 20–30% have died of HIV disease and another 30–40% have AIDS. With the exception of Kaposi's sarcoma, hemophiliacs with HIV disease have manifestations of disease similar to those of other populations with HIV. Chronic liver disease due to hepatitis C and occasionally hepatitis B is another problem; approximately 10–20% of patients die of cirrhosis. Hepatic transplantation is an option for the HIV-negative patients, because it cures both liver disease and hemophilia.

15. What is the hemophilia center?

The United States is divided into 10 regions, each of which has a federally and state-funded hemophilia center. All hemophiliacs are invited to have their care overseen by the center. All hemophiliacs are encouraged to learn home factor transfusion to expedite prompt treatment of bleeding. New patients with hemophilia should be referred to one of these centers.

BIBLIOGRAPHY

 1. Blanchette VS, Vorstman E, Shore A, et al: Hepatitis C infection in children with hemophilia A and B. Blood 79:285, 1991.
 2. Brettler DB, Forsberg AD, Levine PH, et al: The use of porcine factor VIII concentrate (Hyate:C) in the treatment of patients with inhibitor antibodies to factor VIII. Arch Intern Med 149:1381, 1989.
 3. Colman RW, Hirsh J, Marder VJ, Salzman E (eds): Hemostasis and Thrombosis: Basic Principles and Clinical Practice, 3rd ed. Philadelphia, Lippincott-Raven, 1994.
 4. Eyster MR, Gill RM, Blatt PM, et al: Central nervous system bleeding in hemophiliacs. Blood 51:1179, 1978.
 5. Hilgartner MW: Hemophiliac arthropathy. Adv Pediatr 21:139, 1975.
 6. Hoffman R, Benz EJ, Shattil SJ (eds): Hematology: Basic Principles and Practice, 2nd ed. New York, Churchill Livingstone, 1995.
 7. Kasper CK: Incidence and course of inhibitors among patients with classic hemophilia. Thromb Diath Haemorrh 30:264, 1973.
 8. Kasper CK: Postoperative thromboses in hemophilia B. N Engl J Med 289:160, 1973.
 9. Kim HC, McMillan CW, White GC, et al: Purified factor IX using monoclonal immunoaffinity technique: Clinical trials in hemophilia B and comparison to prothrombin complex concentrates. Blood 79:568, 1992.
10. Ludlam CA: Treatment of haemophilia. Br J Haematol 101(Suppl):S13–S14, 1998.
11. Mannucci PM: Desmopressin: A nontransfusional form of treatment for congenital and acquired bleeding disorders. Blood 72:1449, 1988.
12. White G, MacMillan C, Kingdon H, et al: Recombinant factor VIII. N Engl J Med 320;166, 1989.

21. ACQUIRED FACTOR DEFICIENCIES

Jerry B. Lefkowitz, M.D., and Todd M. De Boom, M.D.

LIVER DISEASE

1. Which procoagulant (clot-forming) factors are produced in the liver?
The liver synthesizes all procoagulant proteins except von Willebrand factor (VWF), which is synthesized in megakaryocytes and endothelial cells.

2. How does liver disease affect the synthesis, circulating levels, clearance, and use of procoagulant factors?
In liver disease, the following may occur:
1. Decreased synthesis of procoagulant factors
2. Increased synthesis of acute phase reactants, i.e., factor VIII and fibrinogen
3. Synthesis of qualitatively abnormal clotting factors
4. Decreased clearance of fibrin split products (FSP)
5. Decreased clearance of active or inactive products of coagulation reactions
6. Increased utilization of procoagulant factors

3. Discuss the effect of liver disease on the vitamin K-dependent coagulation proteins.
The vitamin K-dependent gamma-carboxylation step, which converts the precursor coagulation proteins (factors II, VII, IX, and X) to their functional forms, occurs in hepatocyte microsomes. With liver disease, improper use of vitamin K or premature release of proteins by diseased parenchymal cells may result in hypocarboxylated or uncarboxylated (des-gla) vitamin K-dependent coagulation factors. These improperly carboxylated forms are not functional. In addition,

the overall synthetic capacity of the diseased liver is compromised, and the absolute amount of normal coagulant proteins is decreased. (See also the section on vitamin K.)

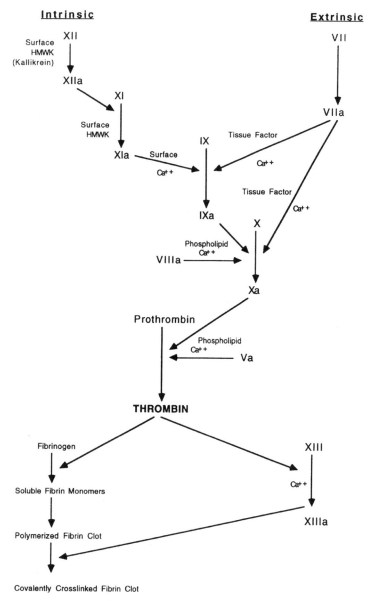

Intrinsic and extrinsic coagulation pathways.

4. Why may patients with early liver disease present with an isolated prolonged prothrombin time (PT)?

As depicted in the figure in question 3, factor VIIa is a key enzyme in the extrinsic pathway of coagulation. This pathway is evaluated in vitro by the PT. Because factor VII has the shortest half-life of the procoagulant proteins, patients with early liver disease may present with an isolated prolonged PT.

5. Discuss the dysfibrinogenemia of liver disease.

Normally, hepatocyte enzymes function to remove sialic acid sidechains from large molecules. With hepatocyte injury, this function is diminished, and the fibrinogen molecule develops an excessively high content of sialic acid. These altered fibrinogen molecules may be dysfunctional and may contribute to the hemorrhagic symptoms of liver disease. However, not all patients with liver disease produce abnormal fibrinogen molecules.

6. What is the thrombin time (TT)? Why is it prolonged in some patients with liver disease?

The TT is a test performed by adding thrombin to citrated plasma and measuring the time to clot formation. This test is sensitive to levels of fibrinogen, to inhibitors of fibrin clot polymerization (especially FSP), and to heparin. The abnormal fibrinogen produced by the diseased liver may not polymerize properly when cleaved to fibrin monomer and thus may act to prolong the TT. In addition, impaired hepatic clearance of FSP can result in high circulating levels of FSP, as reflected in a prolonged TT.

7. Discuss the changes in levels of factor VIII and fibrinogen in liver disease.

These proteins are acute phase reactants and show increased plasma concentrations with stress. However, late in the course of liver disease or with accompanying disseminated intravascular coagulation (DIC), the levels of fibrinogen and factor VIII may be normal or decreased.

8. Decreased levels of coagulation proteins, increased levels of FSP, dysfunctional fibrinogen, and possibly DIC may contribute to the hemorrhagic diathesis of liver disease. Quantitative and qualitative platelet abnormalities are also contributory. Why then do some patients with liver disease manifest a thrombotic tendency?

The liver also synthesizes plasminogen and physiologic anticoagulants, such as protein C, protein S, and antithrombin III (ATIII). For individual patients, decreases in these fibrinolytic and anticoagulant proteins may be more significant than decreases in procoagulant proteins involved in clot formation.

9. Summarize the coagulation test abnormalities associated with chronic liver disease.

PT, activated partial thromboplastin time (aPTT): prolonged
TT: prolonged or normal
Factors V, VII, IX, and X; ATIII; plasminogen: decreased
Factor VIII, fibrinogen: increased, normal, or decreased
FSP: increased or normal
Bleeding time: prolonged or normal

10. How are the acquired deficiencies of liver disease treated?

Treatment of acquired factor deficiencies in liver disease poses a challenging problem. Hemostatic abnormalities in liver disease are quite complex and sometimes confounded by other intercurrent medical problems such as renal failure or DIC. Factor replacement with fresh frozen plasma (FFP) is the treatment of choice in the actively bleeding patient. If fibrinogen levels fall below 75–100 mg/dl, cryoprecipitate also should be used. Vitamin K supplementation may be beneficial, but its effectiveness depends on residual hepatic synthetic capacity. The use of vitamin K-dependent factor concentrates (factor IX concentrates or prothrombin complex concentrates [PCC]) is **contraindicated** in liver disease because of reported thromboembolic phenomena in patients with liver disease after PCC infusions. Due to the multifactorial nature of the coagulopathy of liver disease, the complete normalization of all coagulation parameters may be impossible.

VITAMIN K: DEFICIENCY STATES AND ANTAGONISTS

11. List the forms and sources of vitamin K.

Vitamin K is a fat-soluble naphthoquinone. Vitamin K_1 (phytonadione), which is obtained through dietary intake, occurs naturally in fruits and vegetables. Vitamin K_2 (menaquinone) is synthesized by bacteria in the human digestive tract. Vitamin K_3 (menadione) is available as a synthetic, water-soluble preparation.

12. What is the function of vitamin K?

Vitamin K is a necessary cofactor for the gamma-carboxylation of glutamic acid residues in the amino terminal region of the following coagulation proteins: factors II, VII, IX, and X, protein C, and protein S. The carboxylation enzyme system is localized to the hepatocyte microsomes. The uncarboxylated (des-carboxy or des-gla) forms of these coagulation proteins are not functional.

13. List several causes of vitamin K deficiency that result in decreases in the functional levels of the vitamin K-dependent coagulation proteins.

As a fat-soluble compound, vitamin K requires bile salts for absorption from the gastrointestinal tract. Obstruction of the biliary system or other causes of malabsorption (e.g., pancreatic insufficiency, dysentery, celiac disease, Crohn's disease, blind loop syndrome, short-bowel syndrome, cystic fibrosis) may lead to deficiency. Malnutrition or unsupplemented intravenous hyperalimentation also can result in deficiency. Because the vitamin is produced in part by intestinal bacterial flora, prolonged antibiotic therapy, which may lead to gut sterilization, has been implicated as a cause of deficiency. Infants in the neonatal period often have low levels of vitamin K-dependent coagulation factors due to either (1) immaturity of the synthetic capacity of the neonatal liver or (2) a true state of vitamin K deficiency. It is common practice in the United States to administer vitamin K at birth.

14. What are the clinical and laboratory findings in vitamin K-deficient patients?

Patients with vitamin K deficiency may present with an unexplained bleeding diathesis. Laboratory findings include prolonged PT and aPTT. Assays for factors II, VII, IX, and X show decreased functional levels. Vitamin K deficiency must be differentiated from other causes that decrease the levels of vitamin K-dependent coagulation factors (e.g., liver disease, ingestion of warfarin compounds [see question 16]).

15. How is vitamin K deficiency treated?

In the actively bleeding patient, transfusion with FFP is the initial treatment of choice. Administration of vitamin K compounds usually takes between 4 and 24 hours to have an effect on levels of the vitamin K-dependent proteins. In neonates and pregnant women, the preferred form of vitamin K replacement is phytonadione. In malabsorption syndromes, some physicians prefer the water-soluble form of menadione. However, high doses of menadione have been associated with hepatic injury and hemolytic anemia.

16. Which compounds act as antagonists to vitamin K and cause decreases in the functional levels of vitamin K-dependent proteins? Discuss the uses of these compounds.

Warfarin sodium and its derivatives are antagonists of vitamin K. Therapeutic oral anticoagulation with warfarin is a common cause of decreases in both the antigenic and functional forms of vitamin K-dependent proteins. Drug interactions and intentional or accidental overdose are causes of warfarin toxicity. Less commonly, intentional or accidental poisoning with so-called superwarfarin preparations results in severe and potentially life-threatening decreases in vitamin K-dependent factors. Superwarfarins such as brodifacoum or difenacoum are the active ingredients of commercially available rodenticides.

17. What are the clinical and laboratory findings in warfarin toxicity or rodenticide (superwarfarin) poisoning?

The patient presents with a bleeding diathesis (e.g., hematuria, gingival bleeding, soft-tissue hematomas, gastrointestinal hemorrhage and/or intracranial bleeding). Most patients do not have a prior bleeding history. Laboratory testing reveals a prolonged PT and a prolonged aPTT. Specific factor assay factors show depressed levels of factors II, VII, IX, and X. Serum assays for warfarin are negative in cases of superwarfarin poisoning. To confirm superwarfarin poisoning, specific tests for brodifacoum, difenacoum, or their congeners can be performed at a reference laboratory.

18. Why is it important to distinguish poisoning with rodenticide from toxicity with therapeutic warfarin?

The half-life of warfarin is approximately 36–42 hours, whereas the half-life of rodenticides is measured in weeks. Unlike acute warfarin toxicity, appropriate therapy in cases of rodenticide poisoning may require months of vitamin K replacement.

19. What is the therapy for warfarin toxicity or rodenticide poisoning?

In the actively hemorrhaging patient with warfarin toxicity, factor replacement in the form of FFP is the treatment of choice. In patients not actively bleeding, administration of vitamin K1 usually shows an effect on levels of functional coagulant proteins within 4–24 hours. Vitamin K, as an antagonist to warfarin, increases the difficulty in returning the PT to a therapeutic level. Thus, many physicians prefer to treat patients receiving warfarin for therapeutic anticoagulation with FFP, especially if warfarin therapy is to be reinstituted after the toxic episode. As with all human-derived blood products, the risk of transmission of infectious agents through infusion of FFP must be weighed against the benefits of treatment.

The treatment of rodenticide poisoning is more of a problem. Because of the long half-life of these agents, prolonged therapy with vitamin K is often necessary. Concomitant administration of barbiturates has been suggested to shorten the time course (secondary to inducement of the hepatic microsomal enzyme system). Patients must be watched closely over a period of months for any recurrent bleeding symptoms. Actively bleeding patients should receive FFP.

In both warfarin toxicity and rodenticide poisoning, the efficacy of treatment should be evaluated with frequent monitoring of the PT.

ACQUIRED FACTOR INHIBITORS

20. What is a factor inhibitor?

Factor inhibitors are acquired circulating anticoagulants, which typically are antibodies that inhibit the function of a specific coagulation protein. Usually inhibitors occur in patients with congenital factor deficiencies after exposure to factor concentrates or FFP (alloantibodies). However, inhibitors also may occur in patients with no history of factor deficiency (autoantibodies). This chapter addresses only the autoantibodies (no prior history of factor deficiencies).

21. In the acquired setting, what are the different types of inhibitors?

Two types of inhibitors are identified in patients with no history of congenital factor deficiency:

1. Antibodies that specifically inhibit or neutralize the functional activity of a coagulant protein. Usually these antibodies are of the IgG class, but occasionally IgM and IgA inhibitors are reported in the literature.

2. Paraprotein (monoclonal immunoglobulin or immunoglobulin fragment) produced in such diseases as multiple myeloma, Waldenström's macroglobulinemia, and some cases of lymphoma. By virtue of their nature and high plasma concentration, these paraproteins tend to bind nonspecifically to anything circulating in the plasma. Formation of noncovalent paraprotein/coagulaton protein complexes interferes with the function of the latter.

22. Against which coagulation factors have specific inhibitors been identified?

Acquired inhibitors (autoantibodies) to factors VIII and V are among the most common. Inhibitors of VWF have been reported in many patients with no history of hereditary disease. Inhibitors of factor I (fibrinogen), factor II (prothrombin), factor VII, factor X, and factor XI have been reported but are exceedingly rare. In nonhemophiliacs, inhibitors of factor IX are also extremely rare.

23. What are the clinical conditions associated with spontaneous coagulation factor inhibitors?

Rheumatoid arthritis

Regional enteritis

Systemic lupus erythematosus

Myasthenia gravis

Scleroderma

Pregnancy and the immediate postpartum period

Hematologic and nonhematologic malignancies

Various dermatologic diseases (e.g., psoriasis, pemphigus vulgaris, erythema multiforme, exfoliative dermatitis)

Infections

Drug therapy (e.g., penicillins, sulfa drugs, chloramphenicol, aminoglycoside antibiotics, phenothiazines, phenytoin, arsenicals)

Advancing age (elderly patients account for a large fraction of those with no associated disease)

24. How do patients with acquired inhibitors clinically present?

Patients with acquired factor inhibitors usually present with bleeding symptoms ranging from soft-tissue hematomas to life-threatening intracranial hemorrhages. Factor inhibitors should be included in the differential diagnosis for patients with bleeding symptoms and no previous history of bleeding. The diagnosis of a factor inhibitor, especially a factor VIII inhibitor, represents a possible life-threatening medical condition that requires close patient follow-up along with rapid intervention at any signs of hemorrhage.

25. What is the natural history of a factor inhibitor?

Because factor VIII inhibitors are the most common, they are the best studied of all acquired coagulation factor inhibitors. Approximately 12–40% of patients with a factor VIII inhibitor die from hemorrhage. Patients with inhibitors for 1 year or longer have a greater likelihood of dying from bleeding complications. Without treatment, acquired factor VIII inhibitors may spontaneously remit in postpartum patients and in patients with no underlying conditions.

Factor V inhibitors are the second most common acquired antibody inhibitor. Bleeding problems are more variable than with factor VIII inhibitors. Factor V inhibitors have a high rate of spontaneous remission.

Antibody inhibitors to fibrinogen (factor I) are rare. However, paraprotein inhibitors to fibrin clot polymerization are more common. The clinical severity of the bleeding diathesis parallels the course of the underlying disease, with higher circulating levels of paraprotein predisposing to bleeding problems. Most patients with paraproteinemias **do not** develop hemorrhagic problems; significant bleeding is more commonly associated with IgM or IgA dysproteinemias.

Inhibitors to VWF are rare, but antibody inhibitors arising in patients with no underlying condition typically remit spontaneously. Paraprotein inhibitors to VWF can occur; bleeding problems respond to treatment of the underlying disease state.

Acquired factor XI inhibitors are also rare but deserve mention because some case reports suggest that they are not associated with hemorrhage but with an increased incidence of thrombosis.

The remainder of reported factor inhibitors are rare, and the natural course of the disease process is not well delineated.

26. How are acquired factor inhibitors diagnosed in the clinical laboratory?

Depending on which specific factor is inhibited, the aPTT, PT, or both may be prolonged (see figure with question 3); aPTT and/or PT mixing studies with normal plasma show no significant correction. Specific factor assays can demonstrate the presence of an inhibitor.

27. How are inhibitors quantitated?

The most common method in the United States is a Bethesda titer. By definition, an inhibitor plasma that contains 1 Bethesda unit of antibody per milliliter will neutralize 50% of factor activity in an equal volume of pooled normal plasma after incubation of the mixture at 37° C for 2 hours. In other words, 1 Bethesda unit results in the inactivation of 50% of factor activity in a sample; 2 Bethesda units result in the inactivation of 75% of factor activity; 3 Bethesda units result in the activation of 87.5% of factor activity, and so on. Quantitation of acquired factor VIII inhibitors presents a special problem. Acquired factor VIII inhibitors may show complex kinetics in their reactions with factor VIII. As a result, it is quite possible for a patient to have a high-titer inhibitor, measurable levels of factor VIII, and at the same time serious bleeding. Bethesda titers in such patients should be viewed as estimates of inhibitor potency.

28. How are inhibitors treated?
Treatment for factor VIII inhibitors is tailored for the severity of bleeding and the potency of the inhibitor. Minor soft-tissue bleeds may respond to conservative measures such as immobilization or compression of the affected area. Minor or moderate bleeding with a low-titer inhibitor (< 5 Bethesda units) may respond to desmopressin (DDAVP), which may stimulate adequate increases in factor VIII levels to control bleeding. Severe bleeding requires more aggressive intervention. Depending on the potency of the inhibitor and the kinetics of its reaction with factor VIII, first-line treatment typically involves attempting to overwhelm inhibitors with transfusions of human plasma-derived or recombinant sources of factor VIII. Severe bleeding in a patient with an inhibitor titer less than 5 Bethesda units may respond to an initial bolus of 50–100 U/kg of factor VIII, followed by a drip of 1000 U/hr. High-titer (> 10–20 Bethesda units) inhibitors may not respond well to treatment with high doses of factor VIII concentrate; in an emergent situation, however, it is worthwhile to try infusions of human factor VIII. Factor VIII inhibitors show a significant degree of species specificity, and purified concentrate of porcine factor VIII has been used successfully to treat bleeding with high-titer or refractory low-titer inhibitors. It is important to obtain a Bethesda titer against porcine factor VIII before treatment.

If no clinical response is obtained with either human or porcine factor VIII, several other treatment options exist. Prothrombin complex concentrates (PCC) or factor IX concentrates, containing a mixture of the vitamin K-dependent coagulation factors, may be used in an attempt to "bypass" the factor VIII inhibitory activity. Recombinant human factor VIIa concentrate also possesses "factor VIII-bypassing activity" and has been found to be effective treatment in some patients refractory to plasma-derived products. Unfortunately, the use of PCC, factor IX concentrate, and recombinant human factor VIIa concentrate are not without risks, including scattered reports of DIC and thromboembolic phenomena, especially when administered in high or frequent successive doses. Currently, there is no accepted laboratory test for monitoring such bypass therapy, and the response must be assessed clinically.

If patients are refractory to administration of the above agents, other treatment modalities designed to lower or suppress inhibitor titers may be required. These include plasmapheresis with plasma exchange, plasmapheresis with staph-A columns to absorb the antibody inhibitor, immunosuppressive therapy, and intravenous immunoglobulin. All of these treatments have been used with some success. In many cases, infusions of factor VIII combined with one or more of these therapies has been successful in treating refractory bleeding problems. Short-term administration of immunosuppressive drugs, alone or in combination with cytotoxic agents such as cyclophosphamide and vincristine, also has successfully eradicated inhibitor antibodies.

The treatment of factor V inhibitors usually is less problematic than that of factor VIII inhibitors. Many patients with factor V inhibitors do not exhibit bleeding symptoms, and the rate of spontaneous remission is high. Bleeding symptoms in patients with acquired factor V inhibitor have been successfully treated with FFP infusions, immunosuppressive therapy, and/or platelet transfusions. Platelets contain approximately 20% of the whole blood factor V. The use of platelet transfusions, however, is not without drawbacks. It is possible to sensitize the recipient to platelet and HLA antigens. Once sensitized, the patient may become refractory to further use of platelet transfusions.

The treatment of paraprotein inhibitors usually is aimed at the underlying disease. In acute bleeding problems, plasmapheresis with plasma exchange has been used successfully to lower the level of the circulating paraprotein.

29. What is the lupus anticoagulant? What is its significance?

The term lupus anticoagulant refers to a group of antiphospholipid antibodies that act to inhibit in vitro clot-based coagulation assays. The name lupus anticoagulant is a misnomer. The term was originally coined as descriptive because the first patients had systemic lupus erythematosus (SLE) with bleeding symptoms. Since these first reports, it has become apparent that lupus anticoagulants are not usually associated with bleeding unless concomitant hemostatic abnormalities are present. Additionally, many patients with the lupus anticoagulant do not have SLE.

A very small subset of patients with SLE and the lupus anticoagulant present with hypoprothrombinemia (low levels of factor II) and bleeding symptoms. These patients apparently have an antibody that clears factor II from the circulation.

The lupus anticoagulant is one of the most common causes of an isolated, prolonged aPTT. In recent years it has become apparent that the lupus anticoagulant is more frequently associated with thrombosis and the hypercoagulable state. Further information about the lupus anticoagulant is found in chapter 22.

MISCELLANEOUS

30. List two major mechanisms that result in acquired factor deficiencies in the patient with trauma.

1. Dilutional coagulopathy resulting from large infusions of stored bank blood, packed red blood cells, or crystalloid solutions

2. DIC (reviewed in chapter 16)

31. How is dilutional coagulopathy treated?

Dilutional coagulopathy is treated with transfusions of FFP. A rule of thumb is to provide one unit of FFP for every 5 units of whole blank blood or packed red blood cells. This approximation should be modified in the face of any complicating clinical conditions. In addition, actively bleeding patients with platelet counts < 50,000/mm^3 or fibrinogen levels < 75–100 mg/dl necessitate transfusion of platelet concentrates and cryoprecipitate, respectively.

32. Which factor deficiency has been associated with primary systemic amyloidosis? How is it treated?

Isolated acquired deficiency of factor X, which has been described in a number of patients with amyloidosis, is due to specific adsorption of factor X to amyloid fibrils. Transfusions of factor concentrate are not effective treatment. Treatment must be directed at the underlying disease.

BIBLIOGRAPHY

1. Galloway B: The laboratory response to the trauma patient. Trauma Q 3:63–69, 1997.
2. Hultin MB: Acquired inhibitors in malignant and nonmalignant disease. Am J Med 91(Suppl 5A):95–135, 1991.
3. Kemkes-Matthes B, Bleyl H, Matthes KJ: Coagulation activation in liver diseases. Thromb Res 64:253–261, 1991.
4. Kessler CM: Factor VIII inhibitors—An algorithmic approach to treatment. Semin Hematol (Suppl 4):33–36, 1994.
5. Kunkel LA: Acquired circulating anticoagulants. Hematol Oncol Clin North Am 6:1341–1357, 1992.
6. Ludlam CA, Morrison AE, Kessler C: Treatment of acquired hemophilia. Semin Hematol 31(Suppl 4):16–19, 1994.
7. Mammen EF: Coagulation abnormalities in liver disease. Hematol Oncol Clin North Am 6:1287–1299, 1992.
8. Martinez J, Palascak JE, Kwasniak D: Abnormal sialic acid content of the dysfibrinogenemia associated with liver disease. J Clin Invest 61:535–539, 1978.
9. Routh CR, Triplett DA, Murphy MJ, et al: Superwarfarin ingestion and detection. Am J Hematol 36:50–54, 1991.
10. Suttie JW: Recent advances in hepatic vitamin K metabolism and function. Hepatology 7:367–376, 1987.

22. THE HYPERCOAGULABLE STATE

Richard A. Marlar, Ph.D., and Dorothy M. Adcock, M.D.

1. What is the hypercoagulable state?

The hypercoagulable state (sometimes called the prothrombotic state) is a catch-all phrase for a group of poorly defined abnormalities associated with clinical laboratory tests (abnormal genetic tests of factor V_{Leiden}, prothrombin-20210 polymorphism; decreased protein C, antithrombin, or protein S; homocysteine and/or thrombocytosis) or clinical conditions (malignancy, pregnancy, or postoperative state) that increase the patient's risk for developing thromboembolic complications (deep venous thrombosis [DVT], pulmonary embolus [PE], arterial thrombosis, myocardial infarction, stroke). Also included are patients with recurrent thrombosis who have no recognizable predisposing factor(s).

2. What causes the hypercoagulable state?

The list of causes of hypercoagulability is growing, but they may be classified as genetic, acquired, or physiologic. Each of these groups can be subdivided into a variety of categories, including environmental, pathologic, social, or iatrogenic. The acquired conditions are usually secondary to some underlying clinical condition, disease process, or life decision. When several abnormalities occur simultaneously, the chance of developing thrombosis is enhanced. The underlying mechanisms of the hypercoagulable state are due to excessive initiation of the hemostatic systems and/or loss of the regulatory systems. These factors induce thrombus formation in a number of different ways, such as activation of the coagulation system, downregulation of the endogenous coagulation regulatory mechanisms, induction of vascular injury, or endothelial cell perturbation. All of the mechanisms inducing thrombosis involve components of plasma, blood cells, and blood vessels.

Partial List of Causes of Hypercoagulability

GENETIC	ACQUIRED	PHYSIOLOGIC
Antithrombin deficiency	Surgery	Age
Protein C deficiency	Trauma	Gender
Protein S deficiency	Pregnancy	
Activated protein C resistance	Immobilization	
Hyperhomocysteinemia	Hyperhomocysteinemia	
Prothrombin-20210	Smoking	
Dysfibrinogenemia	Obesity	
Plasminogen deficiency	Antiphosphopholipid syndrome	
	Malignancy	

3. What aspects of the hemostatic mechanism are involved in the hypercoagulable state?

All mechanisms of hemostasis appear to be involved in the hypercoagulable state. The platelet and/or endothelial cell plays a role in acquired abnormalities (thrombocytosis, stasis or vascular injury), whereas the coagulation and fibrinolytic systems have been shown to be involved in hereditary hypercoagulability. Abnormalities of the coagulation system largely involve regulatory mechanisms (naturally occurring anticoagulants) that are associated with hereditary thrombotic disease. The endothelial cell is currently a "black box" with respect to regulation of hemostasis and the hypercoagulable state. A considerable amount of work still needs to be completed to determine the role of the endothelial cell as a pivotal component of the hemostatic system.

4. Is the pathophysiologic basis for the acquired hypercoagulable states known?

The mechanisms for activation of the coagulation system, loss of regulatory systems, and hypofibrinolysis are unknown in the majority of acquired cases. Physiologic phenomena (pregnancy and the postpartum period) as well as pathologic abnormalities (atherosclerosis, malignancy, nephrotic syndrome, myeloproliferative disorders) are associated with hypercoagulability. Iatrogenic or drug interaction complications (prosthetic devices, surgery, oral contraceptives, estrogen therapy) also contribute to the induction of the hypercoagulable state. It appears that multiple mechanisms must be aberrant to induce the hypercoagulable state in many of these disorders. Currently, a number of new laboratory tests assessing coagulation activation (prothrombin fragments 1 and 2 [F_{1+2}] and thrombin-antithrombin complex [TAT]) are under evaluation to confirm the clinical suspicion of a hypercoagulable state and in some cases to diagnose a prothrombotic condition before clinical complications develop. Unfortunately, the potential diagnostic advantage of many new tests has not been fully demonstrated and probably will not provide significant predictive value for determining the hypercoagulable state. Within the next few years the best opportunity to assess the prothrombotic state will reside in the ability to determine the total potential for the development of thrombosis by understanding the different thrombotic risks and their interactions.

5. Explain the concepts of thrombotic risk factor and risk potential.

During the past 5–10 years, a number of risk factors (genetic defects and acquired conditions) have been recognized in individuals and families with a notable history of venous thrombosis, suggesting a cause/effect relationship. A thrombotic **risk factor** is defined as any condition (acquired or inherited) that causes a greater-than-normal chance for developing thrombosis. Acquired factors may be due to acute or chronic conditions and may involve environmental, physiologic, social, or pathologic factors. The combination of factors and the severity necessary to cause thrombosis are currently unknown. The table in question 2 contains a partial list of suspected acquired factors that, when dovetailed with the inherited abnormalities, increase the risk of thrombotic complications. The concept of thrombotic risk for development of a thrombotic event has led to the "multi-hit" theory, in which genetic, acquired, and physiologic factors play a major role. This concept parallels the risk-factor concept of coronary disease: a patient with thrombosis or hereditary thrombosis has at least one and probably more genetic risk factors and at least one acquired risk factor, thereby increasing the potential for developing thrombosis. Such factors include the well-known abnormalities of factor V_{Leiden} (activated protein C [APC] resistance), protein C, protein S, and antithrombin as well as the less understood abnormalities of the untranslated region of factor II and homocysteine-related methylene tetrahydrofolate reductase (MTHFR).

Each factor has a different **risk potential**, which is defined as the ability or capacity to contribute to the thrombotic etiology. The extent of the risk potential varies depending on the factor and its interaction with other factors. Most factors interact in a synergistic manner to cause a significant increase in risk that is greater than the additive effects of the individual factors. Multiple genetic risk factors with varying risk potentials occur in more severely affected individuals and families. In addition, acquired factors (e.g., surgery, pregnancy, hormonal therapy, antiphospholipid syndrome, smoking, nutrition) and physiologic factors (age and gender) contribute in a synergistic manner with genetic factors to the overall risk potential for each person. Genetic risk factors remain throughout the person's life, but the risk potential may increase with age. Acquired factors increase the risk periodically and may be controlled by the patient's behavior. Genetic and acquired factors are synergistic, substantially increasing the thrombotic potential at any given time in the patient's life. For example, if the only risk factor is inherited protein C deficiency, the likelihood of thrombosis appears to be low. However, if several underlying acquired risk factors are present (pregnancy, vascular injury, and inflammation), the risk of thrombosis increases with each additional factor.

6. What is hereditary thrombotic disease?

Hereditary thrombotic disease (HTD or thrombophilia) represents a group of abnormalities in which a patient has recurrent thrombotic complications and a positive family history of thrombosis due to a genetic defect(s) associated with coagulation, fibrinolysis, or their regulatory systems. The first such deficiency, antithrombin, was diagnosed in the early 1960s. Several other deficiencies have been described, and much has been learned about the hereditary nature of thrombotic disease. At least eight inherited abnormalities have been confirmed, and several more are now suspected of causing HTD. About 40–50% of the causes of HTD are still unknown.

7. What is the prevalence of the most common inherited deficiencies?
    Excellent evidence indicates that numerous genetic abnormalities in coagulation-related proteins and various polymorphisms (involving hemostatic and nonhemostatic proteins) are inherited causes of HTD. A polymorphism is defined as a less common variant within a gene that is present in more than 5% of the population. The most common known deficiencies are APC resistance (factor V_{Leiden}), hyperhomocysteinemia, and prothrombin polymorphism at base pair 20210. Antithrombin, protein C, and protein S deficiencies are relatively rare. In 40–50% of people with apparent HTD, the inherited cause has not been established. This large group may represent deficiencies associated with suspected factors or as yet unrecognized abnormalities (other polymorphisms and endothelial cell functional defects).

Prevalence of Genetic Abnormalities in the Normal Population

FACTOR	PREVALENCE
Protein C	200–500 per 100,000
Protein S	200–1000 per 100,000
Antithrombin	20–50 per 100,000
Factor V_{Leiden}	4%
Methylene tetrahydrofolate reductase	4–5%
Prothrombin-20210	2%

8. How is HTD transmitted?
    All of the genetic abnormalities and polymorphisms associated with the known causes of HTD are transmitted by autosomal inheritance. The apparent incomplete penetrance is due to the interaction of the abnormality with other genetic and acquired risk factors for thrombosis.

9. Describe one classic high-risk potential case and one classic low-risk potential case of HTD.
    1. **High-risk potential case.** A 26-year-old woman presents with DVT involving the lower left extremity without a precipitating cause. History reveals a previous DVT after her first pregnancy at age 23. Her mother also had a "clotting problem" and died (probably of PE) at the age of 37 after multiple hospitalizations and treatment with "blood thinners." The patient's brother had died 5 years previously of massive PE. This presentation is typical of the classic form of HTD. Approximately 90–95% of patients with HTD present with venous thrombosis involving the deep venous system of the lower extremity with or without PE. Thromboembolic complication may occur spontaneously or in relation to some underlying event (risk factor), such as surgery, trauma, or pregnancy. Most patients with HTD have their first thrombotic episode between the ages of 18 and 45; about 75–85% have had a clot by the age of 50. Symptoms usually do not manifest until after puberty (age 15). Most patients have multiple episodes of thrombosis and a positive family history. Currently, patients in the age range of 18–45 years are usually evaluated for a hypercoagulable state or HTD after the first episode of thrombosis. In the case presented above, the patient and other family members were found to have protein S deficiency and were treated accordingly.
    2. **Low-risk potential case.** A 63-year-old man develops DVT (his first episode) after a long plane trip from Europe. The clinician rules out cancer and other medical causes. The patient

has no personal or family history of thrombosis. He was evaluated for partial thromboplastin time (PTT), antithrombin, protein C, protein S, and APC resistance. All were within normal range except APC resistance (ratio value of 1.7; normal = > 2.3). The abnormal APC resistance test triggered reflexive genetic testing for factor V_{Leiden}. The patient was heterozygous for factor V_{Leiden} polymorphism. He was treated with low-molecular-weight heparin on an outpatient basis and oral anticoagulant therapy (international normalized ratio [INR] = 2–3) for 1 year.

10. What is the lupus anticoagulant?

The lupus anticoagulant (LA) is an acquired autoimmune disorder in which autoantibodies against phospholipid-protein complexes develop. LA is more accurately described as antiphospholipid syndrome (APS), because it is in fact a multimechanism disorder with a variety of presentations. LA manifests in vitro with prolongation of phospholipid-dependent coagulation tests but paradoxically causes thrombosis in approximately 30% of patients. Therefore, LA is considered a hypercoagulable disorder. In vivo, LA interferes with either coagulation regulatory mechanisms or causes perturbation of the endothelial cell to incite thromboembolic complications. The term "lupus anticoagulant" is a true misnomer. The term "lupus" was applied because this abnormality was first described in patients with systemic lupus erythematosus (SLE). The term "anticoagulant" comes from the laboratory artifact of prolonged coagulation tests, typically demonstrated as a prolonged activated partial thromboplastin time (aPTT). LA may prolong other phospholipid-dependent assays, including prothrombin time (PT) and dilute Russell's viper venom time (dRVVT). LA is not exclusive to patients with SLE; it also is found in a variety of other situations (viral infections, antibiotic and phenothiazine usage, and otherwise normal individuals). It is seen in 1–2% of the general population.

11. What are the laboratory diagnostic criteria for LA?

The diagnosis of LA is based on the following criteria:
1. Prolongation of a phospholipid-dependent coagulation assay
2. Demonstration of a nonspecific coagulation inhibitor
3. Demonstration that the inhibitor is phospholipid-dependent

The phospholipid-dependent assay most commonly used to screen for the LA is the aPTT. This assay is normal in some cases, and assays that use lower phospholipid concentrations, such as the dRVVT and kaolin-clotting time, may be necessary to identify some patients with LA. To determine the presence of an inhibitor, plasma mixing studies should be performed. To demonstrate phospholipid dependency, phospholipid is added to the sample; neutralization of the inhibitor, as shown by a platelet neutralization procedure (PNP) or other manufactured assays, is a positive result. Heparin contamination must be excluded because heparin mimics the presence of an inhibitor. In conjunction with the coagulation tests, the patient's serum should be assayed for anticardiolipin (aCL) or anti-phosphotidylserine (aPS) antibodies. The presence of aCL, aPS, or a positive PNP in conjunction with prolonged aPTT is the basis for the diagnosis of LA or APS.

12. How is LA treated?

The treatment of LA is controversial and can be difficult. Patients with diagnosed LA but no underlying thrombotic complications should not be treated. Patients who develop venous thrombosis should be treated in the standard fashion recommended for venous thrombosis. Monitoring of heparinization may be difficult because of the initially prolonged aPTT. Heparin therapy should be monitored by a heparin assay or thrombin time. Monitoring of oral anticoagulant therapy using the INR also may be difficult because some PT reagents are sensitive to LA. Some experts advocate maintaining the INR in the 3–3.5 range, whereas others suggest using factor X activity levels. Patients presenting with arterial thrombosis should be treated with aspirin and/or oral anticoagulant therapy. If the hypercoagulable state is difficult to control, prednisone may be used in conjunction with other anticoagulant therapy.

13. Explain APC resistance and factor V$_{Leiden}$.

The protein C system involves several plasma and cellular proteins that help to regulate the coagulation system. Protein C in its active form (APC) inactivates factors Va and VIIIa, the two rate-limiting cofactors of coagulation. Abnormalities of the protein C system (such as protein C deficiency, protein S deficiency, and thrombomodulin defect) may lead to increased risk for developing thrombosis. A unique polymorphism in the factor V molecule also increases the risk for thrombosis by decreasing the rate of factor V inactivation by APC (termed APC resistance). This polymorphism, genetically termed factor V$_{Leiden}$, is a G-to-A substitution at position 1691 in the factor V gene; the amino acid arginine is changed to glutamine at position 506. Its prevalence is 4% in the general Caucasian population but very low in Asian, African, and Native American populations. Homozygotes are at significant risk for developing thrombosis at an early age (average age: 26 years), whereas heterozygotes are at a lower risk and develop thrombosis at a later age (average age: 63 years). Patients with APC resistance are treated with standard protocols of heparin and warfarin.

14. How does homocysteine induce thrombosis?

Homocysteine (HC) is a thiol-containing amino acid that is metabolized to either methionine or cysteine. Chronically elevated levels of HC have been associated with an increased risk of thrombosis and atherosclerosis. Elevated levels have been attributed to both genetic and acquired causes. The mechanism of HC-induced vascular disease involves interference with endothelial cell function, including increased levels of tissue factor (increased procoagulant activity), decreased expression of thrombomodulin and protein S (decreased anticoagulant activity), decreased fibrinolytic response, and increased platelet adhesion. Increased plasma levels of HC may be seen in patients with poor nutrition or several known genetic mutations or polymorphisms. One of the most common polymorphisms is a thermal labile variant of methylene tetrahydrofolate reductase (MTHFR). This homozygous polymorphism, affecting 4% of the general population, is a C-to-T mutation at 677 bp in the MTHFR gene. This MTHFR polymorphism reduces the function of the enzyme by 50% and increases plasma HC levels in patients with poor diet. The risk potential for MTHFR is small but may contribute to increased risk when coupled with poor diet. In the majority of cases the increased levels of plasma HC can be reduced with daily folate supplement.

15. What is the 3'-untranslated prothrombin-20210 polymorphism?

A unique polymorphism in the 3'-untranslated region of the prothrombin gene appears to increase the risk of thrombosis at least two-fold. The mechanism is currently unknown but may be due to a longer half-life of the prothrombin mRNA, leading to elevated plasma levels of prothrombin. Currently the only method to test for prothrombin-20210 is genetic analysis of the patient's DNA with polymerase chain reaction (PCR). Such patients are treated with heparin and oral anticoagulant therapy for venous thrombosis.

16. When is the optimal time to perform a work-up for a patient in whom HTD is suspected?

The best time to make a definitive diagnosis of HTD is when the patient is asymptomatic and off all anticoagulation medication. However, most patients develop thrombosis before work-up or receive long-term anticoagulation therapy. For cost-containment purposes and to avoid the chance of obtaining erroneous results, laboratory evaluation should *not* be performed (1) during early postthrombotic periods, (2) when the patient is symptomatic, or (3) when the patient is taking heparin or warfarin therapy. Testing during these periods may mask true results because of consumption or assay artifact. The confirmation of a hereditary abnormality can be made only after two abnormal values are obtained in the patient during an asymptomatic and untreated state and similar values are identified in two other family members. The laboratory abnormalities must cosegregate with the thrombotic complications. When all criteria are met, the patient and family can be diagnosed with a hereditary deficiency. If only the patient can be evaluated, a tentative diagnosis should be established.

17. What factors should be tested in patients with suspected HTD?

The best way to evaluate a patient with hypercoagulability due to HTD is to order assays in a cost-effective manner, starting with the most common deficiencies (see table on following page). Acquired causes of hypercoagulability must be ruled out before any testing is started. The most common acquired abnormalities are APS, malignancy, and myeloproliferative disorders. The cause of hypercoagulability is found in only about 50–60% of cases. The other 40–50% will remain undiagnosed until research testing demonstrates the relevant deficiencies and their relative importance. The collection and preparation of blood or serum for subsequent testing is crucial. The blood draw must be nontraumatic, and the sample must be prepared as rapidly as possible. The sample should be platelet-free (< 10,000/μl) and rapidly frozen for subsequent testing.

18. How are results interpreted for diagnosis of HTD?

The diagnosis of HTD can be complicated by a number of causes (underlying disease, acquired abnormalities, laboratory artifact). Interpretation must be made with caution. All acquired causes of abnormal coagulation values (e.g., liver disease, disseminated intravascular coagulation, thrombosis, APS or LA, malignancy) must be eliminated before evaluation. A definitive diagnosis should never be made in a patient who is anticoagulated or has acquired abnormalities. If all known acquired causes of an abnormal value are eliminated and a hereditary basis is still suspected, the abnormal value must be confirmed on a second sample and in family studies. Cosegregation of thrombosis and the deficiency must be confirmed. If the patient is the only family member who can be tested, only a tentative diagnosis should be assigned. The controversy associated with testing family members is discussed in question 21.

19. What is the treatment for HTD?

Treatment should address the type of thrombotic event and the site of thrombosis rather than the deficiency. In general, for DVT and PE the first thrombotic event should be treated with unfractionated or low-molecular-weight heparin, followed by 3–6 months of oral anticoagulant therapy. The second event is also treated with heparin, followed by 6–12 months (or longer) of oral anticoagulant therapy. The third and subsequent events are usually treated with lifelong oral anticoagulant therapy. In rare cases of protein C or protein S deficiency, the complication of warfarin-induced skin necrosis has been observed when large loading doses of warfarin are used without concurrent heparin. All treatment regimens are highly individual and must be adjusted to the location, type, and past history of thrombosis. Patients at increased risk for thrombosis (e.g., surgery, pregnancy) with a known deficiency or history of thrombosis should be treated prophylactically. However, some evidence suggests that the risks of anticoagulation may outweigh the benefits of prophylactic treatment. The bottom line is that prophylactic treatment must be considered on an individual basis.

CONTROVERSIES

20. Should a cost-effective or complete evaluation of hypercoagulability be performed?

The laboratory evaluation of hypercoagulability has changed significantly in the past few years and continues to change on a regular basis as more defects and polymorphisms associated with venous thrombosis are identified. In addition, numerous factors previously associated with HTD have been reevaluated and found to involve little actual risk or to have an extremely low incidence in the population (i.e., tissue plasminogen activator [tPA], heparin cofactor II, and plasminogen). A wide variety of tests can be performed in the evaluation of the hypercoagulable state, but it may be cost-prohibitive to evaluate all suspected deficiencies (cost = approximately $1500), whereas a cost-effective approach to testing costs about $400. We have designed testing panels that identify the most common and clinically relevant defects; the panel differs with age. Using this cost-effective approach, we can identify 60% of cases, whereas a complete work-up of all known factors identifies only 63% of defects. With both methods, patients are treated in an identical fashion.

Cost-Effective vs. Complete Work-up for Hypercoagulability

COST-EFFECTIVE WORK-UP		COMPLETE WORK-UP
UNDER 60 YR	OVER 60 YR	
LA and APS	LA and APS	LA and APS
Antithrombin	APC resistance	Antithrombin
Protein C	Homocysteine	Protein C
Protein S	Prothrombin-20210	Protein S
APC resistance		APC resistance
Homocysteine		Homocysteine
Prothrombin-20210		Prothrombin-20210
		Plasminogen
		Fibrinogen
		Heparin cofactor II
		Euglobulin lysis time
		tPA/PAI

LA = lupus anticoagulant, APS = antiphospholipid syndrome, APC = activated protein C, tPA = tissue plasminogen activator, PAI = plasminogen activator inhibitor.

21. Should family members of patients with HTD undergo a work-up?

For: The diagnosis of a deficiency state in an asymptomatic family member can pinpoint the potential increased thrombotic risk for each family member. He or she can then be educated about the deficiency and thrombotic signs. In addition, the diagnosis helps in genetic counseling and family planning.

Against: The asymptomatic family member is subsequently labeled for life with a deficiency, even though he or she remains asymptomatic. Insurance companies may not insure a patient with this preexisting condition.

The current consensus is to perform a work-up for family members because it offers the opportunity to educate, to treat during high risk procedures, to eliminate acquired risk factors, and to assess individual risk of thrombosis.

22. Should unaffected deficient members of a family with a history of thrombosis be treated prophylactically?

Prophylactic treatment of asymptomatic family members with HTD is controversial. A number of physicians currently treat asymptomatic patients with known deficiencies with prophylactic heparin when they undergo increased-risk procedures (surgery). The routine daily prophylactic treatment of an asymptomatic family member is usually not recommended because of inherent risks of long-term oral anticoagulation. This approach is highly individualized; the physician and patient make the final decision. In families with a history of life-threatening thrombosis, consideration may be given to prophylactic treatment of asymptomatic family members.

BIBLIOGRAPHY

1. Adcock DM, Fink L, Marlar RA: A laboratory approach to the evaluation of hereditary hypercoagulability. Am J Clin Pathol 108:434–449, 1997.
2. Bertina RM: Introduction: Hypercoagulable states. Semin Hematol 34:167–169, 1997.
3. Brandt JT, Triplett DA, Alving B, Scharrer I: Criteria for the diagnosis of lupus anticoagulants: An update. On behalf of the Subcommittee on Lupus Anticoagulant-Antiphospholipid Antibody of the Scientific and Standardization Committee of the ISTH. Thromb Haemost 74:1185–1190, 1995.
4. Dahlback B, et al: Activated protein C resistance as a basis for venous thrombosis. Am J Med 101:534–540, 1996.
5. Esmon NL, Smirnov MD, Esmon CT: Thrombogenic mechanisms of antiphospholipid antibodies. Thromb Haemost 78:79–82, 1997.

6. Florrel S, et al: Inherited thrombotic disorders: An update. Am J Hematol 54:53–60, 1997.
7. Guba SC, Fink LM, Fonseca V: Hyperhomocysteinemia: Emerging and important risk factor for thromboembolic and cardiovascular disease. Am J Clin Pathol 105:709–722, 1996.
8. Kyrle PA, Stumpflen A, Hirschl M, et al: Levels of prothrombin fragment F1+2 in patients with hyperhomocysteinemia and a history of venous thromboembolism. Thromb Haemost 78:1327–1331, 1997.
9. Mannucci P, et al: Inherited thrombophilia: Pathogenesis, clinical syndromes, and management. Blood 187:3531–3544, 1996.
10. Marlar RA, Adcock DM: Thrombotic threshold trait: Concept of a multi-hit theory for hereditary thrombotic disease. Clin Hemost Rev 12:12–13, 1998.
11. Poort SR, Rosendaal FR, Reitsma PH, Bertina RM: A common genetic variation in the 3'-untranslated region of the prothrombin gene is associated with elevated plasma prothrombin levels and an increase in venous thrombosis. Blood 88:3698–3703, 1996.
12. Rodeghiero F, et al: Epidemiology of inherited thrombophilia: The VITA Project. Thromb Haemost 78:636–640, 1997.
13. Rosendaal FR: Risk factors for venous thrombosis: Prevalence, risk, and interaction. Semin Hematol 34:171–187, 1997.
14. Rosendaal F, et al: The Leiden Thrombophilia Study (LETS). Thromb Haemost 78:631–635, 1997.
15. Thomas DP, et al: Hypercoagulability in venous arterial thrombosis. Ann Intern Med 126:638–644, 1997.

23. NEUTROPENIA

Russell C. Tolley, M.D.

1. What is the definition of neutropenia?

Neutropenia is a neutrophilic granulocyte count—or absolute neutrophil count (ANC)—of less than 1500/mm³. The ANC is calculated by multiplying the total white blood cell (WBC) count by the percentage of band neutrophils and segmented neutrophils:

$$\text{ANC} = \text{WBC count} \times (\% \text{ bands} + \% \text{ segmented neutrophils}) \times 0.01$$

Neutrophil counts of less than 2000/mm³ are uncommon, but some normal individuals of Yemenite Jew or African descent may have counts as low as 1000/mm³ with no apparent disease.

2. What is the risk of infection with neutropenia?

Generally speaking, the lower the neutrophil count, the higher the risk of infection. In studies of bone marrow transplantation, the risk of infection rises dramatically when the ANC falls below 500/mm³. However, the risk of infection also varies with the nature of the primary disease process and the duration of neutropenia. Usually, neutropenia from marrow hypoplasia (due to chemotherapy, aplastic anemia, or other causes of marrow failure) has the greatest risk for infection. Neutropenia associated with a cellular marrow (chronic idiopathic neutropenia in adults, chronic benign neutropenia of infancy, or hypersplenism) usually has less risk of infection.

3. How do infections in acute and chronic neutropenia differ?

In acute neutropenia, *Staphylococcus aureus, Pseudomonas aeruginosa, Escherichia coli,* and *Klebsiella* sp. are common causes of infection, which often presents as sepsis. Patients with severe chronic neutropenia and autoimmune neutropenia, however, have recurrent sinusitis, stomatitis, gingivitis, and perirectal infections but usually do not become septic.

4. How are neutropenias classified?

Like anemias, neutropenias can be classified into categories of (1) decreased production, (2) sequestration from the circulating pool to marginated or tissue pools, (3) increased destruction or utilization, or (4) a combination of the above. Because techniques of measurement are cumbersome and not easily available, most authors divide the neutropenias into two categories: acquired or intrinsic.

5. What are the causes of acquired neutropenia?

Drug-induced neutropenia

Marrow-infiltrating disorders

Benign familial neutropenia

Chronic idiopathic neutropenia

Isoimmune neutropenia

Increased margination of WBCs

Infection with human immunodeficiency
  virus (HIV)

Postinfectious neutropenia

Nutritional deficiencies

Chronic benign neutropenia
  of childhood

Autoimmune neutropenia

Metabolic diseases

Immunologic abnormalities

Chronic acquired neutropenias also can be subdivided into those with splenomegaly (Felty's syndrome, congestive splenomegaly, Gaucher's disease, sarcoidosis, and other infectious diseases) and those without splenomegaly (chronic idiopathic neutropenia, benign familial neutropenia, and chronic benign neutropenia of childhood).

6. How do drugs cause neutropenia? Which agents cause neutropenia most often?

A history of chemotherapy is easily obtained, but many other therapeutic agents may cause neutropenia. The mechanism can involve direct marrow destruction (as with many chemotherapy agents), immune-mediated damage to neutrophil precursors in the bone marrow, or peripheral destruction or clearance of neutrophils. Fortunately, most drug-related neutropenias are due to dose-dependent suppression of bone marrow. After the offending agent is stopped, return of the neutrophil count to normal usually occurs within a few days, preceded by monocytosis (as in the recovery of the neutrophil count after chemotherapy). On rare occasions, chloramphenicol may cause a dose-independent aplastic anemia. The drugs that most commonly cause neutropenia include:

Phenothiazines (chlorpromazine, promazine)

Antithyroid agents (propylthiouracil, methimazole)

Ethanol

Antibiotics (chloramphenicol, semisynthetic penicillins, sulfonamides)

Meprobamate (tranquilizer)

Nonsteroidal antiinflammatory drugs

Antiepileptics (carbamazepine, phenytoin)

Analgesics (salicylates, dipyrone, aminopyrine)

7. What are the common causes of postinfectious neutropenia?

Neutropenia can be seen after **viral infections**, a common cause in children. Viral diseases such as hepatitis A and B, influenza, Kawasaki disease, measles, rubella, and varicella have been implicated; the neutropenia can last for weeks. HIV infection, usually in later stages, can cause neutropenia in both adults and children and is usually associated with a hypercellular marrow. **Nonviral agents**, such as staphylococcus, mycobacterium tuberculosis, and rickettsiae, also can cause neutropenia. Brucellosis and tularemia have been associated with low neutrophil counts, and any cause of sepsis can be associated with a severe neutropenia. Increased utilization and margination probably account for low neutrophil counts in the case of sepsis. A low neutrophil count in streptococcal pneumonia is a poor prognostic sign. The mainstay of therapy is treatment of the underlying infection.

8. What are the characteristic findings in neutropenia associated with HIV infection?

Neutropenia is seen in more than 70% of patients with acquired immunodeficiency syndrome (AIDS) and is usually associated with a hypercellular marrow and a late myeloid arrest in the WBC precursors. Both hypersplenism and antineutrophil antibodies can be found in many patients.

9. What is benign familial leukopenia? What ethnic populations are usually involved?

Benign familial leukopenia is characterized by a mild neutropenia (2100–2600/mm³) with no increased risk of infection. This disorder is seen in several ethnic groups, including Yemenite Jews, West Indians, and people of African descent. The bone marrow biopsy appears normal; this finding represents a genetic variation in the regulation of the circulating neutrophil counts.

10. What is seen on the peripheral blood smear in individuals with neutropenia due to a bone marrow-infiltrating process?

If the bone marrow is infiltrated with either infection or metastatic cancer, other findings from the physical examination and history often lead to a diagnosis. In many patients, however, the peripheral smear shows a myelophthisic picture, with an increase in percentages of immature cell forms from all lines (reticulocytes, nucleated red cells, myeloid precursors, and giant platelets). This condition is sometimes indicative of a marrow infiltrated with metastatic carcinoma or, more rarely, an infectious agent such as mycobacterium.

11. Lack of which vitamins can cause neutropenia?

Vitamin B_{12} or folate deficiency can cause neutropenia with or without anemia. The bone marrow biopsy shows megaloblastic changes with ineffective myelopoiesis. Neutropenia and anemia associated with a meagloblastic bone marrow have been seen in the DIDMOAD syndrome (diabetes insipidus, diabetes mellitus, optic atrophy, deafness). In this syndrome hematologic abnormalities have been responsive to thiamine.

12. Deficiency of which heavy metal can cause isolated neutropenia?

Nutritional deficiency of copper and inherited deficiency of transcobalamin II have been known to cause ineffective myelopoiesis, megaloblastic changes in the marrow, and neutropenia.

13. What are the characteristics of chronic benign neutropenia of infancy and childhood?

Chronic benign neutropenia of childhood is a "chronic state of mature neutrophil depletion with a compensatory increase in immature granulocytes in the bone marrow analogous to erythroid hyperplasia in hemolytic anemia."[8] This disease occurs in the first 3 years of life, with 90% of cases occurring before the age of 14 months. Infection is a common presenting symptom, but the relationship is unclear because infections in this age group are common. Neutrophil counts are characteristically normal at birth, yet less than 500/mm^3 at presentation. The majority of patients have detectable antineutrophil IgG antibodies that react with neutrophils, suggesting an immune mechanism. Immunosuppressive therapy is effective. Most of the infections are easily treated during the neutropenia, and some infants still can mount a neutrophil response. Although an unusual patient remains neutropenic into the adult years, 95% recover by 4 years of age. The bone marrow is normo- or hypercellular. High-dose intravenous gamma globulin, steroids, and granulocyte colony-stimulating factor (G-CSF) can be effective in raising the neutrophil count but are rarely indicated because of the usually benign nature of this disorder. Effective and expedient treatment of infections is the mainstay of therapy. Care must be taken not to confuse this diagnosis with more severe causes of neutropenia in infancy.

14. What is chronic idiopathic neutropenia?

Along with benign familial neutropenia and chronic benign neutropenia of childhood, chronic idiopathic neutropenia is a chronic neutropenia not usually associated with splenomegaly. The diagnosis is applied to neutropenias that do not fit into other categories. Age of onset is quite variable, and neutrophil counts are usually between 200 and 500/mm^3. A normal to increased number of immature granulocytes can be found in the bone marrow (suggesting arrested maturation). Antineutrophil antibodies are usually absent, G-CSF concentrations are usually normal, and cytogenetic analysis of the marrow is normal. A neutrophil response to stimuli can still be seen, and the clinical course is often mild.

16. What are the immune causes of neutropenia?

Even though immune mechanisms are implicated in cases of neutropenia that have been called idiopathic, a few causes of immune neutropenia are well established. Isoimmune neutropenia occurs in newborn infants when antibodies are transferred from the mother to the infant. Autoimmune neutropenia due to neutrophil-associated antibodies can occur at any time, from childhood to old age. Immunologic abnormalities such as hyper- or hypogammaglobulinemia, T-cell defects, and natural killer-cell abnormalities, as well as other autoimmune diseases, can cause neutropenia in childhood. Patients usually present with frequent infections and hepato-splenomegaly. Many have a family history of neutropenia. Severe cases have been treated with allogeneic bone marrow transplanation.

T-gamma lymphocytosis is a disorder in which clonal proliferation of lymphocytes is associated with a normocellular marrow, maturational arrest in neutrophils, and peripheral neutropenia. Although the course of this disease may be benign, some individuals have been successfully treated with gammaglobulin.

17. What is the treatment for isoimmune neutropenia in newborns?

Isoimmune neutropenia in newborns is identical in pathogenesis to Rh hemolytic disease: prenatal sensitization to neutrophil antigens with subsequent IgG antibodies that cross the placental barrier to the newborn. The disorder occurs in 0.2% of births. The newborn may be asymptomatic or present with sepsis. Antineutrophil antibodies are usually detected in both the infant's and mother's serum. Bone marrow biopsy performed on the infant is normocellular and displays a late maturational arrest. Neutropenia usually resolves in 12–15 weeks, although on rare occasions it lasts as long as 6 months. Appropriate antibiotics are the usual treatment; intravenous gamma globulin also has been used successfully.

18. What are the causes of autoimmune neutropenia?

Autoimmune neutropenia can be (1) isolated (i.e., the only hematologic abnormality), (2) secondary to other autoimmune diseases such as rheumatoid arthritis or systemic lupus erythematosus, or (3) related to immune mechanisms triggered by infections or drugs. The neutropenia is moderate to severe, with hypercellular marrow and late myeloid maturational arrest. Hepatosplenomegaly is seen in about half of the patients, and presentation can be at any age. Neutropenia can be associated with a concurrent idiopathic thrombocytopenia purpura (ITP) or hemolytic anemia. Various antineutrophil antibodies of the IgG or IgM type may be detected, and, as in some cases of chronic idiopathic neutropenia, immune complexes have been found. Patients with rheumatoid arthritis, neutropenia, and splenomegaly have Felty's syndrome, a complex autoimmune disorder. Methotrexate treatment sometimes decreases the levels of antineutrophil antibody and concurrently increases the neutrophil count. Other patients with a severe autoimmune neutropenia (ANC < 500/mm^3) and recurrent infections can be treated with intravenous gamma globulin or steroids. Cytotoxic therapy has been used in other immune neutropenias as well as in rheumatoid arthritis. Splenectomy provides no lasting benefit.

19. Which metabolic diseases are associated with neutropenia?

Neutropenia has been seen in patients with ketoacidosis and hyperglycemia, hyperglycinuria, orotic aciduria, methylmalonic aciduria, and glycogen storage disease type Ib. Hypothyroidism may cause neutropenia. Treatment focuses on the underlying disease whenever possible.

20. What are the causes of neutrophil margination? Is it related to acute respiratory distress syndrome (ARDS)?

Complement activation clearly can cause acute and chronic neutropenia due to increased adherence and aggregation in endothelia. Etiologies such as hemodialysis, membrane oxygenators, severe burns, and transfusion reactions have been implicated. Paroxysmal nocturnal hemoglobinuria also generates complement-mediated neutrophil destruction. Lung dysfunction and pulmonary infiltrates have been seen in some patients, suggesting that the neutrophil may play a role in the pathogenesis of ARDS. This theory, however, has not been proved.

21. What is hypersplenism? How is it treated?

Splenomegaly from any cause can produce neutropenia, usually in association with mild thrombocytopenia and anemia. Splenic sequestration and increased peripheral utilization are proposed mechanisms. Predisposition to infection is variable, although usually it is not severe enough to cause symptoms. Splenectomy increases the blood counts but should be reserved for patients with recurrent severe infections.

22. What are the intrinsic causes of neutropenia?

Dyskeratosis congenita is an X-linked disorder characterized by integument abnormalities in association with mild neutropenia or, in some cases, pancytopenia. The bone marrow is hypocellular. Kostmann syndrome (infantile agranulocytosis) is an inherited disorder that presents in infancy with recurrent severe infections and neutropenia. Bone marrow examination reveals myeloid hypocellularity with an arrest at the promyelocyte stage. Bone marrow culture reveals G-CSF–dependent colony growth. This previously fatal disorder responds well to G-CSF in vivo. Shwachman-Diamond-Oski syndrome presents in the first decade of life with neutropenia, metaphyseal dysplasia, and pancreatic insufficiency. Severe, sometimes fatal, infections occur in over half the patients. Chediak-Higashi syndrome is the rare inherited syndrome of oculocutaneous albinism, progressive neurologic impairment, and giant granules in many cells, including neutrophils. Severe neutropenia is also seen. The syndrome of agranulocytosis, lymphoid hypoplasia, and thymic dysplasia is known as reticular dysgenesis. The bone marrow is hypoplastic with few myeloid precursors, and all patients die in infancy unless treated with bone marrow transplant. Cyclic neutropenia is a dominantly inherited disorder of variable expression with neutropenia that recurs about every 15–35 days. The course of the disease tends to be benign, although recurrent infections can be severe and may cause death. Age of presentation is variable, and the marrow is hypoplastic during episodes of neutropenia. Furthermore, isolated neutropenia can be seen in other states of marrow failure, such as refractory anemia, aplastic anemia, and Fanconi's anemia.

23. What is the work-up for neutropenia?

If the patient is without symptoms, physical findings, or historical data that merit further evaluation, clinical observation is the best approach. This is especially true if the patient has a recent history of a viral infection or discontinues a medicine known to cause neutropenia. Complete blood counts must be done twice weekly for 6 weeks if cyclic neutropenia is suspected. In children, the most common causes of isolated neutropenia are benign, and isolated neutropenia is rarely the presentation of malignancy at any age. If thrombocytopenia or anemia is present, if the patient presents with infection, or if the neutropenia persists, bone marrow aspiration and biopsy should be performed. Serum immunologic evaluation, assessment of levels of antineutrophil antibody, and a work-up for collagen vascular disease may then be merited.

24. How is neutropenia managed?

Management of infection is of major concern in the neutropenic patient. Many of the inflammatory signs of infection may not be present because of the inability to mount a neutrophil response. Therefore, the combination of fever and neutropenia usually requires immediate use of broad-spectrum antibiotics. The organisms that cause infection are usually from the gastrointestinal tract and the skin, and therapy should be aimed at gram-negative as well as gram-positive organisms. Intravenous gammaglobulin and steroids have had limited usefulness in some instances of inmmune-related neutropenia, and both G-CSF and allogeneic bone marrow transplantation have been used successfully in certain cases of severe chronic neutropenia.

BIBLIOGRAPHY

1. Coates T, Baehner R: Leukocytosis and leukopenia. In Hoffman R, Benz EJ, Shattil SJ, et al (eds): Hematology: Basic Principles and Practice, 2nd ed. New York, Churchill Livingstone, 1995.
2. Dale DC: Immune and idiopathic neutropenia. Curr Opin Hematol 5:33–36, 1998.
3. Dale DC, Guerry D, Wewerka JR, et al: Chronic neutropenia. Medicine 58:128, 1979.
4. Fronteira M, Myers AM: Peripheral blood and bone marrow abnormalities in the acquired immunodeficiency syndrome. West J Med 147:157, 1987.
5. Hammond WP, Price TH, Souza LM, Dale DC: Treatment of cyclic neutropenia with granulocyte colony-stimulating factor. N Engl J Med 320:1306, 1989.
6. Kyle RA: Natural history of chronic idiopathic neutropenia. N Engl J Med 302:908, 1980.
7. Welte K, Boxer LA: Severe chronic neutropenia: Pathophysiology and therapy. Semin Hematol 34:267–278, 1997.
8. Wright DG, et al: Human cyclic neutropenia: Clinical review and long-term follow-up of patients. Medicine 60:1, 1980.

24. MYELODYSPLASTIC SYNDROMES

Jeanette Mladenovic, M.D.

1. Name the components of the triad that suggests the clinical diagnosis of myelodysplastic syndrome (MDS). *reduction of cellular elements in blood*

The hematologic constellation of chronic refractory cytopenia, bone marrow with increased cellularity, and dysmyelopoietic abnormalities in bone marrow precursors is sufficient to presume the clinical disorder of MDS.

2. Which categories of diseases are included in MDS? What are the diagnostic criteria for each subgroup?

The widely accepted classification of MDS proposed by the FAB (French-American-British) group parallels the classification of leukemias. The classification is based on morphologic criteria that include the numbers of myeloblasts and ring sideroblasts in the marrow, the number of circulating blasts and monocytes in the blood, and the presence or absence of Auer rods. The five types of MDS along with their distinguishing diagnostic criteria are listed below.

Myelodysplastic Syndromes

	PERIPHERAL BLOOD		BONE MARROW	
	% CIRCULATING BLASTS	% MONOCYTES	% BLASTS	% RING SIDEROBLASTS
Refractory anemia (RA)	< 1	Not increased	< 5	< 15
Refractory anemia with ring sideroblasts (RAS)	< 1	Not increased	< 5	> 15
Chronic myelomonocytic leukemia (CMML)	< 5	> 10^9/L	≥ 20	Insignificant
Refractory anemia with excess blasts (RAEB)	< 5	Not increased	5–20	Insignificant
Refractory anemia with excess blasts in transformation (RAEB-T)	≤ 5	Not increased	20–30 and/or Auer rods	Insignificant

As can be seen from the above table, the myelodysplastic syndromes consist of five separate entities, many of which have overlapping characteristics that can be distinguished by the predominant blood and marrow characteristics. The importance of this classification can be seen in patient prognosis, indications for therapy, and therapeutic outcomes.

3. Why is the term *myelodysplastic syndrome* misleading?

The term might lead one to believe that the bone marrow is simply abnormal but not neoplastic in nature. This is not the case. The bone marrow in MDS represents the clonal proliferation of an abnormal stem cell. Thus, although a megaloblastic marrow due to B_{12} deficiency might be considered dysmyelopoietic in descriptive terms, it is not a clonal abnormality of the stem cell representing conversion to neoplasia. Older terms for MDS such as "preleukemia" might in fact be more appropriate. Today, however, these groups of entities are most commonly called MDS.

4. Describe the clinical presentation of a patient with MDS.

The clinical presentation of MDS has no specific features. The most common symptomatic presentation is an elderly individual with fatigue, weakness, and exertional dyspnea, often related to anemia. Most patients present asymptomatically with an abnormality noted in the routine peripheral blood count. Splenomegaly and hepatomegaly are seen in only 5–10% of patients. A small percentage of patients may present with infection related to neutropenia, especially when the neutrophil count is below 1000/µl.

5. How frequently are various cytopenias found in MDS?

The most frequent presentation is anemia, which is found in > 85% of patients. This anemia is characterized by hypoproliferation, with an increase in the mean cell volume. There may be acquired hemoglobinopathies (hemoglobin H disease) or enzyme deficiencies (pyruvate kinase) complicating this anemia.

Neutropenia is often accompanied by a monocytosis, which is present in about half of patients with MDS. Thrombocytopenia is found in about 25% of patients at the time of diagnosis, but mild thrombocytosis also may occur. The abnormality in platelets may be accompanied by abnormal platelet function, leading to prolonged bleeding and abnormal in vitro aggregation responses. Often patients have lymphocyte abnormalities such as lymphopenia with decreased numbers of natural killer cells and/or helper leukocytes.

6. What are the peripheral blood smear clues to the diagnosis of MDS?

Because MDS is a disorder of the myeloid stem cell, there may be abnormalities in all three cell lines on the peripheral blood smear. In addition to abnormalities noted in the differential criteria (percentage of circulating blasts and monocytosis), there may be several other findings that suggest a myelodysplastic abnormality. The red blood cells themselves may be macrocytic or may consist of a second population of cells that are hypochromic and coarsely stippled. There may be a number of misshapen cells with nucleated red blood cells, basophilic stippling, and Heinz bodies. Immature white blood cells that usually do not circulate in the peripheral blood may be evident. The nuclear anomaly of Pelger-Huët is frequently seen with bilobed or even ring-shaped nuclei. Cytoplasmic granules may be decreased or absent. The platelets may be abnormal in appearance in addition to number. There may be large platelets, poorly granulated platelets, or circulating fragments of megakaryocytes. In summary, abnormalities in more than one cell are highly suggestive of the diagnosis of MDS, especially in the absence of peripheral circulating blasts.

7. Characterize the marrow abnormalities of MDS.

Marrow cellularity is usually increased but occasionally may be normal or hypoplastic. When there appears to be decreased cellularity, there are still islands of abnormal appearing cells, which are often atypical megakaryocytes. The erythroid series is usually hyperplastic with megaloblasts and apparent nuclear cytoplasmic maturation abnormalities. There are nuclear fragments in stippled erythroblasts with poorly hemoglobinized cells. On staining for iron with Prussian blue, an increase in macrophage iron is usually found. More importantly, however, there is an increased number of erythroblasts that contain siderosomes (cytoplastic ferritin-containing vacuoles), such that these cells are referred to as abnormal sideroblasts. On occasion, these sideroblasts have mitochondrial iron aggregated around the nucleus in a ring shape (thus ringed sideroblast). Ring sideroblasts are most common in acquired refractory sideroblastic anemia. Granulocytic hyperplasia also is frequently observed. Abnormalities of the granulocytes similar to those in the peripheral smear consist of hypogranulation, Pelger-Huët anomalies, and increased numbers of blasts and other early white cell precursors. Megakaryocytes are usually present or increased with micromegakaryocytes often present.

8. What are the most common cytogenetic abnormalities in MDS? How do they influence prognosis?

Up to 50% of patients with MDS may have chromosomal abnormalities. Most often these abnormalities consist of chromosomal losses or gains such as 5q–, 7–, and 8+ abnormalities. None of these abnormalities is unique for classes or subgroups of MDS. The specific structural abnormalities of acute nonlymphocytic leukemia are less common in MDS. In MDS, virtually every chromosome has been affected. In general, the more complex and the greater number of cells that show evidence of chromosomal cytogenetic abnormalities, the worse the prognosis. The exception is the 5q–syndrome associated with refractory anemia, which usually predicts a good prognosis.

9. What do we know of the pathogenesis of MDS?

As noted previously, MDS is a group of clonal disorders. How clonal abnormalities result in cytopenias in MDS is not clear. In vitro studies of hematopoietic colony growth suggest that failure of differentation may be due to abnormal progenitors or growth factor responses. The marrow, however, shows ineffective hematopoiesis with apoptosis in all cell lineages. Nonclonal hematopoiesis may also be present, although the abnormal clone appears to possess the proliferative advantage. The molecular bases of abnormalities in MDS remain to be determined. A number of target genes have been shown to have mutations (*ras, c-fms*), but these have been inconsistent and likely represent only one clue to the puzzle of abnormal myeloproliferation in MDS.

10. Which factors predispose to the development of MDS?

Usually MDS arises without specific or apparent cause. However, patients with MDS have a greater than expected exposure to benzene. Likewise, cancer treatment, especially with alkylating agents and radiation therapy, is an important factor in the predisposition to MDS. Such patients have an overall risk of about 10% in 10 years for the development of MDS with transition to acute nonlymphocytic leukemia. On rare occasions, aplastic anemia and paroxysmal hemoglobinuria will evolve into MDS.

11. Distinguish primary from secondary MDS.

Although abnormalities in the blood are similar, the bone marrow may more often be hypocellular in secondary MDS. The course of secondary MDS is often more rapid, and the presentation more commonly indicates myelodysplastic syndrome in transition to acute nonlymphocytic leukemia. Therapy-related MDS occurs at variable ages, depending on the antecedent exposure to chemotherapy. It is unclear whether some diseases also predispose to MDS (such as multiple myeloma, Hodgkin's disease, other lymphomas, and polycythemia vera). Most patients with therapy-related MDS have clonal chromosomal abnormalities, and three-fourths have more than one chromosomal abnormality at presentation. Often secondary syndromes follow a more aggressive course and appear to respond to therapy less well.

12. How common is leukemic transformation in MDS?

Overall, with earlier recognition of MDS, only about 20% of patients undergo leukemic transformation. This incidence varies with respect to the FAB category. Refractory anemia with ring sideroblasts shows the lowest leukemic transformation (5%), whereas refractory anemia with excessive blasts in transformation undergoes true leukemic transformation up to 50% of the time. Refractory anemia (10%), refractory anemia with excessive blasts (23%), and chronic myelomonocytic leukemia (20%) are in the intermediate range. MDS is a precursor to any of the variants of acute myelogenous leukemia, but not usually to acute lymphatic leukemia.

13. What is the cause of death in patients with MDS that does not evolve into acute leukemia?

About 25% of patients die from infection or hemorrhage. Because this is a disease of the elderly, death from other entities is likely in many patients. Iron overload may occur in patients who undergo frequent transfusions. The clinical appearance of hemochromatosis is more frequent in patients who are HLAA3-positive, suggesting that sideroblastic anemia and transfusion therapy in combination with a genetic predisposition result in hemochromatosis.

14. An elderly woman with refractory macrocytic anemia and splenomegaly is likely to have which MDS?

She probably has the 5q-syndrome. This entity is seen in elderly women who present with refractory macrocytic anemia and who often have a long and uneventful course other than the occasional need for transfusion. Such patients have splenomegaly (up to 50%) with platelets that are normal or increased in number. The region of the break point of the 5q chromosome contains genes for major hematopoietic growth factors, including interleukins 3, 4, and 5, macrophage colony-stimulating factor (M-CSF), granulocyte–macrophage colony-stimulating factor (GM-CSF), and the protooncogene *c-fms*, which is M-CSF receptor. However, how the abnormality in this chromosomal area relates to the clinical presentation of MDS remains to be discovered.

15. Is MDS ever found in children?

Yes. Childhood MDS may be familial and related to an inherited loss of chromosome 7. The loss of chromosome 7 appears to result in loss of a tumor suppressor gene. Approximately one-fifth of children who develop acute monocytic leukemia (AML) have a preceding syndrome similar to adult akylator-induced MDS.

16. A patient with MDS asks if he will need to quit his job in the next year. How should he be answered?

It is important to determine the clinical subclass of MDS that the patient has, because varying overall prognoses coupled with prognostic factors delineate the expected natural history. The best prognosis is usually for refractory anemia and refractory anemia with ring sideroblasts, whereas the worst prognosis is for refractory anemia with excessive blasts and refractory anemia with excessive blasts with transformation. Chronic myelomonocytic leukemia is intermediate (22 months). A simple scoring system consists of assigning 1 point to each of the following: bone marrow blasts > 5%, platelets < 100,000, neutrophils < 2.5 or > 16, and hemoglobin < 10 gm (total possible score 4). The total score correlates with length of survival: $\leq 1 = 62$ months; 2 or $3 = 22$ months; $4 = 8.5$ months. Thus, taking into account the natural history of the patient's disease, a treatment plan can be developed which takes into account the patient's own desires with respect to the immediate and long-term course of action.

17. How should patients with MDS be managed?

Patients with MDS require close follow-up initially, often every 2–4 weeks until the course of the disease is determined. Initial trials with high-dose folate and cobalamin are warranted, regardless of the serum levels. Likewise, since pyridoxine-responsive anemias may resemble refractory anemia with ringed sideroblasts, a prolonged trial of pyridoxine may occasionally result in a diminution of transfusion requirements. Red cell transfusions should be used as clinically indicated.

Growth factors may be useful in some patients with neutropenia and/or anemia. Erythropoietin has resulted in an increase in hemoglobin levels in approximately one-fifth of patients, regardless of erythropoietin levels. G-CSF and GM-CSF may increase the neutrophil count and function in many patients (as high as 80%), but this must be balanced against the potential risk of hastening the conversion to AML (one-fifth of patients may show increased myeloblasts with therapy). Patients who least need growth factors (those with milder cytopenias) appear to be most responsive to them.

Progressive thrombocytopenia requiring platelet transfusions is one indication for more aggressive therapy. Low-dose cytarabine with or without growth factors appears to be the least toxic treatment to improve counts in older patients but has not improved overall survival. Differentiation agents (i.e., retinoic acid) have not proved effective.

18. Should high-dose chemotherapy be considered?

Chemotherapeutic regimens used to treat AML are most effective in younger patients. While they may induce remission in 50% of treated individuals, the remission, and thus survival, is usually short-lived (six months).

19. How has chemotherapy fared in MDS?

Low-dose chemotherapy or conventional chemotherapy has proved ineffective in changing the overall survival. However, the use of intensive chemotherapy coupled with bone marrow transplantation on some occasions may be appropriate. These aggressive approaches should be considered in young patients who have undergone leukemic transformation. Therapy-related MDS does not preclude use of this approach. Because up to 40% of patients may die during aggressive chemotherapy, the overall intention to treat must consider the high possibility of mortality.

20. Can MDS ever be cured?

Yes. Allogeneic bone marrow transplantation offers a chance of eradication of this disease and prolonged survival in patients with both primary and secondary MDS. Survival is best in younger patients with fewer blasts and in those who receive HLA identical marrow. Patients with primary MDS are more likely to survive this treatment than patients with secondary MDS. Postponement of transplant until severe cytopenias and resistance to treatment are seen enhances early mortality.

BIBLIOGRAPHY

1. Anderson JE, Goolery TA, Schoch G, et al: Stem cell transplantation for secondary AM: Evaluation of transplantation as initial therapy following induction chemotherapy. Blood 89:2578–2585, 1997.
2. Besa EC: Myelodysplastic syndromes. Med Clin North Am 76:599–617, 1992.
3. Besa EC: Myelodysplastic syndromes. Cancer Therapeutics 1:52–63, 1998.
4. Doll DC, List AF (eds): Myelodysplastic syndromes. Semin Oncol 10:1, 1992.
5. Enright H, Miller W: Autoimmune phenomena in patients with myelodysplastic syndromes. Leuk Lymphoma 24:483–489, 1997.
6. Geissler RG, Schulte P, Ganser A: Clinical use of hematopoietic growth factors in patients with myelodysplastic syndromes. Int J Hematol 64:339–354, 1997.
7. Greenberg PL: In vitro marrow culture studies in the myelodysplastic syndromes. Semin Oncol 19:34, 1992.
8. Griffin JD (ed): Myelodysplastic syndromes. Clin Haematol 15:909, 1986.
9. Heim S: Cytogenetic findings in primary and secondary MDS. Leuk Res 16:43, 1992.
10. Hoagland HC: Myelodysplastic syndromes. The bone marrow factor problem. Mayo Clin Proc 70:673–676, 1995.
11. Kantaryian HM, et al: Treatment of therapy-related leukemia myelodysplastic syndrome. Hematol Oncol Clin North Am 7:81–107, 1993.
12. Koeffler HP: Myelodysplastic syndromes. Semin Hematol 33:87–94, 1996.
13. Mathew P, Tefferi A, Dewarld GW, et al: The 5q syndrome: A single institution study of 43 consecutive patients. Blood 81:1040–1045, 1993.
14. Nowell PC: Chromosome abnormalities in myelodysplastic syndromes. Semin Oncol 19:25, 1992.
15. Tricot G, el: Prognostic factors in the myelodysplastic syndromes: Importance of initial data on peripheral blood counts, bone marrow cytology, trephine biopsy and chromosomal analysis. Leuk Res 16:109, 1992.
16. Vallespi T, et al: Myelodysplastic syndromes: A study of 101 cases according to the FAB classification. Br J Haematol 61:83, 1985.

25. HYPEREOSINOPHILIC SYNDROMES

Russell C. Tolley, M.D.

1. What is an eosinophil and how does it function?

Like neutrophils, eosinophils develop in the bone marrow from pluripotent stem cells and have characteristic red-staining granules that contain a unique perioxidase. Proliferation is controlled mainly by three cytokines: interleukin-3 (IL-3), interleukin-5 (IL-5), and granulocyte-macrophage colony-stimulating factor (GM-CSF). IL-5 is the most specific for eosinophils. Overproduction of one or more of these cytokines has been described in most hypereosinophilic disease states, including overexpression of IL-5 in some malignancies, and overproduction of IL-5 by helper lymphocytes in parasitic infections. A complex interaction with other molecules and endothelial cells then results in proliferation, migration into target tissues, and increased survival resulting in tissue eosinophilia. In the case of parasitic infections, the eosinophils secrete the contents of their cytotoxic granules in the vicinity of parasites, inflicting damage to the cell wall of the organism and subsequently killing them. In other diseases, eosinophilia results in harmful destruction of tissue, subsequent end-organ dysfunction, and possible death.

2. What is eosinophilia?

The absolute level of eosinophils can be obtained by multiplying the percent of eosinophils on the differential by the white blood cell (WBC) count:

$$\text{absolute eosinophil count} = \text{WBC} \times \% \text{ eosinophils} \times 0.01$$

Normal levels do not exceed 350 eosinophils/mm^3; 351 to 1500/mm^3 is considered mild eosinophilia, 1501 to 5000/mm^3 moderate eosinophilia, and >5000/mm^3 severe eosinophilia. Moderate to severe eosinophilia or persistent mild eosinophilia without explanation generally requires further diagnostic studies, including a directed history inquiring about medications, atopic conditions, travel to areas endemic for helminthic infections, and symptoms attributable to an occult malignancy; an examination of the peripheral smear to help rule out a hematologic malignancy; and blood smear, stool, and urine examination to look for parasitic infections.

3. Does the eosinophil count vary over the course of a day?

Yes. The number is lowest in the afternoon and highest in the morning.

4. Which growth factors stimulate the production of eosinophils and how are they closely related?

The most specific growth factor for eosinophils is IL-5, which stimulates the proliferation, differentiation, and subsequent release of eosinophils from the bone marrow. GM-CSF and IL-3 also stimulate the production of eosinophils, but are not specific. Of interest, all three of the genes that encode for these proteins are located in close proximity to each other on the long arm of chromosome 5 and bind to receptors that have similar structures. Subsequent adhesion to and migration between endothelial cells with eventual concentration in end organs involves interaction with many other recently described molecules such as chemokines (chemotactic cytokines). Some of these, such as eotaxins, are highly specific for eosinophils and are potentiated by IL-5. Furthermore, IL-5, as well as IL-3 and GM-CSF binds to tissue eosinophils and increases their survival, thus delineating IL-5 a role not only in proliferation and differentiation of eosinophils, but also in accumulation and increased survival of eosinophils in tissues. Appropriately, IL-5 also is known as eosinophil differentiation factor.

5. What are some of the secondary causes of eosinophilia?

- Allergic states, including hayfever, asthma, and drug reactions, which are associated with elevated serum levels of IgE
- Parasitic diseases
- Vasculitides, including Wegener's granulomatosis, Churg-Strauss syndrome (vasculitis associated with eosinophilia, neuropathy, and asthma), Well's syndrome (eosinophilic cellulitis), Shulman's syndrome (eosinophilic fasciitis), and a number of pulmonary infiltrative disorders, including Löffler's syndrome (eosinophilic pneumonia)
- Malignancies such as Hodgkin's disease, non-Hodgkin's lymphoma, and (more rarely) carcinoma, as well as acute myeloblastic leukemia, myeloproliferative disorders, and myelodysplastic states with eosinophilic differentiation
- Collagen vascular diseases and autoimmune disorders, including rheumatoid arthritis, dermatomyositis, and periarteritis nodosa, which may be confirmed through serologic tests (serum complement levels, antinuclear antibodies) or tissue biopsy

6. Is there a way to remember the secondary causes of eosinophilia?

The acronym NAACP is useful:

Neoplasm
Allergies
Asthma
Collagen vascular disease
Parasites

Obviously, this acronym does not identify every possible cause, but it does include the more common causes.

7. Which parasitic diseases cause eosinophilia?

Schistosomiasis is a major source of infection outside the United States and a common cause of eosinophilia. Filariasis, trichinosis, hookworm and Ascaris infection, visceral larva migrans, and strongyloidiasis also can cause marked eosinophilia. Two nonhelminthic protozoans, *Isospora belli* and *Dientamoeba fragilis*, can cause enteric disease. Disseminated *Strongyloides stercoralis* hyperinfection has been fatal in some people on corticosteroids (as used in hypereosinophilic syndrome, a primary disorder), and the diagnosis often requires serology in order to ensure that *S. stercoralis* infection is not present before steroids are prescribed.

8. What are the most common causes of eosinophilia in the United States?

Allergic and hypersensitivity reactions are the most common underlying causes of eosinophilia in adults. Visceral larva migrans due to *Toxocara canis* also is common in children.

9. How do children get visceral larva migrans?

Children may contract visceral larva migrans after eating dirt infected with eggs of nematodes, whose natural host is the dog (*Toxocara canis*) or cat (*Toxocara cati*). The larvae then migrate through the gastrointestinal tract to tissues, causing an illness characterized by fever, intense eosinophilia, wheezing, pneumonitis, and hepatosplenomegaly. If reinfection is prevented, the disorder may be self-limiting.

10. Name some commonly used drugs that cause eosinophilia.

Sulfonamides, iodides, nitrofurantoin, phenytoin, and aspirin may cause elevated eosinophil counts.

11. What is the hypereosinophilic syndrome (HES)? How is it treated?

Idiopathic HES is a primary disorder of unknown etiology. In the past it often has been confused with the truly malignant condition eosinophilic leukemia, a variant of type M4 acute myelogenous leukemia associated with the characteristic inversion abnormality of chromosome 16. Most patients with hypereosinophilic syndrome have no chromosomal abnormalities or abnormalities not associated with acute myelogenous leukemia. It is associated with serious morbidity; some past reviews of untreated patients show a 3-year survival rate of only 12% and a median survival of 9 months. However, a more recent review from 1989 suggests a prolonged survival, with 80% of patients surviving 5 years and 42% surviving > 10 years.

HES is characterized by white blood cell counts between 15,000 and 150,000/mm^3, marked eosinophilia on differential with up to 70% eosinophils, and increased eosinophils and eosinophil precursors on marrow examination. Fever, anemia, and hepatosplenomegaly also are commonly seen. Prominent cardiac findings, including emboli from mural thrombi, abnormal EKGs, congestive heart failure, murmurs, and left ventricular hypertrophy, may be observed, along with pulmonary abnormalities and neurologic dysfunction. Importantly, eosinophilias that involve only specific organs, such as eosinophilic pneumonia, eosinophilic gastritis, eosinophilic fasciitis, and eosinophilic cellulitis, should be ruled out because they do not involve the multiple organs as seen in hypereosinophilic syndrome and do not lead to the secondary cardiac damage that causes much of the morbidity and mortality of HES.

Many patients succumb to a progressive endomyocardial fibroelastosis, the etiology of which is thought to be eosinophilic infiltration of tissues with resultant tissue damage. Therapy consists of decreasing the eosinophilia with either corticosteroids or hydroxyurea; more recently interferon-alpha has been used with success. If necessary, cytotoxic agents such as vincristine and chlorambucil may be used. The advent of corticosteroid and cytotoxic therapy has been mainly responsible for the increased survival rates in patients with HES; some patients now live for decades with the disease.

12. How is HES diagnosed?

Patients with no underlying disorder known to cause eosinophilia, persistence of eosinophilia > 1,500/mm^3 for 6 months, in association and otherwise unexplained underlying organ dysfunction fall into the category of HES. Male predominance is 9:1. Secondary disorders of eosinophilia **must** be ruled out.

13. Which pulmonary disorders are associated with hypereosinophilia?

As mentioned above, parasitic infections and HES may produce pulmonary infiltrates and eosinophilia. Fungi such as *Coccidioides* or bronchopulmonary aspergillosis, a disorder of asthmatic patients, may cause hypereosinophilia. Bronchopulmonary aspergillosis tends to produce segmental and central pulmonary infiltrates, with eosinophils in the sputum as well. *Coccidioides* present with fever, pulmonary infiltrates, arthralgias, and erythema nodosum. Hypersensitivity reactions to molds in grain dust (farmer's lung), allergic granulomatosis (vasculitis with features of polyarteritis nodosa and pulmonary infiltrates), and sarcoidosis (suggested by hilar adenopathy on roentgenogram) are associated with eosinophilia.

Chronic eosinophilic pneumonia (Löffler's syndrome) is a debilitating illness of unknown etiology with fever, weight loss, and the presence of eosinophilia in the blood and/or sputum. The lung infiltrates promptly disappear with corticosteroid treatment.

14. Can eosinophilia be inherited?

Yes. Hereditary eosinophilia is generally a mild, rare disorder that is usually associated with an autosomal dominant pattern and a benign clinical course.

15. What causes the damage in patients with eosinophilia?

Damage results both from the mass effect of eosinophilic infiltration of tissue and from proteins liberated when eosinophils degranulate. The most important protein released appears to be major basic protein (MBP), which is cytotoxic. MBP may be demonstrated in sputum of patients with asthma or in serum of patients with eosinophilia. Leukotriene C4 is produced and its metabolites mediate vascular permeability, mucous secretion, and smooth muscle contraction. Eosinophil peroxidase also induces cell death and subsequent tissue damage.

16. What are Charcot-Leyden crystals?

These characteristic crystals are found in the cytoplasm of eosinophils and in the extracellular environment when degranulation occurs. They are thought to contain lysophospholipase and to be inert once they are formed.

17. Explain the relationship between eosinophilia and leukemia.

Eosinophilia is associated with both acute lymphocytic leukemia and acute myelogenous leukemia. Eosinophilia associated with acute lymphocytic leukemia is a poor prognostic factor and a t(5,14)(q13;32) transformation. Alternatively, eosinophilic patients with type M4 acute myelogenous leukemia (AML) with Inv(16) have a favorable prognosis. AML has been called eosinophilic leukemia in the past and, as noted above, has been confused with the nonmalignant hypereosinophilic syndrome.

18. What is eosinophilia-myalgia syndrome (EMS)?

EMS was first identified in 1989. Patients present with a variety of symptoms, but all patients have myalgias and most have eosinophilia. EMS can be debilitating, with ultimate development of sclerodermalike skin lesions and peripheral neuropathies. Eosinophil counts are modestly elevated but may be as high as 36,000/dl. EMS bears a striking resemblance to toxic oil syndrome as well as other hypereosinophilic syndromes.

19. What causes EMS?

The exact cause is still unknown. The greatest association appears to be with the identification of a novel amino acid consisting of two L-tryptophan molecules. This compound was created in the manufacturing process of L-tryptophan but only at selected manufacturing sites. Some people who develop EMS demonstrate abnormal tryptophan metabolism. It may be that both impurities in the manufacturing process and abnormal metabolism are required for development of the syndrome.

BIBLIOGRAPHY

1. Larson RA, Williams SF, Le Beau MM, et al: Acute myelomonocytic leukemia with abnormal eosinophils and inv(16) or t(16;16) has a favorable prognosis. Blood 68:1242, 1986.
2. Naiman JL, Oski FA, Allen FH, Diamond LK: Hereditary eosinophilia: Report of a family and review of the literature. Am J Hum Genet 16:195, 1964.
3. Olsen EGJ, Spry CJF: The pathogenesis of Löffler's endomyocardial disease, and its relationship to endomyocardial fibrosis. Prog Cardiol 8:281, 1979.
4. Rothenberg ME: Eosinophilia. N Engl J Med 338:1592, 1998.
5. Varga J, Uitto J, Jimenez SA: The cause and pathogenesis of the eosinophilia-myalgia syndrome. Ann Intern Med 116:140, 1992.
6. Weller PF: The immunobiology of eosinophils. N Engl J Med 324:110, 1991.
7. Weller PF, Bubley GJ: The idiopathic eosinophilic syndrome. Blood 83:2759, 1994.

III. Malignant Hematology

26. ACUTE LEUKEMIA: CLASSIFICATION AND LABORATORY EVALUATION

Mitchell A. Bitter, M.D.

1. What are the findings in the complete blood cell count (CBC) and leukocyte differential in patients with acute leukemia (AL)?

AL is typically associated with cytopenias in the CBC and blasts in the peripheral blood film. The most constant findings are anemia and thrombocytopenia. Thrombocytopenia is seen in over 90% of cases, with severe thrombocytopenia ($< 50 \times 10^9$/L) in more than half. In about half of patients, the white blood cell count (WBC) will be normal or low, and the absolute neutrophil count is low in over half of cases. Peripheral blood blasts are usually identified in acute myelogenous leukemia (AML) but are variable in number. Often blasts are not identified in the 100-cell count but may be seen if the blood film is scanned at low power.

2. What information is needed from the laboratory before therapy is initiated in patients with suspected AL?

When a patient with suspected AL is evaluated, hematopathologists and hematologists must address three questions. In order of importance:

1. Is it really AL?
2. Is it AML or acute lymphoblastic leukemia (ALL)?
3. How should the leukemia (AML or ALL) be subclassified?

The importance of the first question is self-evident. Because therapy differs significantly in AML and ALL, the second question is clinically important (see chapter 27). The modalities used to make this distinction are addressed below. Once a firm diagnosis of AML or ALL has been made, subclassification (see below) is undertaken to provide prognostic information; in some circumstances it influences the choice of therapeutic regimen.

3. Which benign conditions are sometimes mistaken for AL in the bone marrow? In the blood film?

The diagnosis of AL is **not** based primarily on examination of the blood film. Rather a diagnosis of AL should be made only after examination of the bone marrow. Both a bone core biopsy and aspirate should be obtained.

In a well-processed specimen, the diagnosis of AL is generally not difficult. Occasionally, benign disorders may be difficult to distinguish from AL. The best examples are (1) florid megaloblastic anemia (may be confused with erythroleukemia) and (2) suppressed bone marrows with superimposed infections (e.g., in the alcoholic with pneumonia).

In the peripheral blood film, myelophthisic anemias (anemias due to marrow infiltration), including disseminated tuberculosis or fungal infection, may show a picture of cytopenias and immature mononuclear cells. In these disorders, however, blasts are not generally prominent.

The inexperienced morphologist may have difficulty in distinguishing reactive lymphocytoses, such as in mononucleosis syndromes, from AL. The morphologic findings that help to distinguish between blasts and reactive lymphocytes are illustrated below.

AL is almost always associated with thrombocytopenia, which is severe ($< 50 \times 10^9$/L) in $> 50\%$ of cases. Although thrombocytopenia is not uncommon in mononucleosis syndromes, it is usually mild. A diagnosis of AL should be reconsidered in the face of a normal or near normal platelet count.

Morphologic Features of Reactive Lymphs and Blasts

	BLAST	REACTIVE LYMPH
Size	Large	Large
Nuclear/cytoplasmic ratio	Higher	Lower
Nucleoli	May be prominent	May be prominent
Chromatin	Fine	Clumped

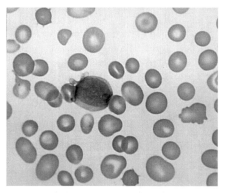

Myeloblast. Myeloblasts are generally 2–4 times the size of red blood cells. Their chromatin is finely granular, and 1–3 nucleoli are often seen. The nuclear to cytoplasmic volume ratio is generally high (relatively little cytoplasm is seen). Granules or Auer rods may be present in the cytoplasm (not shown). (See also Fig. 7, Color Plates).

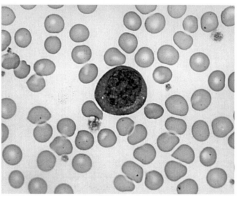

Reactive lymph. Like the myeloblast, the reactive lymph may be a large cell, and a nucleolus may be seen (not shown). Granules may even be present in the cytoplasm (not shown). The reactive lymph is distinguished from the blast by its coarser chromatin (note the clumped chromatin) and its somewhat lower nuclear to cytoplasmic ratio. (See also Fig. 5, Color Plates.)

4. How is AML distinguished from ALL?

As discussed above, after a definitive diagnosis of AL is made, the choice of a therapeutic regimen depends on whether the leukemia is ALL or AML. The two most important modalities used to distinguish AML from ALL are morphologic examination and cytochemistry. Both are low cost and may be performed rapidly. In difficult cases, more costly and time-consuming studies may be required.

In about 80–90% of cases the distinction between AML and ALL can be readily made by the experienced morphologist. Morphologic differences between myeloblasts and lymphoblasts are illustrated below. In some cases, however, morphologic distinction is difficult or impossible. Furthermore, even the experienced morphologist is occasionally surprised when a case that was thought to be AML turns out to be ALL and vice versa. Therefore, at a minimum, myeloperoxidase or Sudan black B stains, which are positive in blasts of AML, should be performed to confirm the morphologic impression in any new AL. These stains are rapid and can be performed within an hour, if need be, on either blood (if blasts are present) or marrow aspirate. The following modalities, useful in difficult cases, are performed regularly in many institutions:

1. Immunophenotyping by flow cytometry or immunocytochemistry for lymphoid and myeloid antigens

2. Detection of terminal deoxynucleotidyl transferase (TdT), a nuclear protein seen in > 95% of ALL and 15% of AML

3. Cytogenetics, which show different abnormalities in AML versus ALL

4. Immunoglobulin and T-cell receptor gene rearrangement studies

The results of cytogenetic and gene rearrangement studies are generally not back in time to influence initial therapy.

Features of Myeloblasts and Lymphoblasts

	MYELOBLAST	LYMPHOBLAST
Size	Large	Smaller
Amount of cytoplasm	More	Less
Nucleoli	Conspicuous	Often inconspicuous
Granules	Frequent, fine	Uncommon, coarse
Auer rods	Observed in 50%	Absent
Myeloperoxidase	Positive	Negative

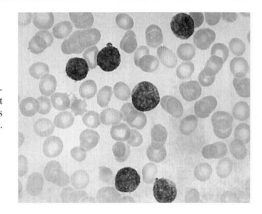

Lymphoblasts. Compared with myeloblasts, lymphoblasts are smaller (cell size 1½–3 times that of the red blood cells). They have inconspicuous nucleoli, coarser chromatin, and scant cytoplasm.

5. How is ALL subclassified?

After a diagnosis of AL is made and it is determined to be ALL (see question 11 for AML subclassification), the disorder is subclassified in a number of ways. Subclassification provides prognostic information and may be used to stratify patients to receive different therapeutic regimens. Subclassification is based on:

1. Clinical parameters such as age, blood counts, and performance status (see chapter 28)
2. Morphology of the blasts
3. Immunophenotype of the blasts
4. Pattern of cytogenetic abnormalities

6. Is morphologic classification of ALL prognostically significant?

According to the French-American-British (FAB) system, ALL is classified into three subtypes (L1, L2, and L3) based on the morphology of the blasts. In adults, the great majority of ALLs are L1 and L2. The distinction between L1 and L2 has, at best, minor prognostic significance. A small number of cases (~ 3–5%) are L3. These patients have a disorder that overlaps with Burkitt's lymphoma, and although they represent an uncommon subtype, they are important to distinguish for therapeutic purposes.

7. Is immunologic classification clinically significant?

In myeloid cells, lineage (i.e., neutrophil versus eosinophil) and stage of maturation (i.e., blast versus promyelocyte) can often be determined by morphology. This is not true for lymphocytes. You cannot generally tell a T cell from a B cell by morphology, and only gross stages of maturation are morphologically distinguishable—lymphoblast versus lymphocyte. Therefore, lineage and stage of maturation are determined by the reactivity of the malignant population with a number of antibodies to cell surface constituents, using either flow cytometry or immunocytochemistry.

ALL is subclassified into a number of immunologic categories. An abbreviated listing is given below. In univariate analysis, these groups differ in prognosis. However, immunologic phenotype is sometimes correlated with other prognostic factors. For instance, patients with T-cell ALL often have a high WBC, which is associated with poorer prognosis. Immature B-lineage ALL in the elderly is often associated with the t(9;22) (Philadelphia chromosome), which portends a dismal prognosis (see below). Therefore, in multivariate analyses, the prognostic importance of immunologic classification is diminished.

Immunologic Classification of ALL

SUBTYPE	MAJOR MARKERS	FREQUENCY (%)
B-precursor (common ALL)	TdT+, CD19+, CD10+	75
T-ALL	TdT+, CD7+, Cytoplasmic CD3+	20
B-ALL	CD19+, SIg+	5

TdT = terminal deoxynucleotidyl transferase, SIg = monoclonal surface immunoglobulin.

8. What are the clinical and laboratory features of T-cell ALL?

Patients with T-ALL are often teens and young adults with a male predominance. In more than 50%, the leukemic population in the thymus forms a mediastinal mass. Patients tend to have a high WBC, often over 50×10^9/L.

9. For prognosis and therapeutic decision making, what is the most important cytogenetic abnormality in ALL?

By far the most important cytogenetic abnormality in adult ALL is the t(9;22) (Philadelphia chromosome). This reciprocal translocation between the long arms of chromosomes 9 and 22 brings together the *abl* protooncogene (9q34) and the *bcr* gene (22q11). A fusion gene is formed that encodes an abnormal protein, which is important in leukemogenesis.

This translocation is most strongly associated with chronic myelogenous leukemia (95% of patients). However, it also present in 20–30% of adults with ALL, and over half of all ALL in the elderly may be associated with the t(9;22). The presence of this translocation may identify patients with little chance (0–20%) of long-term remission after conventional ALL chemotherapy. The t(9;22) is associated with immature B-lineage in most cases. This association may account for the poorer prognosis of immature B-lineage ALL compared with T-cell ALL, which has been observed in some studies of adult ALL. This clinically important genetic rearrangement may be detected by molecular genetic methods in addition to traditional cytogenetics.

10. Overall, which clinical and laboratory findings are most important in determining prognosis in ALL?

Because ALL is most commonly seen in children, more is known about prognostic factors in children than in adults. Although a number of factors bear on prognosis, the most important in children are age, WBC, cytogenetics, and response to initial chemotherapy. In adults, WBC, cytogenetics, and response to chemotherapy are important, as are factors relating to the ability of the patient to withstand induction chemotherapy, such as age and performance status.

11. How is AML subclassified?

Like ALL, AML is subclassified based on (1) clinical parameters, (2) morphology, and (3) cytogenetics. Immunologic subclassification is less important than in ALL. Marker studies are most useful in distinguishing minimally differentiated AML (M0) from ALL, and in identifying myeloid lineages that do not express myeloperoxidase, such as acute megakaryoblastic leukemias (M7).

12. Is morphologic classification of AML clinically important?

According to the FAB system, AML is subclassified morphologically into the eight types listed below. These subtypes have some clinical differences, such as the propensity of monoblastic leukemia (M5) to infiltrate tissues; however, with the exception of acute promyelocytic leukemia (APL, M3), treatment is generally the same for all FAB subtypes.

Classification of AML

M0	AML with minimal differentiation	M4	Acute myelomonocytic leukemia
M1	AML without maturation	M5	Acute monocytic leukemia
M2	AML with maturation	M6	Acute erythroleukemia
M3	Acute promyelocytic leukemia	M7	Acute megakaryoblastic leukemia

It is critical to diagnose APL correctly and to differentiate it from other subtypes of AML. APL accounts for about 10% of patients with AML. At presentation approximately 70% of patients with APL have laboratory evidence of disseminated intravascular coagulation (DIC), which is often exacerbated by the initiation of conventional chemotherapy. In the past, patients with APL and DIC had a high mortality rate during induction chemotherapy; however, patients who survived induction chemotherapy had an excellent chance of long-term disease-free survival. Recently it has been shown that patients respond well to all-trans-retinoic acid (ATRA), which may induce complete remission in most patients with far less toxicity than conventional chemotherapy (although some patients may develop a life-threatening pulmonary syndrome). Because remissions induced by ATRA alone are not durable, current protocols combine ATRA with conventional chemotherapeutic agents.

13. What do the abnormal promyelocytes in APL look like?

As discussed below, APL is associated with a particular chromosomal translocation and molecular genetic rearrangement. However, because of the prolonged turnaround time of cytogenetic studies, the diagnosis of APL is often a morphologic one, with cytochemistry and immunologic markers serving as useful adjuncts.

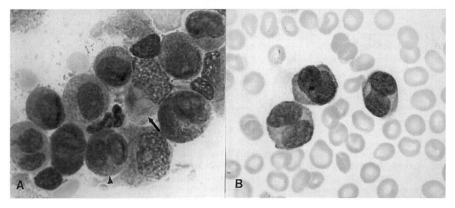

A, Hypergranular acute promyelocytic leukemia (M3). The arrowhead indicates an abnormal promyelocyte showing the typical bilobed nucleus. The arrow shows a degenerating cell with numerous Auer rods in its cytoplasm. B, Microgranular acute promyelocytic leukemia (M3V). Like the hypergranular promyelocytes depicted in A, these cells from a patient with the microgranular variant of APL show the typical bilobed nuclei. However, the heavy cytoplasmic granulation observed in the hypergranular form is not observed in the microgranular variant. Such cases are easily mistaken for monocytic leukemia by the inexperienced morphologist. (See also Fig. 8, Color Plates.)

In the most common form of APL, Wright-stained smears of the leukemic cells show lobated or kidney-shaped nuclei with the cytoplasm stuffed with scarlet-staining granules. Auer rods are prominent, and many may be seen in a single cell. About 25% of APL cases are more difficult to recognize because the granules are below the limit of resolution of the light microscope. Therefore, the cells often appear agranular. These "microgranular" APLs must be recognized by their nuclear features alone. Many of these cases are misdiagnosed as other forms of AML. Patients with microgranular APL have the same problems with DIC as do patients with the more common form of APL, and they respond well to ATRA.

14. Which cytogenetic abnormalities in AML are favorable and which are unfavorable?

Cytogenetic abnormalities are detected in about 80% of cases of AML. Several of them are correlated with clinical findings and prognosis. Three cytogenetic abnormalities have been considered by many to be prognostically favorable. The t(15;17) is specific for APL; in some centers, all or nearly all patients with APL have had this abnormality. The clinical findings of APL are discussed above and in chapter 27. The t(8;21) and certain abnormalities of chromosome 16, including a pericentric inversion (the inv[16]), have been considered to be favorable. These patients have had extremely high rates of complete remission (> 90%); however, remissions may not be particularly durable (in contrast to the t[15;17]). In some studies, but not in others, patients with the inv(16) have had an extremely high incidence of central nervous system relapse.

Many studies have shown that deletions involving the long arms of chromosomes 5 and 7 are associated with therapy-related AML (t-AML). In some studies, 60–80% of t-AMLs are associated with these abnormalities. T-AML and deletions involving the long arm of chromosomes 5 and 7 are considered to augur a poor prognosis.

BIBLIOGRAPHY

1. Bitter MA, LeBeau MM, Rowley JD, et al: Associations between morphology, karyotype and clinical features in myeloid leukemias. Hum Pathol 18:211–255, 1987.
2. Borowtiz MJ: Acute lymphoblastic leukemia. In Knowles DM (ed): Neoplastic Hematopathology. Baltimore, Williams & Wilkins, 1992, pp 1295–1314.
3. Cheson BD, Cassileth PA, Head DR, et al: Report of the National Cancer Institute-sponsored workshop in definitions of diagnosis and response in acute myeloid leukemia. J Clin Oncol 8:813–819, 1990.
4. Glass JP, Van Tassel P, Keathing MJ, et al: Central nervous system complications of a newly recognized subtype of leukemia: AMML with a pericentric inversion of chromosome 16. Neurology 37:639–644, 1987.
5. Larson RA, Williams SF, LeBeau MM, et al: Acute myelomonocytic leukemia with abnormal eosinophils and inv(16) or t(16;16) has a favorable prognosis. Blood 68:1242–1249, 1986.
6. Leith CP, Willman CL: Prognostic markers in acute leukemia. Curr Opin Hematol 3:329–334, 1996.
7. Lestingi TM, Hooberman AL: Philadelphia chromosome-positive acute lymphoblastic leukemia. Hematol Oncol Clin North Am 7:161–175, 1993.
8. Samuels BL, Larson RA, LeBeau MM, et al: Specific chromosomal abnormalities in acute nonlymphocytic leukemia correlate with drug susceptibility in vivo. Leukemia 2:79–83, 1988.
9. Schiffer CA, Lee EJ, Tomiyasu T, et al: Prognostic impact of cytogenetic abnormalities in patients with de novo acute nonlymphocytic leukemia. Blood 73:263–270, 1989.
10. Taylor CG, Stasi R, Bastianelli C, et al: Diagnosis and classification of the acute leukemia: Recent advances and controversial issues. Hematopathol Mol Hematol 10:1–38, 1996.
11. Vahdat L, Maslak P, Miller WJ Jr, et al: Early mortality and the retinoic acid syndrome in acute promyelocytic leukemia: Impact of leukocytosis, low-dose chemotherapy, PMN/RAR-α isoform and CD13 expression in patients treated with all-*trans*-retinoic acid. Blood 84:3843–3849, 1994.
12. Warrell RP, Frankel SR, Miller WH, et al: Differentiation therapy of acute promyelocytic leukemia with tretinoin (all-*trans*-retinoic acid). N Engl J Med 324:1385–1393, 1991.

27. ACUTE MYELOGENOUS AND LYMPHOCYTIC LEUKEMIAS

Barbara W. Grant, M.D.

1. Describe the laboratory features that indicate acute leukemia.

Blast cells are found in the peripheral blood of 85% of patients presenting with acute leukemia. Over 80% of patients also have **anemia** and **thrombocytopenia**. Although the white blood count (WBC) is elevated in over half of patients with acute leukemia, approximately 15% will have a normal WBC, and 33% of patients will present with **neutropenia**.

2. What is the differential diagnosis of pancytopenia or isolated neutropenia?

In addition to acute leukemia, pancytopenia or neutropenia may be caused by bone marrow replacement by other hematologic malignancies such as lymphoma and myelodysplastic syndromes. The bone marrow in aplastic anemia is severely hypocellular, and patients often present with marked pancytopenia. Other causes of pancytopenia or neutropenia include hypersplenism, autoimmune diseases, HIV infection, drug toxicity, and vitamin B_{12} and folate deficiencies.

3. The French-American-British (FAB) classification lists eight different subtypes of acute myelocytic leukemia. List at least three of these subtypes.

Acute myeloblastic leukemia with minimal differentiation	M0
Acute myeloblastic leukemia without maturation	M1
Acute myeloblastic leukemia with maturation	M2
Hypergranular acute promyelocytic leukemia	M3
Acute myelomonocytic leukemia	M4
Acute monocytic leukemia	M5
Erythroleukemia	M6
Acute megakaryoblastic leukemia	M7

4. Name clinical features that distinguish acute monocytic leukemia from the other subtypes.

Monoblasts tend to infiltrate extramedullary tissues, especially the gums, skin, and central nervous system.

5. If the pathologist reports that the bone marrow stains for myeloperoxidase and Sudan black stain are positive, which kind of acute leukemia should be suspected—acute myelocytic leukemia (AML) or acute lymphocytic leukemia (ALL)?

AML. Myeloblasts stain Sudan black positive and myeloperoxidase positive. Lymphoblasts are negative for these two stains but may be positive for periodic acid-Schiff (PAS).

6. Which FAB subtype is most associated with disseminated intravascular coagulation (DIC)?

Acute promyelocytic leukemia (APL), presumably because when released the granules contained in promyelocytes when released can trigger the coagulation cascade.

7. Should allopurinol be started before therapy in patients with both AML and ALL?

Yes. Hyperuricemia may occur in either form of acute leukemia. It may be more common in ALL because of rapid lysis of blasts that may result in renal insufficiency without adequate hydration and allopurinol therapy.

8. What factors predispose to so-called tumor lysis syndrome?

- High white blood cell count
- Hyperuricemia
- Elevated LDH
- Impaired renal function
- Sepsis
- Dehydration

9. Describe the leukostasis syndrome. How is it managed?

Patients with an exceptionally high WBC (generally > 100,000) may develop a syndrome resulting from blasts aggregating in the capillaries. The most common manifestations are cardiopulmonary with acute respiratory insufficiency and a pulmonary edema or pneumonia-type symptoms; and central nervous system (CNS) manifestations, including headache and occasional progression to a strokelike syndrome. This medical emergency requires rapid reduction of the WBCs by leukapheresis, chemotherapy, and sometimes CNS radiation. For reasons that are not entirely clear, this syndrome is seen in AML, ALL, and chronic myelogenous leukemia (CML) but very rarely in chronic lymphocytic leukemia (CLL).

10. Which chemotherapeutic drugs are most often used in the treatment of AML?

Cytosine arabinoside (ARA-C) together with an anthracycline, usually daunorubicin or idarubicin.

11. Which drugs are typically used in the treatment of ALL?

The most commonly used drugs include vincristine, prednisone, daunorubicin, intrathecal methotrexate, and L-asparaginase. Maintenance therapy usually includes 6-mercaptopurine and methotrexate.

12. What are important prognostic factors in AML, and how do they affect treatment?

Evaluation of factors present at diagnosis that affect the duration of remission has led to appreciation that the specific clonal chromosomal changes seen in each malignancy can be used to evaluate the patient's prognosis. Treatment is said to be "risk-stratified" when patients are assigned to therapy depending on the cytogenetics of their leukemia. Dose-intense therapy with autologous or allogeneic transplant in first remission may be recommended for medium- to high-risk patients, whereas standard induction and post-remission therapies are curative over half of the time in low-risk patients. Increasing age and/or a history of previous chemotherapy or of myelodysplastic syndrome decreases the chance of long remission. Overall, the remission rate for adults < 60 is 70–80%.

13. List the poor risk factors in ALL.

- Increasing age after 10 years
- WBC count > 15,000
- Male sex
- Presence of the Philadelphia chromosome
- Leukemic involvement of CNS
- L3 morphology

14. What is the cure rate in childhood ALL and adult ALL?

In children, the complete remission rate is generally in excess of 90% and the cure rate at 5 years is at least 50%; patients who complete 2.5–3 years of maintenance therapy without relapse have a > 80% chance of cure. Adults have a 25% disease-free survival; with more aggressive regimens, a 35–40% 5-year survival is possible.

15. When should bone marrow transplantation be considered in adult ALL or adult AML? What are the results?

Dose-intense therapy with bone marrow transplantation should be considered at the time of the first relapse or the second remission in either ALL or AML. For patients at high risk of relapse, transplantation during the first remission improves the cure rate. Over 60% of patients with leukemia under age 30 years transplanted in first remission are cured, whereas 30–40% of patients transplanted at first relapse or second remission are cured.

16. What are potential sites of relapse in ALL?

The bone marrow, CNS (meninges), and testes are the most common sites. The primary reason relapse may occur in the CNS and testes is that chemotherapy does not achieve very high concentrations in these tissues. Prophylaxis of the testes is not generally performed because of the sterilizing potential and the lack of data supporting its efficacy in improving the cure rate.

17. Do patients with AML usually require prophylactic central nervous system (CNS) therapy?

No. Patients with AML rarely develop meningeal leukemia compared with patients with ALL.

18. How should leukemic involvement of the CNS be managed?

Typically, it is managed by using intrathecal chemotherapy via lumbar puncture or an Ommaya reservoir. Cytosine arabinoside or methotrexate are administered, usually twice a week, until the CSF is cleared of blasts. If a systemic complete remission is achieved, intrathecal treatments are continued monthly. Intrathecal hydrocortisone and radiation therapy also may be used.

19. What factors predispose to renal failure in acute leukemia?

Hyperuricemia	Intravenous x-ray contrast material
Sepsis	Renal infiltration by leukemia
Drug toxicity (e.g., aminoglycosides)	

20. In patients with leukemia, should chemotherapy be avoided until neutropenia resolves?

No. Patients need to be treated based on the presence of leukemia in the bone marrow, not based on peripheral neutropenia.

21. Should management of patients with neutropenia (< 500 absolute neutrophil count) include reverse isolation?

No. There is no proof that reverse isolation decreases the risk of infection.

22. Is granulocyte colony-stimulating factor (G-CSF) safe to use in patients with acute leukemia?

Yes. Colony-stimulating factors support the production of normal granulocytes in patients with AML and ALL and have not caused leukemic progression. The clinical benefit of such factors in treating leukemic patients depends on the regimen used.

23. When a patient with neutropenia has a fever, should systemic antibiotics be administered even though there is no obvious source of infection?

Yes. Once a neutropenic patient is febrile, it is appropriate to start antibiotics rather than wait for the cultures to come back positive. The sooner antibiotics are initiated, the better the chance of reversing an episode of sepsis or other serious infection.

24. What characteristic of acute promyelocytic leukemia (APL) makes retinoic acid effective treatment?

Ninety-nine percent of patients with APL have a balanced translocation between chromosomes 15 and 17 that results in production of a chimeric fusion protein involving the retinoic acid receptor. All-trans-retinoic acid (ATRA) differentiates leukemic promyelocytes into mature cells, and treatment with ATRA during induction or maintenance improves disease-free survival in such patients.

25. When should platelet transfusions be given to patients with leukemia?

Patients with platelet counts lower than 10,000 should receive prophylactic platelet transfusions to prevent bleeding. Patients with higher counts who are bleeding also should be transfused.

26. When should human leukocyte antigen (HLA) typing be performed and in which types of acute leukemia?

HLA typing should be performed for patients < 50 years old who have either ALL or AML at the time of diagnosis. HLA typing is performed to identify sibling or unrelated donors for bone marrow or stem cell transplantation.

27. Define the following forms of bone marrow transplantation: syngeneic, allogeneic, and autologous.

Syngeneic transplant refers to bone marrow or other cells transplanted from an identical twin. Allogeneic refers to a nonidentical donor who is otherwise HLA compatible, and autologous transplants are done using the patient's own cells.

28. What is a chloroma?

A chloroma is an unusual tumor composed of granulocytic malignant cells. Chloromas are so named because of the green color myeloperoxidase gives the cut surface of these tumors. Chloromas sometimes develop before the hematologic presentation of AML or CML.

BIBLIOGRAPHY

1. Bennett JM, Catovsky D, Daniel M, et al: Proposed revised criteria for the classification of acute myeloid leukemia. Ann Intern Med 103:626–629, 1985.
2. Cheson BD, Cassileth PA, Head DR, et al: Report on the National Cancer Institute Sponsored Workshop on Definitions of Diagnosis and Response to Acute Myeloid Leukemia. J Clin Oncol 8:813–819, 1990.
3. Clarkson B, Ellis S, Little C, et al: Acute lymphoblastic leukemia in adults. Semin Oncol 12:169–179, 1985.
4. Clift RA, Buckner CD: Marrow transplantation for acute myeloid leukemia. Cancer Investigation 16:53–61, 1998.
5. Cohen LF, Balow JE, Magrath IT, et al: Acute tumor lysis syndrome: A review of 37 patients with Burkitt's lymphoma. Am J Med 68:486–491, 1980.
6. Cuttner J, Meyer R, Ambinder EP, Young T-H: Hyperleukocytosis in adult leukemia. In Bloomfield CD (ed): Chronic and Acute Leukemias in Adults. The Hague, Martinus Nijhoff, 1985, pp 263–282.
7. Heckman KD, Weiner GJ, Davis CS, et al: Randomized study of prophylactic platelet transfusion threshold during induction therapy for adult acute leukemia: 10,000/µl versus 20,000 µl. J Clin Oncol 15:1143–1149, 1997.
8. Hoelzer D, Thiel E, Loffler H, et al: Prognostic factors in a multicenter study for treatment of acute lymphoblastic leukemias in adults. Blood 71:123–131, 1988.
9. Omura G, Raney M: Longterm survival of adult acute lymphoblastic leukemia: Follow-up of a Southeastern Cancer Study Group Trial. J Clin Oncol 3:1053–1058, 1985.
10. Tallman MS, Andersen JW, Schiffer CA, et al: All-Trans-Retinoic acid in acute promyelocytic leukemia. N Engl J Med 337:1021–1028, 1997.
11. Terpstra W, Lowenberg B: Application of myeloid growth factors in the treatment of acute myeloid leukemia. Leukemia 11:315–327, 1997.
12. Yates J, Glidewell O, Wiernik P, et al: Cytosine arabinoside with daunorubicin or Adriamycin for therapy of acute myelocytic leukemia: A CALGB study. Blood 60:454–462, 1982.

28. CHRONIC LYMPHOCYTIC LEUKEMIA

Robert S. Kantor, M.D.

1. Define chronic lymphocytic leukemia.

Chronic lymphocytic leukemia (CLL) is a malignant proliferation of small lymphocytes that tend to accumulate in the bone marrow, peripheral blood, lymph nodes, spleen, and liver. CLL is an indolent disease with a natural history usually measured in years.

2. Which type of lymphocyte is malignant in CLL?

Although a rare form of T-cell CLL exists, nearly all cases arise from relatively well-differentiated B lymphocytes. Some investigators use the term "chronic lymphocytic leukemia" to refer to the general category of indolent lymphocytic leukemias, of which there are several (see question 14). In this chapter CLL refers specifically to B-cell chronic lymphocytic leukemia.

3. How common is CLL?

CLL is the most common type of leukemia, accounting for 30% of all cases. The incidence is 3.9 and 2.0 per 100,000 in men and women, respectively. Ninety percent of patients are over age 50, although rare cases in children do occur.

4. What is the etiology of CLL?

The etiology of CLL is unknown. Although a direct mode of inheritance has not been established, first-degree relatives of patients with CLL carry a three times normal risk of developing CLL or other lymphoid malignancies. Neither radiation nor retroviruses have been identified as a cause of CLL.

5. Discuss the common symptoms of CLL.

Approximately 25% of patients are asymptomatic and diagnosed as a result of routine clinical or laboratory examination. Those who are symptomatic commonly present with nonspecific complaints such as fatigue and malaise even in the absence of anemia. Specific symptoms such as early satiety or bleeding and bruising can be attributed to splenomegaly and thrombocytopenia, respectively. Occasionally, patients present with infection or have noted lymph node enlargement.

6. What is the significance of fever in patients with CLL?

In the absence of infection, fever is rare in CLL, whereas fever is a common constitutional symptom in other lymphoid neoplasms.

7. Describe the physical findings in CLL.

Lymphadenopathy is present in 80% of patients. Cervical, supraclavicular, and axillary nodes are most commonly involved. The lymph nodes are usually mobile and nontender and have a rubbery feel. The spleen is enlarged 50–70% of the time, and hepatomegaly is present in < 50% of patients. Petechiae and bruising are uncommon. Rarely, massive lymphadenopathy may produce extremity lymphedema and biliary, renal, or upper airway obstruction.

8. What are the peripheral blood findings in CLL?

Lymphocytosis is universal, and the absolute lymphocyte count usually exceeds 15×10^9/L at diagnosis. Granulocytopenia, anemia, and thrombocytopenia are common. The peripheral blood smear reveals an abundance of relatively normal-appearing small lymphocytes. (See Figure 10, Color Plates).

9. What is a "smudge cell"?

CLL lymphocytes tend to rupture during preparation of the peripheral smear. Thee ruptured forms have a distinct appearance known as smudge cells. (See Figure 10, Color Plates). The presence of smudge cells should always raise suspicion for CLL.

10. Describe the bone marrow in CLL.

The marrow is always involved. Either focal or diffuse infiltration can be seen on core biopsies. The extent of marrow infiltration directly correlates with prognosis.

11. Patients with CLL are predisposed to infection. What immunologic defects are associated with CLL?

Granulocytopenia due to marrow infiltration is almost always present. Hypogammaglobulinemia is present 75% of the time; the degree directly correlates with clinical stage and risk of infection. Functional abnormalities in B cells and T cells can be demonstrated in virtually all patients.

12. Why do anemia and thrombocytopenia occur in CLL?

The primary reason is disruption of normal marrow hematopoiesis by the infiltrating lymphocytes. Splenomegaly, when present, causes sequestration of normal blood cells. Autoimmune hemolytic anemia or autoimmune thrombocytopenia may develop and can be particularly troublesome.

13. How is CLL diagnosed?

The history, physical examination, peripheral blood counts, and lymphocyte morphology are usually sufficient to diagnose CLL in the clinical setting. Published criteria for the diagnosis of CLL require peripheral blood lymphocytosis along with either evidence of of marrow infiltration or documentation of B-cell markers (usually by flow cytometry) on the peripheral blood lymphocytes. The bone marrow biopsy and peripheral blood B-cell markers need be studied only when the diagnosis is uncertain or in a research setting.

14. What is the differential diagnosis of CLL?

Several indolent lymphocytic malignancies are related to CLL, including prolymphocytic' leukemia, Waldenström's macroglobulinemia, leukemic phase of lymphomas, hairy cell leukemia, T-cell CLL, adult T-cell leukemia, large granulocytic leukemia, and cutaneous T-cell lymphoma. Small lymphocytic lymphoma (diffuse, well-differentiated lymphoma) is often diagnosed on lymph node biopsies obtained from patients with CLL. This type of lymphoma is histologically identical to CLL. The distinction between the two entities depends simply on the presence or absence of peripheral blood involvement.

15. How is CLL distinguished from related disorders?'

Clinical and morphologic findings are usually sufficient. However, the diagnosis can be confirmed by determining the immunologic phenotype of the malignant lymphocytes using flow cytometry analysis. (See chapter 30, questions 16 and 17 for a discussion of flow cytometry.) Flow cytometry uses monoclonal antibodies to identify cell surface antigens that are unique to an individual type of lymphocyte (e.g., normal cell, CLL cell, T-helper cell).

16. What are the flow cytometry findings in CLL?

A B-cell phenotype is documented by the presence of the cell surface antigens termed CD19, CD20, and CD21. The antigen called CD5 is normally found only on T lymphocytes. However, the diagnosis of CLL is confirmed when CD5 is paradoxically expressed on the same cells that express the above B-cell markers. Flow cytometry has significantly increased our understanding of lymphoid malignancies and is now widely available.

17. What is the natural history of CLL?

The natural history can be determined by the clinical stage of the disease. Patients may be assigned a stage based on the clinical findings and blood counts. A bone marrow biopsy is not necessary to determine the clinical stage. Clinical stage correlates well with expected survival. The Rai and Binet staging systems are commonly encountered.

Rai Staging System for Chronic Lymphocytic Leukemia

STAGE	FINDINGS	MEDIAN SURVIVAL (MONTHS)
0	Lymphocytosis ($> 15 \times 10^9$/L)	> 150
I	Lymphocytosis plus lymphadenopathy	100
II	Lymphocytosis plus splenomegaly	70
III	Lymphocytosis plus anemia (Hgb < 11/gm/dl)	19
IV	Lymphocytosis plus thrombocytopenia (platelet count < 100×10^9/L)	19

In stages II–IV, lymphadenopathy may be present or absent; in stages III–IV, splenomegaly may be present or absent. Anemia and thrombocytopenia due to an autoimmune syndrome should not be used to determine stage.

18. Are there any other prognostic factors in CLL?

Yes. Other factors that adversely influence survival include disease progression, extensive or diffuse marrow infiltration, a rapid lymphocyte doubling time, and the presence of chromosomal abnormalities on karyotype analysis. The degree of peripheral lymphocytosis does not correlate well with prognosis.

19. At what white blood cell count should treatment be initiated?

This is a trick question. The absolute white blood cell count alone never influences treatment decisions. The white blood cell count can sometimes reach very high levels (e.g., $> 500 \times 10^9/L$) in asymptomatic patients.

20. If that is true, then when should patients be treated?

As with other indolent lymphoid malignancies (e.g., hairy cell leukemia, low-grade lymphoma), treatment is indicated only when symptoms occur. It has been clearly established that treatment of asymptomatic patients with these disorders does not result in improved survival compared with those treated later when symptoms occur. Asymptomatic patients who are treated are exposed to unnecessary risks of chemotherapy.

Specific indications for treatment include recurrent infection, symptomatic or unsightly lymphadenopathy, and symptomatic splenomegaly, anemia, or thrombocytopenia. Constitutional symptoms, such as fatigue and malaise, occasionally necessitate treatment. Hemolytic anemia and immune thrombocytopenia are exceptions; both require therapy whether or not symptoms occur.

21. What is the optimal treatment for CLL?

Optimal treatment has not yet been defined. Several treatments can control the disease; however, remissions, whether complete or partial, are usually short-lived. Alkylating agents such as chlorambucil (Leukeran) or cyclophosphamide (Cytoxan) are typically administered with or without prednisone as initial therapy. Combination chemotherapy is tried next. Recently, the nucleoside analogs fludarabine (Fludara) and 2-chlorodeoxyadenosine (Leustatin or 2-CdA) have been shown to be highly effective in patients refractory to combination chemotherapy.

22. How effective are the alkylating agents?

About 60% of patients improve with chlorambucil or cyclophosphamide (either agent alone or with prednisone). Ten percent of these responses are complete (disappearance of all measurable disease) and the remaining 50% are partial.

23. What can be done when CLL is resistant to alkylating agents?

Combination chemotherapy such as cyclophosphamide, vincristine (Oncovin), and prednisone (COP regimen) or doxorubicin (Adriamycin) plus COP (CHOP regimen) result in transient improvement about 50% of the time with very few complete responses.

24. What is the role of the nucleoside analogs?

Fludarabine and 2-CdA interfere with adenosine metabolism, leading to intracellular accumulation of toxic metabolites and resultant cell death. Both drugs produce complete response rates of 15% and partial response rates of 50% in patients resistant to standard chemotherapy. They are significantly less toxic than standard chemotherapeutic agents. Both drugs are presently under investigation in previously untreated patients and for use in combination with alkylating agents.

25. Are there any other effective therapies for CLL?

Yes. Radiation is useful for localized symptomatic lymphadenopathy. Biologic treatments such as interferon and interleukin have activity and are being investigated.

26. How are hemolytic anemia and immune thrombocytopenia managed in patients with CCL?

Immune hemolysis and thrombocytopenia often may be managed without chemotherapy. Prednisone is usually effective. Splenectomy may be required for cases refractory to steroids.

27. What is the cause of death in patients with CLL?

Because CLL is generally a disease of the elderly, 30% die of unrelated causes. Fifty percent die of infection, 15% from complications of therapy, and the remainder from hemorrhage, hemolysis, or vital organ infiltration.

28. Can CLL be cured?

A rare patient under the age of 50 may be cured with high-dose chemotherapy plus radiation therapy, followed by HLA-matched, sibling donor, bone marrow transplantation. However, even though long disease-free intervals are often achieved with standard therapy, CLL is not considered to be a curable disease. It remains to be seen whether the use of fludarabine or 2-CdA as early or initial treatment or in combination with standard therapies can improve the long-term prognosis. Regardless, it is apparent that the natural history of CLL may be significantly improved by these new agents.

BIBLIOGRAPHY

1. Beutler F, Lichtman MA, Coller BS, Kipps TJ (eds): Williams Hematology, 5th ed. New York, McGraw-Hill, 1995.
2. Foon KA, Rai KR, Gale RP: Chronic lymphocytic leukemia: New insights into biology and therapy. Ann Intern Med 113:525, 1990.
3. Foon KA, Todd RF: Immunologic classification of leukemia and lymphoma. Blood 68:1, 1986.
4. Keating MJ, Kantarjian H, Talpaz M, et al: Fludarabine: A new agent with major activity against chronic lymphocytic leukemia. Blood 74:19, 1989.
5. Lee RG, Bithell TC, Foerster J, et al (ed): Wintrobe's Clinical Hemotology. Philadelphia, Lea & Febiger, 1993.
6. Piro LD, Carrera CJ, Beutler E, Carson DA: 2-Chlorodeoxyadenosine: An effective new agent for the treatment of chronic lymphocytic leukemia. Blood 72:1069, 1990.
7. Rai KR, Sawitsky A, Cronkite EP, et al: Clinical staging of chronic lymphocytic leukemia. Blood 46:219, 1975.
8. Tefferi A, Phyliky RL: A clinical update on chronic lymphocytic leukemia. I. Diagnosis and prognosis. Mayo Clin Proc 67:349, 1992.
9. Tefferi A, Phyliky RL: A clinical update on chronic lymphocytic leukemia. II. Critical analysis of current chemotherapeutic modalities. Mayo Clin Proc 67:457, 1992.

29. CHRONIC MYELOGENOUS LEUKEMIA

David Ospina, M.D.

1. Define chronic myelogenous leukemia (CML).

CML is one of the myeloproliferative syndromes (that include polycythemia vera, essential thrombocythemia, and agnogenic myeloid metaplasia and myelofibrosis). These syndromes result from a clonal expansion of hematopoietic progenitor cells. Characteristically, leukocytosis with elevated granulocytes and basophils is present, but the erythrocytes and platelet counts also may be increased. CML frequently progresses to a fatal blast crisis. The Philadelphia chromosome is present in more than 90% of patients and is virtually diagnostic.

2. Describe the Philadelphia chromosome.

The Philadelphia chromosome is a balanced translocation (9:22)(q34;q11). The protooncogene *c-abl* on the long arm of chromosome 9(q34) is transposed to a region on chromosome 22(q11) called the breakpoint cluster region or *bcr*. The result is fusion gene *bcr-abl*. The product of *bcr-abl* is an abnormal tyrosine kinase that may suppress apoptosis, induce cell proliferation, and promote cell growth independent of extracellular growth factors.

3. What are the clinical characteristics of a patient with CML?

CML may present in individuals between 15 and 80 years old with the highest incidence in the 5th and 6th decades of life. Because of routine blood testing, almost one-half of patients are asymptomatic; the other half have signs and symptoms of anemia. Splenomegaly with left upper quadrant pain and early satiety is frequently seen, and hepatomegaly is present in 10–40%. Very rarely patients will present with a WBC of > 500,000/cm (see Figure 9, Color Plates) and complaints suggestive of a hyperviscosity syndrome. Constitutional symptoms such as weight loss, anorexia, fevers, and chills also may be present. Infection and bleeding complications are unusual in the early phase.

4. List the phases of CML and their prognostic importance?

1. Untreated, the **chronic phase** has a median duration of 3.5–5 years before it evolves to a blast phase.

2. The **accelerated phase** is a transitional phase toward a blastic transformation, characterized by an increase in the peripheral and bone marrow blast counts. The accelerated phase may be suspected when the percentage of basophils in blood increases above 20%, with a thrombocytopenia < 100,000/cm. Approximately 75% of patients go through this phase; if left untreated, the median survival is 1–4 years.

3. **Blast phase** resembles acute leukemia, and survival is 3–6 months. Generally, patients are typed as having acute myelogenous leukemia, but lymphocytic and mixed (bi-phenotypic leukemia) types are not uncommon.

5. What are the hematologic laboratory features of CML?

The WBC is usually > 25,000/cm and the differential shows granulocytes in all stages of maturation from blasts to mature granulocytes. Basophils are elevated, and eosinophils also are increased, but to a lesser degree. An abrupt increase in basophils signals an accelerated phase. The platelet count is elevated in half of patients; thrombocytopenia may be seen but also may indicate progression to an accelerated phase. The bone marrow is hypercellular with blast counts ≤ 10% in the chronic phase.

6. What serologic findings may be present in CML?

Leukocyte alkaline phosphatase (LAP) activity is reduced in nearly all patients. Serum levels of B_{12}, transcobalamin, uric acid, and LDH are frequently elevated.

7. What prognostic features are important in chronic phase CML?

For patients in chronic phase the age, spleen size, platelet count, and percentage of peripheral blasts are of prognostic importance. The acquisition of other somatic mutations (clonal evolution) and a quantitative increase of *bcr-abl* expression (determined by polymerase chain reaction[PCR]) may indicate disease progression.

8. What is the standard of care for patients with CML?

Interferon alpha (IFN-α) is now widely accepted as standard therapy. Randomized studies of IFN-α vs. conventional chemotherapy (hydroxyurea or busulfan) have shown that IFN-α induces complete hematologic responses in 70–80% of patients (vs. 70% with conventional chemotherapy). IFN-α also prolongs survival (72 months vs. 52 months) and induces a higher cytogenetic response (30% vs. 5%).

9. What is considered to be conventional chemotherapy for CML?

Both hydroxyurea and busulfan were the treatment of choice before IFN. Both are less costly than IFN and orally administered. Both drugs have a hematologic response rate better than 70% with a median duration of 35–50 months. Virtually no patient achieves cytogenetic response, and cure is unheard of.

10. What is IFN-α and its effect on CML cells?

Interferon is a family of glycoproteins that are produced by most cells in the body; IFN-α is mainly produced by leukocytes or lymphoid cells as a response to a viral infection. The mechanism of action in CML is unclear, but there is evidence of an antiproliferative effect, promotion of natural killer cell cytotoxicity, and normalization of lymphocyte-activated killer cell activity (immune-modulation).

11. How long would you treat a patient with IFN-α before declaring it a therapeutic failure?

The median time to achieve a hematologic remission is 6–8 months, and for cytogenetic responses the median time is 22–24 months. Thus, treatment with IFN must be given for several months before calling it a failure. The time to a hematologic response may be shortened by the use of a cytotoxic drug such as hydroxyurea in combination with IFN during the first few weeks.

12. What are the important prognostic variables with IFN-α treatment?

Patients who have a hematologic improvement and achieve a major cytogenetic response have an improved survival (80% at 4 years vs. 40–60% in noncytogenetic responders). Pretreatment characteristics associated with better survival include good performance status, small spleen size, normal hemoglobin, low leukocyte count, and low percentage of circulating blasts and basophils.

13. Which are the main side effects of INF-α?

Acute toxicity. Flulike symptoms (fever, chills, and anorexia) may be reduced by starting at 50% of the required dose and escalating to a full dose over 1–2 weeks, and also by administering the IFN at bedtime and using acetaminophen as needed.

Late toxicity. The most common side effects are chronic fatigue, neurotoxicity, weight loss, and bone pain.

Because of the side effects, up to one-fourth of patients discontinue the treatment.

14. Is there a treatment for CML that may be considered curative?

The only treatment that may be considered curative (but is still unproven) is dose-intense chemotherapy with HLA-matched sibling bone marrow transplantation, a treatment that may result in long-term survival. In some studies the survival curves seem to have reached a plateau, suggesting a long-term control of the disease. The 7-year disease-free survival reached 60% in some studies, and further follow-up is needed to determine whether cure is possible.

15. When should allogeneic bone marrow transplant (BMT) be considered for a patient with CML?

Allogeneic BMT should be considered for all patients < 60 years old with an HLA-matched donor. BMT in chronic phase is most successful, compared with the accelerated or blastic phases. For unknown reasons the outcome is better if transplant is done during the first year after diagnosis.

16. What is the graft-versus-leukemia effect? Is it prognostic in CML?

The graft-versus-leukemia effect was first noted when recipients of unrelated donor BMT developed developed and then survived the complications of graft-versus-host disease (GVHD). In this group individuals rarely, if ever, suffered a relapse. It is believed that donor T-cell or activated killer cells recognize the recipient leukemia cell as foreign and mediate an antileukemic reaction. Several studies have shown that patients who develop chronic GVHD have a lower risk of relapse, suggesting that a graft-versus-leukemia effect is beneficial in controlling the disease.

CONTROVERSIES

17. Compared with conventional chemotherapy, is treatment with IFN cost-effective?

IFN is an expensive drug and may cost from $500–$2000 a month during induction. On the other hand, hydroxyurea may cost from $150–$200/month. A cost-effectiveness study comparing the two agents (hydroxyurea and IFN) showed that IFN is cost-effective and estimated a cost decrease of $34,800 per quality-adjusted year of life saved for patients treated with IFN.

18. Does the combination of IFN with a cytotoxic drug have a better outcome compared with IFN alone?

The issue is still debatable, but a French trial comparing IFN with IFN plus cytarabine suggests an increase in the rate of cytogenetic response and a prolongation of the median survival for patients in chronic phase CML.

BIBLIOGRAPHY

1. Enright H: Biology and treatment of chronic myelogenous leukemia. Oncology 11:1295–1299, 1997.
2. Enright H, Davies SM, DeFor T, et al: Relapse after non–T-cell depleted allogeneic bone marrow transplantation for chronic myelogenous leukemia: Early transplantation, use of an unrelated donor, and chronic graft-versus-host disease are protective. Blood 88:714–720, 1996.
3. Gale RP, Hehlmann R, Zhang MJ, et al: Survival with bone marrow transplantation versus hydroxyurea or interferon for chronic myelogenous leukemia. Blood 91:1810–1819, 1998.
4. Goldman JM, Szydlo R, Horowitz MM, et al: Choice of pretransplant treatment and timing of transplantation for chronic myelogenous leukemia in chronic phase. Blood 82:2235–2238, 1993.
5. Kantarjian HM, Smith TL, O'Brien S, et al: Prolonged survival in chronic myelogenous leukemia after cytogenetic response to interferon-alpha therapy. Ann Intern Med 122:254–261, 1995.
6. Kattan MW, Inoue Y, Giles FJ, et al: Cost-effectiveness of interferon-alpha and conventional chemotherapy in chronic myelogenous leukemia. Ann Intern Med 125:541–548, 1996.
7. Patel T, Roychowdhury DF: Interferon alpha-2b and cytarabine in chronic myelogenous leukemia. N Engl J Med 337:1634–1635, 1997.
8. Sokal E, et al: Prognostic discrimination in "good-risk" chronic granulocytic leukemia. Blood 63:789–799, 1984.
9. The Italian Cooperative Study Group: Interferon alpha-2a as compared with conventional chemotherapy for the treatment of chronic myelogenous leukemia. N Engl J Med 330:820–825, 1994.

30. HAIRY CELL LEUKEMIA

Robert S. Kantor, M.D.

1. What is hairy cell leukemia (HCL)?

HCL is a malignant disorder of well-differentiated B lymphocytes. HCL is a chronic leukemia; its cell of origin is similar to that of chronic lymphocytic leukemia (CLL). The clinical presentation of HCL, however, is quite distinct. HCL was first described in 1958 and was then referred to as leukemic reticuloendotheliosis.

2. Name the three most characteristic features of HCL.

1. Pancytopenia   2. Bone marrow infiltration   3. Splenomegaly

3. Who gets HCL?

HCL is generally a disease of elderly men, although it has been reported in persons in their early 20s. The median age of onset is 50 years, and 75% of patients are men.

4. How important is HCL?

HCL is a rare disease. Only 600 cases per year are diagnosed in the United States, accounting for 2% of adult leukemia. HCL is quite important, however, because research into this rare disorder has broadened our understanding of immunology and led to the development of effective new drugs that are useful in HCL and other lymphoproliferative disorders.

5. What causes HCL?

The cause of HCL is unknown. Radiation exposure has been associated with HCL, but this remains controversial. There have been isolated familial occurrences; one involved three siblings, all with the HLA A1, B7 haplotype. The retrovirus HTLV-II has been implicated in two atypical cases of T-cell HCL.

6. Why is the disease called "hairy" cell leukemia?

The hairy cell is like no other cell encountered in the peripheral blood and is usually easy to recognize on a Wright-stained smear. (See Figure 11, Color Plates.) Hairy cells are mononuclear with abundant pale cytoplasm. Cytoplasmic projections (pseudopods or microvilli) give the cells their hairy appearance.

7. Describe the clinical features of HCL.

The presenting symptoms of HCL are directly attributable to the cytopenias and splenomegaly.

Clinical Features of HCL

CLINICAL FEATURES	INCIDENCE (%)
Weakness, fatigue	80
Fever, night sweats	20
Early satiety, weight loss	25
Infection*	20–30
Hemorrhage, bruising	20–30
Abdominal pain	20–30
Lymphadenopathy	0–5
Petechiae, ecchymoses	20–30
Hepatomegaly	15
Splenomegaly	90

* Although most infections are produced by typical gram-positive cocci and gram-negative rods, there seems to be a predisposition to atypical mycobacterial infections such as *Mycobacterium avium-intercellulare*.

8. How are these findings different from CLL?

Actually, almost any of the signs and symptoms listed in the table above can be seen in CLL. However, lymphadenopathy almost always accompanies such findings in CLL but is rarely (< 5%) encountered in HCL.

9. Why is the term *hairy cell leukemia* a misnomer?

Only 10–15% of patients with HCL are actually leukemic (WBC count > 10×10^9/L). The majority of patients are leukopenic. The laboratory findings are described below:

Laboratory Features of HCL

LABORATORY FINDINGS	INCIDENCE (%)
Leukocytosis	10–15
Leukopenia	65
Granulocytopenia	75
Monocytopenia	90
Anemia	80
Thrombocytopenia	80
Pancytopenia	50
Hairy cells visible on blood smear	85
Elevated liver function tests	10
Monoclonal paraprotein	1–3

10. What are the typical bone marrow features of HCL?

First, a "dry tap" is often encountered on attempting to aspirate the marrow because of fibrosis, which can be demonstrated by silver reticulin staining of the core biopsy. Second, the hairy cells have a "fried egg" appearance because of a halo of clear cytoplasm around the nuclei and distinct cellular borders. The marrow can be either focally or diffusely infiltrated.

11. Describe the TRAP stain. How is it important?

Tartrate-resistant acid phosphatase (TRAP) staining is extremely useful in distinguishing HCL from other similar disorders. Incubation of normal lymphocytes and those of other hematologic disorders with tartrate renders these cells unstainable for acid phosphatase. Hairy cells are resistant to tartrate inhibition (owing to acid phosphatase isoenzyme 5) and readily take up acid phosphatase stain. TRAP activity, once thought to be pathognomonic for HCL, is now known to be rarely present in other lymphoproliferative disorders and thus somewhat limits the usefulness of this test.

12. Name three causes of the pancytopenia often seen in HCL.

1. Disruption of marrow hematopoiesis by HCL infiltration
2. Splenic sequestration of circulating blood cells
3. Dilutional effect of increased plasma volume (which accompanies splenomegaly)

13. How is HCL diagnosed?

The history, examination, and laboratory findings are extremely important. The diagnosis is confirmed by morphologic identification of hairy cells in the blood, marrow, or spleen. TRAP staining, electron microscopy, and flow cytometry (see below) help distinguish HCL from other lymphoproliferative diseases.

14. What is the differential diagnosis of HCL?

Hairy cells are not found in any other disorder. Atypical forms of HCL do exist and must not be confused with other related disorders. The differential diagnosis includes CLL, prolymphocytic leukemia, large granular lymphocytic leukemia, splenic lymphoma with villous lymphocytosis, monocytoid B-cell lymphoma, and the malignant histiocytic syndromes.

15. How is HCL separated from these disorders?

Usually morphology alone is enough. TRAP staining can help, but recall that this is not entirely specific. Electron microscopy is helpful to identify the cytoplasmic projections but is expensive and not available outside major centers. Flow cytometry analysis of circulating or marrow lymphocytes is the most specific, cost-effective test available.

16. What is flow cytometry?

Lymphocytes express cell-specific surface antigens that can be readily identified with fluorescent-labeled monoclonal antibodies (MoAbs). Each type of lymphocyte (e.g., hairy cell, normal cell, CLL cell) expresses a unique set of cellular antigens, thus allowing MoAb identification. A flow cytometer passes individual MoAb-labeled cells through a column where fluorescence is quantified, thus immunologically identifying each individual cell.

17. Why is flow cytometry so important?

Flow cytometry has significantly increased our understanding of HCL and related disorders by generating a complete, reproducible immunologic profile of each such disease. This technique is now available in most major medical centers. When the cellular antigens termed CD11c, CD22, CD25, and B-Ly7 are identified by flow cytometry, the diagnosis of HCL is assured.

18. Define the natural history of untreated HCL.

Ten percent of patients will have a benign course and never require therapy. Most patients, however, develop progressive pancytopenia and splenomegaly, thus requiring intervention. The median survival for untreated patients is about 5 years.

19. When is treatment for HCL required?

Generally, patients are observed until infection, symptomatic cytopenias, or splenomegaly occurs.

20. How is HCL treated?

The treatment of HCL has dramatically changed during the past several years. Splenectomy, once the mainstay of therapy, is now virtually contraindicated because of the availability of several highly effective new drug therapies. Treatment options include splenectomy, recombinant human interferon alpha (IFN-α), and the two nucleoside analogues deoxycoformycin (DCF) or 2-chlorodeoxyadenosine (2-CdA). Chemotherapy, hormones, steroids, and radiation are rarely effective.

21. What can splenectomy accomplish?

Splenectomy improves blood counts in 98% of cases owing to removal of splenic sequestration and reduction in plasma volume. However, most patients develop progressive pancytopenia within 1 year on account of progressive marrow disease. Splenectomy is associated with significant perioperative morbidity and a long-term risk of recurrent pyogenic infection. Pneumococcal vaccination should be administered to all patients who are under consideration for splenectomy.

22. Is interferon alpha effective?

Yes. About 70% of patients improve, but complete responses (normal blood counts, < 5% hairy cells in the marrow, and no splenomegaly) are rare. IFN-α is administered subcutaneously for 1 year. Toxicity is significant, and most patients relapse within 1 to 2 years after stopping therapy. Subsequent courses usually lead to drug resistance.

23. How effective are the nucleoside analogues?

Very. These new drugs interfere with adenosine metabolism, leading to intracellular accumulation of toxic metabolites and resultant cell death.

DCF (Pentostatin) induces complete responses in about 60% of patients and partial improvement in 25%. Most of the complete responses are long-lasting. DCF is administered intravenously every other week for 3–6 months. It is highly immunosuppressive with serious infections observed in about one-third of those treated.

2-CdA (Leustatin) induces complete responses in 90% with the remainder experiencing near-complete responses. These remissions (whether complete or partial) are long-lasting, with only a rare patient resistant to therapy or relapsing. 2-CdA is administered via a single 7-day infusion. The only toxicity is culture-negative fever in about 40% of patients.

24. Can HCL be cured?

The initial results with DCF and 2-CdA suggest a curative potential for HCL. Both drugs have produced complete remissions lasting up to 12 years at the time of this writing. Hundreds of patients have now been treated with 2-CdA. Of the 90% complete responders, only 10% have relapsed. Only time will tell if these long-term remissions will translate into cures. Regardless, it is apparent that the natural history of HCL has been significantly improved by these new therapeutic modalities.

BIBLIOGRAPHY

1. Alexander SD, Spiers TD, Moore D, et al: Remissions in hairy-cell leukemia with pentostatin (2′-deoxycoformycin). N Engl J Med 316:825, 1987.
2. Beutler E, Lichtman MA, Coller BS, Kipps TJ (eds): Williams Hematology, 5th ed. New York, McGraw-Hill, 1995.
3. Bouroncle BA, Wiseman BK, Doan CA: Leukemic reticuloendotheliosis. Blood 13:609, 1958.
4. Foon KA, Todd RF: Immunologic classification of leukemia and lymphoma. Blood 68:1, 1986.
5. Golomb HM, Fefer A, Golde DW, et al: Update of a multi-institutional study of 195 patients with hairy cell leukemia treated with interferon alfa-2B. Proc Am Soc Clin Oncol 6:215, 1990.
6. Lee RG, Bithell TC, Foerster J, et al (eds): Wintrobe's Clinical Hematology. Philadelphia, Lea & Febiger, 1993.

7. Piro LD, Carrera CJ, Carson DA, Beutler E: Lasting remissions in hairy-cell leukemia induced by a single infusion of 2-chlorodeoxyadenosine. N Engl J Med 322:1117, 1990.
8. Saven A, Piro LD: Treatment of hairy cell leukemia. Blood 79:1111, 1992.

31. NON-HODGKIN'S LYMPHOMA: CLASSIFICATION AND PATHOLOGY

Mitchell A. Bitter, M.D.

1. In a patient with several enlarged lymph nodes, which lymph node should be biopsied?

As a general rule, the largest lymph node should be chosen for biopsy. It is always a temptation to biopsy a smaller, superficial node if it is more easily accessible. However, in some cases, the smaller node may not show diagnostic findings and thereby delay diagnosis or even result in an erroneous diagnosis. A common fallacy holds that inguinal lymph nodes should not be biopsied because they may show nonspecific, confusing, histologic changes that may obscure the correct diagnosis. However, if an inguinal node is the largest node and does not predate the patient's illness, it should be chosen for biopsy.

2. What kind of lymph node biopsy should be performed? How should a tissue specimen be handled before it gets to the laboratory if lymphoma is suspected?

Unless a lymph node is massive and cannot be removed in toto for technical reasons, all lymph node biopsies should be excisional (rather than incisional). The tissue should be delivered without delay to the pathology department **without fixation**. If the tissue is placed in fixative, microbiologic cultures and special studies such as molecular genetic tests and cytogenetics cannot be performed. Furthermore, immunologic marker studies are severely limited.

3. What is the role of fine-needle aspiration (FNA) and needle biopsy in the diagnosis of lymphoma?

In FNA, cells of an enlarged lymph node are aspirated using a needle, smeared onto a slide, and examined cytologically. In addition, material may be submitted for immunophenotyping (see below). For biopsy of lymph nodes and masses that are not easily accessible (e.g., in the abdomen and retroperitoneum), needle biopsy may be performed under computed tomography (CT) guidance. These less invasive techniques are of great use in confirming relapse of a previously diagnosed lymphoma and are adequate for initial diagnosis in many cases. Some hematopathologists favor excisional biopsy of peripheral lymph nodes over FNA in initial diagnosis because biopsy provides more information for histologic classification and more tissue for special studies (see below).

4. What is the purpose of lymphoma classification?

In the clinical setting, lymphoma classification is based on the observation that the pathologic features of a lymphoma are useful in predicting (although imperfectly) the clinical behavior and response to therapy of a lymphoma. Lymphoma subtype is factored into a number of clinical decisions including: Should the lymphoma be treated at all? If so, should it be treated for cure or palliation? What is the regimen most likely to be effective? What is the overall prognosis?

5. What is the Working Formulation?

A number of systems of lymphoma classification are used in clinical practice. Each system uses different terminology, which has led to great confusion among clinicians and pathologists. In 1982, the Working Formulation, which is based on a National Cancer Institute (NCI) study of over 1,000 cases of lymphoma, was proposed to "translate" the terminology of one classification system into another and thus facilitate evaluation of the results of clinical trials. The Working Formulation was not intended to supplant the classification systems already in use. However, over the years, that is exactly what happened. The Working Formulation has become the most widely used system of lymphoma classification in the United States and Canada.

The Working Formulation divides lymphomas into three broad categories: low, intermediate, and high grade. However, many clinicians consider two broad categories of lymphomas: indolent lymphomas, which generally are not curable, and aggressive lymphomas, which may be treated for cure. As a generalization, low-grade lymphomas of the Working Formulation roughly correspond to the former and the intermediate and higher grade lymphomas roughly correspond to the latter.

Working Formulation (Simplified)

GRADE	% IN ADULTS
Low	
Diffuse, small lymphocytic	4
Follicular, predominantly small cleaved cell	23
Follicular, mixed small cleaved and large cell	8
Intermediate	
Follicular, predominantly large cell	4
Diffuse, small cleaved cell	7
Diffuse, mixed small and large cell	7
Diffuse, large cell	20
High	
Large cell immunoblastic	8
Lymphoblastic	4
Small noncleaved	5
Miscellaneous	10

6. What is the Revised European American Lymphoma (REAL) classification?

The recently proposed REAL classification is a listing of all lymphoma entities that hematopathologists can recognize using a combination of morphology and other modalities, such as immunophenotyping, cytogenetics, and molecular genetics. It does not separate lymphoma into broad categories by grade (low, intermediate, and high) as the Working Formulation does. Some clinicians view the REAL classification as overly complex and not useful clinically. Many hematophatologists counter that a number of distinct clinicopathologic entities are not included in the Working Formulation. If such entities are not recognized in a lymphoma classification, we will not learn about their clinical behavior and response to various therapies.

7. How reproducible is the morphologic classification of lymphoma?

Many clinicians are surprised to learn of the poor reproducibility of some aspects of lymphoma classification even among expert hematopathologists. Hematopathologists recognize follicular versus diffuse architecture (approximately 90% reproducibility), but reproducibility of the specific lymphoma subtype is poor. In one study, among expert hematopathologists, interobserver agreement ranged from 21–65%, depending on the observers and the classification system. Moreover, some expert hematopathologists agreed with themselves only slightly more than half of the time (range for different experts: 53–93%).

Placing this information into perspective, how certain can the oncologist be of the histologic classification of a lymphoma rendered by the pathologist? Obviously the answer depends on the pathologist. In general, however, pathologists are good at making the most important histologic distinction in terms of therapeutic decisions—low grade versus intermediate or high grade. Other major distinctions that influence choice of a therapeutic regimen—for instance, distinction between lymphoblastic versus small noncleaved cell lymphoma—are reproducible by expert hematopathologists, especially if immunologic marker studies are available. However, some distinctions are poorly reproducible; for instance, is a follicular lymphoma small cleaved cell type or mixed small cleaved and large cell type? Fortunately, most poorly reproducible distinctions are less important in clinical decision-making.

In general, lymphoma diagnosis and classification are best made by pathologists with a great deal of experience in the field. However, many distinctions are irreproducible even among expert hematopathologists. Therefore, if a local pathologist calls a given case a follicular small cleaved cell lymphoma and the national "expert" calls it a follicular mixed small cleaved and large cell lymphoma, do not assume that the local pathologist is "wrong" and the expert is "right."

8. What is immunophenotyping?

Immunologic marker studies are widely used to characterize malignant lymphomas. These studies may be performed using flow cytometry or by immunohistochemistry. The former technology utilizes a semiautomated instrument that rapidly measures up to three fluorescence signals (up to three antibodies) on a large number of cells and correlates these measurements with other parameters, including cell size.

The technique of immunohistochemistry demonstrates the binding of antibodies to the lymphoma cells on microscope slides and allows the pathologist to correlate visually the pattern of antibody staining with the histology and cytology of the lymphoma. Either technique may be used to characterize a lymphoma, and each has relative advantages and disadvantages.

9. What clinically useful information is derived from immunologic marker studies of lymphomas?

In some institutions, comprehensive and costly panels of antibodies are used to characterize every new case of malignant lymphoma. These studies can be useful in helping to answer a number of clinically important questions.

1. **Is a malignant tumor a lymphoma or a poorly differentiated carcinoma?** In some cases, it may be difficult or impossible to determine whether a tumor is a lymphoma or a carcinoma by microscopic examination alone. In such cases, antibodies that recognize lymphoid cells (such as CD45) and epithelial cells (such as cytokeratin) may be very useful.

2. **Is an atypical lymphoid proliferation malignant, or is it an unusual reactive lesion?** In difficult cases, the demonstration of clonality (for instance, all abnormal cells express kappa light chain rather than the normal mixture of both kappa- and lambda-positive cells) indicates that a given proliferation is malignant rather than reactive. Lymphoma cells also may fail to express antigens present on normal B or T cells or express combinations of antigens not observed in normal cells.

3. **How should the lymphoma be classified?** Because many subtypes of non-Hodgkin's lymphoma have characteristic immunophenotypic profiles, immunophenotyping can be a useful adjunct to improve the accuracy and reproducibility of morphologic classification. For instance, in a difficult case, if the immunophenotype is consistent with the proposed morphologic diagnosis, that diagnosis can be made with greater confidence. Alternatively, if the immunophenotype is inconsistent with the tentative morphologic diagnosis, that diagnosis should be reconsidered. Immunophenotyping also may be used to subclassify a lymphoma within a given histologic group. For instance, is a large cell lymphoma of T or B lineage? The possible significance of this distinction is addressed below.

10. Is it clinically important whether a large cell lymphoma has a T- or B-cell phenotype?

This issue is not resolved. Early studies indicated that this distinction did not influence patient outcome. More recently, some studies have suggested that immunophenotype in large-cell lymphoma is important. Some groups report shorter disease-free survival for T-cell diffuse large-cell lymphoma than for B-cell lymphomas showing similar histology. More definitive information awaits the results of large-scale prospective studies, which are under way.

Other immunophenotypic information has been reported by some to influence prognosis in large cell lymphoma. Lack of expression by the lymphoma of major histocompatibility complex

(MHC) class I and class II antigens has been reported to be associated with shortened survival. Data correlating the percentage of proliferating cells (as determined by staining with the proliferation-associated marker Ki-67) with clinical outcome in large-cell lymphoma have yielded conflicting results.

11. What are immunoglobulin and T-cell gene rearrangement studies?

These studies, which employ the techniques of molecular biology, have been introduced into clinical diagnosis over the past decade.

Early in maturation, lymphoid cells rearrange their immunoglobulin (B cells) and T-cell receptor genes (T cells). This process allows the cells to generate enough different antigen recognition molecules to respond to the antigens that will be encountered over a lifetime. Each cell reconfigures its antigen recognition genes in a slightly different way. Therefore, the size and electrophoretic mobility of rearranged antigen receptor genes will differ for each cell after restriction endonuclease digestion. In addition, the mobility of each will differ from the unrearranged antigen receptor genes of nonlymphoid cells. The mobility of the unrearranged genes is termed **germline**. Because the mobility of each rearranged DNA fragment differs, no distinct bands, other than germline (contributed in part by nonlymphoid cells in the sample), are seen in Southern blots.

Lymphomas are derived from neoplastic transformation and proliferation of a single cell, which occur after the cell has rearranged its antigen receptor genes. All of its progeny have identical antigen receptor gene configurations and therefore identical electrophoretic mobility. This clone is seen as a new distinct band (other than germline) after electrophoresis. Current methodology can detect rearranged bands contributed by as few as 2–5% clonal cells.

The polymerase chain reaction (PCR) can be used to amplify immunoglobulin and T-cell receptor gene rearrangements and to detect clonality in some lymphomas. It is less labor-intensive than Southern blotting.

12. How are immunoglobulin and T-cell gene rearrangment studies used in lymphoma diagnosis?

In clinical practice, immunoglobulin and T-cell receptor gene rearrangement studies are used (1) to assess clonality and thereby help to determine if a given proliferation is malignant and (2) to assign lineage. A prominent rearranged band (a strong band in a position other than germline) indicates the presence of a significant clone and supports a diagnosis of non-Hodgkin's lymphoma. Faint rearranged bands contributed by small populations of clonal cells need to be interpreted individually in conjunction with clinical and other laboratory information to determine the clinical significance and biologic potential of the clone.

Immunoglobulin and T-cell rearrangement studies may be helpful in uncommon cases in which immunophenotypic studies are unable to assign lineage (T versus B). The presence of clonal immunoglobulin gene rearrangement without T-cell receptor rearrangement supports B lineage, whereas clonal T-cell receptor rearrangement without immunoglobulin rearrangement supports T lineage.

13. What are the most important cytogenetic abnormalities in non-Hodgkin's lymphoma (NHL)?

Three cytogenetic abnormalities are strongly associated with particular types of NHL. The most common recurring translocation in NHL is the t(14;18) (reciprocal translocation between chromosomes 14 and 18), which is seen in approximately 80% of follicular lymphomas and 20% of diffuse large-cell lymphomas. Several groups have investigated the prognostic significance of the t(14;18) in diffuse large cell lymphoma. Although some groups report a lower rate of complete remission or shorter disease-free survival, other studies have failed to confirm these results.

The t(8;14) is strongly associated with small noncleaved cell lymphoma, including Burkitt's lymphoma. It also may be seen in large cell and large cell immunoblastic lymphomas, particularly in HIV-infected patients.

Although not entirely specific, the t(11;14) is strongly associated with a relatively newly recognized form of malignant lymphoma known as mantle cell lymphoma. Most examples of this lymphoma are intermediate grade, but most are not curable. They are generally classified as diffuse, small cleaved cell lymphomas using the Working Formulation.

14. What are the most important molecular genetic rearrangements in NHL?

The three cytogenetic abnormalities described above result in genetic rearrangements involving specific genes. Not only are these rearrangements critical in lymphomagenesis, but molecular genetic tests that identify these abnormalities may be used for diagnosis and for rare tumor cell detection in a variety of specimens.

The t(14;18) brings the *BCL-2* (B-cell leukemia/lymphoma-2) gene (18q21) under the regulatory influence of the immunoglobulin (Ig) heavy chain gene (14q32), resulting in overproduction of the *BCL-2* protein in tumor cells. PCR-based tests have been shown to be useful in detecting lymphoma in the bone marrow of these patients, particularly after therapy. The t(8;14) causes inappropriate expression of the *myc* protooncogene (8q24), and the t(11;14) results in disregulation of the *BCL-1* (PRAD1, Cyclin D1) gene (11q13). Recently, rearrangements of the protooncogene *BCL-6* have been found in about 40% of diffuse large B-cell lymphomas.

15. In NHL, what information is more important in determining therapy, histologic classification (grade) or stage? In Hodgkin's disease?

In part because of the unpredictability of spread in NHL, it is generally treated with chemotherapy. The choice of chemotherapeutic regimen depends to a large extent on the subtype (grade) of the lymphoma. Therefore, in NHL, grade is more important than stage.

Because Hodgkin's disease generally spreads in a predictable fashion from one node group to the next, nonbulky localized disease in adults can be treated with radiotherapy. Advanced-stage disease is treated with chemotherapy. The chemotherapeutic regimen does not depend on the histologic subtype of Hodgkin's disease. Moreover, stage for stage, survival in advanced-stage disease is probably similar for all histologic subtypes. Therefore, in Hodgkin's disease, tumor stage is more important than grade in determining therapy.

BIBLIOGRAPHY

1. Berard CW, Bloomfield C, Bonadonna G, et al: Classification of non-Hodgkin's lymphomas. Reproducibility of major classification systems. Cancer 55:91–95, 1985.
2. Harris NL, Jaffe ES, Stein H, et al: A revised European-American classification of lymphoid neoplasms: A proposal from the International Lymphoma Study Group. Blood 84:1361–1392, 1994.
3. Koeppen H, Vardiman JW: New entities, issues, and controversies in the classification of malignant lymphoma. Semin Oncol 25:421–434, 1998.
4. LeBeau MM: Chromosomal abnormalities in non-Hodgkin's lymphomas. Semin Oncol 17:20–29, 1990.
5. Sheibani K: Immunohistochemical analysis of lymphoid tissue. In Knowles DM (ed): Neoplastic Hematopathology. Baltimore, Williams & Wilkins, 1992, pp 197–213.
6. Skarin AT, Dorfman DM: Non-Hodgkin's lymphomas: Current classification and management. CA Cancer J Clin 47:351–372, 1997.
7. Sklar J: Antigen receptor genes: Structure, function, and techniques for analysis of their rearrangements. In Knowles DM (ed): Neoplastic Hematopathology. Baltimore, Williams & Wilkins, 1992, pp 215–244.

32. LOW-GRADE NON-HODGKIN'S LYMPHOMA

Peter C. Raich, M.D., FACP

1. The classification systems for malignant lymphomas seem confusing. How do the low-grade (indolent) non-Hodgkin's lymphomas fit into the overall scheme of malignant disorders involving the lymphatic system?

A number of classification systems for the non-Hodgkin's lymphomas (NHL) have been proposed and used over the past four decades, including those by Lukes, Butler, and Hicks (1966); Lennert (1967); Lukes and Collins (1974); the Kiel classification (1978); the Working Formulation (1982); and, most recently, the Revised European American Lymphoma (REAL) Classification Project (1994). The REAL Classification was tested in 1400 patients with lymphoma from around the world. This study confirmed that diagnoses can be made more accurately and clinically relevant than with previous systems. The REAL Classification divides the lymphoproliferative disorders into five clinical disease categories:

1. Chronic leukemia/lymphoma
2. Nodal or extranodal lymphoma
   - Indolent (low-grade)
   - Aggressive
3. Acute leukemia/lymphoma
4. Plasma cell disorders
5. Hodgkin's disease

The table below compares the major low-grade lymphoma and leukemia types within the REAL Classification and the Working Formulation:

Comparison of the REAL Classification and the Working Formulation for Low-grade Lymphoproliferative Disorders

REAL CLASSIFICATION	WORKING FORMULATION
Chronic leukemia/lymphoma	
Chronic leukemia/lymphoma, B and T-cell type	Small lymphocytic lymphoma/CLL
Lymphoplasmacytoid lymphoma/WM	Small lymphocytic, plasmacytoid
Prolymphocytic leukemia, B- and T-cell type	Small lymphocytic, plasmacytoid
Large granular lymphocytic leukemia	Small lymphocytic leukemia
Hairy cell leukemia	Hairy cell leukemia
Indolent lymphomas	
Follicle center cell lymphoma, follicular, small cell type (grade I)	Follicular, predominantly small cleaved cell
Marginal zone lymphoma, B-cell: 1. Extranodal (MALT) 2. Nodal (monocytoid) 3. Splenic	Small lymphocytic, diffuse, small cleaved cell or mixed small and large cell

CLL = chronic lymphocytic leukemia, WM = Waldenström's macroglobulinemia, MALT = mucosal-associated lymphatic tissue.

2. What are the recommended tests for evaluating (staging) a low-grade lymphoma?

Malignant lymphomas should be considered in the differential diagnosis of enlarged lymph nodes or spleen and also in patients with unexplained fever, weight loss, pruritus, or superior vena cava syndrome. Tests for diagnostic confirmation and staging of NHL include:

- Lymph node biopsy and histologic assessment
- History: presence of B symptoms (fever, night sweats, weight loss ≥ 10%), previous or current immunosuppressive illness (AIDS, organ transplant), previous radiation or chemotherapy
- Clinical assessment of adenopathy

- Radiologic studies: chest radiograph, chest CT scan (if chest radiograph abnormal), abdominal/pelvic CT scan
- Laboratory tests: complete blood count with differential and platelets, alkaline phosphatase, lactate dehydrogenase (LDH), uric acid, creatinine
- Optional procedures: bone marrow aspiration and biopsy (required for intermediate and high-grade NHLs), abdominal ultrasound (if obstruction suspected), bone scan and bone x-rays (if symptoms warrant), CNS CT or MRI (if neurologic symptoms present), splenectomy (if enlarged with cytopenias precluding chemotherapy)

3. What is meant by the stage of a low-grade lymphoma?

Patients with NHL are staged according to the Ann Arbor system originally developed for Hodgkin's disease. This schema emphasizes the distribution of nodal disease sites, the presence of disease above or below the diaphragm, the existence of systemic (B) symptoms, and the presence of extranodal disease.

4. Is there a better way than anatomic stage to predict the response to treatment and survival of patients with NHL?

The International Index prognostic factor model is useful specifically for patients with aggressive NHLs; however, a revised staging system for low-grade lymphomas, incorporating additional prognostic factors besides anatomic distribution of disease, has been developed by the National Cancer Institute:

Stage I: Localized nodal or extranodal disease; roughly equivalent to Ann Arbor stage I disease.

Stage II: Two or more nodal sites of disease or localized extranodal involvement plus draining nodes with *none* of the following characteristics present: Karnofsky performance status < 70, B symptoms, any mass > 10 cm in diameter, serum LDH > 500 IU or three or more extranodal sites of disease.

Stage III: Stage II plus any of the poor prognostic features mentioned above.

5. How important are immunophenotyping and chromosome analysis in the classification of NHLs?

Although an impressive amount of information is available about immunologic, genetic, and other molecular markers, they have little bearing on clinical management of the NHLs. Histologic subtype remains the most significant prognostic determinant; immunologic and molecular markers are most useful within this framework of more definitive identification of the various histologic subtypes. Genetic changes frequently involve genes controlling cell growth or sites of immunoglobulin heavy and light chain genes, especially on chromosomes 2, 14, and 22. The table below summarizes the most important immunophenotypic and genetic findings for the NHLs.

Summary of Immunophenotypic and Genetic Findings in Non-Hodgkin's Lymphomas

LYMPHOMA SUBTYPE	PAN-B	SIg	CD5	CD10	CD23	PAN-T	TdT	CYTOGENETIC FINDINGS
Small lymphocytic	+	+	+	–	+	–	–	+12; 13q14; 14q+
Follicular center cell	+	+	–	+	+/–	–	–	t(14:18) (*bcl*-2)
Marginal zone	+	+	–	–	–	–	–	+3
Diffuse large B-cell	+/–	+/–	–	–/+	+/–	–	–	t(14:18) *bcl*-2; 3q27 (*bcl*-6)
Mantle cell	+	+	+	–	–	–/+	–	t(11;14) (cyclin D1)
Small noncleaved cell	+	+	-	+	–	–	–	t(2;8); t(8;14); t(8;22) (c-*myc*)
Peripheral T-cell	–	–	+	–	–/+	+	–	t(2;5)
Lymphoblastic	–/+	–	+/–	–/+	–/+	+/–	+	Multiple

Pan-B = pan B-cell markers such as CD19, CD20; pan-T = pan T-cell markers such as CD2, CD3, CD7; SIg = surface immunoglobulin staining; TdT = terminal deoxynucleotidyl transferase.
+ = positive; – = negative; +/– = often positive but may be negative; –/+ = often negative but may be positive.
From Skarin AT, Dorfman DM: Non-Hodgkin's lymphomas: Current classification and management. Ca Cancer J Clin 47:351, 1997.

6. How common are the low-grade lymphomas? What is the most frequent subtype?

Overall, the NHLs make up about 3% of all cancers in the United States. Approximately 25% of NHLs are made up of the low-grade subtypes. Among these, the follicular and MALT (marginal zone) lymphomas are the most common (22% and 8%, respectively).

7. What is meant by *indolent* lymphomas?

The natural history of indolent lymphomas is measured in years (median survival: 6–8 yr). They respond readily to treatment, although they are seldom truly cured. Even in complete clinical remission, clonal excess (lymphocytes with abnormal immune or genetic markers) has been found in the blood of one-third of patients with NHL. Within the REAL classification, the indolent lymphomas include grade I follicle cell lymphoma and the more recently described marginal zone lymphomas.

8. What are follicle cell lymphomas?

Follicle cell lymphomas correspond to the term follicular lymphoma under the Working Formulation. They present primarily with widespread lymphadenopathy, showing a nodular (follicular) pattern of lymph node pathology and maintaining a superficially "normal" nodal architecture. Grade I follicle cell lymphoma (follicular small cleaved-cell lymphoma in the Working Formulation) is the most common indolent lymphoma. (See Figure 12, Color Plates.) Grade II and III follicle cell lymphomas (follicular mixed and follicular large cell) are grouped within the aggressive lymphomas (see chapter 33).

9. What are marginal zone B-cell lymphomas?

This recently identified entity was previously classified as small lymphocytic lymphoma under the Working Formulation. Characteristic histologic findings include a so-called "inverted follicular" appearance due to expansion of neoplastic monocytoid B-cells (lighter staining cells surrounding darker-staining normal germinal centers), which reverses the picture found in normal lymph node follicles. They afflict primarily older patients (median age: 65 years).

10. What are the so-called MALT lymphomas?

When marginal zone lymphomas involve mucosal extranodal sites, such as the GI tract, they are called mucosal-associated lymphatic tissue (MALT) lymphomas. Recent studies have shown an association between gastric low-grade MALT lymphomas and *Helicobacter pylori* infection in more than 90% of cases. Complete remission of the gastric lymphoma after eradication of *H. pylori* infection has been observed in 60–70% of cases.

11. What are the other types of marginal zone lymphomas?

When marginal zone lymphomas involve the lymph nodes, they are called monocytoid B-cell lymphomas, whereas those presenting primarily with massive spleen enlargement without lymphadenopathy are called splenic marginal zone lymphomas. The latter frequently exhibit associated diffuse bone marrow involvement, circulating abnormal lymphocytes with villous cytoplasmic projections, and a low level of paraproteinemia. Many patients previously described with primary malignant lymphoma of the spleen may fall into this category.

12. Is mantle cell lymphoma a low-grade lymphoma?

Although some references may list this type of NHL under the low-grade lymphomas, it is better placed within the aggressive lymphomas, because it responds poorly to therapy and has a survival period that is much shorter than patients with low-grade lymphomas (see chapter 33).

13. Why are the low-grade lymphomas approached differently from the aggressive lymphomas when it comes to treatment?

Low-grade lymphomas generally have an indolent course but are seldom cured, even with aggressive combination chemotherapy. Deferring initial treatment, as long as the patient is relatively asymptomatic, has no adverse effect on ultimate survival ("watchful waiting"). Treatment is geared to the goal of improving and preserving the quality of life by controlling symptoms due to lymphoma with minimal treatment-induced side effects and toxicity.

14. How are patients with localized NHL treated?

Localized (stage I and II) disease represents 15% of all low-grade lymphomas. It may be an exception to the general rule of incurability of NHLs. Regional radiation therapy with 35–45 Gy has led to 65–84% 5-year relapse-free survival rates, with the best overall survival in younger patients. The addition of chemotherapy has not been shown to improve these results and is not recommended.

15. What is the best way to start treatment in symptomatic Stage III and IV low-grade lymphomas?

Any treatment that reduces the tumor burden and thereby improves symptoms is associated with improved quality of life as long as the toxicity is kept low. Little evidence indicates that one chemotherapy agent is better than another in accomplishing these goals. Usually treatment is begun with an alkylating agent, such as chlorambucil or cyclophosphamide. The addition of prednisone is helpful in improving associated cytopenias and may improve general tolerance to the alkylating agent. A popular regimen also adds vincristine (cyclophosphamide, vincristine, and prednisone or CVP). Monitoring of blood glucose during initiation of prednisone is advised in elderly patients with a potential for hyperglycemia. Patients with large tumor burden or elevated uric acid need to be started on allopurinol. More aggressive combination regimens, such as cyclophosphamide, doxorubicin, Oncovin (vincristine), and prednisone (CHOP), are generally reserved for aggressive lymphomas or low-grade patients who have relapsed after initial milder regimens.

16. What about the role of newer agents such as fludarabine and 2CdA?

These newer drugs have shown promise in the initial management of low-grade lymphomas. Both fludarabine and 2CdA (2-chlorodeoxyadenosine) have shown complete remission rates of 50–80%, at times maintained for several years. Presently they are the treatment of choice for second-line therapy and may replace the initial use of alkylating agents. One advantage of these agents is that frequently only a brief course of treatment is necessary for producing a prolonged response. A word of caution is in order, however. 2CdA especially is known to reduce CD4+ lymphocytes and has been associated with increased susceptibility to opportunistic infections.

17. What is Richter's syndrome or transformation?

This term is applied to the development of an aggressive lymphoma, usually of diffuse large B-cell type, in patients with a history of low-grade lymphoma or chronic lymphocytic lymphoma. These new lymphomas tend to be more aggressive than de novo large cell lymphomas and respond poorly to treatment. A change in the patient's clinical course (i.e., rapid development of adenopathy) may signal Richter's transformation. Biopsy is generally performed to document transformation.

CONTROVERSIES

18. Does the addition of interferon improve the outlook for patients with low-grade lymphomas?

Although remissions can be obtained in low-grade lymphomas with interferon-alfa-2a alone, this agent is used primarily as an adjunct to chemotherapy. Several prospective, randomized trials have examined the role of interferon-alfa when added to combination chemotherapy in patients with advanced low-grade NHL. These studies found significant prolongation of remission; however, only one trial that continued maintenance interferon observed a significant prolongation of survival and a higher overall response rate. This benefit has to be weighed against the not insignificant toxicity of interferon, especially when given over a prolonged period. One approach is to initiate therapy, including interferon, but to consider discontinuation after maximum response has been obtained in patients who experience debilitating fatigue and malaise.

19. Is radiation therapy helpful in the treatment of advanced low-grade lymphomas?

Although the treatment of choice for stage I and II low-grade lymphomas is radiation therapy, its use for treatment of advanced disease is controversial. In a study from Stanford University, patients randomized to single-agent chemotherapy, combination chemotherapy, chemotherapy plus total nodal irradiation, involved field radiation, or low-dose total-body irradiation showed no differences in relapse-free survival or overall survival. Although not generally used for patients with advanced lymphoma, radiation may be considered for patients with residual bulky disease following chemotherapy.

20. What about high-dose therapy with stem cell rescue?

Although high-dose chemotherapy with or without total-body irradiation appears to have promise in selected patients with aggressive lymphomas and leukemias, its potential role in the treatment of low-grade lymphomas remains controversial. It is tempting to increase dose intensity since standard approaches have not led to significantly increased survival or cure. Ongoing trials are evaluating the role of high-dose therapy vs. standard therapy, but the long natural history of the disease has not allowed meaningful conclusions at this time. Until more definitive results are available, such high-dose regimens should be administered only within an approved clinical trial.

BIBLIOGRAPHY

1. Andersen JW, Smalley RV: Interferon alfa plus chemotherapy for non-Hodgkin's lymphoma: Five-year follow-up. N Engl J Med 329:1821, 1993.
2. Cole BF, Solal-Céligny P, Gelber RD, et al: Quality-of-life-adjusted survival analysis of interferon alfa-2b treatment for advanced follicular lymphoma: An aid to clinical decision making. J Clin Oncol 16:2339, 1998.
3. Freedman AS, Nadler LM: Non-Hodgkin's lymphoma. In Holland JF, Frei E, Bast RC, et al (eds): Cancer Medicine, 4th ed. Baltimore, Williams & Wilkins, 1997, pp 2757–2795.
4. Harris NL, Jaffe ES, Stein H, et al: A revised European-American classification of lymphoid neoplasms: A proposal from the International Lymphoma Study Group. Blood 84:1361, 1994.
5. Longo DL: The REAL classification of lymphoid neoplasms: One clinician's view. PPO Updates 9:1, 1995.
6. Neubauer A, Thiede C, Morgner A, et al: Cure of *Helicobacter pylori* infection and duration of remission of low-grade gastric mucosa-associated lymphoid tissue lymphoma. J Natl Cancer Inst 89:1350, 1997.
7. Non-Hodgkin's Lymphoma Classification Project: Effect of age on the characteristics and clinical behavior of non-Hodgkin's lymphoma patients. Ann Oncol 8:973, 1997.
8. Raich PC: The spleen in lymphoproliferative disease. In Bowdler AJ (ed): The Spleen: Structure, Function and Clinical Significance, 2nd ed. Totawa, NJ, Humana Press, 1998.
9. Shipp MA, Mauch PM, Harris NL: Non-Hodgkin's lymphoma. In DeVita VT, Hellman S, Rosenberg SA (eds): Cancer—Principles and Practice of Oncology, 5th ed. Philadelphia, Lippincott-Raven, 1997, pp 2165–2220.
10. Skarin AT, Dorfman DM: Non-Hodgkin's lymphomas: Current classification and management. Ca Cancer J Clin 47:351, 1997.
11. Thieblemont C, Bastion Y, Berger F, et al: Mucosa-associated lymphoid tissue gastrointestinal and non-gastrointestinal lymphoma behavior: Analysis of 108 patients. J Clin Oncol 15:1624, 1997.

33. AGGRESSIVE AND HIGHLY AGGRESSIVE NON-HODGKIN'S LYMPHOMA

David S. Hanson, M.D.

1. What are the most notable epidemiologic features of the non-Hodgkin's lymphomas (NHLs)?

Approximately 53,600 patients in the United States were diagnosed with NHLs in 1997. They remain lethal diseases; approximately 26,000 people died of NHLs in the U.S. in 1997. Although these numbers are relatively small, lymphomas show a steady age-dependent increase in incidence and are the most common cancer in adults aged 20–40. As such, they account for a large number of years of life lost. Consequently, NHLs rank fourth in economic impact among cancers in the U.S. Certain lymphoid neoplasms are more likely to occur in specific age groups. The aggressive lymphomas are the most common cancer in young adults, but the average age of onset is still 56. In contrast, Burkitt's, lymphoblastic, and diffuse large B-cell lymphoma are the most common lymphomas of childhood. Congenital and acquired immunodeficiencies are associated with the development of NHLs. A combination of chronic antigen stimulation and immune dysregulation seems to predispose patients to developing aggressive or highly aggressive NHLs. These lymphomas may be associated with Epstein-Barr virus (EBV) infection.

2. Specifically, which histologies are included in the aggressive and highly aggressive categories?

Aggressive Lymphomas
(untreated survival measured in months)

B-cell neoplasms	T/NK cell neoplasms
Diffuse large B-cell lymphoma	Anaplastic large cell lymphoma
	Peripheral T-cell lymphomas

Highly Aggressive Lymphomas
(untreated survival measured in weeks)

B-cell neoplasms	T/NK cell neoplasms
Precursor B-lymphoblastic leukemia/lymphoma	Precursor T-lymphoblastic leukemia/lymphoma
Burkitt's lymphoma	Adult T-cell lymphoma/leukemia (HTLV1+)

These diseases are grouped by their tendency to grow rapidly and disseminate. Their prognosis is unfavorable unless multiagent, combination chemotherapy or chemotherapy plus irradiation induces a sustained, complete remission. In general, if remission is sustained 2 years beyond completion of treatment, the likelihood of cure is high.

3. What is the usual clinical approach to staging a patient with an aggressive or highly aggressive lymphoma?

Staging involves a careful history and physical examination with attention to "B" symptoms (weight loss, fevers, night sweats). The physical examination should emphasize all lymph node regions (throat, neck, supraclavicular, axillary, and inguinal regions) as well as careful abdominal and neurologic examinations. Laboratory examination generally includes a complete blood count (CBC) with erythrocyte sedimentation rate (ESR) and evaluation of hepatic function, including alkaline phosphatase and measurement of lactic dehydrogenase (LDH). Renal function, electrolytes, and uric acid levels can be very important both before and during treatment. Radiographic studies often include a chest radiograph, chest/abdominal/pelvic computed tomography (CT) scanning, and possibly bone and/or gallium scanning. Patients with abnormal neurologic exams or patients at high risk for CNS involvement may require evaluation with magnetic resonance imaging (MRI). Bilateral bone marrow biopsies with aspirations provide important information in staging patients with lymphomas.

4. Why is staging of lymphoma important?

Staging is important prognostically and for making treatment decisions. For example, the patient with the prototype aggressive NHL, diffuse large cell lymphoma (DLCL), who has early-stage disease can be successfully treated with an abbreviated course of chemotherapy plus irradiation, whereas a patient with more advanced disease is treated with 6–8 courses of multiagent, combination chemotherapy. In addition, bone marrow involvement or highly aggressive histology may increase the risk of CNS involvement.

5. What pretreatment characteristics are associated with improved survival in patients with aggressive NHL?

- Younger age at diagnosis
- Lack of systemic B symptoms
- Superior performance status
- Normal serum (LDH)
- Normal serum B_2 microglobulin
- Number of nodal sites
- Lack of extranodal involvement
- Tumor bulk: mass < 10 cm
- Localized vs. advanced disease

6. Describe the general treatment approach for patients with aggressive and highly aggressive NHLs.

Most patients are treated with multiagent, combination chemotherapy with curative intent. Patients with early-stage aggressive NHL often can be treated with a brief course of chemotherapy followed by involved-field radiation therapy. Patients with more advanced disease commonly are treated with multiple cycles of doxorubicin-based combination chemotherapy with the intent of achieving a complete remission (CR). Patients are treated two or more cycles beyond CR (usually 6–8 cycles). Certain histologies mandate special treatment approaches. Burkitt's lymphoma requires aggressive combination chemotherapy with CNS prophylaxis. Lymphoblastic lymphoma is treated with a protracted series of treatments identical to those for acute lymphoblastic leukemia (induction, consolidation, and maintenance).

7. Name the usual sites and treatment approaches for patients with extranodal aggressive lymphomas.

- **Orbit and globe:** although aggressive lymphomas of the orbit are uncommon, combined modality therapy can be sight-sparing. Involvement of the eye itself is commonly associated with CNS involvement.
- **Bone:** patients are staged and generally treated with combined modality therapy.
- **Stomach:** resection may be appropriate if tumor burden is low and surgery is followed by chemotherapy. If a total gastrectomy is required, resection is usually not attempted and patients are treated with chemotherapy followed by radiation.
- **Testis:** inguinal orchiectomy often results in removal of all gross disease. Additional chemotherapy is required to achieve long-term survival. Testicular lymphoma cannot be treated solely with chemotherapy, as the testis is a sanctuary site.
- **CNS:** primary CNS lymphoma is almost always an aggressive B-cell lymphoma. Lesions usually are parenchymal and can be multifocal in about one-third of cases. Leptomeningeal involvement is also present in one-third of cases, although autopsy studies show a much higher frequency. Diagnosis generally requires stereotactic biopsy, because the majority of patients will not have an associated systemic lymphoma. Treatment is multimodal involving systemic and intrathecal chemotherapy and radiation therapy. Long-term survival is rare.

8. What is the most common aggressive lymphoma?

Diffuse large cell lymphoma (DLCL) is the most common aggressive NHL; approximately one-third of all lymphomas diagnosed in the U.S. are DLCL. Approximately 40% of patients with this histology enjoy long-term, disease-free survival.

9. What are the similarities and differences among the Burkitt's lymphomas?

Burkitt's lymphomas are the very aggressive small, noncleaved cell NHLs. (See Figure 13, Color Plates.) Endemic or African Burkitt's lymphoma is associated with Epstein-Barr virus (EBV) and the t(8;14) chromosomal translocation. The most common sites of involvement are the jaw and the orbit. Survival can be prolonged by treatment with cyclophosphamide. A sporadic form of Burkitt's lymphoma occurs in the U.S. and elsewhere in the world. The t(8;14) chromosomal translocation is commonly observed; however, this form is rarely associated with EBV. In contrast to African Burkitt's, the abdomen, GI tract, and bone marrow are most often involved. Treatment requires multiagent, combination chemotherapy and CNS prophylaxis.

10. Which highly aggressive lymphoma is also an acute leukemia?

Lymphoblastic lymphoma is also known as the precursor B- or precursor T-lymphoblastic leukemia/lymphoma. Patients commonly present with mediastinal masses, although involvement of the peripheral blood and/or bone marrow is seen. Such masses can become quite large and cause significant clinical problems, including superior vena cava syndrome (SVC), pleural and pericardial effusions, and pericardial tamponade. This is most often a disease of adolescent and young adult males.

11. Which very aggressive lymphoma is most strongly associated with a viral etiology?

Adult T-cell lymphoma/leukemia (ATL/L) is probably caused by the human T-cell leukemia virus type 1 (HTLV-1). The disease was described initially in Japan, but it is also endemic in the Caribbean. Patients present with a constellation of lymphadenopathy, organomegaly, hypercalcemia, bone lesions, and CNS involvement. Response to combination chemotherapy is usually poor; recent research efforts have been focused on monoclonal antibody treatments using radiolabelled immunoconjugates.

12. What are the clinical characteristics of the acquired immunodeficiency syndrome (AIDS)-related lymphomas?

AIDS- or human immunodeficiency virus (HIV)-related lymphomas are usually B-cell malignancies of the large cell or large cell immunoblastic and small noncleaved cell types. In addition to involvement of multiple lymph nodes, the lymphomas frequently involve extranodal sites. Patients whose initial complication of HIV infection is lymphoma are the best candidates for multiagent, combination chemotherapy. Although many patients respond to therapy, HIV increases the risk of cytopenias and infections. Primary CNS lymphoma tends to occur late in the setting of HIV infection. Patients are generally palliated with corticosteroids and radiation therapy, but survival remains short.

13. Are other immunodeficiency states associated with the development of lymphoma?

Congenital and acquired immunodeficiency states may predispose patients to the development of NHLs. States associated with the development of NHLs include ataxia-telangiectasia, Wiskott-Aldrich syndrome, severe combined immunodeficiency, common variable immunodeficiency, and X-linked lymphoproliferative syndrome. Autoimmune disorders, such as Hashimoto's thyroiditis and Sjögren's syndrome, may predispose patients to mucosa-associated lymphoid tissue (MALT) lymphomas. Thyroiditis also may result in aggressive B-cell lymphomas. Patients with nontropical sprue have an increased risk of enteropathy-associated T-cell lymphoma. Rheumatoid arthritis and systemic lupus erythematosus patients also may be at increased risk for contracting NHL, but their therapy often includes immunosuppressive treatment that can also predispose them to NHLs. Finally, patients who are immunodepressed as a result of organ transplantation have at least a 25-fold higher relative risk of developing a NHL. Of note, patients who can tolerate tapering of their immunosuppressive regimen may experience dimunition in their lymphoma, although this approach as sole treatment is rare.

BIBLIOGRAPHY

1. Blayney DW, et al: The human T-cell leukemia lymphoma virus associated with American adult T-cell leukemia/lymphoma. Blood 62:401, 1983.
2. Coleman CN, et al: Treatment of lymphoblastic lymphoma in adults. J Clin Oncol 4:1628, 1986.
3. Connors JM, et al: Brief chemotherapy and involved-field radiation therapy for limited stage aggressive lymphoma. Ann Intern Med 107:25, 1987.
4. Fisher RI, et al: Comparison of standard regimen (CHOP) with three intensive chemotherapy regimens for advanced non-Hodgkin's lymphoma. N Engl J Med 328:1002, 1993.
5. Harris NL, et al: A revised European-American classification of lymphoid neoplasms: A proposal from the International Lymphoma Study Group. Blood 84:1361, 1994.
6. Magrath IT, et al: An effective therapy for both undifferentiated (including Burkitt's) lymphomas and lymphoblastic lymphomas in children and young adults. Blood 63:1102, 1984.
7. National Cancer Institute Sponsored Study of Classifications of Non-Hodgkin's Lymphomas. Summary and description of a working formulation for clinical usage. Cancer 49:2112, 1982.
8. Yums JJ, et al: Distinctive chromosomal abnormalities in histologic subtypes of non-Hodgkins lymphomas. N Engl J Med 307:1231, 1982.

34. CUTANEOUS LYMPHOMAS

Jill Lacy, M.D.

1. Primary lymphomas of the skin comprise a heterogeneous group of tumors. What are the three major categories of cutaneous lymphomas?

1. Mycosis fungoides (MF)/Sézary syndrome complex (more recently termed cutaneous T-cell lymphoma [CTCL]): a low-grade T-cell lymphoma consisting predominantly of small lymphocytes that home to the skin and display the immunophenotype of mature helper (CD4+) lymphocytes.

2. T-cell lymphomas consisting of large cells, described as anaplastic, large cell, immunoblastic, or pleomorphic. These peripheral T-cell lymphomas often express an aberrant immunophenotype with loss of pan-T-cell antigens.

3. B-cell lymphomas that display the spectrum of histopathologies encountered in nodal lymphomas.

2. What is the natural history of CTCL?

CTCL is an indolent low-grade lymphoma, and most patients survive for years if not decades. However, the overwhelming majority of patients cannot be cured; thus, many ultimately die of complications related to lymphoma.

3. How do patients with CTCL typically present?

Before a definitive diagnosis of CTCL, most patients give a history of years of an intermittent pruritic eczematous skin disorder often misdiagnosed as eczema or other benign processes. This phase is referred to as the premycotic phase. As the disease progresses, eczematous lesions evolve into erythematous, indurated plaques, described as the plaque phase, at which time a definitive pathologic diagnosis on skin biopsy is usually possible. Most patients (70%) are diagnosed in the plaque phase.

4. Discuss the major pathologic features of CTCL.

CTCL is an epidermotropic tumor. Characteristic pathologic features include a bandlike infiltrate of atypical lymphoid cells in the upper dermis. Pautrier's abscess, a small collection of atypical lymphoid cells within the epidermis, is an important histologic feature that helps to confirm the diagnosis.

5. Describe the evolution and spread of CTCL.

Typically, plaque lesions increase in number and size to involve an increasing percentage of the body surface area. The plaques also increase in thickness, evolving into nodules or tumors that often ulcerate and become secondarily infected. As the disease progresses, lymph node involvement occurs, and overt visceral dissemination is present in most patients in the terminal stages of the disease. Although any visceral site may be involved with CTCL, common sites include bone marrow, liver, lung, and spleen.

6. Give the two major causes of death in patients with CTCL.

1. Progressive lymphoma, frequently after transformation to an intermediate- or high- grade T-cell malignancy
2. Infection secondary to breakdown of the normal skin barrier

7. The staging system recently adopted for CTCL is a modified TNM system based on the extent and nature of skin involvement (T), nodal involvement (N), visceral metastases (M), and blood involvement (B). Describe the categories of skin involvement.

T1: limited plaques (plaques involving < 10% of body surface area)
T2: generalized plaques

T3: cutaneous tumors
T4: generalized erythroderma

8. What is the importance of staging in CTCL?

Stage is a predictor of prognosis and influences treatment-related decisions. Over 90% of patients with stage I disease are alive at 5 years. In contrast, less than 50% of patients with stage IV disease survive 2 years. With respect to treatment, patients with disease limited to the skin can usually be managed with various topical therapies, whereas patients with visceral involvement may require systemic chemotherapy.

9. What is Sézary syndrome?

Sézary syndrome is a variant of CTCL in which patients present with or develop diffuse erythema of the skin (generalized erythroderma) in association with the presence of circulating malignant T cells or Sézary cells (> 10%) in the peripheral blood. Intense pruritus is characteristic of the generalized erythroderma and often results in severe excoriations and ulcerations. Approximately 15% of patients with CTCL actually present with Sézary syndrome.

10. What is the general approach to the treatment of patients with CTCL?

Because the major manifestations of CTCL are confined to the skin until the late stages of the disease, the approach to treatment has been the use of various skin-directed treatments to control cutaneous symptoms. The use of systemic chemotherapy in early-stage disease has not been shown to affect outcome and, thus, is not routinely used in initial management of CTCL.

11. What is an appropriate staging work-up in patients diagnosed with CTCL?

The initial staging evaluation should include a thorough physical examination, with special attention to assessing the extent of skin involvement and the presence of palpable lymph nodes. The peripheral blood should be examined carefully for the presence of circulating Sézary cells, and a chest radiograph should be obtained. Routine staging computed tomographic (CT) scans, bone marrow biopsies, and liver biopsies are not necessary unless signs and symptoms suggest visceral involvement.

12. Describe the topical therapies that are effective in the treatment of CTCL.

1. **Radiation therapy.** Because CTCL is exquisitely radiosensitive, radiation therapy is an effective treatment for control of cutaneous disease. Two types of radiation therapy are used. Electron beam radiation delivers a superficial dose of radiation and can be used to treat the total skin surface. Toxicities are limited to the skin (e.g., erythema, desquamation, hair loss, damaged

sweat glands) and usually subside after completion of therapy. Electron beam therapy is highly effective treatment for superficial cutaneous disease; the overall response rate to total skin electron beam therapy is nearly 100% (including complete and partial responders); > 90% of patients with limited plaque involvement attain complete remission. Traditional orthovoltage radiation is used to treat small fields ("spot" radiation) to control specific symptomatic tumors or thick plaques requiring more penetrating radiation.

2. **Topical chemotherapy.** The topical application of nitrogen mustard or carmustine (BCNU) is effective therapy for patients with plaque-stage disease. Treatment is applied daily to the entire skin until disease clearance (often 6–12 months), followed by maintenance therapy for 1–2 years. Toxicities include hypersensitivity reactions and secondary skin cancers with long-term usage.

3. **Psoralin ultraviolet A (PUVA) photochemotherapy.** PUVA therapy involves exposure to long-wave UVA light after oral ingestion of methoxypsoralen, a photosensitizing drug that covalently binds DNA and causes cell death after activation by UVA light. Treatment is given 3 times/week until disease clearance is achieved, followed by a tapering maintenance regimen. As with other topical therapies, results are best in patients without tumors or thick plaques. Acute toxicities include pruritus and "sunburn"; the major long-term complication is the development of secondary skin cancers.

13. What is photophoresis? What is its role in the treatment of CTCL?

Photophoresis (or extracorporeal photochemotherapy) is form of systemic therapy that involves the administration of oral methoxypsoralen followed by extracorporeal circulation of the blood with exposure of leukocytes to long-wave UVA light before reinfusion. This therapy is most effective in patients with erythroderma and/or Sézary syndrome.

14. What is the role of systemic chemotherapy in the treatment of CTCL?

Although systemic chemotherapy results in objective responses in approximately two-thirds of patients with CTCL, it is not curative. Furthermore, the addition of systemic chemotherapy to topical therapies does not improve the efficacy of topical therapy alone. Thus, the role of systemic chemotherapy is limited to palliation of symptoms that cannot be controlled with topical therapy. Patients with advanced cutaneous disease, symptomatic nodal or visceral involvement, or Sézary syndrome can derive palliation from various single agents or combinations of drugs, including alkylating agents, methotrexate, etoposide, doxorubicin, prednisone, bleomycin, cis-platinum, and fludarabine. In addition, multidrug chemotherapy regimens are appropriate in the setting of transformation to a high-grade T-cell lymphoma.

15. Is interferon effective in the treatment of CTCL?

Yes. Interferon has good activity against CTCL, including disease refractory to other therapies. The combination of PUVA with interferon is highly effective in preliminary studies and is a promising new treatment strategy.

16. What novel systemic therapies have been used recently in the treatment of CTCL?
- Retinoids
- Interleukin-2 (IL-2) fusion toxin
- Cyclosporine
- Monoclonal antibodies

17. How do the B- and T-cell lymphomas of the skin, excluding mycosis fungoides, usually present?

Patients with nonmycosis fungoides cutaneous lymphoma usually present with skin nodules, tumors, or plaques that are reddish or violaceous in color.

18. Is the approach to the work-up and management of nonmycosis fungoides lymphomas of the skin different from the approach to extracutaneous lymphomas?

No. Although the nonmycosis fungoides cutaneous lymphomas comprise a heterogeneous group of tumors, they are best managed by the same principles that guide the management of typical extracutaneous non-Hodgkin's lymphoma. Thus, patients should have an adequate biopsy to confirm the diagnosis, with immunophenotyping, if possible, and a complete staging evaluation, with a body CT scan and bone marrow biopsies. The appropriate treatment modality (radiation, chemotherapy, or both) is dictated by the pathologic subtype and grade as well as the stage. Thus, a patient with an intermediate-grade diffuse large-cell lymphoma of the skin should be treated with multidrug chemotherapy. In contrast, a patient with a low-grade follicular small cleaved cell lymphoma restricted to the skin (stage I) should be treated with involved field radiation therapy.

BIBLIOGRAPHY

1. Abel EA, Sendagorta E, Hoppe RT, Hu CH: PUVA treatment of erythrodermic and plaque-type mycosis fungoides: 10-year follow-up study. Arch Dermatol 123:897–901, 1987.
2. Abel EA, Wood GS, Hoppe RT: Mycosis fungoides: Clinical and histologic features, staging, evaluation, and approach to treatment. CA Cancer J Clin 43:93–115, 1993.
3. Axelrod PI, Lorber B, Vonderheid EC: Infections complicating mycosis fungoides and Sézary syndrome. JAMA 267:1354–1358, 1992.
4. Bunn PA Jr, Lamberg SI: Report of the committee on staging and classification of cutaneous T-cell lymphoma. Cancer Treat Rep 63:725–728, 1979.
5. Diamandidou E, Cohen PR, Kurzrock R: Mycosis fungoides and Sézary syndrome. Blood 88:2385–2409, 1996.
6. Edelson R, Berger C, Gasparro R, et al: Treatment of cutaneous T-cell lymphoma by extra-corporeal photochemotherapy: Preliminary results. N Engl J Med 316:297–303, 1987.
7. Hoppe RT, Abel EA, Deneau DG, Price NM: Mycosis fungoides: Management with topical nitrogen mustard. J Clin Oncol 5:1796–1803, 1987.
8. Jones GW, Hoppe RT, Glatstein E: Electron beam treatment for cutaneous T-cell lymphoma. Hematol Oncol Clin North Am 9:1057–1076, 1995.
9. Kaye FJ, Bunn PA, Steinberg SM, et al: A randomized trial comparing combination electron-beam radiation and chemotherapy with topical therapy in the initial treatment of mycosis fungoides. N Engl J Med 321:1784–1790, 1989.
10. Kuzel TM, Roenigk HH, Samuelson E, et al: Effectiveness of interferon alpha 2A combined with phototherapy for mycosis fungoides and the Sézary syndrome. J Clin Oncol 13:257–263, 1995.
11. Lambert WC: Premycotic eruptions. Dermatol Clin 3:629–645, 1985.
12. Wieselthier JS, Koh HK: Sézary syndrome: Diagnosis, prognosis, and critical review of treatment options. J Am Acad Dermatol 22:381–401, 1990.
13. Wood GS, Burke JS, Horning S, et al: The immunologic and clinicopathologic heterogeneity of cutaneous lymphomas other than mycosis fungoides. Blood 62:464–472, 1983.

35. MULTIPLE MYELOMA

Jeffrey V. Matous, M.D.

1. What is multiple myeloma?

Multiple myeloma is a disease that results from the clonal proliferation of malignant B-cells (plasma cells) at various stages of differentiation. It is almost always accompanied by the presence in the serum and/or urine of monoclonal immunoglobulin or immunoglobulin fragments (IgG, IgM, IgA, IgD, IgE, or kappa/lambda light chains), because the clone synthesizes a specific immunoglobulin that has either a kappa or lambda light chain—i.e., is light-chain restricted.

2. What is important about the biology of multiple myeloma?

Controversy exists as to the cellular origin of myeloma, which is thought to be an early hematopoietic stem cell disorder (at least as far back as pre-B cells), because plasma cells are incapable of differentiation. Several cytokines, such as IL-6, Il-1, Il-3, and TNF-B, may be important in the proliferation and differentiation of malignant B-cells.

3. What is the epidemiology of multiple myeloma?

In the United States approximately 14,000 cases are diagnosed annually. Multiple myeloma makes up about 1% of all cancers, and its incidence (~ 1/100,000) may be increasing. It is commonly believed that myeloma is a disease of the elderly, but the mean age for myeloma in both men and women is about 61 years. Over one-third of myeloma cases are diagnosed in patients < 60 years. Only 3% of cases occur in patients < 40 years. The incidence is highest in African-American males.

Risk factors for the development of myeloma include previous diagnosis of a monoclonal gammopathy (monoclonal gammopathy of undetermined significance [MGUS]), exposure to radiation or petroleum products, and possibly genetic predisposition.

4. What are characteristic clinical presentations of multiple myeloma?

Patients with advanced stages of myeloma have many or most of the following clinical features:

- Plasmacytosis of the bone marrow
- Anemia
- Lytic bone lesions
- Renal abnormalities
- Hypercalcemia
- Infections
- Elevated monoclonal (M) proteins in the serum and/or urine

Panhypogammaglobulinemia also may be present at diagnosis. The combination of **bone pain and anemia** always must raise the suspicion of myeloma.

5. How does one diagnose multiple myeloma?

Because malignant B-cell disorders such as myeloma may be quite heterogeneous, diagnostic criteria that help to distinguish myeloma from other clonal abnormalities of mature B and plasma cells have been developed. One example is the Durie and Salmon diagnostic system:

Major Criteria

1. Plasmacytomas on tissue biopsy
2. Bone marrow plasmacytosis ≥ 30%
3. Monoclonal immunoglobulin spike in serum (by electrophoresis) of > 3.5 g/dl for IgG, > 2.0 g/dl for IgA, or kappa or lambda light chain excretion of > 1.0 g/day on a 24-hour urine collection by electrophoresis and immunofixation

Minor Criteria

a. Bone marrow plasmacytosis between 10% and 30%
b. Monoclonal immunoglobulin spike present, but less than that mandated by the major criteria
c. Lytic bone lesions
d. Depressed levels of normal immunoglobulins

Any one of the following set of criteria confirms the diagnosis:

- Any two major criteria
- Major criterion 1 plus minor criterion b, c, or d
- Major criterion 3 plus minor criterion a or c
- Minor criteria a, b, and c or a, b, and d

To properly evaluate a patient for possible myeloma, the following diagnostic tests are indicated:

- Skeletal survey to screen for lytic bone lesions
- Bone marrow biopsy and aspirate, complete blood count
- 24-hour urine collection for protein electrophoresis and immunofixation
- Serum protein electrophoresis and immunofixation
- Determination of serum calcium, creatinine, quantitative immunoglobulins, uric acid

It is important to understand that the presence of a monoclonal immunoglobulin protein or M-protein in the serum is **not** sufficient to make a diagnosis of myeloma. It is relatively common to find M-proteins in the serum; they are stable and occur without other signs of myeloma. This is referred to as monoclonal gammopathy of undetermined significance (MGUS). Other B-cell lymphoproliferative diseases may produce M-proteins. Examples are: chronic lymphocytic leukemia (CLL), Waldenström's macroglobulinemia, lymphoma, amyloidosis, and a disease known as smoldering myeloma.

6. How is multiple myeloma staged?

Most staging systems estimate tumor burden. The Durie-Salmon staging system is used most often. Stage is ascertained by the level of M-protein, number of lytic lesions, degree of anemia, and serum calcium level (I, II, and III from lower to higher tumor burden). Patients are further divided based on normal (A) or abnormal (B) serum creatinine.

Perhaps more important than assessing myeloma tumor burden is recognizing certain other prognostic factors, such as the level of B2-microglobulin (level > 4 mg/ml is worse) and the plasma cell labeling index (a reflection of plasma cell DNA synthesis; higher is worse). For example, myeloma patients with a normal B2-microglobulin level and plasma cell labeling index treated with standard therapy have a median survival of 6 years. Certain karyotypic findings, such as the deletions of chromosome 13 or 11q abnormalities, indicate a poor outcome for such patients with myeloma. Samples of the bone marrow at presentation are increasingly submitted for karyotypic analysis.

7. What are plasmacytomas?

Plasmacytomas are solid tumors of monoclonal plasma cells similar to those found in the bone marrow. They may be solitary (i.e., diagnostic criteria of myeloma not met) and may occur in either bone or soft tissue. Approximately one-half of patients diagnosed with a solitary plasmacytoma of the bone will develop multiple myeloma. Solitary plasmacytomas are treated with radiotherapy.

8. What clinical problems may be encountered in patients with multiple myeloma?

Hypercalcemia. Hypercalcemia occurs in up to one-third of myeloma patients through a variety of mechanisms. Symptoms include polyuria, constipation, confusion, nausea and vomiting, and lethargy. Therapy must be instituted promptly with fluids, diuresis, and bisphosphonates such as pamidronate.

Lytic bone lesions. Radionuclide bone scans do not show the lytic lesions of myeloma, and plain films are less sensitive than magnetic resonance imaging (MRI) in detecting early lytic lesions. Attention to sites of impending pathologic fracture is imperative. The regular administration of bisphosphonates may be effective in decreasing or delaying skeletal-related complications such as pain or fracture. At times, preventive orthopedic surgery is indicated to prevent a disabling fracture. **Pain must not be undertreated.**

Renal complications. Renal failure results from any combination of the following in myeloma patients: light chain deposition, hypercalcemia, hyperuricemia, infections, plasma cell infiltration, or amyloid protein deposition.

Infections. Myeloma patients are immunocompromised. Reasons include: suppression of normal immunoglobulins, T-cell cell mediated immune defects, and the immune suppressing effects of the therapy. Where possible, immediate treatment of any suspected infections is required. Vaccinating such patients is rarely successful.

Neurologic disease. First, spinal cord compression should be suspected in any myeloma patient with severe back pain and/or any neurologic signs or symptoms. An MRI should be done promptly and therapy instituted immediately (radiation, dexamethasone, and rarely surgery) if cord compression is found. Second, paraproteins may infiltrate peripheral nerves and cause sensory and motor neuropathies.

9. What various therapies are used to treat multiple myeloma?

Presently, all therapy of multiple myeloma is considered palliative—with the possible exception of allogeneic stem cell transplantation, curative therapy does not exist.

For decades, treatment with the oral alkylating agent melphalan in combination with prednisone (MP) was the standard of care. On average, this regimen extends survival in myeloma patients from 7–9 months to about 30 months. It is well tolerated, even in elderly patients.

Several attempts have been made to improve MP. Strategies usually involve adding or substituting different drugs, such as vinca alkaloids (vincristine or vinblastine), cyclophosphamide, bleomycin and carmustine (BCNU), or doxorubicin. In most clinical situations, combination chemotherapy treatment with several of these drugs results in a higher response of tumor shrinkage and, in selected patient populations, prolonged survival.

One inherent difficulty posed by myeloma cells is their tendency to develop resistance to standard chemotherapy drugs. Resistance is often mediated by the multidrug resistance (MDR) gene, which encodes for a glycoprotein that effectively "pumps out" certain chemotherapy drugs. Other forms of drug resistance exist. Sometimes resistance may be overcome by increasing the dose(s) of the chemotherapeutic agents. Normally, the dose of chemotherapy drugs is limited by the ability of the patient's own bone marrow to recover from the myelotoxic effects of the drugs. Higher, myeloablative doses of chemotherapy and sometimes irradiation may be used to treat myeloma. Hematopoietic stem cells (which have been previously collected from the patient or another donor) are administered immediately following therapy in order to rescue the patient's marrow from the myeloablative doses. Autologous (patient's own stem cells) stem cell transplantation is most often used in multiple myeloma to support more intensive therapy. It has been shown to be highly effective both in newly diagnosed patients and in those with recurrent disease, significantly extending the median survival compared to standard-dose chemotherapy treatment alone. Younger patients may be considered for allogeneic (donor stem cells) transplantation.

Another strategy to overcome drug resistance in myeloma is presently being tested. It involves agents that inhibit gene products that directly mediate drug resistance given with chemotherapy drugs. The efficacy of this approach has not yet been proved.

BIBLIOGRAPHY

1. Durie BGM, Salmon SE: Clinical staging system for multiple myeloma: Correlation of measured myeloma cell mass with presenting clinical features, response to cell mass with presenting clinical features, response to treatment, and survival. Cancer 36:842–854, 1975.
2. Greipp PR, Lust JA, O'Fallon M, et al: Plasma cell labeling index and b2-microglobulin predict survival independent of thymidine kinase and C-reactive protein in multiple myeloma. Blood 81:3382–3387, 1993.
3. Bataille R, Harousseau JL: Multiple myeloma. N Engl J Med 336:1657–1664, 1997.
4. Berenson JR, Lichtenstein A, Porter L, et al: Long-term pamidronate treatment of advanced multiple myeloma patients reduces skeletal events. J Clin Oncol 16:593–602, 1998.
5. Tricot G, Barlogie B, Jagnath S, et al: Poor prognosis in multiple myeloma is associated only with partial or complete deletions of chromosome 13 or abnormalities involving 11q and not other karyotype abnormalities. Blood 86:4250–4256, 1995.
6. Alexanian R, Dimopoulos M: The treatment of multiple myeloma. N Engl J Med 330:484–489, 1994.
7. Gahrton G, Tura S, Ljungman P, et al: Allogeneic bone marrow transplantation in multiple myeloma. N Engl J Med 325:1267–1273, 1991.
8. Attal M, Harousseau JL, Stoppa AM, et al: Autologous bone marrow transplantation versus conventional chemotherapy in multiple myeloma: A prospective, randomized trial. N Engl J Med 335:91–97, 1996.
9. Boccadoro M, Pileri A: Diagnosis, prognosis, and standard treatment of multiple myeloma. Hematol Oncol Clin North Am 11:111–131, 1997.
10. Kyle RA: Monoclonal gammopathy of undetermined significance and solitary plasmacytoma: Implications for progression to overt multiple myeloma: Hematol Oncol Clin North Am 11:71–87, 1997.

36. HODGKIN'S DISEASE

David H. Garfield, M.D., Kelly C. Mack, R.N., M.S.N., A.O.C.N.

1. Who gets Hodgkin's disease?

Although Hodgkin's disease (HD) may occur at any age, the classic bimodal age distribution shows one peak at 20–29 years (mainly of the nodular sclerosis [NS] histology) and a second peak at 60 years or older (mainly of the lymphocyte-depleted [LD] histology). Despite male predominance in children under age 10 years, the sex distribution becomes nearly equal at the two age peaks. In the United States, Caucasians account for more than 90% of all cases. The disease is also associated with small family size, high standard of living, and high level of maternal education. The incidence is increasing in whites and males and is 3/100,000 annually. The incidence is decreasing in females.

2. What cells are found in biopsies of patients with Hodgkin's disease?

The minority of cells (1%) include Reed-Sternberg (RS) cells and RS variants, which are considered to be the malignant cells. Host inflammatory cells comprise the background (90+% of all cells seen) and include lymphocytes, macrophages, granulocytes, and eosinophils. These cells appear in response to cytokines liberated by RS cells.

3. What is the Reed-Sternberg cell?

Reed-Sternberg (RS) cells are giant cells with two or more nuclear lobes and huge eosinophilic, inclusionlike nucleoli. The classic RS cell has a symmetrical, mirror-image nucleus that creates the "owl-eye" appearance. (See Figure 14, Color Plates.) They are altered B-cells, clones of neoplastic cells that, by secreting cytokines, not only cause the symptoms of Hodgkin's disease, but also promote their own growth and evade immune surveillance. Classic RS cells produce at least 12 cytokines. IL-1, IL-6, and/or tumor necrosis factor (TNF) could account for the "B" or other constitutional symptoms. The eosinophils of mixed cellularity Hodgkin's disease (MC) could be produced by IL-5 and the fibrosis of nodular sclerosing Hodgkin's disease (NS) by transforming growth factor beta (TGF-β) and/or platelet-derived growth factor. The lymphopenia in lymphocyte-depleted Hodgkin's disease (LD) could be produced by TNF or TGF-β. Lymphocyte and histiocyte (L&H) cells, which are RS variants, may not produce these cytokines and growth factors, explaining why lymphocyte-predominant Hodgkin's disease (LP) is usually asymptomatic and slow-growing. Variants or precursors of RS cells can also be identified. The lacunar cell, a small variant of the RS cell, is seen in nodular sclerosis histology. It is an artifact of cell fixation. L&H cells are seen most often in LP.

RS cells and variants, which have the phenotype of activated lymphoid cells, express antigens Ki-1 (CD30), Leu-M1 (CD15), HLA-DR, Tac (CD25), and T9 (transferrin receptor). Leukocyte common antigen (LCA or CD45), which is absent in most cases of Hodgkin's disease, helps to distinguish Hodgkin's disease from non-Hodgkin's lymphoma (NHL). L&H cells, on the other hand, are CD30- and CD15-negative but CD20- and CD45-RA-positive.

4. Are Reed-Sternberg cells found only in Hodgkin's disease?

No. RS cells have been seen rarely in other types of cancer (e.g., breast and lung cancer, melanoma); they also have been seen in certain inflammatory states (e.g., myositis, infectious mononucleosis). RS cells are diagnostic for Hodgkin's disease only in the proper **histologic** setting. The diagnosis cannot be made without the presence of RS cells. However, the disease may be diagnosed in the bone marrow without Reed-Sternberg cells in the appropriate **clinical** setting.

5. Describe the four histologic types of Hodgkin's disease, incidence, and classic clinical presentations.

The original classification by Lukes et al. of the histopathology of Hodgkin's disease has been revised according to the Rye classification:

1. In **lymphocyte-predominant** Hodgkin's disease (5–10%), the affected tissue consists primarily of small lymphocytes and benign epithelioid histiocytes. Two subtypes, nodular (80%) and diffuse (20%), are seen. Classic RS cells are rare, but the unusual variants, lymphocytic and histiocytic (L&H), are prominent. It may be confused with non-Hodgkin's lymphoma (NHL). The median age is in the mid 30s. The male-to-female ratio is 3:1. It most commonly presents in peripheral nodes and spares the mediastinum. Patients most often present with early-stage disease; 75% are stages I, II. Ninety percent of all patients are alive 10 years after diagnosis. Late relapses are most common with LP. The cause of death is often other cancers.

2. **Nodular sclerosis** (NS) is the most frequent (40–60%) histologic type in the United States. Hematoxylin and eosin stains show eosinophilic collagen bands of varying width surrounding

blue lymphoid nodules. (See Figure 15, Color Plates.) Some cells may seem to be sitting within a cleared area. These are lacunar variants of the RS cell. NS has been subdivided into grades I (80%) and II (20%). Grade II, which shows areas of lymphocytic depletion or numerous pleomorphic RS giant cells, has a worse prognosis than grade I upon relapse. The background cells of NS are lymphocytes, eosinophils, histiocytes, neutrophils, and plasma cells; necrosis is common. Most RS cells are lacunar and abundant in number rather than classic type. The peak incidence is in adolescents and young adults. The disease usually presents above the diaphragm, especially the mediastinum.

3. **Mixed cellularity** is the second most common type (15–30%). Classic RS cells are seen, along with reactive histiocytes, eosinophils, neutrophils, plasma cell, small lymphocytes, and small foci of necrosis. There is usually only focal or partial involvement of lymph nodes. The infiltrates are diffuse and numerous. Classic RS cells are numerous, with the same background cells as in NS. It is seen at any age with no early adult peak. It is less common in the mediastinum, and more common in the spleen and abdominal nodes.

4. **Lymphocyte-depleted** disease (less than 1%), as the name suggests, is characterized by depletion of lymphocytes, hypocellularity, and, frequently, fibrosis and focal necrosis. Classic RS cells are numerous, but there are few inflammatory cells. LD is most common in older patients, people with AIDS, and third-world countries. It often presents in an advanced stage. Before immunophenotyping studies were available, many cases were, in reality, large cell NHLs, often of the anaplastic type. This variant may be associated with a febrile wasting syndrome, presenting often with subdiaphragmatic involvement and bone-marrow infiltration, but without peripheral nodes. The response rate is the same as those with the other three types of HD.

Immunophenotyping is only an adjunct. It is not always necessary to perform except in difficult cases.

6. What causes Hodgkin's disease?

The cause is unknown. Investigators have long argued that Hodgkin's disease may not even be a malignancy. The clustering of childhood cases and cases within families suggests an infectious etiology. A viral etiology has been proposed, and DNA of the Epstein-Barr virus (EBV) has been found in RS cells of some patients with Hodgkin's disease (NS—40%, MC—70%). Subsequent studies have disputed these theories.

Although chromosomal translocations are common in NHL and are thought to play a role in pathogenesis, no consistent chromosomal abnormalities (except hyperdiploid RS cells) can be demonstrated in Hodgkin's disease. The majority of RS cells have immunologic gene rearrangement and are clonal.

7. How does the clinical presentation of Hodgkin's disease differ from that of non-Hodgkin's lymphoma?

Hodgkin's disease commonly presents as cervical adenopathy, which may remain isolated or spread to contiguous lymph-node groups. NHL does not present with this characteristic contiguous spread. Generalized lymphadenopathy is a rare presentation for Hodgkin's disease but is commonly seen in NHL, especially low-grade.

When found above the diaphragm, Hodgkin's disease is often limited to the supradiaphragmatic area. If first identified only below the diaphragm (unusual), the disease is more often widely disseminated. Similar statements are **not** true for NHL.

Hodgkin's disease may present in the adolescent or young adult as a large mediastinal mass. High-grade histologies of NHL may have similar presentations.

Bulky abdominal adenopathy, especially in the mesentary, or involvement of Waldeyer's ring suggests NHL rather than Hodgkin's disease.

8. What signs or symptoms may suggest the diagnosis of Hodgkin's disease?

Patients with Hodgkin's disease may complain of generalized pruritus and, rarely, may describe lymph node pain with alcohol ingestion. Generally patients are anergic; thus, they do not respond to normal skin antigens such as mumps and candida. If previously positive for tuberculosis skin tests, they may become negative.

9. What are B symptoms in the staging of Hodgkin's disease?
B symptoms, which are specific and prognostic, include:
- Unexplained fever of 101° F (38.5° C) or higher
- Drenching night sweats
- Loss of more than 10% of body weight in the previous 6 months

10. Describe the staging evaluation and classification of a patient with Hodgkin's disease.

Recommended Steps for Staging Evaluation of Patients with Hodgkin's Disease

History and examination
  B symptoms: weight loss > 10% during previous 6 months, documented fever, night sweats
  Detailed physical examination

Radiology
  Plain chest radiograph
  Computed tomography (CT) of thorax, abdomen, and pelvis

Hematology
  Full blood count
  Erythrocyte sedimentation rate
  Bone marrow biopsy, bilateral (unless clinical stage [CS] IA or IIA)

Biochemistry
  Tests of liver function
  Albumin, lactate dehydrogenase (LDH), calcium

Other imaging techniques
  Isotope scanning
    Gallium: usually, especially with mediastinal or periaortic disease
    MUGA (multiple-gated acquisition blood-pool scan): only if Adriamycin is being considered and
      there is a question of heart disease

Under special circumstances
  Magnetic resonance imaging (MRI)
  Bipedal lymphangiogram (LAG): only if pathologic staging (PS) is contemplated
  Technetium bone scan: if bone metastases suspected (unusual)

In 1989 an international interdisciplinary committee modified the Ann Arbor staging classification. This modification, called the Cotswold recommendations, gives due importance to computed tomography scans and other imaging modalities in defining the extent of disease.

Cotswold Staging Classification (Modified Ann Arbor)

STAGE	FEATURES
I	Involvement of a single lymph node region or lymphoid structure (e.g., spleen, thymus, Waldeyer's ring)
II	Involvement of 2 or more lymph node regions on the same side of the diaphragm. The mediastinum is a single site; hilar lymph nodes are lateralized. The number of anatomic sites should be indicated by a subscript (e.g., II_3).
III	Involvement of lymph node regions or structures on both sides of the diaphragm. III_1: with or without splenic, hilar, celiac, or portal nodes III_2: with paraaortic, iliac, or mesenteric nodes

Table continued on following page.

Cotswold Staging Classification (Modified Ann Arbor) (Continued)

STAGE		FEATURES
IV		Involvement of extranodal site(s) beyond that designated E
	A	No symptoms
	B	Fever, drenching sweats, weight loss
	X	Bulky disease
		> $^1/_3$ widening of mediastinum
		> 10 cm maximal dimension of nodal mass
	E	Involvement of a single extranodal side, contiguous or proximal to known nodal site
	CS	Clinical stage
	PS	Pathologic state

11. What are the current views regarding staging laparotomy?

Occult Hodgkin's disease is discovered at laparotomy in at least 25% of patients with only supradiaphragmatic disease on clinical evaluation. The controversy about staging laparotomy can be eased by the philosophy that laparotomy should be avoided unless the findings will change treatment significantly.

Staging laparotomy is to be considered:

For patients with clinical stage I, II, and III$_1$A disease when radiation therapy alone is being considered. Such patients, however, may benefit from combined modality treatment if excessive splenic (> 4 nodules) or upper periaortic nodes are found at laparotomy.

Staging laparotomy is not recommended:

1. For patients with clear CS IIIB or IV disease who are scheduled for chemotherapy.
2. For patients with a bulky mediastinal mass (> $^1/_3$ the diameter of the chest); they benefit most from combined modality treatment.
3. For patients with isolated high right cervical or nonbulky mediastinal involvement with nodular sclerosing Hodgkin's disease who may be managed by mantle or subtotal nodal radiation alone. If CS IA, LP, only above diaphragm, mantle radiotherapy may be sufficient. This also may apply to LP, CS IIA.
4. For CS IA females and CS IIA females ≤ 26 years of age with limited nodal disease. CS IA patients with LP may be candidates for radiotherapy alone, avoiding staging laparotomy since occult infradiaphragmatic involvement is seen in only 4% of patients. The remainder of CS IIA and all CS IB and IIB (80% of all CS I and II patients) have a risk of approximately 30%.

12. What treatment modalities are available for Hodgkin's disease? What are the current recommendations?

The three treatment modalities available for Hodgkin's disease are radiation therapy, combination chemotherapy, and combined modality treatment (CMT = radiation and chemotherapy). The current recommendations for the various stages are as follows:

Stage IA/IIA	Mantle or subtotal nodal irradiation; mantle irradiation for LP
Stage IB/IIB	Combination chemotherapy and/or mantle or extended-field radiotherapy, depending on whether CS or PS as well as other prognostic features
CS III$_1$A	Combination chemotherapy with or without extended-field radiotherapy
CS III$_2$A	Combination chemotherapy
Bulky mediastinal disease	CMT
Stages IIIB/IV	Combination chemotherapy

13. Describe the four different fields of radiation used in Hodgkin's disease.

 1. **Mantle** is for above the diaphragm only, used most often with LP.

 2. **Subtotal nodal or lymphoid radiation** consisting of mantle and spade fields is commonly used for stages IA, IIA, and PS IB and IIB.

 3. **Total nodal or lymphoid radiation** consisting of mantle and inverted-Y fields is used for stages IIB and IIIA (rarely, if ever, used for either).

 4. **Involved-field radiation** is only for sites of known disease and is commonly used in combination with chemotherapy.

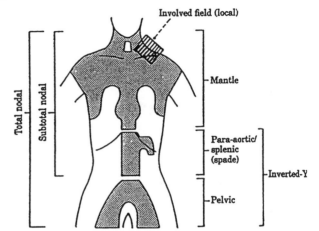

Radiation fields used in Hodgkin's disease.

14. Is the chemotherapy used in Hodgkin's disease the same regardless of stage?

The choice of chemotherapy should be individualized to the patient and stage of disease. Patients who desire to preserve fertility should avoid MOPP (the combination of nitrogen mustard, Oncovin, prednisone, and procarbazine). Patients receiving CMT for bulky mediastinal disease should avoid ABVD (the combination of Adriamycin, bleomycin, vinblastine, and dacarbazine) because of the added pulmonary and cardiac toxicity of radiation combined with bleomycin and Adriamycin. Newer studies are attempting to identify less toxic regimens of combination chemotherapy to be used with involved-field radiation for lower-stage (I and II) disease. In general, ABVD is now preferred over MOPP when chemotherapy is given.

Common Chemotherapeutic Regimens Used in Hodgkin's Disease

REGIMEN	RECOMMENDED DOSE (mg/m^2)*	ROUTE	CYCLE DAYS†
1. MOPP			
Mechlorethamine	6	Intravenous	1 and 8
Oncovin (vincristine)	1.4 (maximum: 2.0)	Intravenous	1 and 8
Procarbazine	100	Oral	1–14
Prednisone	40	Oral	1–14
2. ABVD			
Adriamycin (doxorubicin)	25	Intravenous	1 and 15
Bleomycin	10	Intravenous	1 and 15
Vinblastine	6	Intravenous	1 and 15
Dacarbazine	375	Intravenous	1 and 15
3. MOPP–ABVD in alternating monthly cycles	As for MOPP and ABVD above		

Table continued on following page.

Common Chemotherapeutic Regimens Used in Hodgkin's Disease (Continued)

REGIMEN	RECOMMENDED DOSE (mg/m²)*	ROUTE	CYCLE DAYS†
4. MOPP–ABV hybrid Sometimes used when dacarbazine not readily available (6 cycles, every 28 days, total)			
Mechlorethamine	6	Intravenous	1
Vincristine	1.4 (maximum: 2.0)	Intravenous	1
Procarbazine	100	Oral	1–7
Prednisone	40	Oral	1–14
Doxorubicin	35	Intravenous	8
Bleomycin	10	Intravenous	8
Vinblastine	6	Intravenous	8
5. ChlVPP (For patients with better prognosis, i.e., LP or older patients)			
Chlorambucil	6	Oral	1–14
Vinblastine	6	Intravenous	1 and 8
Procarbazine	100	Oral	1–14
Prednisone	40	Oral	1–14

* Per square meter of body surface area.
† Each cycle lasts 28 days; 6 cycles recommended for 1 through 5.

15. What can be done for the patient who relapses after primary treatment?

If the primary treatment is radiation therapy, the patient should receive combination chemotherapy. Of patients salvaged with chemotherapy after radiation therapy, 50% can be cured with the initial regimen.

If the patient relapses after combination chemotherapy, the interval from treatment to relapse should be considered. Some investigators argue that patients who relapse more than 1 year after treatment is completed may not have received dose-intensive therapy. Such patients may be treated with the same regimen that they initially received. Patients who relapse less than 1 year after treatment should be considered to have aggressive disease and receive a regimen of drugs different (non–cross-resistant) from the initial regimen.

16. When should a bone marrow transplant be considered in the treatment of Hodgkin's disease?

Autologous bone marrow transplantation has been used as salvage therapy for patients with one prior chemotherapy regimen who have subsequently relapsed. Long-term responses are seen in 20–40% of patients. This form of therapy may be considered more in patients who relapse early (< 1 year) after finishing primary chemotherapy and are younger.

17. How can one tell when a patient is cured of Hodgkin's disease?

People who are disease-free for more than 10 years after therapy may be considered cured. Patients who live disease-free for 5 years should have normal life expectancy. Recurrence is rare after 15 years. The risk of death from Hodgkin's disease is 17% at 15-year follow-up; the risk of death from other causes at 15-year follow-up is also 17% but increases sharply thereafter, especially in patients treated from 1960–1982. The major causes of death in the latter group are mainly secondary malignancies and cardiac events.

18. Which patients have the highest rate of relapse?

Relapse cannot be predicted accurately in Hodgkin's disease. Poor prognostic factors, however, have been identified. Tumor bulk and stage appear to be the most important prognostic factors. Of interest, the presence of a residual radiographic abnormality is not associated with a greater relapse rate; thus the importance of a pretherapy gallium scan. The presence of B symptoms (generally signifying greater tumor burden) is a poor prognostic factor. Low hematocrit and high LDH also have been associated with a higher rate of relapse. The histopathology has been suggested to have prognostic significance but should **not** guide the choice of therapy.

19. Is Hodgkin's disease an AIDS-defining illness?

No. Although it is the most common non–AIDS-defining cancer, the prevalence may be secondary to the high incidence of Hodgkin's disease in the group of people acquiring the AIDS virus (young adults).

20. What are the complications of therapy for Hodgkin's disease?

1. **Hypothyroidism**, manifested by a rising TSH, is seen in 30% of patients treated with mantle radiation therapy (see figure with question 13) and correctable by replacement therapy. It is more common when radiotherapy is started ≤ 30 days after lymphangiogram (LAG). Thyroid-stimulating hormone (TSH) levels should be followed yearly for 5 years after radiotherapy, especially in children.

2. **Sterility** is seen in women after pelvic radiation. MOPP is the most likely chemotherapy to cause sterility in men. MOPP or alkylator-containing regimens produce sterility in women 50% of the time and 80% of the time in men. Fifteen percent to 25% of men given ABVD develop sterility.

3. **Pneumonitis** is seen after mantle radiation and/or bleomycin or bleomycin and carmustine (BCNU). There may be immediate pneumonitis with radiotherapy or "recall" with chemotherapy, usually Adriamycin, anytime after radiotherapy.

4. **Cardiac toxicity.** Accelerated coronary atherosclerosis may be seen with mediastinal radiotherapy, especially in younger patients. "Recall" may occur with chemotherapy given after radiotherapy, leading to a cardiomyopathy.

5. **Aseptic necrosis of femoral and humoral heads** is associated with prednisone in MOPP chemotherapy.

6. **Infectious and immunologic complications.** There is an increased incidence of herpes zoster. Postsplenectomy sepsis is a problem mainly with patients receiving curative radiotherapy, then relapsing and receiving chemotherapy. Pneumovax vaccination should be given at least 10 days before splenectomy. Immune suppression may last many years after therapy.

7. **Secondary neoplasms**
   (1) Acute nonlymphocytic leukemia occurs 3–10 years after treatment in 2–10% of patients treated with a combination of MOPP and radiation. The 12-year estimate of leukemia development after treatment is 1.3% for chemotherapy alone, 10.2% for radiation plus MOPP, 0% for radiation plus ABVD, and 4.8% for radiation plus other regimens. This is seen more when therapy is given after the age of 40.
   (2) NHL may develop, usually with high-grade B-cell tumors. This is believed to be secondary to chronic immune deficiency from treatment of the disease.
   (3) Epithelial tumors and sarcomas are known to develop in patients treated for Hodgkin's disease, especially in radiated fields. Younger women and smokers have an increased incidence of breast cancer and lung cancers, respectively, when the mediastinum is radiated.

8. **Neurologic complications** may include peripheral neuropathy after vincristine therapy and myelopathy after radiotherapy. Transverse myelitis and Lhermitte's sign may be seen as well.

At 15 years and later, death from complications, including second cancers, cardiovascular events, and late infections, greatly exceed the deaths from Hodgkin's disease.

21. Describe the appropriate follow-up of patients after completion of treatment.

Most relapses occur within the first 3–4 years after therapy. Treated individuals should be followed every 2 months for the first year, every 3 months for the next 2 years, every 6 months until year 5, and then yearly. Appropriate procedures during follow-up may include:

- History and physical examination at each visit
- Complete blood count with sedimentation rate at each visit
- Chemistry panel every 6 months for 4 years
- Chest radiograph yearly for 5 years
- TSH yearly for 5 years
- Sterility testing before and after treatment if desired by the patient

BIBLIOGRAPHY

1. Armitage JO: Bone marrow transplantation in the treatment of patients with lymphoma. Blood 73:1749, 1989.
2. Bodis S, et al: Clinical presentation and outcome in lymphocyte-predominant Hodgkin's disease. J Clin Oncol 15:3060–3066, 1997.
3. Brain MC, Carbone PP: Current Therapy in Hematology/Oncology, 5th ed. Philadelphia, B.C. Decker, 1995.
4. DeVita VT, Mauch PM, Harris NL: Hodgkin's disease. In Devita VT, Hellman S, Rosenberg SA: Cancer: Principles and Practice of Oncology, 5th ed. Philadelphia, J.B. Lippincott, 1997, pp 2242–2283.
5. Hoffman R, Benz EJ Jr, Shattil SJ, et al: Hematology: Basic Principles and Practice, 2nd ed. New York, Churchill Livingstone, 1995.
6. Hoppe RT: The contemporary management of Hodgkin's disease. Radiology 169:297, 1988.
7. Longo DL, Young RC, Wesley M, et al: Twenty years of MOPP chemotherapy for Hodgkin's disease. J Clin Oncol 4:1295, 1986.
8. Mauch P, et al: Patterns of presentation of Hodgkin's disease. Cancer 71:2062–2071, 1993.
9. Schwartz RS: Hodgkin's disease—Trials for a change (editorial). N Engl J Med 337:495–496, 1997.
10. Urba WJ, Longo DL: Hodgkin's disease. N Engl J Med 326:678, 1992.
11. Williams SF, Farah R, Golomb HM: Hodgkin's disease. Hematol Oncol Clin North Am 3:1–368, 1989.

IV. General Care of the Cancer Patient

37. CARCINOGENESIS

Douglas Y. Tamura, M.D., and George E. Moore, M.D., Ph.D.

1. How is carcinogenesis defined?

The alteration of normal cells into malignant cells is almost always a multistage evolution of genetic and epigenetic alterations that eventuate in cells that escape the normal growth constraints of the host.

2. What are the stages of carcinogenesis?

The multistage process may include the following:

1. Mutation/activation may involve unconstrained factors of cell growth and multiplication, advantageous metabolic patterns, oncogenes, inactivated suppressor gene functions, and autonomy from cell-cell controls.

2. Selective clonal growth usually occurs from a single cell with a new growth advantage which permits further mutations.

3. Selection of additional "malignant features" allows progression from benign hyperplasia to autonomous neoplastic growth.

4. Clonal cancers developing from mutations with varying mosaics of genetic and functional activities become even more autonomous from dependence on hormones and other host factors.

5. Additional changes promote the ability to invade and metastasize—the establishment of individual and groups of cells at distal sites.

Note: The stages outlined above are not necessarily distinct and each stage probably includes multiple alterations of antigenicity, regulatory enzymes, and inappropriate expression of growth factors and other centers of genome activation.

3. What are the classes of carcinogens?

Physical agents	Infectious agents	Chronic inflammation
Chemical compounds	Foreign body reactions	Genetics

Carcinogens may also be divided into:

Inherited genetic defects

Social agents such as tobacco and alcohol

Occupational exposures such as benzenes, vinyl chloride, and asbestos

Radiation exposure

Contaminants of the food chain such as aflatoxin B

Immunosuppressive agents

Foreign body reactants such as asbestos fibers

Chronic inflammation such as ulcerative colitis

Iatrogenic agents such as cancer chemotherapeutic drugs, radiation, and estrogens given to pregnant women that caused vaginal cancers in their daughters

Infectious agents such as viruses, bacteria, and parasites

4. In addition to chimney sweep's cancer (scrotal carcinoma), what are other historical causes of cancers?

There were and continue to be many "causes" of cancers with and without known biologic rationale.

Many different microorganisms, various soil conditions, water contaminants, and dietary substances such as smoked fish, raw fish, and spices have been thought to cause cancers without proof.

Thyroid tumors developed in the trout of certain streams; a problem that was immediately solved by the addition of iodine to the water (an observation with direct relevance to humans).

The observation of nasal and oral cancers from snuff and chewing tobacco was made centuries ago. Cigarette smoking causes more deaths than all other known carcinogens combined.

Women who pointed their paint brushes dipped in uranium salts by twirling them between their lips and then painted the numbers on watches developed horrible carcinomas and sarcomas of the mouth and jaws (1915 to 1925). Pioneers in the use of radiation developed skin cancers, lymphomas, and leukemias (1907 to 1945).

The uranium miners in the Schneeberg mountains of Saxony in Europe had increased lung "disorders." Ironically, the minerals were not mined for their radioactivity but for the beautiful colors they imparted to glass.

Many years ago, cancer of the urinary bladder was associated with infestation by the trematode *Schistosoma haematobium.*

Presently, there is a fear of radiation from radon seepage from the ground into homes and schools.

A current noncause of cancer is exposure to electromagnetic fields (EMF).

5. How are carcinogens identified?

Most human carcinogens such as tobacco and vinyl chloride have been identified first by clinical observation.

Fruit flies (*Drosophila*), molds (*Neurospora*), bacteria, round worms, and a variety of experimental animals have been used as test subjects. Cultured human and rodent cells have been very useful in studies of carcinogenesis but are less applicable for screening purposes. Various routes of delivery and extended application of potential carcinogens to animals may be required.

The complexity of such assays can be understood when one considers that some carcinogens are metabolites while others require growth-promoting agents, hormones, and specific exposures that may be limited to specific cells of specific species at specific ages with and without additional "promoting" agents.

The Ames test is an assay of mutagenesis in bacteria. It is a valuable screening test but has limited in direct significance for human carcinogenesis.

6. Discuss the roles of oncogenes and tumor suppressor genes in carcinogenesis.

These families of regulator genes—oncogenes are positive growth regulators and tumor suppressor genes are negative regulators—are subject to genetic segregation, deletion, mutation, and alterations of expression.

About 100 oncogenes and 6 or 7 tumor suppressor genes have been identified. Both can be carried, activated, or inactivated by viruses or viral proteins and both may be altered by mutation, mutational amplification, expression out of sequence, and activation/suppression by translocation to an abnormal chromosomal site.

7. What are examples of oncogenes and tumor suppressor genes in human malignancies?

In Burkitt's lymphoma, the *myc* oncogene is frequently translocated from chromosome 8 to 14. In many neuroblastomas, one of the many *myc* oncogenes is highly amplified. Mutational forms of the *K-ras* oncogene are present in cancers of the colon, bladder, bronchi, and pancreas. Translocations may expose or form critical hybrid transcripts with oncogenes. The well-known Philadelphia chromosome (associated with chronic myelogenous leukemia) is an altered chromosome 22 and brings into juxtaposition the important *bcr* gene and the *c-abl* proto-oncogene from chromosome 9.

The complexity involved in sorting out translocations, deletions, suppression, and activation that take place on multiple chromosomes during *multiple sequential* stages of carcinogenesis numbs the mind.

The first tumor suppressor genes identified were the *Rb* genes, whose deletion from chromosome 13 is associated with retinoblastoma, and the *p53* gene on chromosome 17. Alteration or deletion of *p53* has been detected in nearly 50% of certain human tumors.

Remember, our knowledge of the interactions of these genes is primitive and their exact functions are probably much more complicated than reflected by initial studies, but there is no doubt of their role in human carcinogenesis and the subsequent evolution of malignancies.

8. Discuss the role of infectious agents in carcinogenesis.

Microscopic and submicroscopic infectious agents were thought for many years to cause human cancers without proof. Once viral agents were confirmed as carcinogenic agents in animals, it was predicted that vital human carcinogens would soon be found.

From an historical view, mention should be made of the discovery of sarcoma virus by Roux (1911), papillomavirus by Shope (1933), mouse mammary virus by Bittner (1936), leukemia virus by Gross (1951), polyomavirus by Stewart (1957), papilloma virus type 16, and many others in both plants and animals.

Vital carcinogens include viruses, bacteria, parasites, and perhaps transplanted cells. Burkitt's lymphoma is an example of carcinogenesis by the Epstein-Barr virus (EBV)—a virus capable of immortalizing B-lymphocytes. Human papillomaviruses (HPV) type 6 and 11 are associated with condylomas and HPV types 16, 18, 31, and 32 are associated with carcinogenic transformation of various keratinocytes such as those of the cervix.[7] Human herpes virus 8, associated with Kaposi's sarcoma, is another neoplastic virus that is frequently detectable in asymptomatic individuals, and may require immunosuppression for activation—such as HIV infection.

As molecular assays become available, the detection of many more viral sequences at various stages of carcinogenesis in humans seems reasonable. Other viruses or virus-like organisms will probably be found that transfer critical nucleic acid sequences or otherwise activate carcinogenesis in various cells. For example, it has been hypothesized that infections of stromal cells may transform adjacent myeloma cells.

The *Helicobacter pylori* causes severe gastritis, peptic ulcer disease, and probably causes some gastric cancers. Chronic bacterial infections may play a critical role in malignancies developing at sites of chronic inflammation. Some parasitic infections such as schistosomiasis are also carcinogenic.

Observations of carcinogenesis in rodents injected with human cells has led to the hypothesis that insertion of homologous cells and tissue transplants in humans may be carcinogenic—other than direct injection of occult malignancies.

The occurrence of malignancies at the site of ureteral insertions into the colon is unique. This may represent an abnormal chemical or infectious exposure of the colonic mucosa.

In an era of intense oncologic research, additional agents of initiation and promotion of human carcinogenesis will be found. The exact genes or lesser nucleic acid sequences required for carcinogenic activation and promotion-enhancement will be identified.

9. What are major examples of inherited susceptibilities to cancer, and what types of cancers are associated with these syndromes?

Li-Fraumeni syndrome—cancers of multiple organs

Xeroderma pigmentosa—cancers of the skin and melanoma

Familial polyposis coli—colon cancer

Familial retinoblastoma—uveal melanoma

Cowden's syndrome—cancer of the breast and thyroid

DiGeorge syndrome—leukemia

Some of these traits provide inherent genome instability and increase susceptibility to infectious/environmental agents, whereas others reflect a specific lack of host defenses, including repair mechanisms. Some are single gene defects, but most involve multiple activator and tumor suppressor genes that mutate and promote oncologic change. Carcinogenesis may develop from repetitive DNA sequences subject to unusually high mutation rates that escape host surveillance.

10. Discuss the iatrogenic causes of cancers.

There is a risk of cancer, although low, from diagnostic and therapeutic radiation, from many chemotherapeutic agents such as the alkylating agents and antimetabolites, hormones such as estrogens, growth hormone (which causes leukemia), and even the implantation of iron-dextran. Any intensely biologically active medication must be suspect. For example, the antibiotic metronidazole apparently causes lung adenomas in mice, azidothymidine (AZT) is carcinogenic in rodents, and tamoxifen (a preventative breast cancer agent) causes hepatocellular cancers in rodents and rarely uterine carcinomas in humans.

A dramatic example of medical carcinogenesis was the use of diethylstilbestrol for threatened abortion in many thousands of women whose daughters subsequently developed carcinomas of the vagina and exocervix from ages 7 to 28.

Radioactive thorium dioxide (Thorotrast) provided excellent angiograms but also caused a variety of malignancies.

Foreign bodies such as the metallic replacement of joints and struts for fractured bones and the various meshes have been shown to be carcinogenic in mice, but **not** in humans.

11. What are the effects of immunosuppression on carcinogenesis?

An exception to the long precancerous period—10 to over 30 years—is the rapid progression of cancers in those patients with acquired immunodeficiency syndrome (AIDS) and some with malaria.

Patients on immunosuppressive medication following organ transplantation are also at risk. Explosive cancerous growth occurs. Reversal of the immunosuppression may cause regression of the cancers—a confirmation of the importance of normal regulatory controls.

12. Explain the Delany Clause.

This infamous legislation in 1958 declared that anything added to our food chain that caused cancer in animals (**except tobacco products**) under any circumstance must be excluded—the theory of **zero tolerance**.

Unfortunately, many experimental animals are very susceptible to carcinogens that may, in massive doses, cause cancers, but these assays are not always relevant to humans.

Controversies rage as to the optimal method(s) of testing and the species used for assays. Even the definition of "carcinogen" is inexact. Confounding issues include the age at which the exposure is begun, the route and length of applications, dosage (often at a maximal tolerated level), nutrition, and sex of the animals. The functional activities of the host organs must be considered as well as the burden of "normal" viruses and bacteria in the test animal.

13. Are the recent claims of carcinogenicity associated with "natural" foods reasonable?

It is estimated that 99.9% of carcinogens in our foods are of natural origin. These natural carcinogenic substances include mold toxins such as aflatoxins, certain bracken ferns, cycasin from the cycad nut, mushrooms (pyrrolidine alkaloids), safrol (formerly used to flavor root beer), and even several molecules in coffee. A popular drink in South America, "mate," which is a hot infusion of the leaves of the Ilex tree, has been implicated in cancers of the pharynx and esophagus. Carcinogens have been isolated from both herbal medicines and teas.

In brief, it is impossible to avoid all carcinogens but fortunately most are of only experimental interest rather than significant dangers to humans. Undoubtedly, additional natural and synthetic carcinogens will be identified and will evoke terrifying headlines and rarely some will require preventive action.

14. Are there preventive carcinogenic dietary patterns?

There is no conclusive evidence of carcinogenesis directly attributable to eating habits except obesity, which may accelerate aging of tissues and cells—a lessening of good health. Most information is derived from epidemiologic studies. Obesity has been related to breast cancer, a lack of fiber or stool bulk with colon cancer, the ingestion of hot liquids with pharyngeal and esophageal cancer, and the excessive use of grilled and smoked meat and fish with gastric cancer.

Experimental data suggest various antioxidants may negate or inhibit stage progression of many carcinogens (i.e., asbestos) in experimental animals. Unfortunately, the toxicity of acceptable agents for human use has been excessive. There is a great popular interest in vitamins C and E as preventatives.

Epidemiologic studies have suggested a reduced risk of colon cancer in persons taking aspirin regularly. There are supporting observations of both human and animal tumor inhibition with nonsteroidal antiinflammatory drugs (i.e., aspirin for colon cancer).

Agents that cause cellular differentiation and maturation have been effective preventatives in experimental animals and may have clinical usefulness in the future.

Health food stores continue to advertise untested concoctions and herbs as cancer preventatives and treatment (i.e., the craze for shark cartilage extract without valid evidence).

In brief, lifestyle and dietary patterns that slow aging are probably helpful but unproven preventatives.

15. Do cancers develop at sites of chronic inflammation? Are they associated with some chronic diseases?

Yes to both. Ulcerative colitis, usually after 10 years, is associated with colon cancer. Most cancers of the gallbladder are found with cholelithiasis. Chronic ulcers of the leg from stasis, old burn sites (Marjolin's ulcer), and persistent sinus tracts may evolve into cancers. The recent implication of a bacterial infection (*H. pylori*) with gastritis and gastric cancer is interesting.

In contrast to rodents, humans rarely have malignant reactions to foreign bodies. Asbestosis is an exception, and there is some evidence that other fibers such as glass wool and wood splinters may be dangerous in rare cases. Controversies concerning the actual dangers of low-level asbestos exposure in humans are tainted by social and political imagery and biases*.

Lung cancer or, more accurately, bronchial carcinomas result in part from continuous cellular injury and repair plus exposure to the carcinogens in cigarette smoke. Cigarette smoke is the single greatest preventable carcinogen.

Asiatic people who smoke "cigars" with the smoldering end within the mouth develop oral cancers, as do chewers of betel nut concoctions with tobacco.

The development of skin cancers in Kashmiris at the abdominal site burned by the heated kangri bowl held against it for warmth was reported by missionary brothers in 1900.

* As a personal note from a surgeon oncologist, the emotional diatribes about the dangers of asbestos have departed from any and all scientific data. There has not been the predicted disastrous epidemic of asbestos-related deaths. The billions of dollars spent in removing asbestos from public buildings such as schools has benefited new industry and countless lawyers at the expense of education.

16. Does trauma cause malignancies?

Over the years there have been many claims and counter claims that traumatic injuries cause cancer. There has been no evidence of such causation by single injuries and doubtful evidence of the dangers of repetitious injuries unaccompanied by chronic infection, and repetitive regeneration.

Postulates for trauma-induced cancers were developed in response to compensation claims, and include:
1. Proof of site-specific severe trauma without prior disease
2. Minimal interval before tumor development
3. Diagnosis of an appropriate malignancy
4. Evidence of an evolving tumor without cancer elsewhere

Note: There are millions of fractures and surgical procedures yearly without evidence of related malignancies. Although the cumulative exposure to ionizing radiation, ultraviolet light, and chemicals is probably more dangerous than a single exposure, there is no evidence of increased malignancies of skin areas susceptible to repetitive trauma (i.e., face from shaving, hands, or feet).

17. What are the intervals between exposure to a carcinogen and the development of cancer?

A number of years are required for carcinogenesis in humans. For example, occupational asbestos-related cancers in nonsmokers rarely develop in less than 15 years and more often become evident in 25 to 40 years. Multiple exposures to ionizing radiation may eventuate in skin cancers and leukemia after only a few years, whereas malignancies of connective tissue cells and adeno-carcinomas may take 15–30 years to develop. Smoking-induced cancers often require 15 or more years of exposure. Youthful exposures are more dangerous and the carcinogenic interval is shorter.

Note: Cessation of exposure usually decreases the risk of malignancy.

18. How can we escape exposure to carcinogens?

We can't—even vegetables and fruits touted for optimal diets contain carcinogens. One should minimize exposure to ultraviolet light and ionizing radiation, especially persons with sensitive skin such as those with blonde or red hair, blue eyes, and freckles.

Those with familial risks require identification and regularly scheduled diagnostic procedures such as mammography, colonoscopy, and the inspection of dermal abnormalities.

In the future, some of the genetic factors will be identified and perhaps eliminated by genetic engineering.

19. Why haven't epidemiologic studies of human carcinogenesis been more successful?

Carcinogenesis is complex, may extend over many years, and may progress in only a tiny percentage of the persons at risk. Simple small correlations collected from interview studies and computer analyses are often erroneous. Indeed, the most common epidemiologic study of cancer causation is one denying a prior report.

"Causes" of cancers have many confounders: genetic factors, different target organ/cells, age, sex, pregnancy, multiple carcinogens, multiple "promoting" agents, infectious agents, dosage- and time-related/multiple exposures, and specific alterations of systemic and local immunities.

The list of spurious reports is endless: EMF (electromagnetic fields), cellular phones, radar, caffeine, hair coloring, food additives, cotton clothing, and "new car odor," to name a few.

Assertions of carcinogenesis are subject to emotional, political, and legislative interpretations, which in turn are affected/driven by scientific uncertainties, ambitions, economic gain, and seemingly last of all valid biologic data.

Actually, most if not all human carcinogens were first identified by personal observations. However, confirmation of these observations by epidemiologic studies has been very important.

Environmental factors other than tobacco and ultraviolet light probably cause < 10% of malignancies but 90% of the headlines.

Exposure to infectious agents, environmental factors, and other diverse health factors always evolve and change over the years, which further minimizes the ability of epidemiologic studies to detect causative agents.

20. Why don't we all develop malignancies?

We probably develop "malignant" cells daily but most are so abnormal that they do not survive or cannot successfully generate daughter cells. Others are repaired or destroyed by cellular and humoral defense mechanisms. As we age these defenses are impaired which allows newly generated and dormant malignant cells to establish themselves.

21. How can we prevent or minimize carcinogenesis?

1. Choose cancer-free ancestors
2. Minimize exposure to carcinogens
3. Maintain a nutritious diet with antioxidants
4. Early vaccinations to avoid viral infections (e.g., nearly 100% of children in Taiwan with hepatocellular carcinoma tested positive for the antigen of hepatitis B. A nationwide hepatitis B vaccination program has reduced the carrier rate and probably childhood hepatocellular carcinoma).
5. Excision or other therapies of percancerous lesions
6. Avoid excessive iatrogenic drugs (and hormones) that may sustain or stimulate abnormal cell growth

BIBLIOGRAPHY

1. Ames BN, Gold LS: Too many rodent carcinogens: Mitogenesis increases mutagenesis. Science 249:970–971, 1990.
2. Anderson M, Storm HH: Cancer incidence among Danish Thorotrast-exposed patients. J Natl Cancer Inst 84:1318–1325, 1992.
3. Auvinen A, Makelainen I, Hakama M, et al: Indoor radon exposure and risk of lung cancer: A nested case-control study in Finland. J Natl Cancer Inst 88:966–972, 1996.
4. Chang MH, Chen CJ, Lai MS, et al: Universal hepatitis B vaccination in Taiwan and the incidence of hepatocellular carcinoma in children. N Engl J Med 336:1855–1859, 1997.
5. Druker BJ, Mamon HJ, Roberts TM: Oncogenes, growth factors, and signal transduction. N Engl J Med 321:1383–1391, 1989.
6. Feinstein AR, Horwitz RI, Spitzer WO, et al: Coffee and pancreatic cancer: The problems of etiological science and epidemiologic case-control research. JAMA 246:957–961, 1981.
7. Halbert CL, Demers GW, Galloway DA: The E7 gene of human papillomavirus type 16 is sufficient for immortalization of human epithelial cells. J Virol 65:473–478, 1991.
8. Harris CC: Chemical and physical carcinogenesis: Advances and perspectives for the 1990s. Cancer Res (Suppl 51):5023–5044, 1991.
9. Hay A: Testing times for the tests. Nature 350:555–556, 1991.
10. Ionov Y, Peinado MA, Malkhosyan S, et al: Ubiquitous somatic mutations in simple repeated sequences reveal a new mechanism for colonic carcinogenesis. Nature 363:558–561, 1993.
11. Koeffler HP, McCormick F, Denny C: Molecular mechanisms of cancer. West J Med 155:505–513, 1991.
12. Moore GE, Palmer QN: Money causes cancer, ban it. JAMA 238:397, 1977.
13. Mossman BT, Bignon J, Corn M, et al: Asbestos: Scientific developments and implications for public policy. Science 247:294–301, 1990.
14. Neve EF, Neve A: Kangri-burn cancer. BMJ 2:1255–1256, 1923.
15. Penn I: Depressed immunity and the development of cancer. Clin Exp Immunol 46:459–474, 1981.
16. Shibata T: Detection of *Helicobacter pylori* in biopsy patients with gastric carcinoma. Biomed Pharmacother 51:22–28, 1997.
17. Stone R: News and comments. Science 254:928–931, 1991.
18. Ulfelder H: The stilbestrol-adenosis-carcinoma syndromes. Cancer 38:426–431, 1976.
19. Vogt PK: Cancer genes. West J Med 158:273–278, 1993.
20. Weiss L: Some effects of mechanical trauma on the development of primary cancers and their metastases. J Forensic Sci 35:614–627, 1990.

38. CANCER IN THE ELDERLY

Madeline J. White, M.D.

1. Why is it important to focus on cancer issues in patients over 65 years of age?

Cancer is second only to heart disease as the cause of death in this age group. The risk of cancer continues to rise throughout an individual's life. One-half of all cancers occur in people over 65. This age group is expanding more rapidly than any other in the U.S. population. Life expectancy for someone aged 65 averages about 17–20 years. An 85-year-old woman can expect to live about 7 more years, an 85-year-old man about 5.5 years. This is longer than the two to three year recurrence time of most treatable cancers. Therefore, the 5-year survival rate for various treatments is significant for people > 65 years.

2. Name some common solid tumor types and hematologic malignancies that present in the elderly age group.

Breast, lung, colorectal, prostate, pancreatic, head and neck, bladder, and ovarian cancers are commonly encountered in the older population. Among hematogic malignancies, acute myelogenous leukemia, chronic lymphocytic leukemia, myeloproliferative disorders, lymphomas, and myeloma most commonly present.

3. List some theories as to why cancer is so prevalent in the elderly.

Many theories link oncogenesis and aging:
- Prolonged exposure to carcinogenic agents
- Accumulation of DNA damage over time in various cell lines
- Failure of cellular repair mechanisms
- Loss of tumor suppressor genes with multiple cell divisions
- Decreased immune surveillance

Over a lifetime, all of the above factors may play interweaving roles that allow cells to emerge as malignant clones.

4. How can concurrent problems of aged individuals obscure the diagnosis of cancer?

Almost 50% of cancer patients over age 70 have three or more comorbid conditions. Before suspecting active cancer, the caregiver relies on an accurate history of new symptoms or signs. Below are some confounding situations:
- Poor hearing, cognitive impairment → delivery of a difficult, inaccurate history
- Poor vision → unaware of skin changes
- Arthritis → confusing new bone pain with joint pain
- Chronic constipation, hemorrhoids → failure to report new bowel problems
- Trouble urinating → attributing symptoms to common, benign prostate problems
- Depression → masks or mimics cancer symptoms
- Increased fatigue and decreased exercise tolerance → interpreted as just "getting old"
- Fear of cancer diagnosis → minimizing symptoms, refusing exams
- Multiple complaints → obscuring new problems

Caregivers must be familiar with the patient and able to evaluate prudently new symptoms and signs, especially if a decline in performance status and/or weight loss is documented.

5. What cancer screening tests are recommended in the fit elderly at average risk?

There is not complete consensus as to what tests and what intervals are appropriate for those over 65. Guidelines are available from the American College of Physicians (ACP), the U.S. Preventative Services Task Force (USPSTF), the American Academy of Family Practice (AAFP), the American Cancer Society (ACS), and the American Geriatric Society (AGS).

Below is an overview summarizing several guidelines:
- **Clinical breast exams** can be performed yearly during regular visits. Decreased fibrocystic changes make the exam easier, but widespread hormone replacement therapy in older women may minimize this advantage.
- **Mammography** is recommended annually. The AGS discontinues this at age 85, the ACP at age 75. Other groups recommend it as long as the woman is fit.
- **Pap smears**. If a woman has had regular, normal pap smears before age 65, most groups recommend to stop screening. Some do three more exams at 2-year intervals. If all are normal, screening is discontinued. It is very important to establish if a cervix is present or not. Some elderly women are not accurate regarding their surgical history. If a hysterectomy was done for cancer, vaginal paps are appropriate; otherwise no cervical cancer screening is needed.
- **Digital rectal exams** (DRE). The USPSTF, AAFP, and ACP do not strongly recommend this exam as a good screen for either colorectal or prostate cancer. The ACS recommends it yearly, but the USPSTF says that evidence does not sway them for or against.
- **Prostate specific antigen** (PSA). Controversy continues to rage over the usefulness of this test for screening. In general, older men have less aggressive disease and early detection may not alter their life course. If the test is done, counseling regarding the consequences of both a positive or negative result is necessary.
- **Fecal occult blood** (FOB). Annual tests for those over 50 is the common recommendation. The ACP encourages its use in those who refuse endoscopy.
- **Sigmoidoscopy**. There is controversy regarding invasive screening for colorectal cancer. Sigmoidoscopy, colonoscopy, or air contrast barium enema every 10 years from age 50–70

is the ACP's position. Others suggest sigmoidoscopy alone at 5-year intervals. Patient acceptance is a problem.

6. **What problems may arise in attempting to screen elders, especially the older old?**
   • Many elders do not believe that screening applies to them. It has not been a part of their routine health maintenance. Atrophic tissues make the exams uncomfortable for some.
   • Exams by caregivers of the opposite sex may not be acceptable.
   • Directions can be confusing due to visual, auditory or cognitive impairments.
   • Physical constraints and bowel dysfunction may make FOB collections and bowel preps impossible.
   • Arthritis or orthopnea make exam manipulations difficult.
   • A companion is needed if a procedure requires some sedation.
   • Transportation problems may scuttle a scheduled appointment.
   • Screening procedures outside of a regular office visit require coordination with support staff and the patient's family and friends.

7. **If a diagnosis of cancer is made, how does the approach to care differ for the elderly compared to younger patients?**
   The initial approach to treatment planning should be the same regardless of age. Consider surgery, radiation therapy, chemotherapy, or a combination of modalities appropriate for the tumor and its particular stage. Make modifications to fit the individual's physiologic state and his/her psychosocial perspective. Issues of overall life expectancy, time in therapy, quality of life with treatment vs. cancer symptoms, and the individual's overall life view will enter into the treatment discussion. Older patients may be concerned with costs and burden on other family members. A number of sessions may be necessary to come to a decision regarding the proposed options. Protocol treatments, standard therapies, programs modified for the less fit elderly, as well as palliative or hospice care only, all require a comprehensive plan to best serve the patient's medical, psychological, and social interests.

8. **Will elderly patients tolerate cancer surgery?**
   Although age > 70 is a risk factor for surgery, functional status rather than age determines the successful outcome of cancer surgery. Surgeons know that aging brings diminished function of various organ symptoms:
   • Cardiovascular: decreased maximum heart rate with stress, decreased adrenergic response
   • Pulmonary: decreased vital capacity, decreased maximum oxygen uptake, decreased cough and cilia activity, decreased elasticity
   • Renal: decreased creatinine clearance, decreased maximum urine osmolality, and decreased acidification
   • Skin: decreased wound healing and thinning
   Other non–age-related factors add to the risk:
   • Impaired preoperative functional status
   • Concurrent cardiovascular and/or pulmonary disease
   • Malnutrition
   • Body cavity surgery
   • Dementia
   • Emergent surgery

   Compared to radiation therapy, surgery entails more acute stress to the contracted homeostatic reserve of the elderly patient, but it is usually short term. For common cancer surgeries on the breast, the colon, or the prostate, reviews have shown no increase in morbidity or mortality with age alone. Lung cancer surgery follows the usual guidelines for estimating pulmonary reserve.

9. **What should you monitor if elders are undergoing radiation therapy as part of the treatment?**
   One VA group has looked at the ability of the oldest old to tolerate full dose radiation therapy. Out of 36 patients over 80 years of age, only 5 had treatment interruption. Mucositis was

the limiting toxicity for radiation to the head and neck area; diarrhea the major problem for pelvic irradiation. An older individual cannot tolerate days of poor intake as a younger person can. Close attention to symptom control, weight change, hydration, and nutrition allowed most patients to complete their courses.

Radiation therapy has less acute toxicities compared to surgery, but the need for daily transport and decreased tissue tolerance over the weeks of treatment may decrease compliance. In addition, elders also seem to develop pneumonitis more frequently than younger patients. Overall, newer patterns of short-course, high-dose schedules for palliation may be better suited for limited elders.

10. Are there any chemotherapy agents that should be avoided in the older patient?

No drug is absolutely contraindicated, but some modifications may be needed. Common chemotherapy agents, like many drugs, have not been pharmacologically studied in the elderly. Increased variability in organ function in the older population and concurrent medications make predicting drug bioavailability, volume of distribution, and clearance difficult. Most toxicity and efficacy information in elders comes from trials using standard doses for younger patients. Although changes in gut motility, absorption, splanchnic and hepatic blood flow, lean/fat ratio, and total body water may alter drug pharmacokinetics, the most significant adjustments that need to be made are for decreased glomerular filtration rate and bone marrow reserve. Renally cleared drugs must be modified for creatinine clearance; bone marrow toxic drugs modified for tumor involvement, fibrosis, malnutrition, and high dose regimens. Elders seem to be able to tolerate moderately toxic chemotherapy regimens but show decreased rebound and recovery with aggressive treatments. The use of cytokines is being investigated to overcome this problem.

Below are some observations with common agents in the elderly:
- Methotrexate: must adjust for creatinine clearance < 60 ml/minute
- Bleomycin: increased pulmonary toxicity in elders
- Vincristine: more neuropathy and constipation
- Anthracyclines: avoid if congestive heart failure is present by radionuclide ejection fraction. Coronary artery disease or hypertension alone are not contraindications.
- Paclitaxel: no unusual toxicity in elders
- Cisplatin: some decline in renal function is seen with moderate dose levels, but tolerable. Ototoxicity must be considered.
- 5-Fluorouracil: some see increased diarrhea and mucositis in elders
- Interferon: more neurotoxicity and fatigue

11. How do the elderly handle the side effects of chemotherapy?

- Elders seem to have less nausea and vomiting but tolerate prolonged bouts poorly
- Decreased thirst sensation allows dehydration to develop early
- Medications needed to control pain and nausea may in turn cause other complications.

Narcotics or long-acting benzodiazepines and anticholinergics may cause falls, delirium, urinary retention, blurred vision, and constipation. Nonsteroidal antiinflammatory drugs may comprise renal function.

The caregiver must be aware and sort out symptoms arising from the malignancy itself, from the particular cancer therapy, from concurrent medications, or from ongoing medical conditions. Control of symptoms and avoidance of side effects plays a significant role in the elder patient's ability to continue therapy.

12. Who should care for elders with cancer?

Geriatricians sometimes divide the over 65 population into the young-old (65–74), the old-old (75–84), and the oldest-old (85+). In each bracket, the percentage with functional impairment rises. In a study in New Mexico of the 75–84 age group with newly diagnosed cancer, 12% required assistance with activities of daily living (ADLs), 34% with instrumental activities (IDLs), and 40% had poor recent memory. The oncologist and the oncology nurse will find the primary caregiver, the social worker, the home care agency, the pharmacist, the family, and the friends of the patient all involved in the effort to care for the elder. Communication and coordination from all parties are critical. No one person can meet all the needs.

13. When should advance care directives be discussed?

End-of-life issues should be approached early in the course of cancer evaluation, but the discussion should not be seen as a poor prognostic sign. A cancer diagnosis is not a death sentence or the end of hope. It can be an opportunity to review life goals and to direct end-of-life care even for those with long life expectancy. The medical durable power of attorney or the less formal medical proxy (designated spokesperson) is the most flexible for the changing prognosis as the cancer responds or progresses.

Along with advance care directives, the caregiver should:
• Review the facts and treatment issues
• Establish a prognosis, if possible
• Reinforce a realistic outlook
• Involve family and friends as desired by the patient
• Elicit and answer all questions
• Reassure the patient that care will continue whether the decision is to continue active therapy, to withdraw therapy, or to seek palliation only

CONTROVERSIES

14. Is there age discrimination in referral and treatment of older cancer patients?

The literature says yes. In a survey of female patients with breast and colon cancer, 1993 data show that for women 65 and older compared to younger women fewer were offered adjuvant chemotherapy, equal numbers were offered hormonal adjuvant therapy, and fewer were sent for consultation with medical or radiation oncologists.

On the other hand, they also found that women 65 and older, if offered adjuvant therapy, were more likely to decline it and were more concerned about side effects compared to younger women.

A British study looking at cases of lung cancer discovered that even with good performance status (ECOG 0-1), fewer patients aged 65–74 and 75+ received active initial treatment compared to younger patients:

Age	% Active Treatment
< 65	86
65–74	74
75+	39

Using vignettes describing different stages of cancer, different treatment toxicities, and projected survival benefits, levels of acceptance of treatment were found to be equal for young and old, but that younger patients would tolerate greater toxicity for a smaller survival benefit than older patients.

Conclusion: age alone is not the single determinant of treatment. Caregivers must individualize and give a fair assessment of risks and benefits for their older patients.

15. How does the geriatric adage "start low, go slow" apply to chemotherapy?

Chemotherapy programs are designed to kill the most tumor cells possible on a regular schedule. Multiple drugs are used at maximally tolerated doses. "Start low, go slow" is safer, but allows for early emergence of drug resistance. If the goal of chemotherapy is cure or an increase in quality survival time, the fit elderly should have the option of adequate dose intensity. Clinicians can strategize with cytokines, organ protective agents, and substitution of equally active but less toxic drugs to allow proper dosing when a clear survival advantage is expected.

BIBLIOGRAPHY

1. Balducci L, Lyman GH, Ershler WB (eds): Comprehensive Geriatric Oncology. Buffalo, NY, Harwood Academic Publishers, 1998.
2. Brown JS, Eraut D, Trask C, Davison AG: Age and the treatment of lung cancer. Thorax 51:564–568, 1996.
3. Cohen HJ: Cancer in the older patient. Semin Oncol (Suppl 22):1–35, 1995.
4. Cohen HJ: Oncology and aging: General principles of cancer in the elderly. In Hazzard WR, Bierman EL, Blass JP, et al (eds): Principles of Geriatric Medicine and Gerontology. New York, McGraw-Hill, 1994, pp 77–89.
5. Cortes J, Kantarjian H, O'Brien S, et al: Results of interferon-alpha therapy in patients with chronic myelogenous leukemia 60 years of age and older. Am J Med 100:452–455, 1996.
6. Goodman JS, Hunt WC, Samet JM: A population-based study of functional status and social support networks of elderly patients newly diagnosed with cancer. Arch Intern Med 151:366–370, 1991.
7. Herman CJ, Robertson JM: Preventative geriatrics. In Reuben DB, Yoshikawa TT, Besdine RW (eds): Geriatrics Review Syllabus, 3rd ed. Dubuque, Kendell Hunt, 1996, p 81.
8. Ibrahim NK, Frye DK, Buzdar AU, et al: Doxorubicin-based chemotherapy in elderly patients with metastatic breast cancer. Arch Intern Med 156:882–888, 1996.
9. Kaesberg PR: Oncology. In Reuben DB, Yoshikawa TT, Besdine RW (eds): Geriatric Review Syllabus, 3rd ed. Dubuque, Kendell Hunt, 1996, pp 321–328.
10. Lichtman SM, Zaheer W, Gal D, et al: No increased risk of Taxol toxicity in older patients. J Am Geriatr Soc 44:472–473, 1996.
11. Masetti R, Antinori A, Terribile D, et al: Breast cancer in women 70 years of age or older. J Am Geriatr Soc 44:390–393, 1996.
12. Meyer RM, Browman GP, Samosh ML, et al: Randomized phase II comparison of standard CHOP with weekly CHOP in elderly patients with non-Hodgkin's lymphoma. J Clin Oncol 13:2386–2393, 1995.
13. Newcomb PA, Carbone PP: Cancer treatment and age: Patient perspectives. J Natl Cancer Inst 85:1580–1584, 1993.
14. Phister JE, Cusack BJ: Oncology. In Beck JC (ed): Geriatrics Review Syllabus. William Byrd Press, 1989, pp 204–210.
15. Thomas DR, Ritchie CS: Preoperative assessment of older adults. J Am Geriatr Soc 43:811–821, 1995.
16. Thyss A, Saudes L, Otto J, et al: Renal tolerance of cisplatin in patients more than 80 years old. J Clin Oncol 12:2121–2125, 1994.
17. Yellen SB, Cella DF, Leslie WT: Age and clinical decision-making in oncology patients. J Natl Cancer Inst 86:1766–1770, 1994.
18. Zachariah B, Casey L, Balducci L: Radiotherapy in the oldest old cancer patients: A study of effectiveness and toxicity. J Am Geriatr Soc 43:793–795, 1995.

39. CANCER PREVENTION

Sheila A. Prindiville, M.D., M.P.H., Tim Byers, M.D., M.P.H., and Dennis J. Ahnen, M.D.

1. What is cancer control?

Cancer control is the reduction of cancer incidence, morbidity, and mortality through an orderly sequence of research ranging from the evaluation of interventions and their impact in defined populations to the broad systematic application of the research results.

2. Give an example of a primary preventive intervention.

Primary prevention refers to health promotion and risk reduction in the general population so that invasive cancer does not develop. Examples of primary preventive measures include smoking cessation, diet and lifestyle modification, and micronutrient supplementation.

3. Give an example of a secondary preventive measure.

Secondary prevention is the identification and treatment of asymptomatic persons who already have developed premalignant or early malignant disease in whom the condition has not become clinically apparent. Screening (e.g., mammography, Pap smears, flexible sigmoidoscopy) is a form of secondary prevention.

4. Name the single most avoidable cause of cancer in the United States.

Tobacco. About one-third of the estimated 560,000 deaths due to cancer in the United States each year are directly attributable to cigarette smoking. It is estimated that tobacco use causes 23% of all cancer deaths in women and 42% in men. Smoking is a major cause of cancers of the lung, larynx, oral cavity, and esophagus. Smoking also contributes to cancers of the bladder, kidney, pancreas, and uterine cervix. Nearly 90% of lung cancer is attributable to cigarette smoking. A current smoker of about one pack of cigarettes a day has about a 20-fold increased risk of lung cancer. Environmental tobacco smoke (passive smoking) is a significant cause of lung cancer in nonsmokers as evidenced by the 30–50% increased risk for lung cancer in nonsmokers who live or work with smokers.

5. How soon after smoking cessation does the risk of lung cancer decline?

Within a year of quitting, the risk of heart disease in former smokers is reduced by nearly 50% compared to persons who continue to smoke. Unfortunately, it takes longer for the risk of lung cancer to decline. The benefit of cessation on lung cancer risk becomes apparent after about 5 years and continues to decline with each year of abstinence. However, even after 20 years of abstinence, the risk of lung cancer in former smokers is still about 2 times higher than among people who never smoked.

6. List the four general dietary guidelines recommended by the American Cancer Society to reduce cancer risk.

1. **Choose most of the foods you eat from plant sources**. Eat 5 or more servings of fruits and vegetables each day. Eat other foods from plant sources, such as breads, cereals, grain products, rice, pasta, or beans several times each day.

2. **Limit your intake of high-fat foods, particularly from animal sources**. Choose foods low in fat. Limit consumption of meats, especially high-fat meats.

3. **By physically active: achieve and maintain a healthy weight**. Be at least moderately active for 30 minutes or more each day. Stay within your healthy weight range.

4. **Limit consumption of alcoholic beverages, if you drink at all**. For people who drink alcoholic beverages, limit intake to two drinks a day for men and one drink per day for women.

7. A diet high in fruits and vegetables has been most consistently associated with a decreased risk of which tumors?

Fruits and vegetables have been consistently associated with a decreased risk of cancers at multiple sites. The strongest protective effect has been associated with cancers of the respiratory and gastrointestinal tracts. Fruits and vegetables contain a variety of substances with anticancer effects including micronutrients such as carotenoids, and other bioactive compounds such as phenols, isothiocyanates, and indoles, making it difficult to sort out which component(s) are responsible for the protective effect.

8. What are carotenoids and why are they important in cancer prevention?

Carotenoids are a group of pigments in fruits and vegetables that include alpha-carotene, beta-carotene, lycopene, lutein, and numerous other compounds. They are found in dark yellow and orange fruits and vegetables such as carrots, sweet potatoes, cantaloupe, and leafy dark green vegetables, such as broccoli and spinach. A diet high in fruits and vegetables containing carotenoids has been consistently associated with a decreased risk of cancer.

9. Does beta-carotene prevent lung cancer?

No. The carotenoid, beta-carotene, is an antioxidant found in fruits and vegetables. Eating a diet rich in fruits and vegetables has been consistently associated with decreased risk of lung cancer. In prospective, epidemiologic studies, high serum levels of beta-carotene were associated with a decreased risk of lung cancer. These findings led to three large clinical trials, in which high doses of synthetic beta-carotene were given to subjects at risk for developing lung cancer. Two of these studies found beta-carotene to be associated with a higher risk of lung cancer in cigarette smokers and a third study found no association between beta-carotene supplementation and lung cancer. Thus, clinical trials do not support the notion that beta-carotene can prevent lung cancer, and it may in fact be harmful in cigarette smokers (see table below).

Selected Large-scale Clinical Trials of β-carotene Supplementation and Lung Cancer

TRIAL	POPULATION	INTERVENTION	OUTCOME
Alpha-tocopherol and Beta-carotene (ATBC)	29,133 male Finnish smokers	β-carotene and/or α-tocopherol vs. placebo (2 x 2 factorial design)	18% increase in lung cancer and 8% increase in overall mortality in β-carotene arm
Beta-carotene and Retinol Efficacy Trial (CARET)	18,314 U.S. male and female smokers, former smokers, and asbestos workers	β-carotene and Retinol vs. placebo	28% increase in lung cancer and 17% increase in overall mortality in treatment arm
Physician's Health Study	22,071 U.S. male physicians	β-carotene and/or aspirin vs. placebo (2 x 2 factorial design)	No effect of β-carotene on lung cancer incidence or overall mortality

10. What are cruciferous vegetables and why are they important in cancer prevention?

Cruciferous vegetables include broccoli, cauliflower, and brussels sprouts, whose stems share certain structural features indicated by the reference to a cross in their collective name. Epidemiologic studies have related dietary intake of such vegetables to decreased incidence of certain cancers, particularly lung, stomach, colon, and rectal cancer. Several classes of chemicals are found in cruciferous vegetables, including indoles and isothiocyanates, that inhibit experimental tumors in animals or in vitro. One of these chemicals, sulforaphane, may exert its chemoprotective effect by inducing detoxification enzymes in the liver.

11. Can selenium lower cancer risk?

Possibly. Selenium is an essential mineral used by the body as part of the cellular and tissue defense against oxidative damage. Animal studies suggest a protective role of selenium against various cancers, but human epidemiologic data are inconsistent. In the Nutritional Prevention of Skin Cancer study, a randomized, controlled trial, selenium supplementation did not protect against skin cancer development. Of note, total cancer incidence and the rates of lung, colorectal, and prostate cancer were significantly lower in the selenium treatment arm, suggesting a possible protective effect of selenium. Among the population of Linxian, China, which has a very low intake of several micronutrients, dietary supplementation with a combination of various micronutrients (beta-carotene, vitamin E, and selenium) has been shown to modestly reduce total deaths from cancer (9%) and stomach cancer (21%). Whether this type of intervention would be of any benefit in populations with a typical Western diet is not known. Although excessive selenium supplementation can have serious adverse health effects. the question of whether selenium can prevent cancer warrants further study.

12. Does a diet high in dietary fiber prevent cancer?

Dietary fiber is generally defined as those components of food plants resistant to the enzymes produced by the digestive tract and is divided into two categories, water-soluble and water-insoluble. Evidence suggests that diets high in fiber-containing foods are associated with a reduced risk of cancer, particularly colorectal cancer. Because foods that are high in fiber (fruits and vegetables) also contain other micronutrients and phytochemicals that are potential anticarcinogens and are usually lower in fat, it is not clear if all the protective effect is attributable to dietary fiber. Epidemiologic and animal studies are somewhat inconsistent and information gained from ongoing large-scale, randomized clinical trials may help to clarify the relationship between dietary fiber and cancer.

13. A high-fat diet has been associated with an increased risk of which cancers?

A diet high in fat has been linked to increased risk of various cancers, particularly colon, prostate, and breast. Ecologic studies correlating international rates of cancer and per capita fat consumption have consistently shown higher incidence and mortality rates for colon, prostate, and breast cancer in populations consuming high-fat diets compared to low-fat diets. In addition, studies of populations migrating from low- to high-incidence areas have found that the migrants adopt the cancer rates of the new environment. Experimental studies in animals also support a role for fat in carcinogenesis in that diets high in fat promote tumor growth in animal models. Dietary fat has not been accepted by all as important in the etiology of these cancers, particularly breast cancer. International correlational and migrant studies are subject to confounding because many other factors, including physical activity, reproductive behaviors, and obesity, also differ among these countries. Individuals who consume a low-fat diet typically have other dietary patterns such as a diet high in fruits and vegetables, also associated with protection against cancer. Dietary fat intake is highly correlated with calorie intake, making it difficult to sort out whether it is fat calorie intake that is the major dietary factor affecting cancer risk. Some prospective cohort studies have weakened the support for a relationship between fat and breast cancer and others suggest that other components in red meat besides fat may be responsible for the relationship between colon cancer and fat. Ongoing randomized clinical trials should help clarify these issues.

14. Which cancers are most strongly associated with alcohol ingestion?

Cancers of the oropharynx, esophagus, and larynx are most strongly associated with alcohol ingestion. Cigarette smoking tends to be synergistic with alcohol in the risk for these tumors. For example, individuals who consume more than four drinks per day have a 9-fold increased risk of oral and pharyngeal cancers. Heavy drinkers and smokers have a greater than 36-fold excess risk of these cancers. About 75% of all oral and pharyngeal cancers may be attributed to excess alcohol ingestion and smoking. Alcohol is also associated with hepatocellular carcinoma—deaths from this cancer are about 50% higher in alcoholics. Epidemiologic evidence also supports the role of alcohol in breast cancer, although the magnitude of the risk is small. Drinkers of at least 2 drinks per day have about a 1.3-fold increased risk of breast cancer compared to nondrinkers. Epidemiologic studies suggest that alcohol intake may be associated with an increased risk of rectal cancer. Limiting or eliminating alcohol intake is fundamental to the prevention of alcohol-related cancers.

15. What is the role of physical activity in cancer prevention?

Physical activity may be protective against some cancers, particularly breast and colorectal cancer. Animal studies and epidemiologic studies support an inverse association between physical activity and some cancers. The protective mechanism of physical activity is uncertain. For breast cancer, the protection may be related to effects of physical activity on endogenous hormones. Decreased contact time between bowel mucosa and potential mutagens in the stool due to bowel transit stimulation by physical activity has been proposed to explain the protective effect of physical activity on colorectal cancer. Because physical activity is very difficult to measure accurately and is associated with other factors such as obesity, bias and confounding exist in the epidemiologic data. Thus, it is premature to conclude a causal relationship between physical activity and cancer at the present time.

16. What is the relationship between sunlight exposure and skin cancer?

Skin cancer occurs predominantly in white populations, particularly in fair-complexioned individuals who freckle and burn easily. Skin cancer can be divided into melanoma and nonmelanoma skin cancer (e.g., basal and squamous cell cancers). Skin cancer most often occurs on areas of the body exposed to sunlight; this anatomic pattern is more typical for nonmelanoma skin cancer than melanoma. The incidence of skin cancer is inversely correlated with latitude and is positively related to ultraviolet (UV) radiation. Most nonmelanoma skin cancers are related to cumulative exposure to UV radiation, while melanoma is more related to intense intermittent exposure to UV radiation, accompanied by episodes of blistering, particularly in early life. Preventive measures, including protective clothing, sun avoidance, and sunscreen lotions, may reduce the risk of skin cancer. Although the use of sunscreens may provide some protection against skin cancer, their full efficacy has not yet been established.

17. Infectious agents may have a role in which cancers?

Several viruses have been associated with the development of certain cancers. Recently, the bacterial infection *Helicobacter pylori* has been linked to gastric carcinoma and mucosal-associated gastric lymphoma. Although it is unlikely that humans can be protected from all infectious agents, preventive measures such as vaccines have been developed (hepatitis B) or are being developed (human papillomavirus) to prevent some of these infections.

Selected Human Viruses with Oncogenic Potential

VIRUS	ASSOCIATED TUMOR
Hepatitis B	Hepatocellular carcinoma
Hepatitis C	
Epstein-Barr	Burkitt's lymphoma
	Hodgkin's disease
	Nasopharyngeal carcinoma
Human Herpesvirus 8	Kaposi's sarcoma
Human papillomaviruses 16, 18	Cervical carcinoma
Human lymphotropic virus type I (HTLV-I)	Adult T-cell lymphoma/leukemia

18. Define chemoprevention.

Carcinogenesis of most (if not all) tissues is a multistep process in which multiple discreet molecular and cellular alterations occur over time, resulting in the disruption of normal cell growth and regulation. The long (often greater than 20 years) latent period over which these changes occur provides the opportunity to arrest or reverse this process. Chemoprevention is the use of synthetic, chemical, or natural agents to reverse, suppress, or prevent the carcinogenic process. For example, the nonsteroidal antiinflammatory drug Sulindac has been used as a chemopreventive agent in clinical trials to prevent the development of colorectal adenomas and to cause regression of established adenomas in patients with familial adenomatous polyposis coli who are at very high risk for developing colorectal cancer.

19. Describe the differences in study design between cancer chemoprevention and cancer chemotherapeutic clinical trials.

Chemoprevention trials are larger, more complex, and more delicate than chemotherapeutic trials, because chemopreventive agents are intended for use by large numbers of people, most of whom will never develop cancer. As a result, no significant toxicity is acceptable for a chemopreventive agent. Chemoprevention trials in average-risk populations using the incidence of cancer as the endpoint typically require thousands of patients to be followed for as long as decades. Because such large trials are very expensive, strong epidemiologic data, consistent animal data, and favorable phase I and II clinical trials are required to justify a phase III chemoprevention trial. Identification of high-risk populations and reliable intermediate endpoints can simplify such trials substantially. Some distinctions can be drawn between cancer therapeutic trials and chemoprevention trials as outlined below:

1. **Phase I chemotherapeutic trials** are designed to define the maximal dose that does not cause life-threatening toxicity. The goal of a phase I chemoprevention trial is to define the maximal nontoxic dose of the compound.

2. **Phase II chemotherapeutic trials** are designed to determine if one or more of the tolerated doses of the agent causes objective regression of a cancer. Phase II chemoprevention trials are designed to determine if one or more nontoxic doses of an agent have a biologic effect on the relevant intermediate endpoint (inhibition of prostaglandin synthesis or regression of adenomas in the colon by sulindac, for example).

3. **Phase III chemotherapeutic trials** are controlled studies designed to determine the treatment efficacy of an agent and usually can be completed with hundreds of patients followed from several months to a few years. Phase III chemoprevention trials are designed to determine if an agent can prevent the occurrence of a new malignant lesion and often require thousands of patients and long follow-up.

20. List the qualities of an ideal chemoprevention agent.
1. High therapeutic index (high efficacy/toxicity ratio)
2. Easy to administer (oral or topical administration)
3. Competitively priced
4. Known mechanism of action

No one agent is likely to meet all these criteria, but they need to be kept in mind in the design of clinical trials.

21. What is meant by the terms intermediate endpoint and biomarker?
The use of intermediate endpoints in clinical trials is not a new paradigm in medicine. Clinical investigations in the cardiovascular literature have used intermediate endpoints such as blood pressure and cholesterol measurements for quite some time. In the context of carcinogenesis, an intermediate endpoint is a feature of one or more of the early stages of carcinogenesis that may be used as a surrogate endpoint (in place of cancer itself) for a primary prevention trial. Intermediate endpoints can be histologic (adenomas in the colon, dysplasia in the lung), genetic (*K-ras* or p53 mutations), or biologic (proliferative or apoptotic rate of a tissue). The term biomarker is more general and can be defined as any biologic phenomenon that marks a cellular event. The word biomarker is often used to describe intermediate endpoints but can also be used to describe features that establish the biologic effect of an agent on relevant tissue, regardless of whether the feature is intrinsic to the process of carcinogenesis. For example, inhibition of prostaglandin synthesis can be used as a biomarker of the effects of Sulindac on the colon without knowing whether inhibition of prostaglandin synthesis is essential for any chemopreventive effect(s) of the agent.

22. List the ideal characteristics of an intermediate endpoint marker.
Several characteristics are to be considered when evaluating the potential of a biomarker to serve as an intermediate endpoint in a clinical trial:
1. Differential expression between normal and premalignant epithelium
2. Low rate of spontaneous reversion
3. High association with the eventual development of cancer
4. Reduction or disappearance of the marker indicates control of the disease
5. Modulation by chemopreventive agent being tested
6. Detection in easily accessible samples from healthy individuals
7. Highly sensitive, specific, and reproducible results

23. What preventive interventions are under investigation in the Women's Health Initiative?
The Women's Health Initiative is a 10-year multidisciplinary trial that was initiated in 1993 and includes both dietary and chemopreventive interventions. The effects of (1) a low-fat diet

(20% of calories from fat) and a diet high in fruits, vegetables, and fiber; (2) hormone replacement therapy; and (3) calcium and vitamin D supplementation on the prevention of cancer, cardiovascular disease, and osteoporosis are being studied in approximately 63,000 postmenopausal women. In addition to the randomized clinical trial, another 100,000 women will be followed prospectively for etiologic factors of future disease. Community-based intervention studies will also be implemented to determine effective ways to promote healthy behaviors aimed at preventing cancer, cardiovascular disease, and osteoporosis.

24. Does aspirin prevent colon cancer?

Possibly. There is substantial epidemiologic and animal data that aspirin and other nonsteroidal antiinflammatory drugs (NSAIDs) may prevent colorectal cancer. The mechanism by which NSAIDs exert their protective effect is unknown but may be due to the induction of apoptosis in early neoplastic cells. Clinical trials of NSAIDs in patients with familial adenomatous polyposis coli (who have a very high risk of colorectal cancer) have found that Sulindac decreased the size and number of adenomatous polyps. Whether these findings can be generalized to sporadic adenomas remains to be proven. The Physician's Health Study randomized 22,071 male physicians in the United States to aspirin on alternate days or placebo. The incidence of colorectal cancers in the men on the aspirin was not significantly different from those receiving placebo. The dose of aspirin (325 mg on alternate days) and duration of treatment and follow-up may not have been sufficient to see a protective effect. There are several ongoing clinical trials testing whether aspirin can prevent the development of adenomas in persons who have a prior history of colorectal adenoma or cancer. Recommendations regarding the use of aspirin by the general public for colorectal cancer prevention are premature based on the current scientific evidence and the risk of adverse events (e.g., hemorrhagic stroke and gastrointestinal bleeding) associated with aspirin use.

25. Name two hormonal agents being tested in chemoprevention trials.

Tamoxifen and finasteride. The Breast Cancer Prevention Trial (BCPT) is a large, multicenter chemoprevention study that is testing the ability of tamoxifen, an antiestrogen, to prevent the development of breast cancer in women at increased risk for developing breast cancer. Initial results from this study, which began in 1992, were recently released. More than 13,000 women aged 35 and older were randomized to either tamoxifen or placebo for an average of 4 years. A 45% reduction in breast cancer incidence occurred in the tamoxifen arm compared with the placebo arm (85 vs. 154 cases). Tamoxifen, however, did increase the risk of three rare events: endometrial cancer, pulmonary embolism, and deep venous thrombosis. Women who are at increased risk of breast cancer based on the criteria used for the BCPT now have the option to use tamoxifen for breast cancer chemoprevention. The decision whether or not to take tamoxifen is complex and requires careful consideration of the risk and benefits in consultation with one's personal physician.

Another hormonal agent being tested in a chemoprevention trial is finasteride. Finasteride, a 5-α-reductase inhibitor, blocks the conversion of testosterone to dihydrotestosterone (DHT) in the prostate. DHT is a more potent stimulator of prostate epithelial proliferation than testosterone. The Prostate Cancer Prevention Trial is a large, multicenter chemoprevention study testing the ability of finasteride to prevent the development of prostate cancer in healthy men aged 55 years and older. Eighteen thousand men have been randomized to 5 mg/day of finasteride or placebo for 7 years. At the end of the treatment period, all men will undergo a prostate biopsy with the endpoint of this study being prostate cancer.

BIBLIOGRAPHY

1. The Alpha-Tocopherol, Beta-Carotene Cancer Prevention Study Group: The effect of vitamin E and beta-carotene on the incidence of lung cancer and other cancers in male smokers. N Engl J Med 330:1029–1035, 1994.
2. The American Cancer Society 1996 Advisory Committee on Diet, Nutrition, and Cancer Prevention: Guidelines on diet, nutrition, and cancer prevention: Reducing the risk of cancer with healthy food choices and physical activity. CA Cancer J Clin 46:325–341, 1996.

3. Blot WJ: Alcohol and cancer. Cancer Research 52(Suppl 7):2119s–2123s, 1992.
4. Blot WJ, Li JY, Taylor PR, et al: Nutrition intervention trials in Linxian, China: Supplementation with specific vitamin/mineral combinations, cancer incidence, and disease-specific mortality in the general population. J Natl Cancer Inst 85:1483–1492, 1993.
5. Clark LC, Combs GF, Turnbull BW, et al: Effects of selenium supplementation for cancer prevention in patients with carcinoma of the skin. JAMA 276:1957–1963, 1996.
6. Greenwald P, Cullen JW: The new emphasis in cancer control. J Natl Cancer Inst 74:543–551, 1985.
7. Greenwald P, Kelloff G, Burch-Whitman C, Kramer BS: Chemoprevention. CA Cancer J Clin 45:31–49, 1995.
8. Harras A, Edwards BK, Blot WJ, Ries LA (eds): Cancer Rates and Risks. NIH Publication No. 96–691, 1996.
9. Hennekens CH, Buring JE, Manson JE, et al: Lack of effect of long-term supplementation with beta-carotene on the incidence of malignant neoplasms and cardiovascular disease. N Engl J Med 334:1145–1149, 1996.
10. Omenn GS, Goodman GE, Thornquist MD, et al: Effects of a combination of beta-carotene and vitamin A on lung cancer and cardiovascular disease. N Engl J Med 334:1150–1155, 1996.
11. Schatzkin A, Longnecker MP: Alcohol and breast cancer: Where are we now and where do we go from here? Cancer 74:1101–1110, 1994.
12. Shopland DR, Eyre HJ, Pechacek TF: Smoking-attributable cancer mortality in 1991: Is lung cancer now the leading cause of death among smokers in the United States? J Natl Cancer Inst 83:1142–1148, 1991.
13. Smigel K: Breast cancer prevention trial shows major benefit, some risk. J Natl Cancer Inst 90:647–648, 1998.
14. Thune I, Brenn T, Lund E, Gaard M: Physical activity and the risk of breast cancer. N Engl J Med 336:1269–1275, 1997.
15. Willett WC: Diet and nutrition. In Schottenfeld D, Fraumeni JF (eds): Cancer Epidemiology and Prevention. New York, Oxford University Press, 1996, pp 438–461.

40. CANCER CHEMOTHERAPY: PREVENTION AND MANAGEMENT OF COMMON TOXICITIES

Amy W. Valley, Pharm.D., BCPS, and Laura Boehnke Michaud, Pharm.D.

1. Why is toxicity a major problem in cancer chemotherapy?

The drugs used in cancer chemotherapy are unique in that they have a narrow therapeutic window. The dosage needed for antitumor effect is not much different from the dosage that causes potentially lethal toxicity. Because many of these toxicities are irreversible or life-threatening, emphasis should be placed on prevention, whenever possible. The table below summarizes the major toxicities of the most commonly used antineoplastic agents.

Major Toxicities of Commonly Used Antineoplastic Agents

GENERIC NAME (BRAND NAME)	TOXICITIES
Bleomycin (Blenoxane)	Pulmonary toxicity,* fevers, hypersensitivity reactions (rare), dermatologic toxicity (mucositis, desquamation)
Carboplatin (Paraplatin)	Myelosuppression,* moderate-to-severe N/V
Cisplatin (Platinol)	Nephrotoxicity,* severe N/V, neurotoxicity,* anemia
Cyclophosphamide (Cytoxan) Ifosfamide (Ifex)	Myelosuppression,* hemorrhagic cystitis (Ifosfamide*), moderate-to-severe N/V, SIADH[‡] (Cytoxan)
Cytarabine, Ara-C (Cytosar-U)	Myelosuppression,* mucositis, severe N/V,[†] neurotoxicity,[†] conjunctivitis[†]

Table continued on following page.

Major Toxicities of Commonly Used Antineoplastic Agents (Continued)

GENERIC NAME (BRAND NAME)	TOXICITIES
Dacarbazine (DTIC)	Severe N/V, mild-to-moderate myelosuppression,* flulike symptoms, phlebitis
Daunorubicin (Cerubidine) Doxorubicin (Adriamycin) Idarubicin (Idamycin)	Myelosuppression,* cardiotoxicity,* moderate-to-severe N/V, complete alopecia, vesicants
Etoposide, VP-16 (VePesid)	Myelosuppression,* hypotension with rapid infusion
5-Fluorouracil (Adrucil, others)	Myelosuppression,* mucositis,* diarrhea,* phlebitis
Gemcitabine (Gemzar)	Myelosuppression*
Irinotecan, CPT-11 (Camptosar)	Myelosuppression,* diarrhea,* severe N/V
Methotrexate (Mexate, others)	Myelosuppression,* mucositis,* nephrotoxicity (with high-dose regimens), neurotoxicity (with intrathecal dosing)
Mitoxantrone (Novantrone)	Myelosuppression,* moderate N/V, cardiotoxicity
Nitrogen mustard (Mechlorethamine, Mustargen)	Myelosuppression,* severe N/V
Paclitaxel (Taxol) Docetaxel (Taxotere)	Myelosuppression,* hypersensitivity (Paclitaxel), fluid retention (docetaxel), myalgias, neurotoxicity, complete alopecia
Topotecan (Hycamtin)	Myelosuppression, mild-to-moderate N/V
Vincristine (Oncovin) Vinblastine (Velban) Vinorelbine (Navelbine)	Neurotoxicity (vincristine*), vesicant, SIADH‡, myelosuppression (vinblastine* and vinorelbine* only)

* Dose-limiting side effect(s)
† With high-dose regimens
‡ Syndrome of inappropriate antidiuretic hormone

MYELOSUPPRESSION

2. Do all chemotherapy drugs cause myelosuppression?

In cancer chemotherapy, the dose-limiting side effect (DLSE) is defined as the toxicity that determines the maximal tolerated dose. Although myelosuppression is a common DLSE of antineoplastic agents, a few agents do not produce this effect, such as bleomycin and vincristine. Patient-specific factors also significantly influence the risk for bone marrow toxicity. Empiric dosage reductions of myelosuppressive agents are often made for the first chemotherapy treatment in patients with low baseline white blood cell or platelet counts, diminished bone marrow reserve from prior chemotherapy or radiation therapy, tumor involvement of bone marrow, and impaired capability for drug elimination. The last factor is related to the pharmacokinetic profile of the myelosuppressive agent. For example, if a marrow-toxic drug depends on renal excretion for elimination, the patient with impaired renal function will have higher drug levels and be at increased risk for myelosuppression. When myelosuppressive drugs are used in combination chemotherapy regimens, the dosages are lower than when the drugs are used as single agents to prevent additive toxicity.

3. When should patients be monitored for chemotherapy-induced myelosuppression?

The bone marrow is a common site of toxicity because many chemotherapy agents target rapidly dividing cells, including committed blood cell precursors. Direct stem cell damage is not common, but when it occurs, it is usually related to use of the alkylating agents. Myelosuppression does not usually occur immediately after chemotherapy administration. Blood components that have already been produced by the bone marrow must be consumed before the effect is realized. White blood cells, especially granulocyte precursors, are usually affected to the most significant degree because of their short lifespan (6–12 hours). Platelets (5–10 day lifespan) are also affected but usually to a lesser degree than white blood cells. Erythrocytes have the longest lifespan (120 days) and are affected to the least degree. After chemotherapy, usual nadirs (lowest blood cell counts) occur at 7–14 days, with recovery by 21–28 days. Patients should have a complete blood count (CBC) with differential performed 1–2 weeks after chemotherapy to assess marrow toxicity. Exceptions to this time frame include the nitrosoureas and mitomycin-C, which produce more prolonged patterns of nadir (4–6 weeks) and recovery (6–8 weeks). Planned courses of chemotherapy may be delayed while waiting for blood counts to recover. For a patient to resume chemotherapy safely, a WBC $\geq 3000/mm^3$ or absolute neutrophil count (ANC) of $\geq 1500/mm^3$ and platelets $\geq 100,000/mm^3$ are usually required. The ANC may be calculated by multiplying the percentage of neutrophils (segmented + banded neutrophils) by the total WBC count.

4. What is the most appropriate management for patients who experience myelosuppression?
Marrow suppression is an expected phenomenon in leukemic patients receiving induction chemotherapy. In contrast, myelosuppression is an undesirable side effect in patients receiving chemotherapy for treatment of other malignancies. Most patients with solid tumors do not experience clinically significant myelosuppression after standard-dose chemotherapy. If neutropenia or thrombocytopenia occurs, doses of the myelosuppressive drug(s) may be reduced on subsequent cycles. Patients receiving myelosuppressive chemotherapy must be counseled about signs and symptoms of infection and bleeding and instructed to seek prompt medical attention if they experience these effects.

Neutropenia. Another alternative for patients who experience significant neutropenia (ANC $< 500/mm^3$) is the use of the colony-stimulating factors (CSFs). Granulocyte-CSF (G-CSF) and granulocyte-macrophage CSF (GM-CSF) may be used to maintain full chemotherapy doses and to prevent recurrence of neutropenia. In this setting, the CSFs are usually started the day after chemotherapy ends and are continued throughout the period of neutropenic risk (7–14 days). The use of CSFs in the treatment of established neutropenia is more controversial. To date, no preponderance of data supports routine clinical use of these costly drugs in uncomplicated neutropenia. Patients with neutropenic fever should receive prompt empiric treatment with broad-spectrum antibiotics. The management of infections in immunocompromised patients is covered in another chapter. G-CSF and GM-CSF do not produce clinically significant effects on erythrocyte and platelet precursors.

Thrombocytopenia. Recently, the first CSF to effect platelet recovery has been approved by the Food and Drug Administration. Interleukin-11 (NeuMega) is indicated to prevent thrombocytopenia and reduce platelet transfusions in high-risk patients after myelosuppressive chemotherapy. It does not appear to be effective in the treatment of established thrombocytopenia. In this setting platelet transfusions are indicated for platelet counts $< 10–20,000/mm^3$ or at higher levels if the patient is bleeding. Side effects of interleukin-11 include tachycardia, atrial arrhythmias, and fluid retention, with subsequent weight gain, edema, dyspnea, and pleural effusions.

Anemia. Anemia in cancer patients is often multifactorial. Epoietin alfa (recombinant human erythropoietin) is indicated for the management of chronic cancer- and chemotherapy-related anemia. This CSF should be considered only after ruling out other causes of anemia (e.g., iron deficiency, bleeding, hemolysis). The onset of effect of epoietin alfa is delayed for 1–2 weeks. Significant anemia (hematocrit < 25% or higher if symptomatic) is managed acutely via red blood cell transfusions.

GASTROINTESTINAL TOXICITY

5. How common are nausea and vomiting due to chemotherapy?
An estimated 1–10% of cancer patients refuse or prematurely discontinue chemotherapy because of nausea and vomiting (N/V). With the widespread use of the serotonin-receptor antagonists, this percentage may improve. However, complications of uncontrolled N/V still delay scheduled courses of chemotherapy and significantly impair the patient's quality of life. These complications include anorexia, malnutrition, dehydration, electrolyte and acid-base imbalance, gastrointestinal

mucosal tears, wound dehiscence, aspiration pneumonia, and development of anticipatory N/V. The reported incidence of chemotherapy-induced N/V varies markedly and depends on several factors:

1. **Emetogenic potential** of chemotherapy agent(s) (see table below). Not all chemotherapy agents cause N/V. This factor is the most important determinant of N/V risk.

2. **Dosage** of chemotherapy agent. For example, high-dose cytarabine often produces severe N/V, whereas low-dose cytarabine is associated with a low incidence (see table below).

3. **Method of administration.** For example, doxorubicin given as a rapid intravenous bolus is associated with a moderately high incidence of N/V, but when it is given as a continuous intravenous infusion over 24 hours, the incidence is mild.

4. **Patient-specific factors.** Previous N/V experience with chemotherapy influences the outcome with subsequent treatment regimens. Patients with a history of heavy alcohol use (> 5 mixed drinks/day) have a decreased incidence of N/V.

5. **Use of combination regimens.** Many combination regimens are associated with additive or synergistic N/V.

Relative Emetogenic Potential of Antineoplastic Agents

LEVEL 1: LOW (< 10%)	LEVEL 2: MODERATELY LOW (10–30%)	LEVEL 3: MODERATE (30–60%)	LEVEL 4: MODERATELY HIGH (60–90%)	LEVEL 5: HIGH (> 90%)
Bleomycin	Cytarabine	Aldesleukin	Carboplatin	Carmustine
Busulfan	< 1 gm/m^2	Altretamine	Carmustine	> 250 mg/m^2
Capectitabine	Docetaxel	Cyclophosphamide	≤ 250 mg/m^2	Cisplatin
Chlorambucil	Etoposide (VP-16)	≤ 750 mg/m^2	Cisplatin	≥ 50 mg/m^2
Cladribine	5-Fluorouracil	Cyclophosphamide	< 50 mg/m^2	Cyclophos-
Estramustine	< 1 gm/m^2	(PO)	Cyclophosphamide	phamide
Fludarabine	Gemcitabine	Doxorubicin	> 750 and	$> 1,500$ mg/m^2
Hydroxyurea	L-asparaginase	20–60 mg/m^2	≤ 1500 mg/m^2	Dacarbazine
Interferon alfa	Methotrexate > 50	Daunorubicin	Cytarabine	Mechlorethamine
Melphalan (oral)	and < 250 mg/m^2	Epirubicin	≥ 1 gm/m^2	Streptozocin
Mercaptopurine	Mitomycin -C	≤ 90 mg/m^2	Doxorubicin	
Methotrexate	Paclitaxel	Idarubicin	> 60 mg/m^2	
< 50 mg/m^2	Teniposide	Ifosfamide	Dactinomycin	
Rituximab	Thiotepa	Methotrexate	Irinotecan	
Thioguanine	< 15 mg/m^2	250–1000 mg/m^2	Methotrexate	
Tretinoin	Topotecan	Mitoxantrone	> 1 gm/m^2	
Vinblastine		≤ 15 mg/m^2	Lomustine (CCNU)	
Vincristine			Pentostatin	
Vinorelbine			Procarbazine	

Descriptors and (%) refer to the incidence of moderate-to-severe nausea and vomiting without antiemetics. The above information pertains to conventional doses of chemotherapy and is not applicable to the setting of bone marrow transplantation.

6. How is the most appropriate antiemetic regimen selected?

Several antiemetics are available, and selection depends on desired potency, adverse effects, patient-specific factors, and cost, as described below. In general, all antiemetic regimens are most effective when given to *prevent* N/V. The antiemetic regimen should be started before chemotherapy administration and continued around the clock throughout the period of N/V risk. For most chemotherapy drugs, the period of N/V risk is 24–36 hours. However, there are some exceptions. Cisplatin is associated with a delayed phase of N/V at 48–72 hours after administration. Antiemetic coverage should be provided on a regular schedule throughout this period (3 days after cisplatin). N/V control should be reassessed before each chemotherapy treatment.

1. **Potency.** Using the information presented in the table below and in question 5, the risk for N/V can be estimated for specific chemotherapy regimens. Some antiemetics are effective only against mild-to-moderate emetogens, whereas others are effective against even the most

emetogenic antineoplastics. The more potent antiemetics are not used routinely for all chemotherapy regimens because of adverse effects and/or cost. In general, combination antiemetic therapy is indicated for patients receiving moderately to highly emetogenic chemotherapy regimens.

2. **Adverse effects.** Antagonism of dopamine receptors in the chemoreceptor trigger zone (CTZ) is the mechanism of action for many of the currently available antiemetic agents (e.g., phenothiazines, butyrophenones, metoclopramide). Unfortunately, the antidopamine effects also may lead to extrapyramidal side effects such as dystonic reactions, pseudo-Parkinsonism, and akathisia. Other antiemetics, such as the serotonin-receptor antagonists, lack these side effects.

3. **Patient-specific factors.** For example, patients with anticipatory N/V may benefit from the anxiolytic and amnestic effects of benzodiazepines. Patients less than 30 years of age are at higher risk for extrapyramidal side effects.

4. **Cost.** Although highly effective, the use of serotonin-receptor antagonists is limited by high cost.

Comparison of Antiemetic Agents

CLASS GENERIC (BRAND)	MECHANISM OF ACTION	POTENCY*	ADVERSE EFFECTS	COST†	COMMENTS
Phenothiazines Prochlorperazine (Compazine) Thiethylperazine (Torecan)	Dopamine inhibition at CTZ	Mild to moderate	Mild sedation, anticholinergic effects, EPS	+	Side effects minimal, multiple routes of administration (PO/IV/IM/PR)
Butyrophenones Haloperidol (Haldol) Droperidol (Inapsine)	Dopamine inhibition at CTZ	Mild to moderate	Mild sedation, EPS	+	Low doses effective, less EPS than with antipsychotic doses
Benzodiazepines Lorazepam (Ativan)	Inhibition of cortical input into VC	Mild	Sedation, amnesia, respiratory depression (uncommon)	+	Anxiolytic effects useful in some patients, used to prevent/treat anticipatory N/V
Cannabinoids Dronabinol (Marinol)	Inhibition of cortical input into VC?	Mild to moderate	Sedation, anticholinergic effects, euphoria/dysphoria	++	Appetite stimulation may be useful side effect
Corticosteroids Dexamethasone (Decadron) Methylprednisolone (Solu-Medrol)	Inhibition of cortical input into VC?	Moderate to severe	Short-term effects: insomnia, agitation, mild euphoria, perirectal burning w/IV use	+	Not for long-term use due to side effects
Metoclopramide (Reglan)	5-HT3 inhibition at CTZ and GI tract	Severe	Sedation, EPS (premedicate with Benadryl), diarrhea	+ (PO) ++ (IV)	Combine with corticosteroids against severe emetogens
Serotonin antagonists Ondansetron (Zofran) Granisetron (Kytril) Dolasetron (Anzemet)	5-HT3 inhibition at CTZ and GI tract	Severe	Mild headache, constipation	+++	Combine with corticosteroids against severe emetogens

* Expressed as efficacy against antineoplastic agents of mild, moderate, or severe emetogenic potential.
† Cost per day: + = $0–3.00 (PO), $0–20.00 (IV); ++ = $4.25 (PO), $21–95 (IV); +++ = $26–70 (PO), $96–160 (IV) (source: 1997 Redbook).
CTZ = chemoreceptor trigger zone, VC = vomiting center, 5-HT3 = serotonin type 3 receptors, GI = gastrointestinal, EPS = extrapyramidal side effects.

7. How should mucositis in the chemotherapy patient be prevented and treated?

The gastrointestinal (GI) mucosa is composed of epithelial cells with a high mitotic index and rapid turnover rate, making it a common site of chemotherapy-induced toxicity. The subsequent inflammation or mucositis may lead to painful ulcerations, local infection, and inability to eat, drink, and swallow. The disruption of the GI mucosal barrier also may provide an avenue for systemic microbial invasion. The time course for development and resolution of mucositis often parallels that seen with neutropenia. Agents most commonly associated with mucositis include 5-fluorouracil (5–FU), doxorubicin, and methotrexate.

The most effective means of preventing mucositis is good oral hygiene. Patients at high risk for this toxicity should be evaluated by a dentist before chemotherapy and should be instructed to rinse their mouth frequently with baking soda and salt water or chlorhexidine (Peridex) rinses after chemotherapy. For patients receiving 5-FU treatment, the use of ice (oral cryotherapy) may decrease the risk for mucositis. Once mucositis has developed, treatment is mainly supportive, including use of topical or systemic analgesics and oral hygiene (e.g., rinses described above). Severe cases may require intravenous hydration. Local infections due to *Candida* species and herpes simplex viruses are common. Suspicious lesions should be cultured and appropriate antifungal and/or antiviral treatment instituted. Antifungal therapy may be delivered topically for mild infections (thrush), using clotrimazole (Mycelex) troches or nystatin (Nilstat) oral suspension. For more severe oral or esophageal fungal infections, systemic treatment with oral ketoconazole (Nizoral) or fluconazole (Diflucan) is indicated.

Mucosal damage may occur at any point along the entire length of the GI tract. In the lower portion of the GI tract, this damage may be manifested as diarrhea (mild to life-threatening) and abdominal pain. Support with intravenous fluids and electrolyte supplementation should be initiated promptly in severe cases. Once infectious causes have been ruled out, diarrhea can be treated safely with antispasmodics, such as diphenoxylate/atropine (Lomotil) or loperamide (Immodium). Recently, the somatostatin analog octreotide has been used successfully to treat severe cases of 5-FU-induced diarrhea.

8. A 62-year-old woman with colon cancer has been admitted to the hospital with refractory diarrhea, dehydration, and hypokalemia. She received chemotherapy 9 days before admission. Do any chemotherapy drugs cause significant diarrhea?

The chemotherapy agents most likely to cause diarrhea are 5-fluorouracil (5-FU), irinotecan, and interleukin-2. Both 5-FU and irinotecan are commonly used in colon cancer. 5-FU-induced diarrhea is due to mucositis in the lower GI tract, as described in the previous question. Irinotecan (CPT-11, Camptosar) has even greater potential to cause diarrhea but by different mechanisms. There are two forms of irinotecan-related diarrhea: early and late. Early diarrhea generally occurs during or shortly after administration of the drug in up to 50% of patients (8% grade 3 or 4 in severity). It is often preceded by facial flushing, diaphoresis, and abdominal cramping. It is believed to be a cholinergically mediated process and responds well to atropine, 0.25–1 mg IV × 1. The late form of diarrhea occurs in 90% of patients (30% grade 3 or 4 in severity). The median onset is 11 days after irinotecan administration with a median duration of 3 days. However, the diarrhea is prolonged in some patients, resulting in life-threatening dehydration and electrolyte imbalances. The mechanism is unclear but may be related to high levels of the active metabolite SN-38 in the gut. It is notoriously refractory to standard antidiarrheals, with the exception of high-dose loperamide. Patients are instructed to take two capsules (4 mg) at the first sign of loose stools and to continue one capsule every 2 hours until 12 hours without a bowel movement. This regimen is higher than the usual maximal recommended daily doses of loperamide (16 mg/day) but is highly effective and well tolerated in this setting. High-dose interleukin-2 regimens (600,000 µ/kg/dose) cause diarrhea in 76% of patients, possibly due to bowel edema. This diarrhea may be severe; bowel hemorrhage, infarction, and intestinal perforation have been reported.

9. What treatment strategies can be used to enhance appetite in patients with cancer?

The complications of cancer cachexia are a common cause of death. Malnutrition appears to result from a combination of decreased caloric intake and increased metabolic requirements caused by the tumor. The most common causes of decreased intake include anorexia, chronic nausea, alterations of taste or smell, pain, dysphagia, and depression. Several measures have been used to increase appetite. Clinical studies have shown that megestrol acetate (Megace) a progestational agent, stimulates appetite and produces weight gain in patients with cancer and AIDS. The usual effective dose is 800 mg/day. Because some studies have shown an increased risk for thromboembolism in patients treated with megestrol acetate, the drug should not be used in patients with known thromboembolic disease. Recently, several reports of adrenal insufficiency have been described in patients with cancer and AIDS taking megestrol acetate. Because of these side effects and its high cost, megestrol acetate should be discontinued if no benefit is seen after a 4–8 week trial. Other drugs used for appetite stimulation include the cannabinoid dronabinol (Marinol) and corticosteroids. Cyproheptadine (Periactin) and hydrazine sulfate have failed to show benefit in clinical trials and should be avoided. For patients who experience loss of appetite due to a feeling of persistent abdominal fullness or GI obstruction, metoclopramide (Reglan) or cisapride (Propulsid) may be beneficial. Patients with anorexia due to pain or depression should receive specific treatment for these disorders. Improvement of caloric intake does not address the problem of metabolic alterations caused by the tumor. Consequently, not all patients will benefit from these interventions, especially if they are initiated after cancer cachexia is in the advanced stages.

COMMON ORGAN-SPECIFIC TOXICITIES

10. How can cisplatin-induced nephrotoxicity be prevented?

During the early clinical trials of cisplatin, nephrotoxicity emerged as the dose-limiting side effect. Further experience with the drug has revealed that nephrotoxicity can usually be prevented or minimized with adequate hydration. Like other heavy metals, cisplatin concentrates in the kidneys, where it may cause necrosis of the proximal and distal tubules. These effects are both dose-related and cumulative. Increases in blood urea nitrogen (BUN) and serum creatinine are evident 1–2 weeks after cisplatin administration and usually reverse in 1–2 weeks in time for the next treatment. However, with repeated courses, the nephrotoxicity may worsen or become irreversible. Patients with preexisting renal dysfunction and patients receiving other nephrotoxic drugs are at highest risk.

Cisplatin nephrotoxicity may be prevented by vigorous hydration before, during, and after drug administration. Various regimens have been used successfully. The common factors of these regimens include use of a chloride-containing intravenous hydration solution (0.9% normal saline or dextrose 5%/0.9% normal saline), and maintenance of adequate urine output (≥ 100 ml/hr). The chloride solution is important to maintain the intrarenal cisplatin in its most nontoxic form. Maintenance of adequate urine output may require use of diuretics such as mannitol or furosemide (Lasix). The renal damage also leads to decreased tubular reabsorption of electrolytes. Patients receiving cisplatin require frequent magnesium and potassium supplementations. Adequate antiemetics for control of delayed emesis must be provided (see questions 5 and 6). Dehydration from uncontrolled emesis increases the risk for significant nephrotoxicity. Before each treatment, BUN, serum creatinine, and electrolytes should be reevaluated. Other strategies to prevent cisplatin nephrotoxicity include the use of less nephrotoxic analogs, such as carboplatin, and the use of the chemoprotectant, amifostine (WR-2721, Ethyol). Amifostine is costly and associated with adverse effects such as hypotension during infusion and severe refractory N/V. For prevention of cisplatin-induced nephrotoxicity, its use is usually reserved for high-risk patients. However, amifostine also appears to minimize other chemotherapy-related toxicities, including myelosuppression and possibly neurotoxicity. Further studies will define its ultimate role in cancer therapy.

11. The chronic dose-limiting side effect of doxorubicin is cardiotoxicity. At what total cumulative dose should doxorubicin be discontinued?

The cardiac toxicity of doxorubicin (Adriamycin) is most commonly manifested as congestive heart failure (CHF), which may progress to cardiomyopathy. The cause of the cardiac damage is believed to be formation of free oxygen radicals, induced by doxorubicin-iron complexes. Mortality from this toxicity is as high as 60%. The risk for development of cardiotoxicity depends on several factors. The most important is a total cumulative dosage of 450–550 mm/m^2, when the doxorubicin has been administered as an intravenous bolus every 3–4 weeks. The incidence of CHF below a cumulative dose of 450–550 mg/m^2 is only 0.1–0.2%. However, the incidence increases to 30% for cumulative doses exceeding 550 mg/m^2. Administration of the drug on a weekly basis or as a continuous infusion may safely permit higher cumulative doses, presumably because of the lower peak doxorubicin concentrations in the heart. Other risk factors for doxorubicin cardiotoxicity include age (young children or elderly patients), preexisting cardiac disease, concomitant treatment with other cardiotoxic agents, and prior mediastinal irradiation. Although cumulative dosage determines risk, actual cardiac function determines whether treatment should be discontinued. A baseline left ventricular ejection fraction (LVEF) is usually elevated before doxorubicin administration and monitored throughout treatment. Decreases in LVEF of 10% or more or an LVEF of less than 50% indicates that doxorubicin should be discontinued. Although analogs of doxorubicin (e.g., mitoxantrone [Novantrone], idarubicin [Idamycin]) have less cardiotoxicity than doxorubicin, some degree of cardiotoxicity is associated with their use. The chemoprotectant dexrazoxane (ICRF-187, Zinecard) is an iron chelator that prevents anthracycline-induced cardiotoxicity. It is currently indicated for patients with metastatic breast cancer who have received more than 300 mg/m^2 of doxorubicin. If further studies in other malignancies and early-stage disease confirm lack of a tumor-protective effect, dexrazoxane may become standard therapy for prevention of anthracycline-induced cardiotoxicity. Once cardiotoxicity occurs, the clinical management is the same as for any other type of CHF or cardiomyopathy.

12. Which chemotherapy agents are associated with pulmonary toxicity?

Although several chemotherapeutic drugs are associated with pulmonary toxicity, bleomycin is the most common causative agent. Toxicity appears to result from formation of reactive oxygen metabolites and subsequent inflammatory response in the lung. The initial reaction produces interstitial pneumonitis, which may progress to pulmonary fibrosis and death from hypoxia. The reported incidence of bleomycin pulmonary toxicity varies widely (0–50%) but averages 3–5% in most series. It increases dramatically after a total cumulative dose of 400 units (400 mg) is reached but may occur at any point during therapy or even several months after the last bleomycin dose. Other factors that may increase the risk include concurrent or subsequent use of high oxygen concentrations, prior or subsequent mediastinal irradiation, age > 70 years, and administration of single doses greater than 25 mg/m^2. The onset is insidious, consisting of cough, dyspnea, and occasional fever. Chest radiographic findings are nonspecific, and open lung biopsy may be required to differentiate bleomycin toxicity from other possible causes, such as infection and tumor infiltration. Once toxicity is detected, bleomycin should be discontinued. Despite drug withdrawal, pulmonary symptoms may continue to worsen. Use of corticosteroids may be beneficial, especially if the toxicity is related to a hypersensitivity reaction. Other chemotherapy agents associated with pulmonary toxicity include busulfan, the nitrosoureas (carmustine [BCNU], lomustine [CCNU]), mitomycin-C, methotrexate, and cyclophosphamide.

13. A 55-year-old man with extensive small cell lung cancer is admitted to the oncology service with a possible spinal cord compression. He reports numbness and tingling in his fingers and toes. Which chemotherapy drugs may cause these effects?

Vincristine is the chemotherapy agent most commonly associated with neurotoxicity. The most common manifestation is a peripheral neuropathy, but the spectrum of vincristine neurotoxicity also includes autonomic neuropathy (constipation, abdominal pain, ileus, urinary retention) and cranial nerve palsies (jaw pain, ptosis, optic nerve neuropathy). Initially, the peripheral neuropathy consists of paresthesias in the fingers and toes, accompanied by a decrease and eventual loss of deep tendon reflexes (DTRs). Some patients develop severe neuropathic pain as a consequence of the neuropathy. The most severe cases involve impairment of motor function, including wrist drop, foot drop, gait abnormalities, and even quadriparesis. Vincristine neurotoxicity is reversible if it is detected early and therapy is discontinued. Mild paresthesias are not an indication to stop vincristine therapy. However, if muscle weakness or difficulty with fine hand motions (buttoning the shirt, picking up small objects) occurs, vincristine therapy should be interrupted. Other vinca alkaloids (vinorelbine and vinblastine) are also associated with neurotoxicity but not to the same degree as vincristine.

Cisplatin is also associated with neurotoxicity, including ototoxicity, ocular toxicity, and peripheral neuropathy. The peripheral neuropathy caused by cisplatin is a cumulative dose-related effect (total dose: 300–600 mg/m^2), characterized mainly by sensory loss in a stocking-and-glove distribution. DTRs are usually decreased, but motor neuropathy is not common. The syndrome is usually reversible, but some patients have long-term sequelae. A similar cumulative syndrome is commonly observed in patients treated with paclitaxel (Taxol). High-dose cytarabine (Ara-C) (> 500 mg/m^2/dose) is also associated with severe and potentially fatal neurotoxicity. However, this toxicity is usually characterized by cerebellar and central nervous system alterations rather than peripheral neuropathy. Other neurotoxic antineoplastic agents include hexamethylmelamine (altretamine, Hexalen) and procarbazine (Matulane).

14. Which chemotherapy agents are associated with hypersensitivity reactions?

Like other drugs, almost every chemotherapy agent has been reported to cause at least a few cases of allergic reactions. The chemotherapy drugs most commonly associated with hypersensitivity reactions are bleomycin, L-asparaginase, and paclitaxel (Taxol). Although hyperpyrexia (with fevers up to 42° C) occurs in up to 30% of patients after the first few bleomycin treatments, true hypersensitivity reactions are rare. Nonetheless, the standard of practice at many institutions requires intradermal administration of a 1-unit (1-mg) test dose before the first dose of bleomycin. Patients receiving bleomycin should be premedicated with acetaminophen (Tylenol) to prevent fever. L-asparaginase is associated with the highest incidence of hypersensitivity reactions. The overall incidence is as high as 40% for patients receiving single-agent therapy and 20% for patients receiving combination regimens, which often include corticosteroids. The reactions may occur at any time during treatment but are most likely to occur in the second week of therapy. Test doses are associated with both false-negative and false-positive results and do not predict which patients will be affected. However, some clinicians still recommend a 2-unit test dose before the first dose of L-asparaginase; the test is repeated after any lapse between doses of more than 7 days. Commercially available L-asparaginase is derived from *Escherichia coli*. For patients who experience allergic reactions, an *Erwinia*-derived product is available. Recently, a pegylated formulation of L-asparaginase has been developed. This product is created by covalent attachment of polyethylene glycol to the *E. coli* enzyme, prolonging the half-life of the drug and also reducing the immunogenicity.

In the early development of paclitaxel, hypersensitivity reactions occurred in 84% of patients. Paclitaxel is formulated in a castor oil-based (cremophor-El) vehicle, which is believed to be the cause of hypersensitivity reactions. When patients are premedicated with dexamethasone, diphenhydramine (Benadryl), and an H$_2$-antagonist (such as cimetidine [Tagamet]), the incidence of reactions is significantly decreased but not completely eliminated. The other taxane, docetaxel (Taxotere), does not produce hypersensitivity reactions as commonly as paclitaxel, but it does produce cumulative, dose-related fluid retention. In severe cases, pulmonary edema and pericardial effusions have been observed. This syndrome is best prevented by a 3–5-day corticosteroid regimen.

15. A patient has just experienced extravasation of doxorubicin (Adriamycin). What should be done to prevent or minimize tissue damage?

Vesicants are drugs that can produce tissue necrosis on leakage outside the vein (extravasation). Commonly used antineoplastics with vesicant potential include the anthracyclines (doxorubicin and daunorubicin), mitomycin-C, nitrogen mustard (mechlorethamine), vincristine, and vinblastine. Once extravasation has occurred, several local maneuvers can decrease the extent of tissue damage. For most chemotherapy drugs, the most important intervention is application of ice to the affected area. The exception to this general rule is the application of heat to vinca alkaloid extravasations. Initially, the needle should be left in place, and an attempt should be made to aspirate drug from the site. If nothing can be aspirated, the needle should be removed. If fluid is aspirated, the needle can be left in place for instillation of specific antidotes, if applicable. Otherwise, the specific antidote can be injected locally to the affected area. Use of specific antidotes is controversial and is recommended for only a few chemotherapy agents. Examples include hyaluronidase (Wydase), which facilitates drug dispersion for vinca alkaloids, and sodium thiosulfate, which inactivates nitrogen mustard. Topical application of dimethylsulfoxide (DMSO) may be beneficial in anthracycline and mitomycin-C extravasations. Despite appropriate measures, some patients still develop severe tissue damage and possibly functional loss. The key to management is prevention of extravasations through skilled and careful nursing techniques. Use of central venous catheters should be considered in patients with poor peripheral venous access.

USE OF ADJUNCTIVE PROTECTIVE AGENTS

16. What are chemoprotectants?

Chemoprotectants are agents used to prevent toxicities from cancer chemotherapy. They specifically prevent toxicity in target tissues; they are not rescue agents. As such, CSFs, leucovorin, and antiemetics are not considered to be chemoprotectants. The characteristics of an ideal chemoprotectant are (1) protection against chemotherapy-induced toxicity, (2) lack of interference with the antitumor effects (3) lack of additive toxicities, and (4) cost-effectiveness. Three chemoprotectants are currently available: Mesna (see question 17), amifostine (see question 10), and dexrazoxane (see question 11).

17. Why is mesna given with ifosfamide?

Mesna (2-mercaptoethanesulfonate sodium [Na]) is used to prevent ifosfamide-induced hemorrhagic cystitis. Hemorrhagic cystitis is the DLSE of ifosfamide and occurs to a lesser extent with cyclophosphamide. Both drugs undergo extensive hepatic metabolism. The inactive metabolite acrolein is believed to cause hemorrhagic cystitis by binding to and irritating the epithelial lining of the genitourinary tract. Although toxicity is usually limited to the bladder, the entire genitourinary system is at risk. The clinical spectrum of hemorrhagic cystitis ranges from mild bleeding to life-threatening hemorrhage. Long-term consequences include bladder fibrosis and malignancy. When standard doses are used, cyclophosphamide-induced urotoxicity can be easily prevented with oral hydration (2–3 L/day) and frequent urination to decrease bladder contact time. High-dose cyclophosphamide regimens, as used with bone marrow transplants (BMTs), have a higher risk for bladder toxicity. Preventive regimens vary but include vigorous intravenous hydration, continuous bladder irrigations, mesna, or some combination of these interventions. The incidence of hemorrhagic cystitis is higher with ifosfamide because more acrolein is formed. Mesna is a sulfhydryl compound that inactivates acrolein. Mesna and hydration should always be given with ifosfamide to prevent hemorrhagic cystitis. Because mesna has a shorter plasma half-life than ifosfamide, mesna is usually continued for 8–24 hours after ifosfamide is administered. Once hemorrhagic cystitis occurs after either cyclophosphamide or ifosfamide, treatment consists of discontinuing the drug and intravenous hydration. Mild cases (microscopic hematuria) usually respond to this intervention alone. Several agents (alum, silver nitrate, formaldehyde) have been used in bladder irrigations to treat severe or refractory hemorrhagic cystitis. Most recently the prostaglandins (dinoprost and dinoprostone) have been used with some success. Surgical intervention, including arterial ligation or cystectomy, is indicated for severe, refractory patients.

18. When is leucovorin rescue necessary with methotrexate therapy?

Methotrexate (MTX) is a folic acid antagonist that exerts its antineoplastic action by reversibly binding to the enzyme dihydrofolate reductase. This action depletes cells of reduced folate, which is necessary for numerous biochemical reactions, including formation of precursors required for DNA synthesis. Administration of leucovorin (folinic acid) after MTX supplies normal cells with reduced folate and "rescues" them from methotrexate toxicity. To avoid rescuing cancer cells, it is necessary to wait for 24–42 hours after methotrexate administration before initiating leucovorin. If leucovorin rescue is delayed more than 42 hours, the rescue may not be complete, and toxicity will occur. Leucovorin rescue is usually not necessary for methotrexate doses < 100 mg/m². For methotrexate doses of ≥ 100 mg/m², leucovorin rescue is given in divided doses for 24–72 hours or until methotrexate serum concentrations fall below 0.01–0.05 µM. Leucovorin rescue prevents MTX-induced myelosuppression and mucositis. Another toxicity of high-dose (> 1 gm/m²) MTX is nephrotoxicity from crystallization of MTX in renal tubules. Leucovorin does not protect against this side effect. Aggressive hydration and alkalinization of the urine are crucial to prevention of nephrotoxicity from high-dose MTX.

19. Why is leucovorin used with 5-FU therapy?

Leucovorin is commonly used with 5-FU, especially in the treatment of gastrointestinal malignancies such as colorectal cancer. However, the purpose of leucovorin in this setting is *not* as a rescue agent. The active metabolite of 5-FU (5-FdUMP) exerts its cytotoxic effect by binding reversibly to thymidylate synthetase (TS). This action leads to depletion of thymidine, a necessary ingredient for DNA synthesis. Reduced folate is a necessary cofactor for the binding of 5-FdUMP to TS. Leucovorin is given with 5-FU to maximize enzyme binding and to enhance the anticancer activity of 5-FU. Although efficacy is increased, toxicity in the form of mucositis, diarrhea, and myelosuppression is also increased. As a result, dosages of 5-FU are lower when used with leucovorin than when 5-FU is given alone.

LATE COMPLICATIONS

20. How common are secondary malignancies from chemotherapy agents?

Advances in cancer treatment and chemotherapy have rendered several malignancies curable. As a result, there are increasing numbers of long-term cancer survivors and greater recognition of the late complications of chemotherapy, including secondary malignancies and gonadal dysfunction. The risk of secondary cancers after chemotherapy is difficult to evaluate, because many of the available data come from retrospective case reports. Acute myelogenous leukemia (AML) accounts for over 50% of secondary malignancies. Solid tumors more commonly arise as a late complication of radiation therapy. AML has been reported after successful treatment of Hodgkin's disease, non-Hodgkin's lymphoma, acute leukemias, multiple myeloma, breast cancer, and ovarian cancer. Long-term survivors of Hodgkin's disease who have received radiation therapy and chemotherapy that included nitrogen mustard are the most recognized population; the risk of AML is 17.6% compared with 2.5% for the general population. The risk for AML is highest in the first few years after chemotherapy, with a mean time to diagnosis of 5 years (range: 2–10 years). Chemotherapy-induced AML is usually refractory to standard treatment regimens. The antineoplastic agents most commonly associated with secondary cancer are the alkylating agents (melphalan, chlorambucil, nitrogen mustard, cyclophosphamide) and the nitrosoureas (carmustine [BCNU], lomustine [CCNU]). Recently, the epipodophyllotoxins (etoposide and teniposide) have been linked to secondary acute leukemias. Etoposide-related leukemias occur earlier (30–36 months after treatment) and have a characteristic chromosomal abnormality at 11q23. For curable tumors, the relatively small increased risk for secondary cancer is far outweighed by the benefits of increased survival in large numbers of patients. In less responsive tumors, the risk may not prove acceptable. Secondary malignancies are a particular concern in the setting of adjuvant chemotherapy.

21. Do all chemotherapy agents cause infertility?

Although gonadal dysfunction has been a known toxicity of antineoplastic agents for decades, it has not received must consideration because most patients did not survive long enough to worry about reproductive potential and it is not a life-threatening toxicity. As with secondary malignancies, the alkylating agents are the chemotherapy drugs most often associated with gonadal dysfunction. The risk for infertility is related to sex of the patient, age at exposure, type of chemotherapy regimen, total dose administered, and duration of exposure. In postpubertal males, the primary toxicity appears to be at the lining of the seminiferous tubules, leading to reduced sperm counts, testicular atrophy, and infertility. The effects on sperm numbers and function are often reversible but may take 2–3 years after chemotherapy to recover. The type of chemotherapy regimen is an important determinant of infertility risk. For example, 100% of patients receiving MOPP chemotherapy (mechlorethamine [Mustargen], vincristine [Oncovin], procarbazine, and prednisone) for Hodgkin's disease experience azoospermia, and only 10% of such patients recover spermatogenesis. In contrast, another Hodgkin's disease regimen, ABVD (doxorubicin [Adriamycin], bleomycin, vinblastine, and dacarbazine [DTIC]), produces reversible azoospermia in only 35% of male patients. In women, germ cell toxicity is more difficult to assess because of the inaccessibility of the ovary to biopsy and inability to measure actual germ cell numbers. Chemotherapy appears to induce gonadal dysfunction in women by causing ovarian fibrosis and follicle destruction. The clinical results are amenorrhea and decreased estradiol levels, which lead to menopausal symptoms such as hot flashes and vaginal dryness. Younger women seem to be more resistant to ovarian toxicity and are more likely to recover ovarian function after chemotherapy than older women. Patients with potentially curable cancers should be counseled about the risk of chemotherapy-induced infertility and the use of sperm or oocyte cryopreservation.

BIBLIOGRAPHY

1. Balmer CM, Valley AW: Basic principles of cancer treatment and cancer chemotherapy. In DiPiro JT, Talbert RL, Hayes PE, et al (eds): Pharmacotherapy: A Pathophysiologic Approach, 4th ed. Norwalk, CT, Appleton & Lange, 1998.
2. Berger AM, Clark-Snow RA, Kilroy TJ, et al: Adverse effects of treatment. In DeVita VT, Hellman S, Rosenberg SA (eds): Cancer: Principles and Practice of Oncology, 5th ed. Philadelphia, Lippincott-Raven, 1997, pp 2705–2806.
3. Cazzola M, Mercuriali F, Brugnara C: Use of recombinant erythropoietin outside the setting of uremia. Blood 89:4248–4267, 1997.
4. Chabner BA, Longo DL (eds): Cancer Chemotherapy: Principles and Practice, 2nd ed. Philadelphia, Lippincott-Raven, 1996.
5. Nemunaitis J: A comparative review of the colony stimulating factors. Drugs 54:709–729, 1997.
6. Perry MC (ed): Toxicity of chemotherapy. Semin Oncology 19:453–604, 1993.
7. Tuxen MK, Hansen SW: Neurotoxicity secondary to antineoplastic drugs. Cancer Treat Rev 20:191–214, 1994.
8. Valley AW: Gastrointestinal complications of cancer chemotherapy. In Balmer C, Finley RS (eds): Concepts in Oncology Therapeutics, 2nd ed. Bethesda, MD, American Society of Health System Pharmacists, 1998.

41. CANCER PAIN MANAGEMENT

Amy W. Valley, Pharm.D., BCPS, and Laura Boehnke Michaud, Pharm.D.

I found that when I didn't have pain, I could forget I had cancer.

Terminally ill cancer patient

1. Is cancer pain still a common problem?

Despite an improved understanding of the pathophysiology and management of pain, approximately 60–90% of patients with advanced stages of cancer still suffer from moderate-to-severe pain. Barriers to adequate pain management include poor pain assessment, reluctance of patients to report pain and to take prescribed pain medications, poor narcotic availability, and the health care professional's lack of basic skills in cancer pain management. If the basic principles of cancer pain management are used, it is estimated that over 90% of cancer pain could be controlled.

2. What information is needed to assess pain in patients with cancer?

Of the barriers to adequate pain management listed in question 1, poor pain assessment is one of the most common. The following steps can be used to perform an appropriate pain assessment:

1. **Believe the patient's complaints of pain.** Patients with chronic cancer pain do not necessarily exhibit the usual signs associated with acute pain, such as tachycardia, perspiration, and anxiety. They are more likely to appear depressed.

2. **Perform a careful history and physical examination**, evaluating each site of pain for intensity, quality, variation, and response to prior therapy. Questions that may elicit this information include: Where is your pain? What is the pain like? A dull ache or a sharp stabbing or shooting pain? What makes the pain better or worse? When is the pain at its worst? Does the pain keep you awake at night or keep you from performing normal daily activities? The patient's current analgesic regimen also should be recorded.

3. **Use pain assessment tools to evaluate pain intensity.** The Visual Analog Scale (VAS) consists of a 10-cm line upon which the patient makes a mark that corresponds to the level of pain that he or she is experiencing.

No pain _____ Worst pain imaginable

The Visual Analog Scale.

Patients who are unable to use the VAS may be asked to rate their pain on a scale of 0 to 10. This numerical rating scale uses the same descriptive parameters as the VAS. Patients should be asked to rate their pain at the time of evaluation; they also should be asked about their best and worst pain scores in the past 24 hours or past week. This information provides a reference range to evaluate the efficacy of therapeutic interventions.

4. **Individualize the therapeutic approach.** Continue to reassess pain and side effects frequently as the therapeutic regimen is individualized.

3. How is chronic pain different from acute pain?

Acute pain and chronic pain are two distinct syndromes. Acute pain is usually related to a specific event, has a well-defined onset, and is reversible. Acute pain requires temporary, short-term treatment with agents that provide a rapid onset of action. Untreated chronic pain is usually irreversible and gets worse over time. Such pain requires long-term analgesic management with the principal goal of pain prevention. When analgesics are given routinely to prevent pain, a rapid onset of action is not necessary. Recognition of the differences between acute and chronic pain forms the foundation for the basic principles of cancer pain management. Although patients with cancer may experience acute pain, management techniques are based on the prevalence of chronic pain.

4. What are the basic principles of pain management in chronic cancer pain?

1. **Assess pain and treat the underlying cause, if possible.** Approximately 70% of pain in patients with cancer is directly due to the cancer. Therefore, treating the underlying cause may involve surgery, radiation, or chemotherapy.

2. **Match the analgesic choice to the degree of pain.** See question 5.

3. **Titrate the analgesic regimen to patient response.** Give an adequate trial of the analgesic and maximize dosage before switching to another drug.

4. **Administer analgesic medications on a regular basis** (around the clock) to prevent pain rather than on an as-needed basis. The as-needed schedule requires the patient to experience pain repeatedly before receiving medication and requires larger amounts of analgesics to control pain than an around-the-clock schedule. As-needed dosing is indicated for the management of breakthrough pain during dosage titration.

5. **Use oral medications whenever possible.** Oral administration provides the same degree of analgesia as parenteral administration, facilitates patient independence and home care, and is much less expensive. Drugs with longer durations of action are preferred. Transdermal delivery systems are also an effective option.

6. **Anticipate and treat side effects.** (See questions 15–16.)

7. **Consider adjuvant medications and nondrug measures to maximize efficacy.** (See question 19.)

8. **Be aware of tolerance.** Tolerance is usually manifested as a decrease in the duration of analgesic effect rather than a decrease in the overall degree of analgesia. Tolerance can usually be managed simply by increasing the narcotic dosage. In patients with cancer and increasing pain, advancing disease is more often the reason than tolerance.

5. Do all patients with cancer need narcotics to control their pain?

Although narcotics are one choice for the management of cancer pain, other appropriate options exist. The choice of analgesic should match the degree of pain experienced by the patient. The World Health Organization (WHO) has developed a systematic approach, or pain ladder, to assist in this process. For mild pain (the first step of the ladder), nonsteroidal antiinflammatory drugs (NSAIDs) or acetaminophen (Tylenol) are effective choices. For moderate pain (the second ladder step), products that combine a weak opioid with a nonnarcotic are indicated. The final step of the ladder for severe pain, or pain unresponsive to the previous measures, is the opiate, or narcotic, analgesics. Adjuvant analgesics should be added as needed for specific pain syndromes (see question 19).

6. What is the role of NSAIDs in cancer pain?

The NSAIDs are highly effective agents for cancer pain and act via inhibition of prostaglandin synthesis. This mechanism imparts a ceiling effect, or a maximal dosage above which there is no additional analgesia. NSAIDs are used as single agents to control mild pain and in combination with narcotics to treat moderate-to-severe pain. The NSAIDs are particularly effective for management of cancer pain due to bony metastases. Side effects of NSAIDs include GI irritation and bleeding, antiplatelet effects, and renal toxicity. They must be used cautiously in patients with other risk factors for these complications, such as the elderly. Unlike aspirin, which irreversibly acetylates platelets, the antiplatelet effects of the NSAIDs are reversible on discontinuation of the drug. Nonacetylated salicylates, such as salsalate, have significantly fewer antiplatelet effects.

7. When should Tylox or Tylenol No. 3 be used to treat cancer pain?

The usefulness of combination agents such as Tylox or Tylenol No. 3 in patients with moderate cancer pain is well established. Most products combine a weak opioid, such as codeine, hydrocodone, or oxycodone, with a nonnarcotic, such as aspirin or acetaminophen (Tylenol). Combination products have a ceiling effect imparted by the nonnarcotic component. Currently, because no long-acting forms of combination products are available, dosing is usually at 4–6-hour intervals. Be aware of the amount of acetaminophen and aspirin in these products to avoid chronic overdose (do not exceed 4 gm/day of either product).

8. Why do so many patients with cancer receive morphine instead of other narcotics?

Many opioid analgesics are available for the treatment of pain. When given in equipotent doses, all of these agents provide effective analgesia. Morphine is considered the gold standard for cancer pain treatment for several reasons. It has a reasonable duration of analgesic activity (4–6 hours), and long-acting forms with a duration of 8–12 hours are available. In addition, morphine is formulated in a wide variety of dosage forms (see question 18); it is the most readily available narcotic and one of the least expensive. Analgesics with agonist/antagonist properties, such as pentazocine (Talwin), are not commonly used to treat cancer pain because they are less potent analgesics, may precipitate withdrawal in opioid-dependent patients, and possess undesirable side effects.

9. What is the correct dosage of morphine for cancer pain?

Unlike the nonnarcotic agents, the opiates do not possess an analgesic ceiling. Dosages can be progressively increased, resulting in additional analgesic effects. The optimal dosage of morphine or any other opiate is the dosage that controls pain with minimal side effects. Dosage requirements vary considerably among patients. Opioid-naive patients are usually started at a low dosage, such as 10 mg morphine orally every 4 hr or 30 mg long-acting morphine orally every 12 hr, or an equivalent dosage of another narcotic. One study of long-acting morphine reported that 67% of patients with advanced cancer required a dosage of more than 120 mg/day for pain relief.

10. A 50-year-old woman with metastatic breast cancer is receiving hydromorphone (Dilaudid), 4 mg orally every 4 hr, for pain. Her oncologist wishes to switch to long-acting morphine for dosing convenience. What is an equivalent dosage of morphine?

This patient is currently receiving a total of 24 mg/day of oral hydromorphone. It takes 5 times as much oral hydromorphone to attain the same effects as parenteral hydromorphone because of the first-pass effect through the liver. Thus, the patient is receiving the equivalent of 4.8 mg/day of intravenous hydromorphone (24 mg orally ÷ 5 = 4.8 mg IV). According to the table below, 1.5 mg of parenteral hydromorphone is equivalent to 10 mg of parenteral morphine. Using simple proportions, 4.8 mg of parenteral hydromorphone is approximately equal to 32 mg of parenteral morphine. It takes 3 times as much oral morphine to get the same effect as parenteral morphine. Thus, the patient is receiving approximately 96 mg/day of morphine (32 mg IV × 3 = 96 mg orally). Because the long-acting morphine tablets come in 30-mg tablets, a reasonable regimen is 30 mg orally every 8 hr of long-acting morphine. An as-needed dose also should be provided to cover breakthrough pain during the dosage titration. A reasonable as-needed regimen is to calculate how much morphine the patient receives in a 2-hour period and to administer this amount every 2 hr as needed for pain. The number of as-needed doses should be recorded and used to make future dosage titrations.

Narcotic Analgesic Comparison

DRUG	ONSET* (min)	DURATION[†] (hr)	PLASMA HALF-LIFE (hr)	EQUIANALGESIC DOSES	
				IM (mg)	ORAL (mg)
Codeine (various)	15–30	4–6	3	120	200
Fentanyl (Sublimaze, Duragesic)	7–8	1–2	1.5–6	0.1	N/A
Hydromorphone (Dilaudid)	15–30	4–5	2–3	1.5–2	7.5
Meperidine (Demerol)	10–45	2–4	3–4	75	300
Methadone (Dolophine)	30–60	6–8	15–30	10	20
Morphine (various)	15–30	4–6[‡]	2–3.5	10	30[§]
Oxycodone (Roxicodone, Oxycontin)	15–30	4–6[//]	ND	N/A	20

* Onset of activity is delayed with oral administration.
[†] After IV administration. Duration of action may be longer with oral administration.
[‡] Sustained-release products are available (MS Contin, Roxanol SR) that extend the duration of action to 8–12 hours.
[§] With repeated dosing, the IV:PO ratio is 1:3. Single-dose studies have shown a ratio of 1:6.
[//] Sustained-release oxycodone (Oxycontin) extends duration of action to 8–12 hours.

11. A 70-year-old man with pancreatic cancer has been receiving morphine as an intravenous infusion by patient-controlled analgesia (PCA) pump. He is now ready to go home. What is an equivalent dosage of oral morphine?

PCA pumps allow the patient to activate a hand-held device that delivers a predetermined dosage of medication. To prevent overdosing, the dosage can be repeated only at certain intervals, defined as the lockout interval. In addition, pumps permit delivery of a constant infusion of medication. They have the advantage of prompt delivery of as-needed doses, patient control, and increased nursing convenience. To determine the dosage of morphine that the patient needs, the total daily morphine dosage (constant infusion plus as-needed doses) must be determined and converted to an equivalent dosage of morphine using the table in question 10.

12. What are the advantages and disadvantages of methadone in cancer pain?

Methadone has a long duration of action and is one of the least expensive narcotics available. Its use is limited by poor availability in many pharmacies and by its complex pharmacokinetic profile. The plasma half-life of methadone (15–30 hours) is much longer than the duration of analgesia (6–8 hours). It takes four half-lives (4–5 days) for methadone plasma concentrations to reach steady-state levels. Therefore, when methadone is initiated or when dosage changes are made, a period of 4–5 days must elapse before maximal pain control is seen and efficacy can be fully evaluated. In the meantime, the patient should be covered with as-needed doses of an immediate-acting narcotic with a shorter half-life, such as morphine. More rapid titration leads to accumulation of methadone, which may result in respiratory depression.

13. Why is meperidine (Demerol) *not* a drug of choice for chronic pain control?

Meperidine has a short half-life and duration of analgesia (2–3 hours), which make long-term use inconvenient for the patient. The oral bioavailability of meperidine is also poor (see table in question 10). In addition, meperidine's major metabolite, normeperidine, can produce CNS excitation and is eliminated renally. Tremors, agitation, and seizures have been reported in patients with renal insufficiency who received meperidine.

14. When is a fentanyl patch (Duragesic) an appropriate choice for pain control?

Fentanyl patches are an excellent option for many patients with cancer, especially those who are not able to swallow or who are noncompliant. Each fentanyl patch provides sustained drug release for 72 hours. The onset of action is delayed (12–24 hours until maximal effect), and patients should be covered with as-needed doses of an immediate-acting narcotic, such as morphine, during treatment initiation. Because of the delayed onset, fentanyl patches are difficult to use when rapid titration is necessary. After a patch is removed, fentanyl continues to be released from subcutaneous tissue for an additional 24 hours. Fentanyl patches are sometimes more expensive than long-acting morphine—another reason that morphine is still considered first-line therapy for most patients.

15. How common is respiratory depression in patients with cancer?

Respiratory depression is rarely observed in patients who are tolerant to narcotics or opioid-naive patients with unrelieved pain. Sedation almost always occurs before respiratory depression becomes apparent. Tolerance develops to both respiratory depression and sedation. When respiratory depression occurs, it should be treated with a slow injection of naloxone (0.4 mg diluted in 10 cc normal saline) to avoid severe rebound pain. If the patient was receiving a long-acting opioid (methadone, long-acting morphine, or fentanyl patches), a prolonged naloxone infusion may be necessary.

16. What other side effects are associated with narcotic analgesics?

Sedation is a common side effect during initiation of treatment or after dosage increases. However, tolerance develops to this side effect within a few days to 1 week. In patients who do not develop tolerance but have adequate pain control, a dosage decrease should be attempted. If a dosage decrease cannot be made, addition of a stimulant, such as methylphenidate (Ritalin) or dextroamphetamine, should be considered.

Constipation is one of the most problematic side effects associated with narcotics. Tolerance does *not* develop to this side effect. All patients taking chronic narcotic analgesics also should receive a regular bowel regimen that includes a stool softener and stimulant laxative. The bowel regimen should be titrated to produce a bowel movement every 1–2 days. Lactulose and sorbitol are useful alternatives for refractory patients.

Nausea and vomiting occur in approximately 30% of patients during initiation of narcotic therapy or after dosing increases. Tolerance to this adverse effect develops in 5–10 days. Mild antiemetics, such as oral prochlorperazine (Compazine) or scopolamine patches, are effective for narcotic-induced nausea.

Other less common side effects of the narcotics include urinary retention, bladder spasm, pruritus, orthostatic hypotension, and dry mouth.

17. What are the differences between dependence and addiction?

Dependence is the physical, biologic need for a drug to prevent withdrawal symptoms on sudden discontinuation. Addiction is the psychological craving for a drug. When a physical impairment requires chronic pain control (e.g., cancer), addiction is rarely seen. However, patients with cancer do become physically dependent on narcotics. The distinction between physical dependence and addiction is important because some patients refuse narcotics because of fear of addiction, and some health care professionals wrongly avoid using opioids for the same reason.

18. What analgesic options are available for patients who cannot swallow?

Sublingual and transdermal routes are the simplest and least invasive methods of delivery in patients who are unable to swallow oral medications. Morphine is the narcotic usually used for sublingual administration. The only narcotic available in the transdermal form is fentanyl (see question 14). Morphine and hydromorphone are also available as rectal suppositories.

Continuous intravenous infusions are also an alternative in patients who are unable to swallow. In patients without intravenous access, subcutaneous infusions may be used. The intramuscular route is rarely necessary because so many other less painful administration options exist. In general, parenteral administration is more expensive than the less invasive routes of administration (e.g., oral, sublingual, transdermal). In addition to the cost of the drug, the cost of infusion pumps, nursing care, and associated supplies must be considered.

Epidural or intrathecal administration is another option for patients who are not candidates or who have failed systemic narcotic regimens. The advantages of spinal administration include long duration of action (6–24 hours) and lower incidence of systemic side effects such as sedation and respiratory depression. Disadvantages include the risk for infection and the need for expensive support services and equipment. Patient selection is crucial to make best use of this invasive and costly analgesic option. Because 90% of patients can achieve pain control using basic principles (see question 4) and less invasive routes of administration, spinal administration has a limited role in cancer pain management.

19. What adjuvant analgesics are most useful for managing neuropathic pain and other specific pain syndromes?

Neuropathic pain is characterized by an intense stabbing or shooting quality. The source of such pain is direct damage to nerves, nerve roots, or plexuses from tumor invasion or compression. Antidepressants (e.g., amitriptyline, nortriptyline) and anticonvulsants (carbamazepine) are the most effective adjuvant analgesics for control of nerve pain. They may be used alone for mild neuropathic pain or in combination with narcotics and antiinflammatory agents for moderate-to-severe pain. The necessary doses are often much lower than those required for the treatment of depression or seizures. Corticosteroids also may be helpful in refractory patients. Recently, gabapentin also has produced encouraging results.

Bone pain is common in patients with cancer that has either originated or metastasized to the bone. The usefulness of the NSAIDs is described in question 6. NSAIDs are effective alone in mild bone pain and have synergistic effects with the opioids in moderate-to-severe bone pain. Addition of NSAIDs to narcotic regimens may permit the use of lower narcotic doses and aid in minimizing narcotic side effects. The bisphosphonate drug pamidronate also may produce analgesic effect in bone pain, especially in patients with breast cancer and multiple myeloma.

In addition to their activity in neuropathic pain, corticosteroids are also effective in the treatment of pain due to intracranial pressure and lymphedema.

BIBLIOGRAPHY

1. American Pain Society: Principles of analgesic use in the treatment of acute pain and chronic cancer pain, 2nd ed. Clin Pharm 9:601–611, 1990.
2. Cancer Pain Management Panel: Cancer Pain Management. Clinical Practice Guideline. AHCPR Pub. No. 94–9592. Rockville, MD, Agency for Health Care Policy and Research, Public Health Service, U.S. Department of Health and Human Services, 1994.

3. Cherny NI, Foley KM: Nonopioid and opioid analgesic pharmacotherapy of cancer pain. Hematol Oncol Clin North Am 10:79–102, 1996.
4. Levy MH: Pharmacologic treatment of cancer pain. N Engl J Med 335:1124–1132, 1996.

42. INFECTIOUS COMPLICATIONS OF CHEMOTHERAPY

Richard B. Hesky, M.D., and Patrick L. Moran, M.D.

1. What explains the propensity of cancer patients to develop infections?

Although particular malignancies may be associated with specific infections (e.g., mycobacterial infections in patients with hairy cell leukemia), most cancer patients develop infections as a consequence of neutropenia (< 500 neutrophils), generally following cytotoxic chemotherapy. Both the depth and duration of neutropenia affect the likelihood of infection.

2. What organisms commonly cause infections in neutropenic patients?

Infection in the neutropenic patient can be conceptually divided into waves. The first wave of infection consists of common skin flora (*Staphylococcus aureus* and *Streptococcus*) and enteric gram-negative rods, gut flora (*Pseudomonas, Escherichia coli, Klebsiella*). If neutropenia persists, however, unusual infections such as systemic fungal infections develop, usually in the setting of ongoing antibiotic therapy (the second wave).

3. Can anything be done to prevent infection in the neutropenic patient?

Yes, there are several measures that are of value. First, there is evidence that exposure to fresh fruits and vegetables and even flowers and pepper increases the incidence of infection in patients with profound neutropenia of long duration (e.g., leukemics receiving induction chemotherapy). Prophylactic antibiotics also affect the incidence of infection in neutropenic patients. In patients with lymphoma treated with intensive chemotherapy it has been shown that the addition of trimethoprim-sulfamethoxazole can reduce both the incidence of *Pneumocystis* and gram-negative bacteremia. The quniolone antibiotics have been used similarly. The value of fungal prophylaxis with ketoconazole or fluconazole is controversial and may, in fact, promote the emergence of resistant fungal species. Intravenous immunoglobulin (IgG) may decrease the frequency of infection in select patients with low IgG levels and the use of irradiated cytomegalovirus (CMV)-negative blood products may reduce the incidence of CMV pneumonia in select bone marrow transplant patients.

4. What are the signs and symptoms of infection in the neutropenic patient?

The predominant sign is fever. Unfortunately, the classic signs of infection are frequently absent since exudates, infiltrates, and abscesses all require neutrophils, although a thorough history and physical examination, including special attention to the skin, mouth, perianal areas, and IV catheters may indicate a source of infection. In approximately 50% of cases a source of infection is never defined.

5. When a neutropenic patient presents febrile, what evaluation is warranted?

In addition to a careful history and physical examination, peripheral blood cultures, urine culture, sputum culture (if the patient has a productive cough), and a chest radiograph should be obtained. In the absence of dyspnea, tachypnea, or cough, a chest radiograph is rarely positive, but obtaining a baseline examination is warranted. While it may be helpful to draw blood cultures from each port of any indwelling catheter, a concomitant peripheral culture must be obtained, since catheter cultures are frequently false-positive.

6. What constitutes reasonable initial antibiotic coverage in the febrile neutropenic patient?

Empiric coverage is based on commonly encountered blood cultured isolates in this setting (*Staph.*, *Strep.*, and enteric gram-negative rods). Reasonable choices include a third-generation cephalosporin plus an aminoglycoside; double beta-lactam therapy; monotherapy with a third-generation cephalosporin or imipenem; or triple therapy with a third-generation cephalosporin, an aminoglycoside, and vancomycin. Obviously, therapy is adjusted according to clinical course and culture results.

7. When should antifungal therapy be considered?

If a patient has persistent neutropenia and fever or fever recurs after defervescence, empiric antifungal therapy with amphotericin is warranted. Fluconazole can treat superficial fungal infections such as thrush, but is not adequate therapy for invasive fungal processes in neutropenic patients.

8. How long should antibiotics be continued?

Generally, antibiotics are continued until the patient is afebrile and the absolute neutrophil count (total WBC times the percentage of segmented neutrophils plus bands) is above 500.

9. How should colony stimulating factors (CSFs) be used in the treatment of febrile neutropenia?

First, granulocyte colony-stimulating factor and granulocyte-macrophage CSF have been used prophylactically in select patients likely to develop severe chemotherapy-associated neutropenia. In patients who present with febrile neutropenia, CSFs may speed hematologic recovery but probably do not affect infection-related mortality.

10. Does the presence of a central venous catheter change the management of febrile neutropenia?

Gram-positive infections are more commonly seen in patients with catheters, and vancomycin is frequently included in the antibiotic program in these patients. Generally the catheter need not be removed when it is the suspected source of infection. Removal is warranted when there is an associated abscess (tunnel infection), when the blood cultures are persistently positive despite appropriate antibiotics, or when blood cultures are positive for fungus. Low-virulence organisms, such as bacillus species recovered from blood culture, also mandate catheter removal since they are rarely eradicated.

11. How should pneumonia be managed in the febrile neutropenic patient?

Except for the patient who develops an infiltrate during hematologic recovery, febrile neutropenic patients with pulmonary infiltrates need to be managed very aggressively. The patient who is tachypneic, has a respiratory alkalosis, or is hypoxic specifically needs broad initial antibiotic coverage and early intervention (bronchoscopy or thoracoscopic lung biopsy) to define the etiology of the infiltrate. Diagnostic or therapeutic delay may be fatal.

BIBLIOGRAPHY

1. Buckley RH, et al: The use of intravenous immunoglobulin in immunodeficiency diseases. N Engl J Med 325:100–117, 1991.
2. DePauw BE, et al: Controversies in antibacterial treatment of patients with neutropenia. Cancer Invest 15:37–46, 1997.
3. DeVita VT, Hellman S, Rosenberg SA (eds): Cancer: Principles and Practice of Oncology. 5th ed. Philadelphia, Lippincott-Raven, 1997.
4. Herrman F, et al: Effect of granulocyte macrophage colony-stimulating factor or neutropenia and related morbidity induced by myelotoxic chemotherapy. Am J Med 88:619–625, 1990.
5. Lazarus HM, et al: Infectious emergencies in the oncology patient. Semin Oncol 16:543–560, 1993.
6. Pizzo PA: Management of fever in patients with cancer and treatment-induced neutropenia. N Engl J Med 328:1323–1331, 1993.

43. GASTROINTESTINAL COMPLICATIONS OF CHEMOTHERAPY

Patrick L. Moran, M.D., and Richard B. Hesky, M.D.

1. What other causes of nausea and vomiting should be considered in a cancer patient in addition to chemotherapy?

Other common causes include narcotics and other medications; metabolic disturbances, especially hypercalcemia; bowel obstructions; and liver or brain metastases.

2. Describe the pathophysiology of vomiting in the cancer patient.

This is a complex problem. It is believed to be related to stimuli to the vomiting center, which is located in the medulla. Closely allied to this is the chemoreceptor trigger zone that is sensitive to noxious substances (e.g., chemotherapy). Neurotransmitters, such as dopamine and serotonins, mediate the transmission of stimuli between the chemoreceptor trigger zone and the vomiting center.

3. Name two additional emetic problems in addition to acute chemotherapy-induced emesis.

The first problem is the development of delayed emesis, which occurs 24 hours or more after chemotherapy. This is most common with moderate to high doses of cisplatin or doxorubicin and may be seen in as many as 80% of patients receiving high-dose cisplatin. Treatment consists of dexamethasone plus either metoclopramide or serotonin antagonist.

The second problem is anticipatory emesis, which occurs when nausea and vomiting are experienced prior to the actual chemotherapy administration. This is a difficult problem. The best prevention is to treat nausea aggressively at the onset of therapy; however, it may respond to anxiolytics and behavior modification approaches.

4. How should antiemetic therapy be selected in the cancer patient?

Primary consideration is the emetogenic potential of the chemotherapy agents to be used. A regimen containing high-dose cisplatin will cause nausea in virtually 100% of patients treated, whereas 5-fluorouracil (5-FU) regimens commonly used in colon cancer have little emetogenic potential. The greater the potential for vomiting, the more aggressive the antiemetic regimen should be.

Emetogenic Potential of Common Chemotherapeutic Agents

HIGH	MODERATE	LOW
Cisplatin	Mitomycin-C	Vinca alkaloids
Mechlorethamine	Doxorubicin (low dose)	5-Fluorouracil
Streptozocin	Cytarabine	Etoposide
Dacarbazine	Procarbazine	Bleomycin
Cyclophosphamide	Methotrexate (high dose)	Methotrexate (low dose)
Daunorubicin	Lomustine	Melphalan
Doxorubicin (moderate-high dose)	Methyl (CCNU)	L-Asparaginase
	Carboplatin	Chlorambucil
	Mitoxantrone	Gemcitabine
	Ifosfamide	Taxanes
		Camptothecins

Factors that may increase the likelihood of nausea include previous emesis with chemotherapy, anxiety, history of motion sickness, or severe emesis during pregnancy. Of note, a current or past history of heavy ethanol ingestion decreases the risk of chemotherapy-induced emesis.

5. Which classes of drugs are active as antiemetics?

Phenothiazines act as dopamine antagonists, inhibiting the vomiting center. They are useful in outpatient regimens, causing mild to moderate nausea. Metoclopramide in low doses acts primarily as a dopamine antagonist. Metoclopramide in high doses also acts as a serotonin antagonist, but its use is hindered by side effects.

A new class of medications, the serotonin antagonists, block serotonin receptors peripherally in the gastrointestinal tract as well as centrally in the medulla. These are well tolerated and have proved to be extremely active in the treatment of chemotherapy-related emesis.

Other drugs used in combination with the above medications include benzodiazepines and corticosteroids. For a more thorough discussion of this subject, refer to chapter 42.

6. What is mucositis?

Mucositis is a painful irritation of the oral mucosa produced by the effect of chemotherapeutic drugs on the rapidly dividing cells of the oral epithelium. Drugs commonly associated with mucositis include methotrexate, 5-FU, doxorubicin, and bleomycin.

7. What can be done to prevent mucositis?

It is sometimes unavoidable; however, the onset of severe oral lesions may indicate a need for prompt dosage reduction or discontinuance of therapy. Mucositis related to methotrexate may be ameliorated by the use of oral leucovorin 24 hours after the administration of methotrexate (leucovorin rescue). Cooling of the mucosa with ice chips may reduce the exposure to mucositis-inducing drugs and may be helpful in prevention. A good oral hygiene regimen is important, although mouthwashes containing alcohol or hydrogen peroxide should be avoided.

8. Once mucositis has occurred, how should it be treated?

Mucositis can be extremely painful, and adequate analgesia, including opiate narcotics, is often needed. Yeast or herpes infections can contribute. An appropriate therapy should be instituted if these are suspected. Topical solutions such as KBX (Kaopectate [combination of kaolin and pectin], Benadryl [diphenhydramine], viscous Xylocaine [lidocaine] in a 1:1:1 formulation) may provide temporary relief of pain. Sucralfate, which forms an ionic bond at proteins in an ulcer site, may also be of benefit. Preliminary data indicate that capsaicin is effective in promoting temporary relief of pain from chemotherapy-induced mucositis; further studies are under way.

9. What is a "vincristine belly"?

It is constipation caused by autonomic neuropathy brought on by vincristine. It is especially prominent in elderly patients and can cause severe obstipation and possibly bowel obstruction. The condition can be managed prophylactically with a combination of laxatives and stool softener.

10. A neutropenic patient presents with fever and right lower quadrant abdominal pain with positive peritoneal signs. What are the diagnostic possibilities?

Certainly appendicitis is a consideration. Another entity is typhlitis, which is a potentially necrotizing infection of the cecum. It is best managed with the addition of anaerobic coverage to the broad-spectrum antibiotics and close monitoring for possible surgical intervention. Surgical therapy has been successful and should be considered in patients who have failed medical therapy, especially if there is evidence of free intraperitoneal perforation or clinical deterioration requiring support with pressors or large volumes of fluid.

11. Name three forms of hepatocellular injury possibly related to chemotherapy.

1. Chemical hepatitis
2. Venoocclusive disease, which results from blockage of venous outflow in the small centrilobular hepatic vessels, particularly in patients receiving very high-dose combination chemotherapy
3. Chronic fibrosis, particularly related to chronic oral methotrexate

12. Diarrhea is not a particularly severe complication of infusional 5-FU therapy. True or false?

False. In a patient receiving 5-FU therapy, the complaint of diarrhea must be taken seriously and evaluated carefully. Diarrhea in this situation may become watery or bloody and potentially life-threatening with a risk of dehydration and sepsis. The development of diarrhea should call for careful evaluation, possible temporary cessation of 5-FU therapy, and reinstitution of therapy at a lower dose when appropriate. The somatostatin analogue octreotide has been useful in severe cases of chemotherapy-induced diarrhea. Irinotecan, a new drug active in colon carcinoma, can also cause profound diarrhea that must be managed aggressively with loperamide.

13. Describe the clinical presentation, risk factors, and treatment of antibiotic-associated pseudomembranous enterocolitis.

Clinical features include watery or bloody diarrhea, fever, leukocytosis, and cramping abdominal pain. The primary risk factor is previous antibiotic therapy; however, there is an increasing incidence in patients who have not received antibiotics. It should be considered in immunocompromised patients receiving chemotherapy. Treatment consists of either oral metronidazole or vancomycin.

BIBLIOGRAPHY

1. Berger AM, Barto Shuk LM, Duffy VB, et al: Capsaicin for the treatment of oral mucositis pain. Principles and Practice of Oncology 9:1, 1995.
2. Cascinu S, Fedeli A, Fedeli SL, Catalano G: Octreotide vs. loperamide in the treatment of FU-induced diarrhea. J Clin Oncol 11:148, 1993.
3. Consensus Conference: Oral complications of cancer therapies: Diagnosis, prevention, and treatment. Conn Med 53:595, 1989.
4. DeVita VT, Hellman S, Rosenberg SA (eds): Cancer: Principles and Practices of Oncology, 5th ed. Philadelphia, J.B. Lippincott, 1997.
5. Holland JF, Frie E, Bast RC, et al: Cancer Medicine, 4th ed. Baltimore, Williams & Wilkins, 1997.
6. Keidan RD, Fanning J, Gatenby RA, Weese JL: Recurrent typhlitis, a disease resulting from aggressive chemotherapy. Dis Colon Rectum 32:206–209, 1989.
7. Rittenberg CH, Gralla REJ, Letow LA, et al: New approaches in preventing delayed emesis: Altering the time of regimen initiation and use of combination therapy in a 109 patient trial. Proc Am Soc Oncol 14: 526, 1995.
8. Stewart DJ: Nausea and vomiting in cancer patients. In Kucharczyk J, Stewart OJ, Miller AD (eds): Nausea and Vomiting: Recent Research and Clinical Advances. CRC Press, 1991, p 177.

44. HEMATOLOGIC COMPLICATIONS OF CHEMOTHERAPY

Samer E. Bibawi, M.D.

1. Which organ is most frequently and consistently affected by cancer chemotherapy?

The bone marrow and, secondarily, the peripheral blood cells. As a matter of fact, the suppression is so predictable (according to particular agents used) that peripheral counts are used to guide dosage, mode of administration, and frequency of administration of a particular drug(s).

2. Why does the bone marrow express such sensitivity to chemotherapy compared with other organs?

Chemotherapy exerts its antitumor effect by impairing DNA synthesis in rapidly dividing cells. This effect is not tumor- or organ-specific but rather affects rapidly dividing cells. The fact that cancer cells proliferate uncontrollably makes them an excellent target for the effects of chemotherapy, but this same fact makes rapidly proliferating normal tissues (bone marrow, gastrointestinal mucosa, and hair follicles) highly susceptible to cytotoxic effects.

3. Are neutrophils and platelets more susceptible than red blood cells to chemotherapy?

No. What one sees is a function of the life span of each given cell line. Chemotherapy exerts its toxic effect primarily on the stem cell, the immature precursor cell. Neutrophils have the shortest half-life, about 6 hours, resulting in the most rapid drop. Platelets have a half-life of 5–7 days, so their drop is slower. Mature red cells have the longest half-life of about 120 days, and that is the reason they appear to suffer the least.

4. Why do some people develop more hematologic toxicity than others, despite receiving the same dose of drug(s)?

Factors related to the host may alter the degree of cytopenia, including the patient's age (older people have less marrow reserve and are therefore more likely to develop more cytopenias). Patients who received multiple courses of chemotherapy in the past and those who received radiation to bones (particularly pelvis and vertebrae in adults) have a compromised marrow reserve. Patient compliance (particularly with oral cytotoxics), significant liver or renal disease, and some genetic enzymatic alterations with lack of specific enzymes involved in the metabolism of certain chemotherapeutic agents all may alter drug pharmacokinetics and subsequent hematotoxicity. Nutritional status also may alter drug sensitivity; earlier data suggest that folate depletion may increase the toxicity of chemotherapy.

5. When do counts start to fall? How long does it take before they recover in relationship to chemotherapy?

As a general rule, most chemotherapy drugs lead to a nadir (lowest count) 8–12 days after drug administration, which lasts an average of 2–5 days, followed by prompt recovery. Patients undergoing induction chemotherapy for acute leukemia and those undergoing bone marrow transplant have longer nadir counts. Neutrophil recovery is frequently heralded by a mild monocytosis. Platelet recovery usually follows neutrophils. Occasionally, agents like actinomycin D lead to immune thrombocytopenia (ITP). Some alkylating agents such as busulfan and melphalan lead to a delayed and often prolonged (sometimes lasting for months) pancytopenia, which is usually reversible. The adenosine analogs (e.g., fludarabine and 2-CDA are associated with CD4+ lymphocyte suppression that can last up to 1 year; patients receiving them are susceptible to opportunistic infections (e.g., *Pneumocystis carinii* pneumonia).

6. What is the role of granulocyte colony-stimulating factor (G-CSF) in the treatment of neutropenic fever?

G-CSF has a limited role in the *treatment* of neutropenic fever because once established, profound neutropenia is less likely to respond to G-CSF, with a median shortening of the neutropenic duration by 24–36 hours. When used to *prevent* neutropenia, in which case G-CSF is started 24 hours after the last dose of chemotherapy, it is more effective and has more impact on the neutropenic duration and the incidence of febrile episodes, and it results in significant cost savings because of decreased hospitalizations and antibiotic use. The American Society of Clinical Oncology (ASCO) published guidelines for the use of G-CSF, which include history of febrile and/or prolonged neutropenia, advanced malignancy, extensive prior chemotherapy, preexisting neutropenia, and poor performance status. Note that once begun, G-CSF should be continued until the neutrophil count reaches or exceeds 1,500/mm^3 *and* a minimal duration of 7–10 days' use has been achieved; otherwise counts will drop precipitously if the drug is discontinued.

7. Can chemotherapy lead to significant anemia? If so, what is the mechanism?

Chemotherapy can lead to significant anemia, but unlike neutropenia and thrombocytopenia, it is usually not an acute event (remember that the half-life of red blood cells averages 120 days) but rather a steady and slow, downward drift as long as chemotherapy is being administered. Such anemia is due to continued bone marrow suppression. Some nephrotoxic agents like cisplatin can contribute to anemia by impairing erythropoietin production. Fludarabine is sometimes associated with autoimmune hemolytic anemia that may be severe (with rare fatalities reported) and/or resistant to treatment. Note that cancer patients frequently have multifactorial anemia secondary to the cancer process (a form of anemia of chronic disease, mediated by cytokines like tumor necrosis factor and interferon-γ), marrow infiltration by tumor, gastrointestinal blood loss, or other comorbid conditions.

Patients receiving folic acid antagonists (e.g., methotrexate) and drugs interfering with DNA synthesis (e.g., hydroxyurea) frequently express megaloblastic changes with normal B_{12} and folic acid levels.

8. Is erythropoietin of any value during cancer chemotherapy?

Recent placebo-controlled phase III studies showed that the administration of recombinant human erythropoietin increased hemoglobin levels to a degree that reduced or eliminated transfusion requirements in patients undergoing cancer chemotherapy. Another study evaluated the impact of using erythropoietin on the quality of life in that same patient population and demonstrated a statistically significant increase in mean scores for energy level, daily activities, and overall quality of life. The magnitude of increase in these scores was proportional to the increase in hemoglobin concentration.

9. Has thrombotic thrombocytopenic purpura (TTP) and hemolytic uremic syndrome (HUS) been reported as a complication of chemotherapy?

Yes. A registry to analyze cancer-associated HUS (a syndrome of Coombs' negative hemolytic anemia, consumptive microangiopathy with thrombocytopenia, and renal failure) was established in 1984. When analyzed in 1986, 84 of 85 patients had received mitomycin-C. However, only those patients who received higher doses of mitomycin-C developed HUS; the overall incidence with this drug is close to 10%. Other agents rarely associated with TTP and HUS are cisplatin, bleomycin, and Vinca alkaloids.

TTP and HUS have a high mortality unless recognized and subsequently treated. Urgent plasmapheresis remains the optimal therapeutic modality for this syndrome.

10. What other coagulopathies are associated with chemotherapy?

Drugs like daunorubicin, mithramycin, and bleomycin and camustine (BCNU) can impair platelet function and aggregation leading to a prolonged bleeding time. The precise mechanism of this effect is not known. Affected people are usually asymptomatic but occasionally will manifest mucosal-type bleeding (e.g., gum bleeding, nose bleeds, and petechiae).

L-asparaginase frequently leads to hypofibrinogenemia due to reduced hepatic synthesis of fibrinogen. It usually is of little clinical significance unless the drug is continued. L-asparaginase affects protein synthesis in general and hence may impair synthesis of vitamin K-dependent coagulation factors.

11. What is the threshold for prophylactic platelet transfusion?

Until recently, most physicians transfused cancer chemotherapy patients when their platelets dropped below 20,000/mm³, which was based on anecdotal observations that patients had a higher risk of spontaneous bleeding below this level. Such observations were previously made when aspirin, which at one time was the antipyretic of choice, was used to treat fever in thrombocytopenic patients with acute leukemia. Aspirin's effect on platelets was not yet recognized. In 1997, two randomized studies compared a threshold platelet count of 20,000/mm³ with a count of 10,000/mm³ and found that a threshold of 10,000/mm³ decreased utilization of platelet transfusions with only a small adverse effect on minor bleeding episodes and no statistically significant effect on morbidity or mortality.

12. Are there any delayed hematologic complications related to cancer chemotherapy?

Yes. These include cytogenetic abnormalities with no cytologic changes in the bone marrow (frequently involving multiple chromosomes, with chromosomes 5 and 7 being the most frequently affected), myelodysplastic syndrome, and frank acute leukemia, namely acute myelogenous leukemia. Abnormalities are particularly seen following the use of alkylating agents, e.g., mechlorethamine (nitrogen mustard) and cyclophosphamide. Etoposide (VP-16), a topoisomerase II inhibitor, may lead to secondary leukemia characteristically associated with an 11q23 abnormality, also referred to as mixed-lineage leukemia (MLL) gene. Most secondary leukemias develop 5–7 years after chemotherapy, except for etoposide-related cases, which often occur earlier. The risk drops dramatically after 10 years. The overall incidence of secondary leukemia is 3–12%, depending on the agents used, cumulative doses of chemotherapy, and whether or not irradiation was part of the treatment regimen. Irradiation has an additive effect on the incidence of secondary leukemia.

CONTROVERSIES

13. Do all patients with febrile neutropenia have to be hospitalized for treatment?
For:

Over the past three decades, febrile neutropenia has been viewed as an oncologic emergency requiring prompt hospitalization and parenteral antibiotic therapy for all patients.

Against:

In recent years, a few studies have shown that some febrile neutropenic patients are considered "low-risk" and may be successfully treated as outpatients either with intravenous or potent oral antibiotics. Further randomized studies need to evaluate the safety and efficacy of such an approach, perhaps with a more specific definition of "low-risk" febrile neutropenics.

14. What about neutrophil transfusions for febrile neutropenic patients?
For:

It is extremely hard, if not impossible, to eradicate fungal infections in the absence of neutrophils.

Against:

Recent in-vitro studies show that priming the donor with G-CSF not only increased the number of cells being harvested but also improved chemotaxis, phagocytosis of virulent *Candida* species, and delayed apoptosis compared with nonprimed neutrophils. Phase III studies are currently under way to assess the efficacy of such an approach. Neutrophil transfusions were considered for septic patients with fungal infections not responding to antifungal therapy and whose neutrophil recovery was expected to be delayed. When such transfusions were tried in the past they failed to prove a substantial benefit, primarily because of the short half-life of transfused neutrophils. Neutrophils also may transmit certain infections, such as cytomegalovirus.

BIBLIOGRAPHY

1. Bennett CL, Smith TJ, Weeks JC, et al: Use of hematopoietic colony-stimulating factors: The American Society of Clinical Oncology Survey. The Health Services Research Committee on the American Society of Clinical Oncology. J Clin Oncol 14(9:2511-2520, 1996.
2. Cohen DM, Bhalla SC, Anaissie EJ, et al: Effects of in-vitro and in-vivo cytokine treatment, leucopheresis and irradiation on the function of human neutrophils: Implication for white blood cell transfusion therapy. Clin Lab Haem 19:39–47, 1997.
3. Creaven PJ, Mihich E: The clinical toxicity of anticancer drugs and its prediction. Semin Oncol 4:147–163, 1977.
4. Di Raimondo F, Giustolisi R, Cacciola E, et al: Autoimmune hemolytic anemia in chronic lymphatic leukemia patients treated with fludarabine. Leuk Lymphoma 15:187–188, 1994.
5. Freifeld AG, Pizzo PA: The outpatient management of febrile neutropenia in cancer patients. Oncology 10:599–606;611–612, 1996.
6. Glaspy G: The impact of epoietin alpha on quality of life during cancer chemotherapy: A fresh look at an old problem. Semin Hematol 34:20–26, 1997.
7. Harris JR, Coleman CN: Estimating the risk of second primary tumors following cancer treatment. J Clin Oncol 7:5, 1989.

8. Heckman KD, Weiner GJ, Davis CS, et al: Randomized study of prophylactic platelet transfusion during induction therapy for adult acute leukemia: 10,000/microL versus 20,000/microL. J Clin Oncol 15:1143–1149, 1997.
9. Lesence JB, et al: Cancer associated hemolytic uremic syndrome: Analysis of 85 cases from a national registry. J Clin Oncol 7:781, 1989.
10. Ramsay NKC, Coccia PF, Krivit W, et al: The effect of L-asparaginase on plasma coagulation factors in acute lymphoblastic leukemia. Cancer 40:1398–1401, 1977.

45. COLONY STIMULATING FACTORS

Alka Srivastava, M.D., and Malcolm Purdy, M.D.

GRANULOCYTE AND GRANULOCYTE-MACROPHAGE STIMULATING FACTORS

1. What are colony-stimulating factors?

Bone marrow regeneration is known as *hematopoiesis*. All hematopoietic proliferation originates from stem cells found primarily in the bone marrow. These stem cells circulate with a very low frequency in the peripheral blood. Primitive stem cells capable of regenerating all components of the blood or lineage specific progenitor cells may be grown in culture after being removed from the bone marrow or peripheral blood. The cultured stem cells form colonies in the semi-solid agar that are visually very similar to bacterial colonies, and are named for the type of cell proliferating with the colony, such as granulocyte (neutrophils) colony-forming units (G-CFU). Granulocyte and macrophage colonies (GM-CFU), erythroid colonies (BFU-E), or colonies containing granulocytes, macrophages, monocytes, and erythroid cells (GEMM-CFU).

Hematopoietic cells require the presence of growth factors to initiate and sustain proliferation to mature into blood cells. In response to infection or low numbers of circulating neutrophils, lymphocytes, monocytes, fibroblasts, and other cells in the bone marrow microenvironment release proteins that stimulate the stem cell or lineage specific progenitor cells to increase the number or rate of production of white blood cells, red blood cells (RBCs), or platelets. Among the many bone marrow-stimulating proteins are specific factors that stimulate colonies of G-CFUs or GM-CFUs. These factors have been isolated and are commercially available through the use of genetic recombination. The colony-stimulating factors (CSFs) presently available for clinical use include granulocyte-macrophage colony- stimulating factor (GM-CSF) and granulocyte colony-stimulating factor (G-CSF). Various recombinant forms (glycosolated and nonglycosolated) of these compounds also are available for clinical use. Each has been modified from the native human form to increase the circulating half-life of the compound, thereby allowing the factors to be delivered by subcutaneous and intravenous (IV) routes.

2. What are the biologic effects of G-CSF or GM-CSF?

The CSF binds to specific G-CSF or GM-CSF receptors on the membrane of the hematopoietic stem cell. When the recombinant forms are used clinically, the time to release of mature neutrophils from the stem cell is decreased. Significantly, the maturation time decreases between the promyelocyte stage and mature neutrophil stage. An initial increase in the number of neutrophils in circulation occurs, either from release from the bone marrow or from demargination of the peripheral neutrophil pool; the number of circulating neutrophils after the first several doses are notably increased. Stem cells are released into the peripheral blood the first several days of CSF administration. This process is termed *stem cell mobilization* and is used clinically to obtain large numbers of stem cells for marrow transplant instead of harvesting bone marrow. CSFs modify mature neutrophil function as well. A decrease in neutrophil margination occurs in blood vessels and the generation and release of superoxide from granules and chemotaxis of neutrophils with G-CSF increases. Macrophage functions are enhanced with GM-CSF. The potential clinical benefits of neutrophil and macrophage functioning that results after administering CSFs are under study.

3. What are the clinical effects of administering CSFs?

The total white cell count increases, sometimes dramatically (> 100,000). The cells are predominantly neutrophils and bands. More primitive forms are seen in the peripheral blood as well, such as promyelocytes and blasts. Bone marrow biopsy shows marked proliferation of all myeloid precursors.

The most common side effect from both G-CSF and GM-CSF is bone pain, probably from the expansion of the myeloid (white cell) compartment of the bone marrow. GM-CSF has been associated with low-grade fever. Other systemic symptoms occur with both medications, but are infrequent. A tender macular rash resembling Sweet's syndrome (neutrophilic dermatosis) has been seen. On chronic administration in children splenomegaly, thrombocytopenia, and thinning of hair have been reported. Long-term administration may lead to osteopenia or osteoporosis.

Stimulation from G-CSF or GM-CSF may increase the serum lactate dehydrogenase (LDH), uric acid, or alkaline phosphatase (with normal gamma-glutamyl transpeptidase [GGTP]). Electrolyte abnormalities have been noted (e.g., decreased serum potassium and magnesium), but rarely require electrolyte replacement.

A first-dose effect in a minority of patients occurs with GM-CSF, and includes flushing, hypotension, tachycardia, peripheral oxygen desaturation with symptoms of shortness of breath, and nausea. The effect is not dose-dependent and may occur with re-challenge. The syndrome is more frequent with IV administration then subcutaneous. At high doses (> 20 µg/kg), fluid retention and pleural effusions may occur.

Preclinical studies have raised concerns of whether stimulation of the stem cells increases growth of leukemia or tumor cells (e.g., small cell lung cancer cells) that express the importance. In mobilizing (releasing) stem cells into the circulation, CSFs also may release tumor cells into circulation. Concern about tumor cell release clinically is only of concern in treatments using autologous (the patient's own) mobilized stem cells as rescue for high-dose chemotherapy.

4. How are these agents used to support chemotherapy?

The primary use of G-CSF and GM-CSF has been to prevent anticipated neutropenia associated with chemotherapy. Guidelines for use have been established by several national groups as well as by hospitals and insurers:

1. First-time chemotherapy is likely to produce severe neutropenia in > 40% of patients. Neutropenia of this severity occurs in adults with leukemia and in the autologous transplant setting. It is not seen often in patients with solid tumors such as lung or breast cancer on standard therapeutic regimes.

2. Use of CSFs in the second or subsequent cycles of chemotherapy for patients who develop febrile neutropenia with the first cycle of chemotherapy or who have significant delays in delivering the next cycle of chemotherapy due to neutropenia. The clinician may first consider reducing the dose of chemotherapy for the next cycle. Dose reduction instead of using CSFs to maintain dose intensity has not been demonstrated to improve patient outcome.

3. Using CSFs immediately after completing chemotherapy for adults with leukemia decreases the length of hospital stay and the number of infections. Use of CSFs in pediatric patients with leukemia shows less clear benefit.

4. Avoid starting use of CSFs in patients presenting with neutropenia due to chemotherapy, including patients presenting with or without fever. Randomized studies do not confirm that initiating CSF use after neutropenia is established decreases the length of time a patient is in the hospital or the chance that a patient will require hospital care.

Prophylactic use begins after chemotherapy. The first dose is given 1–2 days days after completing chemotherapy. The therapy is continued through the period of neutropenia until the absolute neutrophil count rises above 10,000 cell/ml. Shorter courses that achieve adequate neutrophil counts are reasonable if the patient is closely monitored.

Guidelines for the Use of G-CSF/GM-CSF in Neutropenic Cancer Patients

INDICATION FOR G-CSF/GM-CSF	STATUS
Severe neutropenia of childhood	Clear benefit
Neutropenia associated with AIDS	Benefit at low doses
Neutropenic fever with first cycle of therapy (intended curative therapy)	Benefit, if dose reduction inappropriate
Stem cell mobilization for autologous transplant	Benefit
Neutropenic fever in more than 40% of cases	Potential benefit, if dose reduction inappropriate
Acute leukemia in an adult, after chemotherapy (curative attempt)	Possible benefit, individual therapy decision
Acute leukemia, with chemotherapy	Not demonstrated to have benefit
Acute leukemia, childhood, after chemotherapy	Clear benefit not demonstrated
Patient presents with neutropenia, fever or no fever	No benefit shown
Improvement in rate of cure with addition after standard chemotherapy	No benefit shown

5. Are CSFs beneficial in treating a patient presenting with chemotherapy-induced neutropenia?

No. Several recent studies have confirmed that initiating CSFs after a patient has presented with chemotherapy-related neutropenia does not reduce the number of infections or admissions for infection despite shortening the time of neutrophil recovery in the blood by two days.

6. Are CSFs useful in treating acute leukemia?

Substantial morbidity occurs during the neutropenia and thrombocytopenia that accompanies induction and consolidation therapy for leukemia. The adult mortality rate within the 28-day period of induction-associated neutropenia is 25%. In most published studies the number of days with severe (< 500/ml) neutropenia using CSFs substantially decreases, ranging from 20 to 7 days. The reduction in the number of days with severe neutropenia must be interpreted as an intermediate marker; benefit to the patient would be either reduced infection or improved survival (the absolute marker of benefit).

Randomized studies using CSFs in leukemia either use the factor to drive the leukemic cells into S phase during chemotherapy delivery or to shorten the duration of neutropenia after chemotherapy. Stimulating the leukemia with CSFs during chemotherapy did not result in an increase in the number of patients entering complete remission. Studies in children with acute lymphoblastic leukemia did not demonstrate a decrease in the number of days in the hospital or in the number of serious infections. Studies in adults, especially those > 55 years old, have shown improvements in morbidity and inconsistent improvements in complete response or overall survival. Shortened hospital stays (by 2–5 days) and variable reduction in the number of fungal infections and severity of infections also have been demonstrated using G-CSF or GM-CSF.

7. How are CSFs used in bone marrow or stem cell transplant?

CSFs mobilize stem cells into the peripheral blood for leukopheresis collection. CSFs increase the number of stem cells circulating in the blood by 100 times baseline level, thereby facilitating adequate collection of stem cells for transplant. Compared to use of unstimulated (no prior use of CSFs) bone marrow for autologous or allogeneic transplant, the number of days to both neutrophil and platelet recovery is significantly reduced.

Use of CSFs after stem cell transplant has demonstrated a modest benefit compared to the use of mobilized peripheral blood stem cells alone. The beneficial effect is greater when unstimulated bone marrow is used instead of mobilized peripheral blood stem cells.

Use of CSFs to harvest allogeneic donor stem cells has demonstrated improved engraftment but is coupled with greater incidence of acute graft-versus-host disease. This usually takes place in a controlled, clinical trial setting.

8. How effective are CSFs in treating AIDS-related neutropenia?

The clinical benefit of CSFs has been demonstrated in patients with AIDS-associated neutropenia resulting from the disease or from medications such as AZT. Small doses (< 20% of the dose used after chemotherapy) may be used. Reduction in neutropenic fever has been demonstrated.

9. How effective are CSFs in treating congenital neutropenia?

CSFs have been shown to be useful in cases of rare, severe chronic neutropenias of childhood, including congenital agranulocytosis, cyclic neutropenia, neutropenia with T lymphocytosis, myelokathexis, and idiopathic neutropenia not of myelodysplastic or neoplastic origin. Improved survival, substantial reduction in severe infections, and improvements in quality of life have been demonstrated.

10. Can CSFs alleviate drug-induced neutropenia?

The usual course of recovery from drug-induced neutropenia is 7–10 days. There are no controlled studies of this topic, because it is an unpredictable event. No available studies demonstrate that the severe neutropenia associated with use of the antipsychotic clozapine may be prevented with CSF use: therefore, using CSFs to facilitate the use of clozapine is not recommended.

11. Are CSFs helpful in treating infections (without neutropenia)?

CSFs have not been released for the treatment of sepsis or infections, but preclinical studies have demonstrated that this may be a future application. In the future, compromised immunity resulting from conditions such as infection with comorbid alcoholism or diabetes mellitus may benefit from CSFs. Diabetic patients with foot ulcers were treated in a double-blind, placebo-controlled study with or without G-CSF. Compared to controls, patients treated with G-CSF had quicker resolution of cellulitis, shorter hospital stay, shorter duration of antibiotic use, and less need for surgery. The authors hypothesize that the increase in neutrophil superoxide generation with G-CSF in diabetic patients may be the mechanism of improvement.

12. Are CSFs a cost-effective measure to improve quality of life?

Most of the concern about use of CSFs relates to the cost of including CSF in therapy. Little data is available as to the quality of life noted by patients with fewer days of hospital stay or fewer days of fever. Using CSFs and CSF-mobilized stem cells instead of bone marrow, overall treatment costs have been reduced in pediatric populations.

13. Is there a difference clinically in using G-CSF or GM-CSF?

Most clinicians believe that no distinct difference exists. The CSF guidelines of the American Society of Clinical Oncology note that there are no comparative trials published that describe a clinical difference between the two factors. The FDA has released G-CSF and GM-CSF for distinct purposes as listed in the package inserts. The spectrum of side effects, the experience of the clinician with the factor, and cost are clinically important aspects to consider.

Experimental evidence shows that G-CSF and GM-CSF have overlapping but not identical stimulation of hematopoiesis. GM-CSF may stimulate macrophages with the future potential of demonstrating a role in modulating macrophages to induced tumor cell recognition and treat parasite or fungal infections. G-CSF may stimulate the primitive stem cell with the future potential of demonstrating interaction with other cell growth factors to enhance production of stem cells, megakaryocytes for platelets, or dendritic cells for immune therapy.

ERYTHROPOIETIN

14. What is erythropoietin and what are its sites of production?

Erythropoietin (EPO) is a glycoprotein hormone that circulates in plasma and regulates RBC production. Natural human EPO is present in two forms depending upon the amount of carbohydrate present: alpha, which contains 31% carbohydrate, and beta, which contains 24% carbohydrate, but they are similar in their biologic and antigenic properties. EPO is produced by cells in the adult mammalian kidney-interstitial cells in the peritubular capillary bed and perivenous hepatocytes in the liver.

The liver is the primary site of production of EPO in the fetus; a gradual shift from the liver to the kidney occurs shortly after birth.

15. What are the target sites of action of EPO?

EPO is known to bind to a specific receptor on the cell surface of erythroid cell membranes. The colony-forming unit-erythroid (CFU-E) is the primary target cell for EPO, and the highest number of EPO receptors are at the stage of development between the CFU-E and the proerythroblast. The burst-forming unit-erythroid (BFU-E), orthochromatic normoblasts, reticulocytes, and mature RBCs lack EPO receptors and are mostly unresponsive to EPO.

The binding of EPO to the receptor causes a sequence of events that leads to internalization of the EPO receptor and increase in transcription and translation activity within the cell. The rapid DNA cleavage in erythroid cells deprived of EPO is an important property of cells undergoing apoptosis. With the addition of EPO, CFU-E cell death is avoided and the CFU-E survives, proliferates, and differentiates into the nucleated erythroid compartment.

16. List and describe the indications for use of EPO.

- **Anemia of end-stage renal disease.** EPO increases hemoglobin and hematocrit levels in patients with chronic renal failure with decreased cardiac output, resting heart rate, and left ventricular hypertrophy. Reduction or elimination of transfusion requirements has been reported. The correction of anemia in such patients has been shown to improve quality of life and is cost-effective in patients who are severely incapacitated by anemia.

  The recommended initial dosage is 20 IU/kg 3 times/week subcutaneously with increases of 20 IU/kg/month to achieve the target hematocrit, up to a maximum recommended dose of 240 IU/kg 3 times/week.

- **Anemia in HIV-infected patients receiving AZT with EPO levels < 500.** Some studies have shown that blood transfusions may be associated with accelerated mortality in patients with AIDS; thus, EPO offers an attractive alternative to reduce or eliminate transfusions. Anemic patients receiving AZT who have low baseline levels of EPO (< 500 IU/L) exhibit significant increases in mean hematocrit levels and a decrease in number of units of blood transfused with a trend towards improved quality of life.

  The recommended initial dosage of EPO is 100 IU/kg IV or subcutaneously 3 times/week for 8 weeks. If response is considered unsatisfactory, dosage may be increased by 50–100 IU/kg. Therapy should be withdrawn after hematocrit rises above 40%.

- **Anemia in patients with bone marrow suppression secondary to cancer chemotherapy.** Anemia associated with cytotoxic chemotherapy results from impairment of erythropoiesis. Serum EPO levels are lower relative to the degree of anemia. Reduction in transfusion requirements, increase in hemoglobin levels, and corresponding increase in overall quality of life have proved the efficacy of EPO in chemotherapy-associated anemia.

  The recommended starting dose is 150 IU/kg administered subcutaneously 3 times/week. If the response is suboptimal after 4 weeks, the dose may be increased to 300 IU/kg 3 times/week. Further dosage increases are unlikely to improve response.

- **Autologous blood donation.** Autologous blood is now the preferred alternative for elective transfusions. EPO therapy results in reduction to exposure to allogeneic blood in anemic patients who donate autologous blood (hematocrit < 39%).

The patients who benefit most from therapy have hematocrit ranging between 33 and 39% and surgical blood losses estimated between 1000 and 3000 ml.

An initial starting dose of 100 IU/kg once/week for 4 weeks with increases up to 600 IU/kg have been recommended to produce evidence of a reticulocytosis. The use of IV iron (100 mg if body weight < 50 kg; 200 mg if body weight > 50 kg) or oral iron supplementation (ferrous sulphate 325 mg 3 times/daily for 21–28 days before surgery) is an appropriate addition to EPO.

- **Therapeutic use in myelodysplastic syndrome (MDS).** The rationale of treating patients with MDS who have high serum EPO levels is to overcome the defective proliferation and maturation of erythroid precursors by increasing serum EPO levels further.

  Factors associated with better response to EPO are:
  - Absence of need for transfusions
  - Endogenous EPO levels < 200 IU/L
  - Absence of ringed sideroblasts
  - Absence of karyotypic abnormalities

Response rates have ranged between 16% and 24% in various trials. Improvement is seen within the first 8 weeks in the majority of responders.

- **Thalassemia.** Trials of erythropoietin in combination with hydroxyurea have shown that the two drugs have an additive effect. The minimum effective dose is 500 IU/kg 3 times/week.
- **Anemia of chronic disease.** Although EPO levels are increased in anemia of chronic disease, the increase is less than that seen in iron deficiency anemia. In general, successful treatment of anemia of chronic disease relies on treatment of the underlying pathology. However, EPO administration does improve hemoglobin levels that result in an improvement in quality of life.
- **Anemia of prematurity.** This anemia is characterized by low hemoglobin and hematocrit with low EPO levels, reticulocytopenia, and bone marrow erythroid hypoplasia. The recommended dosages are 250 IU/kg subcutaneously 3 times/week with oral iron supplements to be continued for 5–6 weeks.

17. Discuss the side-effects associated with EPO therapy.

- **Hypertension.** Clinically significant increases in diastolic blood pressure have been observed in patients with renal disease given EPO and occasional cases of hypertensive encephalopathy have been reported. A positive correlation has been observed between incidence of hypertension and rate of increase in hematocrit in patients receiving erythropoietin; therefore, rapid increase in hematocrit should be avoided. The mechanism is unclear, but may be related to increased blood viscosity and increased peripheral vascular resistance. Most patients can be treated with management of fluid status and antihypertensive medication.
- **Vascular access thrombosis.** Currently, it is not clear if the administration of EPO increases the incidence of vascular access thromboses. Hence, a risk-benefit assessment should be made in each patient and early shunt revision done when necessary.
- **Hyperkalemia.** Although increased serum potassium levels have not been seen in clinical trials, regular monitoring of serum potassium and phosphate levels is recommended during first 3 months of therapy.

18. Is it necessary to provide iron supplementation with EPO?

Stimulation of erythropoiesis by erythropoietin causes a state of relative iron deficiency with decrease in serum iron levels, transferrin saturation, and serum ferritin. To maximize the effect of EPO, oral or IV iron supplementation should be provided to maintain serum iron levels between 80 and 100 μg/dL in all patients.

19. How soon should one expect a response to administration of EPO?

Stimulation of erythropoiesis with EPO is seen with an increase in the reticulocyte count by day 3 of treatment in normal subjects. When a dosage adjustment is necessary, it should be done at intervals of at least 4 weeks. Most patients who respond to EPO normally do so within 3 months after starting therapy.

20. If a patient does not respond to a trial of EPO, what reasons should the clinician look for?
EPO may not be successful because of the following:

1. Iron deficiency is the most common cause of resistance to EPO. Occult blood loss should be ruled out if the patient is already on iron supplements.

2. Acute or chronic infections

3. Occult malignancy

4. Folate or vitamin B_{12} deficiency

5. Ongoing hemolysis

6. Bone marrow fibrosis in patients with chronic renal failure due to secondary hyperparathyroidism

7. Aluminum overload should be considered in patients with chronic renal failure

THROMBOPOIETIN

21. Name the forms of thrombopoietin currently being studied in clinical trials.
There are two forms of thrombopoietin currently being studied: one is recombinant human thrombopoietin, which is the full-length polypeptide; the other is a truncated protein called PEG-conjugated recombinant human megakaryocyte growth and development factor, and contains only the receptor-binding region. This form has been chemically modified by the addition of polyethylene glycol (PEG).

22. How is the production of thrombopoietin regulated?
The liver and kidneys produce thrombopoietin constitutively and release it into circulation. Mature platelets have thrombopoietin receptors and remove thrombopoietin from circulation. In thrombocytopenia, less thrombopoietin is metabolized, resulting in high plasma levels, which then stimulates the marrow to increase megakaryocyte and platelet production. The clinical implications of this are:

1. Platelet transfusions may blunt recovery of megakaryocytes

2. When cytotoxic chemotherapy is administered, the megakaryocytes and their precursors are destroyed. But the platelet count drop is delayed and plasma thrombopoietin concentration does not increase until significant thrombocytopenia occurs. Hence, early treatment with thrombopoietin with chemotherapy is important.

23. Describe the clinical settings in which thrombopoietin may potentially be useful.
- **Chemotherapy-induced thrombocytopenia.** Results from clinical trials of thrombopoietin in patients receiving cytotoxic chemotherapy showed faster return of platelet counts to baseline, higher nadir platelet counts, and a reduction in need for transfusions in patients given thrombopoietin as compared to those receiving placebo or in the same patients during their first cycle of chemotherapy. These effects have been observed with administration of thrombopoietin both before and after chemotherapy.
- **Stem cell transplantation.** Early results from trials of thrombopoietin and G-CSF in myeloablative treatment with stem cell transplantation indicate that thrombopoietin enhances mobilization of peripheral blood progenitor cells. Thus, it may be useful in decreasing the number of aphereses necessary to harvest adequate number of progenitor cells. Another potential use of thrombopoietin is to improve the quality of stem cells or marrow to be used for transplantation.
- **Engraftment failure or delayed platelet recovery.** In patients who do not recover their platelet count and remain transfusion-dependent beyond 30 days, recombinant thrombopoietin has limited activity. In a study of 38 patients with delayed platelet recovery after stem cell transplantation, the administration of thrombopoietin made only 2 patients transfusion-independent.

• **Transfusion medicine.** The clinical trials of thrombopoietin have shown that a single dose of 3 μg/kg may increase the yield of platelets for aphereses in healthy donors by a factor of four. Therefore, if thrombopoietin proves to have an excellent safety profile, it may have important clinical utility in transfusion medicine.

24. Are any side effects associated with the administration of thrombopoietin?
Studies indicate that thrombopoietin is well tolerated. The usual toxicity associated with administration of other cytokines—flulike symptoms (fever, chills, arthralgia, myalgia, bone pain), fatigue, fluid retention, and major organ toxicity—have not been observed.

Thrombotic events have been described infrequently with thrombopoietin; however, the potential of thrombopoietin to potentially increase the activation of platelets is of concern.

BIBLIOGRAPHY

1. Adamson J: Erythropoietin, iron metabolism, and red blood cell production. Semin Hematol 33:5–9, 1996.
2. Anderlini P, Prepriorka D, Champlin R, Korbling M: Biology and clinical effects of granulocyte colony stimulating factor in normal individuals. Blood 88:2819–2825, 1996.
3. Crawford J, Ozer H, Stoller R, et al: Reduction by granulocyte-stimulating factor of fever and neutropenia induced by chemotherapy in patients with small cell lung cancer. N Engl J Med 325:164–170, 1991.
4. Dunn CJ, Markham A: Epoetin beta: A review of its pharmacological properties and clinical use in the management of anemia associated with chronic renal failure. Drugs 51:299–318, 1996.
5. Fisher JW: Erythropoietin: Physiologic and pharmacologic aspects. Proc Soc Exp Biol Med 216:358–369, 1997.
6. Ganser A, Hoelzer D: Clinical use of hematopoietic growth factors in the myelodysplastic syndromes. Semin Hematol 33:186–195, 1996.
7. Goodnough LT, Monk TG, Andriole GL: Erythropoietin therapy. N Engl J Med 336:933–938, 1997.
8. Glough A, Clapperton M, Rolando N, et al: Randomized placebo-controlled trial of granulocyte-colony stimulating factor in diabetic foot infection. Lancet 350:855–859, 1997.
9. Hartmann LC, Tschetter LK, Habermann TM, et al: Granulocyte colony-stimulating factor in severe chemotherapy-induced afebrile neutropenia. N Engl J Med 336:1776–1780, 1997.
10. Hoelzer D: Hematopoietic growth factors—Not whether, but when and where. N Engl J Med 336:1822–1824, 1997.
11. Human granulocyte colony-stimulating factor after induction chemotherapy in children with acute lymphoblastic leukemia. N Engl J Med 336:1781–1787, 1997.
12. Johnson PRE, Liu Yin JA: The role of granulocyte-and granulocyte-macrophage colony stimulating factors in the treatment of acute myeloid leukemia. Br J Haematol 97:1–8, 1997.
13. Kaushansky K: Thrombopoietin. N Engl J Med 339:746–754, 1998.
14. Markham A, Bryson HM: Epoetin alfa: A review of its pharmacodynamic and pharmacokinetic properties and therapeutic use in nonrenal applications. Drugs 49:232–254, 1995.
15. Messmer K, on behalf of the Roundtable of Experts in Surgery Blood Management: Consensus Statement: Using epoetin alfa to decrease risk of allogeneic blood transfusion in the surgical setting. Semin Hematol 33:78–80, 1996.
16. Negrin RS, Stein R, Vardiman J, et al: Treatment of anemia of myelodysplastic syndromes using recombinant human granulocyte colony-stimulating factor with erythropoietin. Blood 82:737–743, 1993.
17. Rachmilewitz EA, Aker M: The role of recombinant human erythropoietin in the treatment of thalassemia. Ann N Y Acad Sci 850:129–138, 1998.
18. Scadden DT: Cytokine use in the management of HIV disease. J Acquir Immune Defic Syndr Hum Retrovirol 16: S23–S29, 1997.
19. Schiffer CA: Hematopoietic growth factors as adjuncts to the treatment of acute myeloid leukemia. Blood 88:3675–3685, 1996.
20. Update of recommendations for the use of hHematopoietic colony-stimulating factors: Evidence-based clinical practice guidelines. J Clin Oncol 4:1957–1960, 1996.
21. Vadhan-Raj S: Recombinant human thrombopoietin: Clinical experience and in vivo biology. Semin Hematol 35:261–268, 1998.
22. Vora M, Gruslin A: Erythropoietin in obstetrics. Obstet Gynecol Surv 53:500–508, 1998.
23. Welte K, Gabrilove J, Brouchud MH, et al: Filgrastim (r-metHuG-CSF): The first 10 years. Blood 88:1907–1926, 1996.
24. Zachee P: Controversies in selection of epoetin dosages—Issues and answers. Drugs 49:536–547, 1995.

46. BIOLOGIC THERAPY OF CANCER

Clay M. Anderson, M.D., and Haleem J. Rasool, M.D.

1. What is biologic therapy?

It is the treatment of cancer aimed at eliciting or taking advantage of an immune response in the body against tumor cells.

2. What are the different types of biologic therapy?

The two major types of biologic therapy are: (1) use of substances such as cytokines, certain bacteria, vaccines, drugs, or gene introduction to stimulate cellular immune response to the cancer and (2) use of specific monoclonal antibodies directed against the tumor antigens.

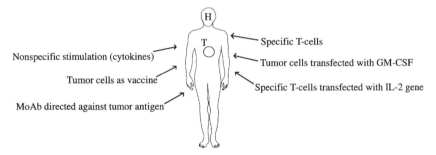

Methods to simulate or mimic host response against a tumor. T = tumor, H = host, GM-CSF = granulocyte-macrophage colony-stimulating factor, IL-2 = interleukin-2, MoAb = monoclonal antibody.

Types of Biologic Therapy

TYPE	EXAMPLES
Cytokines	Interleukin-2, interferon-α, tumor necrosis factor-α
Adoptive immunotherapy	Lymphokine-activated killer cells, tumor-infiltrating lymphocytes
Vaccines	GM2 ganglioside vaccine for melanoma, melanoma cell vaccine for melanoma
Monoclonal antibodies	Anti-CD20 for lymphoma, anti-L^y MoAb-doxorubicin immuno-conjugate for breast cancer

3. How old is the idea of biologic therapy?

In the early 1800s clinicians noted that tumors sometimes regressed in patients with cancer who acquired bacterial infections. This was the beginning of the idea of host reaction as therapy for cancer.

4. When did biologic therapy start in clinical practice?

Clinical research in biologic therapy has been ongoing for almost a century. William B. Coley, a surgeon at Memorial Hospital in New York City from 1892–1936, spent his career creating treatments aimed to attack disease with the body's own defenses. He demonstrated occasional tumor regression. His work was not broadly accepted because the results were unpredictable.

5. Is biologic therapy useful in 1999?

Yes. Interferon-α (IFN-α) is useful in node-positive melanoma, hairy cell leukemia, and chronic myeloid leukemia. Interleukin-2 (IL-2) is routinely used in renal cell carcinoma and melanoma. Bacille Calmette-Guérin (BCG) is used as adjuvant intravesical therapy for noninvasive bladder carcinoma.

CYTOKINES

6. What are cytokines?

Cytokines are small proteins or peptides that occur naturally in mammalian species and have multiple physiologic functions, including modulation of immune function. Lymphokines modulate lymphocyte immune responses, whereas monokines modulate monocyte/macrophage responses. The number of cytokines identified is increasing by the month, yet few have been produced in adequate quantity through recombinant DNA methods and tested clinically for effects against various tumor types.

7. Describe the different types of IFNs.

IFNs come in two types, type A, including IFN-α and IFN-γ, and type B, including IFN-β. Only type A IFNs have come into clinical use in oncology. There are actually dozens of naturally occurring and genetically engineered subtypes of each type, but few have been tested extensively. All IFNs share in common the ability to inhibit viral replication in cells.

8. How do the IFNs work?

IFNs bind specific cell surface receptors, activate kinase cascades, and eventually activate transcription factors that bind to IFN-responsive elements on DNA, thereby causing expression of IFN-inducible genes. Type A IFNs are potent immunostimulants and also have antiproliferative and antiangiogenic properties. Their mechanism of action against cancers in vivo is not known and may depend on route, dose, schedule, and chronicity of administration.

9. What are the accepted indications for clinical use of type A IFNs?

IFN-α has been approved by the Food and Drug Administration (FDA) for treatment of hairy cell leukemia, chronic myelogenous leukemia, and stage III melanoma; it is also used for therapy of low-grade lymphomas, multiple myeloma, and in combination with 5-fluorouracil for recurrent colon carcinoma. IFN-γ is FDA-approved only for treatment of chronic granulomatous disease, but it is also used clinically for renal cell carcinoma.

10. What are interleukins?

Interleukins (ILs) are lymphokines that specifically regulate the lymphocyte immune response, both T-cell and B-cell components. They start, maintain, and dampen the immune response and can cause a switch from cellular (T-helper 1) to humoral (T-helper 2) immune responses or vice versa, depending on their relative quantities.

11. How does IL-2 work?

A product of activated T-cells, IL-2 stimulates the proliferation and enhances the functions of other T-cells, natural killer (NK) cells, and B-cells. NK cells activated by IL-2 develop lymphokine-activated killer (LAK) activity. IL-2–stimulated B-cells generate secretory rather than membrane-associated IgM. Macrophages gain cytolytic maturation and elaborate transforming growth factor beta (TGF-β) upon stimulation with IL-2.

12. Describe the clinical uses of ILs.

The only IL that is used clinically so far is IL-2. IL-1 and IL-4 have been tried, but their clinical utility is limited. IL-3 may be a useful molecule for bone marrow stimulation but has no in vivo or in vitro antitumor activity. IL-5 through IL-15 have been characterized, cloned, and produced. IL-12 and IL-15 have potential utility as antitumor immunity potentiators. IL-11 has been approved by the FDA to improve platelet recovery after chemotherapy. IL-2 has FDA approval for treatment of metastatic renal cell carcinoma and is used frequently with an established track record in treating advanced melanoma. It has shown some activity in hematologic malignancies, including acute myelogneous leukemia and refractory lymphoma. Utility in the posttransplant setting is under investigation.

13. What is tumor necrosis factor alpha (TNF-α)?

Also known as cachexin, TNF-α is a peptide involved in the production and maintenance of the inflammatory response. It is produced primarily by activated T-cells and has multiple effects on monocyte/macrophages, endothelial cells, and other cells throughout the body. It works through a cell surface receptor to produce either death through apoptosis or activation of target cells. In vitro it can kill many tumor targets that express the receptor. In vivo it has potent proinflammatory activity that leads to profound toxicity at therapeutic doses.

14. What are the toxicities of TNF-α?

The toxicity includes fever, malaise, shock, and multiorgan failure. This severe toxicity has limited its clinical use.

15. What are the clinical uses of TNF-α?

Currently TNF-α (in combination with melphalan) is used investigationally for isolated limb perfusion, in the treatment of melanoma and sarcoma.

ADOPTIVE IMMUNOTHERAPY

16. What is adoptive immunotherapy?

It is an approach in which T-cells or other effector cells, stimulated by exposure to tumor cells or antigens ex vivo, are injected into patients to carry out a cell-mediated immune response against the tumor.

17. How can the patient serve as the T-cell donor as well as the recipient for adoptive immunotherapy?

Presumably, tolerance is overcome through the ex vivo stimulation. In addition, if another donor is used, T-cells from one person are generally rejected in another person's body.

18. Does adoptive immunotherapy have a role in cancer treatment?

Although newer ex vivo manipulations may yield improved therapeutic benefit, so far clinical results have not justified the expense and resources necessary for this novel approach.

CANCER VACCINES

19. What is a cancer vaccine?

It is an active immunization intended to induce T-cells or other components of the immune system to recognize and vigorously attack malignant tissue.

20. What are the different types of vaccines?

Types of vaccines currently in clinical tests include whole cell vaccines composed of autologous or allogeneic cells, cell lysate or membrane preparations, purified proteins, carbohydrates, peptides, or antiidiotypic antibodies that mimic the tumor epitopes.

21. Which antigens in the malignant tissue are used for cancer vaccination?

Several categories of antigens can be exploited for this purpose:

1. Proteins and peptides (i.e., fragments of tumor proteins)
2. Gangliosides (e.g., GM2). It has been suggested that patients with melanoma who develop anti-GM2 antibodies after vaccination have a better prognosis.
3. Nucleic acids (DNA and RNA coding for tumor antigens)

22. What are the accepted clinical uses of cancer vaccines in 1999?

Outside clinical research, cancer vaccines currently have no established role. Several different cancer vaccines are under investigation in all phases of clinical trials, but standard clinical use is still in the future.

MONOCLONAL ANTIBODIES

23. What is a monoclonal antibody (MoAb)?

A MoAb is a purified antibody generated against a specific antigen or epitope.

24. How are MoAbs made?

Mice are immunized with purified antigen preparations, tumor extracts, or whole cells. Immunoglobin-producing B lymphocytes from the spleens of the mice are then fused with an immortalized cell line to form hybridomas. Hybridomas can be grown in culture indefinitely and screened for production of the antibody of interest. The hybridoma clones that produce the antibody of interest can be purified and grown in culture in large quantities. Monoclonal antibodies are produced in sufficient quantities for clinical use.

25. How are MoAbs used to diagnose cancer?

Several laboratory techniques use MoAbs to diagnose malignant disorders. The most applicable and widely used technique is flow cytometry, in which the cells are incubated wtih specific MoAbs tagged with different fluorescent molecules directed against certain cell surface markers. The cells are then passed in a thin stream through a laser beam. A computer reads the diffraction of the laser light and interprets the data to assess the presence or absence of different cell surface markers. This technique is helpful in establishing monoclonality as evidence for malignancy as well as cellular phenotypes in most hematologic malignancies and many solid tumors. MoAbs tagged with radionuclides are becoming important diagnostic tools as well.

26. What are the toxicities of MoAbs?

Because MoAbs are foreign antigens, they can produce an antigen–antibody reaction similar to other extrinsic particles. Some patients develop fever, chills, and hypersensitivity reactions that on rare occasions result in anaphylaxis. Organ damage may result from nonspecific binding of the MoAbs to nontumor tissue. When the monoclonal antibody is bound to a toxin or radionuclide, toxicities specific to those agents can be expected.

27. How can the immune response aginast MoAbs be avoided?

The MoAbs currently in clinical use are obtained from mice that have been immunized. Scientists have begun to construct human therapeutic antibodies that should escape immune recognition. In the meantime, scientists are masking the immunogenicity of the murine antibodies, rearranging them into something that more closely resembles human antibodies. They do so by substituting all of the nonessential structures in the mouse antibody with the analogous human counterparts through recombinant DNA methods. This process, called humanization, has yielded antibodies that in initial clinical tests have evaded the human immune system more successfully.

28. Why have the initial studies of monoclonal therapy yielded disappointing results?

Barriers to effective MoAb therapy are many:
- Cross-reactivity of the MoAb with normal antigens
- Expression of the tumor antigen on normal cells
- Binding kinetics of the antibody to the cell surface
- Weak effector mechanisms such as antibody-dependent, cell-mediated cytotoxicity or complement-mediated cytotoxicity
- Large tumor burden
- Circulating tumor antigen, which prevents MoAb from binding to the tumor cell surface

- Modification of the tumor antigen by the tumor cell so that the cell no longer binds the MoAb
- Production of human antimurine antibodies (HAMAs) by the patient, which inactivate the MoAb before it reaches the tumor cell
- Poor uptake of MoAb beyond the first few layers of tumor cells surrrounding capillaries

29. What techniques are used to overcome barriers to monoclonal therapy?
- Generation of Fab (variable region active sites) fragments, which are less likely to generate HAMA, have a longer half-life, and penetrate tumors better
- Conjugation to toxin, drugs, and radionuclides has dramatically enhanced the cytotoxicity of MoAbs

BIBLIOGRAPHY

1. Anderson CM, Tabacof J, Legha SS: Malignant melanoma: Biology, diagnosis, and management. In Pazdur R (ed): Medical Oncology: A Comprehensive Review, 2nd ed. PRR Inc, 1995, pp 493–509.
2. Ben-Efraim S: Cancer immunotherapy: Hopes and pitfalls: A review. Anticancer Res 16:3235–3240, 1996.
3. Figlin RA, Gitlitz J, Belldegrun A: Immunologic approaches to the treatment of cancer [editorial]. Cancer Invest 13:339–340, 1995.
4. Frost JD, Sondel PM: Immunotherapy for infection and malignancy in children with cancer. Adv Pediatr 41:385–415, 1994.
5. Lindner DJ, Kalvakolanu DV, Borden EC: Increasing effectiveness of IFN α for malignancies. Semin Oncol 24 (Suppl 9):99–104, 1997.
6. Old LJ: Immunotherapy for Cancer. Sci Am 275(3):136–143, 1996.
7. Smith RT: Cancer and the immune system. Pediatr Clin North Am 41:841–850, 1994.

47. BONE MARROW TRANSPLANTATION

Jeffrey W. Cronk, M.D., and Maureen Ross, M.D., Ph.D.

1. What is bone marrow transplantation?

The intravenous administration of hematopoietic stem cells to patients is termed bone marrow transplantation. The purpose of transplantation is to reestablish bone marrow function in patients with dysfunctional hematopoiesis due to acquired or inherited disease or toxic insult. Hematopoietic stem cells have traditionally been harvested from bone marrow but more and more commonly are being obtained from peripheral blood. Bone marrow transplantation is now more properly and generically dubbed stem cell transplantation.

2. Who can serve as donors of hematopoietic stem cells?

Hematopoietic stem cells have historically been obtained from a sibling donor who is identical to the patient at the HLA A, B, and Dr loci. Transfer of stem cells from a donor to another person is termed **allogeneic** transplantation. When the donor is a genetically identical individual (an identical twin) the transplant is designated a **syngeneic** transplant. In some instances, stem cells from the patient himself/herself are used; reinfusion of such cells constitutes an **autologous** stem cell transplant. The majority of patients (70%) who are transplantation candidates do not have a suitably HLA-matched family member. The probability of an HLA-matched sibling donor is $1-(3/4)^n$, where n = number of siblings. Alternative donors must be sought for many patients. Choices include volunteer unrelated donors or partially matched family members. Alternatively, some patients undergo transplantation with their own bone marrow (autologous transplantation).

3. What determines whether a patient undergoes an autologous or allogeneic transplant?

The choice between an allogeneic and autologous transplant procedure is dictated by the patient's disease type, disease status (i.e., remission, relapse, bone marrow contamination), age, concomitant medical problems, and donor availability. Allogeneic transplantation is associated with an increased risk of infectious complications and graft-versus-host disease (GVHD), whereas autologous transplantation is associated with an increased risk of disease relapse. Use of alternative allogeneic donors other than HLA-matched siblings has resulted in delayed engraftment, increased risk of graft rejection, and increased incidence of acute GVHD disease. Allogeneic transplantation is the only potentially curative modality for patients with inherited diseases of hematopoiesis or lymphopoiesis and for patients with bone marrow failure states. In malignant diseases such as lymphoma and breast cancer, the majority of patients are treated with autologous transplantation. In acute myelogenous leukemia either allogeneic or autologous transplantation can be performed for patients in remission, although recent gene marking studies have demonstrated that malignant cells within the autologous graft may contribute to relapse.

4. Why are patients treated with chemotherapy or radiation before transplantation?

Before infusion of stem cells, patients are treated with high doses of chemotherapy or a combination of chemotherapy and radiation. The preparative regimen both in autologous and allogeneic transplantation functions to eradicate neoplastic cells. In allogeneic transplantation the preparative regimen is also used to immunosuppress the recipient to prevent destruction of the allograft by residual immunologically active cells in the host, allowing for permanent and functional stem cell engraftment. When immunosuppression is inadequate, graft failure results. The exception is children with severe combined immunodeficiency diseases, who do not require pretransplant conditioning unless immunosuppression is required because of the use of a mismatched donor.

5. Which patients should be considered for stem-cell transplantation?

Stem-cell transplantation can be curative for patients with both malignant and nonmalignant diseases. Nonmalignant diseases of hematopoiesis including aplastic anemia, thalassemia, and life-threatening immunodeficiency disorders are frequently cured by allogeneic or syngeneic stem-cell transplantation. In principle, all genetic disorders of the immunologic and hematopoietic systems can be cured by allogeneic stem-cell transplantation.

Patients with malignant diseases also are candidates for stem-cell transplantation. It represents the only chance for cure for patients with acute myelogenous leukemia, acute lymphoblastic leukemia, non-Hodgkin's lymphoma or Hodgkin's disease who have relapsed despite prior chemotherapy. It is the only curative therapy for patients with chronic lymphocytic leukemia (CLL) and chronic myelogenous leukemia (CML), myelodysplasia, and multiple myeloma. The use of autologous stem-cell transplantation to restore hematopoiesis after the administration of high doses of chemotherapy or chemoradiotherapy is being applied increasingly to solid tumors such as breast cancer, neuroblastoma, and germ cell tumors. Breast carcinoma, either high-risk primary disease or recurrent disease, is now the most common indication for stem-cell transplantation.

6. How are hematopoietic stem cells obtained?

Hematopoietic stem cells are obtained from bone marrow or peripheral blood. Marrow is harvested from the posterior iliac crests of the patient or donor by repeated aspirations under general anesthesia. The number of cells harvested is usually $2–4 \times 10^8$/kg of recipient weight. Except for the development of mild anemia, bone marrow harvesting is generally well tolerated with no significant change in the donor peripheral blood counts.

Peripheral blood stem cells are collected from the peripheral blood of the donor/patient by a procedure called leukapheresis. Mobilization of primitive progenitor cells into the peripheral circulation may be accomplished either by chemotherapy with collection in the bone marrow recovery phase or by administration of hematopoietic growth factors such as granulocyte colony-stimulating factor (G-CSF) or granulocyte-macrophage colony-stimulating factor (GM-CSF). The circulating progenitor cells are collected and concentrated by leukapheresis. Although initially developed for autologous transplantation, interest and experience in allogeneic peripheral blood stem-cell transplantation is growing. Mobilization of volunteer donors is accomplished by growth factors given as a subcutaneous injection for 4–5 days prior to the start of leukapheresis. Immediate side effects of growth factors in normal donors have been minimal; most donors complain only of mild bone discomfort. Ramifications for patient outcome with respect to disease relapse and GVHD remain under intense scrutiny.

7. Why use peripheral blood stem cells rather than bone marrow?

In autologous transplantation, use of peripheral stem cells rather than bone marrow has resulted in decreased duration of neutropenia, decreased duration of platelet transfusion dependence, and a concomitant reduction in length of hospital stay and costs. For certain disease processes, the use of peripheral blood cells rather than marrow also may reduce the level of tumor contamination of the autologous graft. Collection of peripheral blood cells rather than bone marrow obviates the need for general or spinal anesthesia. Bone marrow harvest, on the other hand, yields a sufficient number of stem cells from a single procedure, whereas repetitive leukapheresis of patients on consecutive days is often required to obtain a suitable graft. Although peripheral blood stem-cell transplantation (PBSCT) has essentially replaced bone marrow in the autologous setting, its role in allogeneic transplantation continues to be defined. Skepticism about the feasibility of PBSCT in the allogeneic setting centers predominantly on the increased number of T cells contained in an unmanipulated PBSC graft vs. a bone marrow graft. The PBSC graft contains at least a one log greater number of T cells. T cells are the primary mediators of GVHD, a major cause of morbidity and mortality after allogeneic transplantation. However, T cells also may be the mediators of the so-called "graft versus leukemia/tumor" effect, which is responsible for the decreased relapse rates observed after allogeneic transplantation.

8. What are the major complications of hematopoietic stem-cell transplantation?

In addition to myelosuppression, a number of unique toxicities are encountered after transplantation, including organ toxicities (renal, hepatic, cardiac, and pulmonary) attributable to the high-dose chemotherapy or chemoradiotherapy regimens used as preparation for transplantation, infectious complications resulting from post-transplant prolonged immune dysfunction, and GVHD arising from discrepant donor and recipient antigens.

Up to 20% of patients undergoing transplantation will develop pulmonary toxicity from the preparative regimen. Such patients routinely present with cough, dyspnea, pulmonary infiltrates, and hypoxemia. The exact mechanism of pulmonary toxicity remains unknown, although it appears that a number of chemotherapy agents used in the preparative regimens (e.g., bleomycin and carmustine [BCNU]) are toxic to the pulmonary parenchyma. The addition of total body irradiation also appears to increase the risk of pulmonary toxicity.

Hepatic injury following transplantation frequently presents as veno-occlusive disease of the liver (VOD), which is characterized by hyperbilirubinemia, weight gain (from fluid retention), and tender hepatomegaly. The pathophysiology of veno-occlusive disease is believed to be endothelial cell damage from chemoradiotherapy. The damage promotes the development of hepatic venule thrombosis and fibrosis with resultant hepatic dysfunction and not infrequently multiorgan failure. Treatment is primarily supportive with a mortality rate > 50% in severe VOD.

GVHD, an immunologic reaction of donor T lymphocytes to host tissues, frequently complicates allogeneic transplantation and may result in considerable morbidity. The degree of HLA incompatibility between donor and recipient is the most important factor governing the development of GVHD. GVHD may be divided into an acute and chronic phase. Acute GVHD occurs within the first 100 days following transplantation and typically involves the skin, liver, and gastrointestinal tract. Chronic GVHD occurs more than 100 days after transplantation and may be limited to the skin and liver or involve multiple organs. The prevention and treatment of GVHD is briefly outlined below.

Other complications of transplantation include infertility, graft rejection, cataract formation, and hypothyroidism.

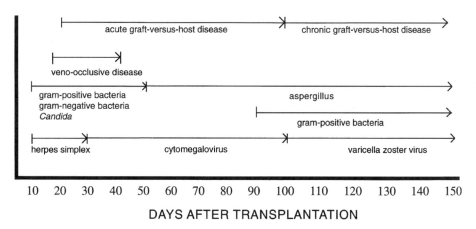

The most common transplant-related complications and their approximate times of occurrence.

9. How is GVHD prevented and treated? What are some of the long-term consequences of GVHD?

Histocompatibility remains the most important determinant of the frequency and severity of GVHD. Nonetheless, without post-transplant immune suppression almost all matched allogeneic transplants will develop severe GVHD, which suggests that minor histocompatibility antigens play a prominent role in its pathogenesis. A combination of methotrexate and cyclosporine (with or without steroids) appears to be the best preventive regimen currently available and reduces the incidence of clinically significant GVHD to approximately 20–30% in HLA-matched sibling stem-cell transplants.

T cell depletion of the donor graft also has been used to decrease the incidence and severity of GVHD. Although a dramatic decrease in the incidence of GVHD with T cell-depleted grafts is evident, this has not resulted in improved survival because of the concomitant increase in both the incidence of graft rejection and relapse.

Treatment options for established GVHD remain poor. High-dose steroids are the most frequently used agents, although other immunosuppressants such as antithymocyte globulin, Imuran, and thalidomide are used in steroid-refractory patients. The long-term consequences of chronic GVHD are varied and depend on the organ systems involved with the immunologic process. Skin findings range from erythema and hyperkeratosis to diffuse fibrosis with resultant contractures and deformity. Obstructive lung disease with chronic pulmonary infections and cholestatic liver dysfunction also are quite common. Ocular and oral manifestations include marked dryness with keratoconjunctivitis and lichen planus. The presence or absence of chronic GVHD is the major determinant of quality of life after allogeneic stem-cell transplant.

10. What are the most frequently encountered infections after hematopoietic stem-cell transplantation? How are these infections prevented and/or treated?

Hematopoietic stem-cell transplantation places the recipient at risk for a number of infectious processes. Increased risk is in part due to the profound immunosuppression induced by the preparative regimen as well as breaches in mucosal integrity. Measures to prevent the introduction of infectious agents often include the use of reverse isolation environments and high-efficiency particulate air filters.

The most common infectious agents encountered within the first 30 days after transplantation include bacteria (both gram-negative and gram-positive), fungus, and herpes simplex. Patients who are both neutropenic and febrile receive empiric antibacterial and/or antifungal coverage that will be tailored to culture results. Recipients of allogeneic transplants often receive prophylactic low-dose amphotericin or fluconazole, acyclovir for herpes simplex prophylaxis, and biweekly immunoglobulin for decreased endogenous antibody production.

Strict attention is paid to decreasing the risk of acquiring primary cytomegalovirus (CMV) infection in patients who are CMV-negative. Blood products for transfusion to CMV-negative recipients are from CMV-seronegative donors and are leukocyte depleted and irradiated to further decrease the risk of CMV infection and the induction of transfusion-mediated GVHD. Patients who are CMV-positive or recipients of a graft from a CMV-positive donor are either treated prophylactically with ganciclovir or are treated preemptively at the first sign of viremia before organ infection is manifested. If CMV pneumonitis occurs, it is treated with a combination of ganciclovir and immunoglobulin. Infections occurring many months to years after transplantation include those secondary to gram-positive bacteria and varicella zoster virus.

11. What is the "graft-versus-leukemia" effect?

Relapse rates after allogeneic stem-cell transplantation are substantially less than after autologous transplant. A portion of relapses in autologous transplant may be attributable to the presence of contaminating cells within the graft. If so, relapse rates after syngeneic transplant should be identical to those of sibling-matched allogeneic transplant. Syngeneic transplant offers little improvement in outcome over autologous transplant, implying that the decreased relapse rates with allogeneic transplant arise from a graft-versus-tumor effect. For example, in CML relapse rates after syngeneic transplant approach 70% versus 10–20% with sibling-matched stem-cell transplant. The graft-versus-leukemia effect appears to be mediated by T cells within the graft; when T cell-depleted bone marrow from HLA-matched siblings is used, relapse rates approximate rates seen with syngeneic transplantation.

Disease	Autologous Stem Cell Relapse Rate	Allogeneic Stem Cell Relapse Rate
AML (1st CR)	35–65%	10–25%
AML (2nd CR)	40–70%	40%
ALL (1st CR)	50%	10%
ALL (refractory)	50–80%	30%
CML (chronic phase)	N/A	10%
NHL/Hodgkin's disease	45%	20%

ALL = acute lymphocytic leukemia, AML = acute myelogenous leukemia, CML = chronic myelogenous leukemia, CR = complete remission, NHL = non-Hodgkin's lymphoma.

Direct evidence of a graft-versus-leukemia effect has recently been demonstrated by the use of donor lymphocytes. In a majority of patients with CML who relapse after allogeneic transplant, durable remissions can be obtained by administration of lymphocytes from the previous donor without addition of chemotherapy or radiation. Encouraging results in CML have prompted investigation of donor lymphocyte therapy in other diseases such as myeloma, lymphoma, CLL, and acute leukemia.

12. What is marrow purging?

One of the proposed disadvantages of autologous transplantation for hematopoietic malignancies or malignancies that involve the bone marrow is the risk of reinfusion of contaminated marrow. Numerous purging techniques are currently under investigation in an attempt to decrease the number of viable tumor cells present in an autologous graft. The techniques often use monoclonal antibodies directed against the malignant cell, exposure of the graft to chemotherapeutic agents, or positive selection of hematopoietic stem cells based on expression of CD34, an antigen present on early hematopoietic stem cells but absent from most tumor cells.

13. What is an umbilical cord-blood transplant, and how does it differ from a peripheral blood stem-cell transplant?

Umbilical cord-blood transplantation has become one of the most vigorously investigated areas in hematopoietic stem-cell transplantation. The presence of hematopoietic stem cells in cord blood has been recognized since 1974. In an umbilical cord blood transplant, progenitor cells are harvested from the cord, HLA typed, tested for infectious disease, cryopreserved (frozen), and reinfused into an appropriate recipient as in peripheral blood stem-cell and marrow transplantation. So far, clinical results in children are extremely encouraging with an apparent diminished risk of GVHD. The lower incidence of GVHD in cord-blood transplants remains incompletely understood, although it is suspected that the immature immune system of the cord blood is less likely to mount an immunologic attack on host antigens. Unanswered questions about cord-blood transplantation include whether adequate numbers of progenitor cells are present in cord blood to engraft larger (adult) recipients and whether the graft-versus-leukemia effect noted with bone marrow or PBSC grafts also will be present with cord-blood grafts. Ongoing investigation of cord-blood transplantation will better help to define its role in stem-cell transplantation and determine if it will be a useful approach to expanding the donor pool for nonrelated transplants.

BIBLIOGRAPHY

1. Baron F, Deprez M, Beguiin Y: The veno-occlusive disease of the liver. Haematologica 82:718–725, 1997.
2. Bearman S: The syndrome of hepatic veno-occlusive disease after marrow transplantation. Blood 85:3005–3020, 1995.
3. Cairo MS, Wagner JE: Placental and/or umbilical cord blood: An alternative source of hematopoietic stem cells for transplantation. Blood 90:4665–4678, 1997.
4. Hann DM: Quality of life following bone marrow transplantation for breast cancer. A comparative study. Bone Marrow Transplant 18:257–264, 1997.
5. Kantrow SP, Hackman RC, Boeckh M, et al: Idiopathic pneumonia syndrome: Changing spectrum of lung injury after marrow transplantation. Transplantation 63:1079–1086, 1997.
6. Lee SJ, Kuntz KM, et al: Unrelated donor bone marrow transplantation for chronic myelogenous leukemia: A decision analysis. Ann Intern Med 127:1080–1088, 1997.
7. Lemoli RM, Bandini G, Leopardig G, et al: Allogeneic peripheral blood stem cell transplantation in patients with early phase hematologic malignancy: A retrospective comparison of short term outcome with bone marrow transplantation. Haematologica 83:48–55, 1998.
8. Mossad SB, Longworth DL, Goormastic M, et al: Early infectious complications in autologous bone marrow transplantation: A review of 219 patients. Bone Marrow Transplant 18:265–271, 1996.
9. O'Marcaugh AS, Cowan MJ: Bone marrow transplantation for inherited diseases. Curr Opin Oncol 9:126–130, 1997.
10. Robinson N, Sullivan KM: Complications of allogeneic bone marrow transplantation. Curr Opin Hematol 1:406–411, 1994.
11. Roy V, Ochs L, Weisdorf D: Late infections following allogeneic bone marrow transplantation: Suggested strategies for prophylaxis. Leuk Lymphoma 26(1-2):1–15, 1997.
12. Serody JS, Shea TC: Prevention of infections in bone marrow transplant recipients. Infect Dis Clin North Am 11:459–477, 1997.
13. Tabbara IA: Allogeneic bone marrow transplantation: Acute and late complications. Anticancer Res 16:1019–1026, 1996.
14. Van Rhee F, Kolb HJ: Donor leukocyte transfusions for leukemic relapse. Curr Opin Hematol 2:423–430, 1995.

48. PRINCIPLES OF RADIATION ONCOLOGY

Brad A. Factor, M.D., and Rachel Rabinovitch, M.D.

1. What is radiation oncology?

Radiation oncology is a specialty of clinical medicine that uses ionizing radiation to treat cancer and occasionally benign disease. The goal of radiation therapy is to eradicate cancer through delivery of a precisely measured dose of radiation to a defined tissue volume with minimal damage to surrounding healthy tissue. Radiation oncologists work closely with surgical oncologists, medical oncologists, and physicians in related disciplines to manage the cancer patient's treatment course.

2. What is the physical basis of radiation therapy?

The types of ionizing radiation used in the treatment of cancer patients include both electromagnetic waves and particulate radiation. The electromagnetic spectrum includes radio waves, infrared light, visible light, ultraviolet light, gamma rays and x-rays. X-rays and gamma rays (high-frequency high-energy waves) are used clinically to treat patients because of their ionizing properties. Using quantum mechanics, gamma rays and x-rays may be represented as particles called photons. Particulate radiation includes electrons, neutrons, alpha-particles, and other heavy ions. Of these, only electrons are widely available for routine clinical use.

3. How does exposure to radiation kill cancer cells?

The classic model of radiation-induced tumor cell death is based on the concept that the accumulation of double-strand DNA breaks leads to the loss of cellular reproduction. Because tumor cells generally lack intact repair mechanisms that normal cells use to repair DNA, they are inherently sensitive to the effects of radiation. On average, after each standard dose of radiation, 63% of tumor cells sustain lethal damage to their DNA molecule. Such damage does not kill the cell immediately, but is considered lethal because the cell dies when it attempts to divide.

Damage to DNA by radiation particles occurs through the direct interaction of particles on cellular DNA or through an indirect mechanism mediated by free radicals. Because the mammalian cell is approximately 80% water, the H_2O molecule is the main source for the production of free radicals. The radiolysis of water produces unstable and thus highly reactive free radicals that diffuse throughout the cell over very short distances to react with cellular macromolecules. It is specifically the interaction of free radicals with cellular DNA that causes cell death. Studies suggest that the indirect mechanism causes approximately 70% of the damage produced by photons (amount of damage from electrons is probably similar). Recently, several other mechanisms have been identified to explain the cytotoxic effects of radiation, including radiation-induced activation of signal-transduction pathways and gene activation, stimulation of growth factor production, and apoptosis (programmed cell death).

4. What is a linear accelerator (or Linac)?

Linear accelerators are treatment machines that have revolutionized the field of radiation oncology. They can selectively create high-energy radiation beams to the specifications of the user. By accelerating an electron beam into a tungsten target, photon beams of various energies can be created (most commonly 6–25 MeV). Alternatively, the same electron beam can be accelerated into a scattering foil rather than the tungsten target to spread the electron beam into a more uniform and clinically useful distribution.

5. What determines whether the radiation oncologist will prescribe electron or photon beam therapy?

Because electrons have both mass and charge, they are highly interactive with the atomic structures of body tissue. However, their useful treatment range is limited to a tissue depth of only a few centimeters because the energy they possess is quickly dissipated through atomic interactions. Electron beam therapy is therefore ideal for treatment of skin cancers and other superficial lesions when it is desirable to minimize dose delivery to underlying tissues. In contrast, because photons have no mass or net charge, they are deeply penetrating beams and are ideal for treatment of tumors or tissues located deep within the body. Photons are used most commonly in clinical medicine because most cancers are located below the body surface.

6. How is the dosage of ionizing radiation expressed?

Absorbed dose is the amount of energy deposited by ionizing radiation per unit mass. The SI unit of absorbed dose is the gray (Gy), which is equal to one joule/kilogram. Doses used in radiotherapy are often expressed in centigrays (one hundredth of a gray = cGy), which is equal to one rad (radiation absorbed dose), a term previously used in older literature. Because certain types of radiation are more biologically damaging than others, a radiation weighting factor (also called quality factor) is multiplied by the absorbed dose to yield the dose equivalent. The dose equivalent is measured in rem (roentgen equivalent man). Because the quality factor for both electrons and photons is equal to one, one cGy equals one rem. The average American receives the equivalent of 300 millirem to the whole body over the course of a year from natural sources. The dose equivalent to skin from a chest film at beam entry is 25 millirem.

7. Is the Cobalt-60 machine antiquated and inferior?

No! Cobalt-60 machines differ from linear accelerators because they house a radioactive piece of cobalt that emits a therapeutically useful photon beam with an average energy of 1.25 MeV. The photons are no different from those created by a linear accelerator, but because of their lower energy, the Co-60 machine has limited application. Low-energy beams in this range are most appropriate for treatment of smaller body parts, such as extremity or head and neck tumors. In fact, in many academic institutions the Co-60 machine is the preferred treatment device for head and neck cancers because of its particular beam characteristics.

8. Why is radiotherapy given in divided doses (fractions), rather than in a single treatment, and what are the "4 R's of radiobiology"?

In classic experiments conducted in the 1920s, investigators in France studied the potential therapeutic use of radiation using the external genitalia of rams as a model of cancer in humans. Spermatogenesis represented the rapidly proliferating cancer cells and scrotal skin represented dose-limiting normal tissue. The investigators observed that it was not possible to sterilize a ram with a single dose of radiation to the testes without producing severe skin damage to the scrotal skin. However, when the total dose was divided into a number of fractions delivered over time, it was possible to sterilize the ram without injuring the overlying skin. The total fractionated dose was actually less than the single dose needed to produce infertility.

The efficacy of dividing a dose into a number of fractions is now understood in terms of radiobiologic principles that have been established in more relevant test systems. Such principles are often referred to as the "4 R's of radiobiology": **r**epair, **r**epopulation, **r**edistribution, and **r**eoxygenation. The repair of sublethal damage and the repopulation of cells between dose fractions explains the increased tolerance of normal tissue to radiation when the dose is divided into numerous smaller treatments. Fractionation improves tumor cell kill by allowing cells to redistribute or move into the radiosensitive phases of the cell cycle (G_2 and M) between fractions, which enhances radiosensitivity with the next treatment. Reoxygenation describes the process through which hypoxic cells in the center of a large tumor become better oxygenated, and therefore more radiosensitive, through the course of a fractionated treatment. As the greater oxygenated and hence more radiosensitive cells located at the periphery of the tumor die, the tumor shrinks and blood vessels within the tumor are decompressed, which increases the blood supply to the previously hypoxic deeper cells, making them more radiosensitive.

9. Is there a standard fractionation regimen?

Yes. In standard fractionation a single dose of 180–200 cGy is delivered once a day, Monday through Friday. Typical curative treatment courses usually require 5–8 weeks of treatment.

10. What is hyperfractionation?

Hyperfractionation halves the usual dose/fraction to 100–120 cGy and increases the daily number of treatment to ≥ 2 fractions. Because long-term side effects of radiotherapy are primarily dependent on the dose per treatment, the goal of hyperfractionation, compared with standard fractionation, is to reduce late side effects. Alternatively, hyperfractionation allows an increase of the total dose delivered to achieve better tumor control while maintaining the same degree of late effects as standard fractionation. Radiobiologic evidence also demonstrates that improved cell kill is achieved when hyperfractionation is used in rapidly growing tumors, and clinical studies have confirmed this in limited tumor sites.

11. Do other fractionation schemes exist aside from standard fractionation and hyperfractionation?

Yes. Accelerated fractionation delivers multiple fractions per day without decreasing the dose/fraction, thereby shortening the overall treatment time. Acute toxicity is significantly higher with this approach, but it is used to reduce repopulation of cancer cells in rapidly proliferating tumors. Hypofractionation delivers single, daily treatments with large doses per fraction and shortens the overall treatment time. The most common clinical application of this technique is in the care of dying patients who require palliation of pain or other distressing cancer symptoms. Patients with a limited life expectancy will not encounter the late complications of treatment, and treatment time is compressed to minimize the inconvenience of therapy. Finally, split-course refers to a course of radiotherapy with a planned treatment break (usually 2 weeks) midway through treatment to allow for resolution of acute toxicity before reinstitution of treatment. It also can be used to evaluate tumor response midway through treatment before completing therapy. This approach has been used in pancreatic, lung, and head and neck cancers.

12. What is the difference between brachytherapy and teletherapy?

All forms of radiotherapy can essentially be divided into two general categories: teletherapy (tele = at a distance) and brachytherapy (brachy = short).

External beam radiotherapy is synonymous with teletherapy. Teletherapy refers to radiation beams that originate outside of the patient. The radiation beam, usually delivered from a linear accelerator, originates ≥ 80 cm from the patient, a distance which allows a more uniform dose distribution over the treatment volume. Brachytherapy describes placement of radioactive substances directly into the tumor tissues within the patient, providing a highly selective but invasive method of delivering radiation while minimizing the dose to surrounding normal tissue.

13. What is the inverse square law?

The inverse square law is an equation that describes the relationship between the intensity of radiation exposure and distance from the radioactive source. As the equation demonstrates ($I \propto 1/d^2$), exposure is inversely proportional to the square of the distance from the source where I is the intensity and d is the distance from the source. For example, doubling the distance from a radiation source would decrease exposure by a factor of four.

14. How is brachytherapy applied?

Brachytherapy is the implantation of radioactive isotopes directly into the body and is used most commonly to treat tumors, although it also has been explored as a technique for preventing cardiovascular restenosis. Treatment delivered through preexisting body cavities (i.e., vagina, esophagus, or blood vessels) is termed **intracavitary brachytherapy**; **interstitial brachytherapy** refers to implantation of sources directly through body tissue. Implanted radionuclides can be left permanently within the tissues at risk (permanent implant) or for a defined period of time and then removed following delivery of the intended dose (temporary implant).

Brachytherapy is a standard curative treatment technique for prostate cancer (temporary or permanent interstitial), cervical cancer (temporary intracavitary), soft tissue sarcomas (temporary interstitial), and can be used to treat esophagus, lung, and head and neck tumors as well.

15. What parameters are used to describe the differences between radionuclides?

Numerous radionuclides are available for clinical use and vary in their activity, half-life, energy, and half-value layer. Activity describes the rate of radioactive decay in units of disintegrations per second. Because a radionuclide is constantly decaying, the activity of the substance is constantly decreasing. Since the dose delivered depends upon exposure over time, the activity must be considered when calculating treatment times. The half-life of the substance describes the time in which the activity of the source decreases by 50%. The half-value layer is used to define the thickness of a given material, usually lead, necessary to absorb 50% of the emitted radiation from a radionuclide.

16. What radionuclides are used most commonly in brachytherapy?

Radionuclide	Half-life	Photon Energy (MeV)	Half-value Layer (mm Lead)
Cesium 137	30 yrs	.662	5.5
Iridium 192	74 days	.38 (average)	2.5
Iodine 125	60 days	.028 (average)	0.025
Palladium 103	17 days	.024	0.02
Gold	2.7 days	.412	2.5

Cesium is used most often for treatment of cervical cancer, and iodine or iridium are the isotopes most appropriate for treatment of prostate cancer and soft tissue sarcomas. High-activity iridium is now commercially available for high-dose rate therapy and can be safely stored in the radiation oncology department.

17. What is high-dose rate (HDR) brachytherapy, and what are some of its advantages over traditional low-dose rate (LDR) brachytherapy?

HDR brachytherapy delivers radiation at dose rates similar to external beam radiotherapy— 2–3 Gy per minute; LDR brachytherapy delivers radiation more slowly at a rate of 0.4–0.8 Gy per hour. Traditional LDR brachytherapy requires several hours or days to deliver an adequate treatment dose, and the patient must be hospitalized over the entire course of treatment for radiation safety monitoring. With HDR brachytherapy, computer-controlled remote afterloading loads a high-intensity source into the patient to deliver an adequate dose in minutes, avoiding several complications associated with LDR brachytherapy—exposure of health care workers to the radiation source, prolonged patient hospitalization, and complications of prolonged bed rest associated with indwelling pelvic implants.

18. How are radiation treatments specified by the physician?

The physician writes a therapy prescription that includes the date, site (e.g., larynx), number of fields or ports (two), field arrangement (left lateral and right lateral), energy (4 MeV), dose per fraction (200 cGy), number of fractions (33), planned total dose (6600 cGy), fractions per day/days per week (1/5), and the appropriate dose distribution as represented by an isodose plan, which is a planar representation of dose through an anatomic cross section displaying varying dose level lines represented by either absolute dose or relative percentages. An isodose plan looks similar to a topographic map, which is a planar representation of a landscape using contour lines of equal elevation. During treatment planning, several dose distribution plans may be generated before the physician selects the most appropriate isodose plan.

19. What are some typical total curative doses of radiation?

Prescribed doses for cancer therapy depend on the radiosensitivity of the primary tumor, the tumor volume (e.g., gross disease vs. microscopic residual), and the radiosensitivity of surrounding normal tissues. Highly radiosensitive tumors such as seminomas can be cured with doses of only 2000–3000 cGy. Lymphomas are also relatively radiosensitive and respond to doses of 2000–4000 cGy. Squamous cell cancers and sarcomas require higher doses, > 6000 cGy in most instances. Cervical cancers, through a combination of treatment techniques, are treated to 8000–9000 cGy with an acceptable complication rate. Adjuvant or postoperative treatment for breast, lung, and rectal cancer when no gross disease remains results in adequate tumor control with 4500–5400 cGy. Although melanomas and renal cell carcinomas are often described as radioresistant, ample literature demonstrates their responsiveness to radiotherapy.

20. What is the most common arrangement of fields?

Field arrangements may include one field or a combination of fields. Two opposing fields are used most commonly (i.e., AP and PA, or right and left lateral) because an adequate dose distribution is achieved with minimal setup. Multiple fields at irregular angles can improve upon the dosimetry obtained from simple treatment techniques. Such treatment plans are more labor intensive and require advanced planning technology not available in all treatment facilities in the United States.

21. What does the term *treatment planning* mean?

Treatment planning describes the process of customizing radiotherapy delivery for each patient. During treatment planning the physician works closely with physicists, dosimetrists, and radiation therapists to accomplish the steps necessary for the patient to receive radiation treatments.

22. What is a simulation?

A simulation is a process performed before a patient's first treatment, during which the precise anatomic area to be treated is established. This complex process includes optimization of patient positioning and specification of beam dimensions and angles, and is performed on a treatment simulator that duplicates the exact geometry and mechanical movements of the treatment machines. The simulator contains an x-ray tube rather than a linear accelerator, and produces diagnostic x-ray pictures that delineate the tissue volume to be treated. Customized immobilization devices may be designed, including face masks or trunk and extremity cradles to provide patient comfort during the treatment process, as well as stabilization to minimize involuntary patient movement. After the patient is appropriately positioned in space relative to the desired treatment beams, multiple measurements are taken, and the patient's skin is tattooed at points where lasers positioned within the walls of the room intersect the patient's skin surface. Since the treatment room contains lasers with geometry identical to those in the simulator, the tattoos allow for precise reproduction of patient position for every treatment.

23. What are beam-modifying devices?

To obtain ideal dose distributions in the treated area, many processes can be performed to modify the treatment beam. Beam-modifying devices are placed within the beam's path anywhere from the origin of the beam within the machine head to the surface of the patient's body. Devices used to modify the beam include blocks, wedges, tissue compensators, and bolus.

Because primary treatment beams are always rectangular as they exit a treatment machine, **blocks** are used to alter the beams' shape into any configuration desired by the physician. The block is custom made for each individual patient and field, and is placed where the beam exits the machine to prevent passage of radiation within the "blocked" area from reaching the patient. Cerrubend, an alloy of lead, is used almost universally as block material because its low melting point easily allows it to be reused. At the thickness used clinically, cerrubend absorbs approximately 97% of a beam's energy. A multileaf collimator, which is made up of multiple pairs of narrow leaves within the machine head, is an alternative to custom-made blocks. The leaves can be programmed selectively for each patient and field to shape the beam just as conventional blocks do, but minimize the physical labor and time required to insert and remove standard blocks for each field.

Wedges are triangular wedges of dose-absorbing metal placed between the beam and patient to compensate for a sloping treated surface. If no modifying devise is used, the thinner part of the body receives more dose than the thicker part. When the thick end (heel) of the wedge is placed parallel to the thinner portion of the treated area, enough dose is absorbed as the beam passes through the heel to cause a uniform dose distribution through the uneven treatment area. Wedges are described by the angle of the wedge, and the most common wedges used are 15, 30, 45, and 60°. **Tissue compensators**, designed to be positioned at a distance from the skin surface, can be used to deliver a more uniform dose to an irregular surface. **Bolus** is a tissue-equivalent material that can be placed directly on the skin to increase the dose delivered to the skin surface.

24. What is a port film?

A port film is an x-ray film taken of the patient in the treatment position on the treatment machine to visually document the anatomy being treated. This tool allows the physician to assess the accuracy of treatment and modify the treatment parameters if necessary.

A port film differs from a diagnostic x-ray film because the picture is generated using high energy x-rays in the therapeutic range, megaelectron volts (MeV), rather than the lower energy range used for diagnostic purposes, kiloelectron volts (KeV). Lower energy x-rays interact with tissue predominantly by the photoelectric effect, which is highly dependent on atomic number; bone and soft tissue, which have very different average atomic numbers, interact differentially with the x-ray beam and can be distinguished easily on a diagnostic x-ray. In contrast, port films appear hazy to the untrained observer. Tissues of varying atomic number interact similarly with the higher energy x-rays, causing soft tissue and bone to be less easily distinguishable on a port film.

25. What does a patient experience during and after radiation therapy?

Nothing! During the delivery of radiation (which usually lasts less than 3 minutes), the patient experiences nothing except the sound of the treatment machine ticking. The patient cannot feel the beam and does not experience pain, temperature change of the skin, or any other sensation. During or after external beam radiotherapy the patient is not radioactive, does not glow in the dark, and, contrary to popular opinion, does not obtain any super powers.

26. What are some short-term and long-term side effects of radiotherapy?

The effects of radiation on tissue depend on the body site treated, the total dose prescribed, and the time frame over which the dose is delivered. Acute effects usually begin 2–3 weeks into treatment and subside within 6 weeks of therapy completion. Acute effects depend more on the dose delivered and time frame of delivery than on the inherent fractionation sensitivity of the tissues treated. Depending on the body region treated, acute radiation effects may include fatigue, skin erythema or desquamation, mucositis, odynophagia, hair loss, nausea, diarrhea, and bone marrow suppression.

Delayed effects of radiation, which generally occur at least 6 months after therapy has ended, depend more on the inherent fractionation sensitivity of tissues and are usually irreversible. Radiation is responsible for late effects of cancer therapy only when the toxicity occurs within the previously irradiated area. Delayed radiation toxicity includes atrophy to any lining epithelia, cataracts, permanent hair loss, stenosis of treated organs (esophagus or vagina), bone hypoplasia (when a growing child is treated), memory deficits, hormonal dysfunction, and interstitial fibrosis of the treated tissues.

27. What is tolerance dose or TD5/5 and TD50/5?

The TD5/5 is the dose of radiation expected to cause severe complications in the treated tissue in no more than 5% of treated patients within 5 years, which is considered an acceptable threshold for toxicity. Radiation oncologists generally attempt to limit doses to this level for a given tissue. Similarly, the TD50/5 is the dose at which 50% of treated patients are expected to experience severe toxicity within the target organ at 5 years. Such terms are used to express relatively the radiotolerance of various body tissues. The minimal tolerance dose (TD5/5) for various organs expressed in cGy ranges from the testes (100), ovary and lens of the eye (600), lungs and kidneys (2000), to the heart (4000), brain (6000), and muscle, bone, and cartilage (> 7000).

28. What is palliative radiation?

Rather than curing the disease process, palliative radiation is intended to improve a patient's quality of life by relieving distressing symptoms or preventing tumor-related complications. The dose per fraction is generally larger (i.e., 300–800 cGy) and the number of fractions less (i.e., 5–10) than standard fractionation. Bone pain secondary to metastases is the most common pain syndrome requiring treatment in cancer patients, and typical palliative doses for bone pain range between 800 cGy in a single fraction and 3000 cGy in 10 fractions.

29. What is conformal radiotherapy?

Conformal or 3D therapy uses new developments in computer technology. Patients undergo a CT scan of the body area to be treated in a specified treatment position. Information from the

CT scan is downloaded into a treatment planning computer, where the body is reconstructed in three dimensions. The entire simulation process takes place in virtual reality, with the ability to maneuver various beam angles, energies, and blocks until an optimal plan is achieved, all without having the patient present. Because of the enhanced ability to differentiate the location of the target tumor from surrounding normal structures, beam configurations can conform more tightly to the tumor site, reducing dose and therefore toxicity to healthy adjacent organs. This technology allows treatment of tumors to higher doses than previously possible.

30. What is stereotactic radiosurgery?

Stereotactic radiosurgery (SRS) of the brain delivers a single high-dose fraction to an intracranial target within submillimeter accuracy. In SRS a halo is affixed to the patient's skull to serve the dual purpose of strict immobilization and act as an external reference system. Anatomic information obtained from CTs and MRIs is used to reconstruct the skull and intracranial contents in three dimensions, creating reference coordinates (x, y and z) for any given point within the brain relative to the extracranial frame. Using multiple radiation arcs with beam apertures of millimeters, SRS delivers high doses of radiation to target intracranial tissues, keeping the dose to adjacent brain tissue at an absolute minimum. This technique serves as an alternative to surgery in the treatment of brain arteriovenous malformations (AVMs), and its use is currently being investigated for the treatment of several malignant and benign intracranial lesions, including high-grade gliomas, single and multiple brain metastases, and craniopharyngiomas.

BIBLIOGRAPHY

1. Cox JD (ed): Moss' Radiation Oncology: Rationale, Technique, Results, 7th ed. St. Louis, Mosby, 1994.
2. Perez CA, Brady LV (eds): Principles and Practice of Radiation Oncology, 3rd ed. Philadelphia, Lippincott-Raven, 1998.
3. Steel GG: Basic Clinical Radiobiology, 2nd ed. New York, Oxford University Press, 1997.

49. RADIATION ONCOLOGY: THERAPEUTICS

Rachel Rabinovitch, M.D., and Brad A. Factor, M.D.

1. What is the role of radiation therapy (XRT) in early-stage breast cancer?

Over the past three decades, numerous randomized trials have proved the equivalency of mastectomy to lumpectomy followed by breast XRT for treatment of early breast cancer. Appropriately selected women compromise nothing (i.e., local control, disease-free survival, or overall survival) by opting for therapy that preserves the breast. Guidelines for choosing patients appropriate for breast conservation include tumors < 5 cm (T_1–T_2), no evidence of multifocality on physical exam or mammography, and a breast size that will accommodate tumor resection and result in a cosmetically satisfactory outcome. Contraindications include pregnancy, collagen vascular disease, and prior XRT to breast tissue. Tumor within axillary lymph nodes following a lymph node dissection does not limit a woman's local treatment options. Breast XRT generally requires 5–6½ weeks of daily outpatient treatment lasting less than 15 minutes.

2. Is there ever a role for XRT following mastectomy for breast cancer?

Yes. The traditional purpose of chest-wall XRT following mastectomy is to decrease the risk of local failure (LF), i.e., chest wall recurrence. Patients with T > 5 cm, positive mastectomy margins, and/or ≥ 4 positive axillary lymph nodes are considered to be at sufficient risk for local chest wall failure to benefit from chest-wall XRT. Recently published studies from Europe and Canada have indicated that chest-wall XRT not only decreases LF but also improves long-term cancer-free survival rates. Patients with even a single positive axillary lymph node and no other high-risk factors benefited from therapy. These trials are widening the range of patients thought to benefit from adjuvant chest-wall radiotherapy.

3. How do you treat noninvasive breast cancer (ductal carcinoma in situ [DCIS])?

Mastectomy has been the gold standard for treatment of DCIS, yielding a 99.9% cure rate. Based on the effectiveness of lumpectomy and breast irradiation (lump/RT) for **invasive** breast cancers, this approach was applied to patients with DCIS and had surprising results. Unlike invasive breast cancers in which multiple studies have proved the equivalence of mastectomy to lump/RT, these treatment choices for DCIS result in failure rates of 0.1% and 10%, respectively. The poorer disease-free survival rate with breast-conserving therapy does **not** translate into decreased survival; nearly all patients can be salvaged upon recurrence with a mastectomy. Women should therefore be advised of the differences between these two treatment approaches and allowed to participate in the decision-making process.

The NSABP (National Surgical Adjuvant Breast Project) performed a randomized trial for patients with DCIS, comparing lumpectomy alone with lump/RT. The addition of RT resulted in significantly better local control rates (93% vs. 84%). Physicians experienced in treating DCIS have followed many women with favorable subtypes of DCIS treated with lumpectomy only with control rates similar to lump/RT series. Favorable DCIS is generally defined as tumors detected by mammography, measuring < 2.5 cm, having negative margins following resection, and being of low or intermediate grade. A randomized trial comparing lumpectomy with lump/RT in this subset of favorable DCIS will likely take place in the near future.

4. Is XRT to the axilla as effective as an axillary dissection for breast cancer?

For a clinically normal axilla—one in which lymph nodes (LNs) are not palpable—XRT and surgery are equally effective in preventing regional tumor recurrence. Although XRT is less morbid than an axillary node dissection (AND), the latter is the most common approach used in the United States because it provides prognostic information by identifying the number of lymph nodes involved with tumor. If recommendations for adjuvant therapy will be affected by the **number** of positive axillary lymph nodes, then an AND is performed both to treat the axilla and to obtain pertinent prognostic information.

At times, adjuvant therapy is determined by the knowledge that at least one LN is involved with tumor, rather than determination of the total number. Use of a sentinel LN biopsy is ideal in this situation, which carries minimal morbidity and provides the tumor status of the "sentinel" LN. If negative, no further axillary therapy is considered necessary, although this has not been confirmed yet in a randomized trial. If positive, axillary radiation is given to assure long-term control of tumor within the axilla. Axillary radiation results in ipsilateral long-term lymphedema in less than 5% of patients if an AND has not been performed and is not associated with the uncomfortable numbness and range-of-motion difficulties associated with an AND.

5. What is the standard treatment for limited-stage small cell lung cancer?

The designation of "limited stage" to a patient with small cell lung cancer specifically indicates the ability to include all of the patient's known disease within a reasonable XRT portal. Numerous randomized trials along with two meta-analyses have proved that the addition of XRT to chemotherapy for limited-stage small cell lung cancer improves not only control of the disease within the chest, but overall survival as well.

Chest XRT should be initiated early in the course of treatment in order to maximize its benefit. The most common side effects of chest XRT include esophagitis, fatigue, and mild skin changes. Because small cell tumors are more radiosensitive than non-small cell tumors, moderate doses of radiotherapy are generally prescribed (i.e., 4500–5400 cGy).

6. Is there any value in treating "inoperable" or locally advanced lung cancer?

Yes! Although surgery is ineffective in treating the majority of T_4N_{2-3} lung cancers, XRT plays a key role in controlling thoracic disease. Trials published over the past two decades have further demonstrated that the addition of systemic therapy to chest XRT improves local control and 2-year survival rates. This aggressive combined modality approach has the most benefit in patients < 70 years of age, without anemia, good performance status, and with weight loss comprising < 10% of ideal body weight. The outcome for treated patients is still poor, with 2-year survival rates of approximately 25%. National trials are investigating the potential benefit of adding surgical resection following chemoradiotherapy in locally advanced patients. Nevertheless, treatment results in improved survival rates when compared with supportive care.

7. Is adjuvant XRT appropriate following resection of non-small cell lung cancer?

Thoracic XRT improves local control whenever postresection pathology demonstrates positive hilar/mediastinal lymph nodes or positive margins. Prevention of tumor progression within the chest is valuable to prevent symptoms of hemoptysis and postobstructive pneumonia. The standard dose is 5000 cGy delivered in 5 weeks. A recent meta-analysis found that the survival of patients treated with postoperative thoracic XRT was actually inferior to those who were not irradiated. The reason for this finding is not obvious, but may be related to antiquated and inferior radiation techniques used many decades ago in the studies analyzed, resulting in cardiopulmonary morbidity.

8. Is a total laryngectomy necessary for patients with advanced laryngeal cancer?

No. A randomized trial published by the Veterans Administration compared total laryngectomy followed by XRT with neoadjuvant chemotherapy (5-FU/cisplatin) for three cycles followed by definitive XRT in partial responders. Although the patterns of failure differed between the two arms, overall survival was the same. Single-institution results of XRT alone also yield comparable results. To determine which approach is optimal, an ongoing RTOG trial is comparing XRT alone, XRT and concomitant chemotherapy, and neoadjuvant chemotherapy with XRT.

9. What are the short- and long-term side effects of head and neck radiation therapy?

The primary tumor site and stage of a head and neck cancer determine the nodal and mucosal regions that require treatment. Irradiated skin becomes indurated and erythematous, and may progress to dry or moist desquamation. Mucous membranes can similarly develop painful ulceration called mucositis. Such changes are temporary and are treated symptomatically with lanolin-based salves, topical anesthetics, and oral narcotics. The most irritating long-term side effect is xerostomia to varying degrees, depending on the treatment volume and dose delivered to the salivary glands. The use of pilocarpine (Salagen) is now FDA-approved for treatment of XRT-induced xerostomia. Three randomized trials have proved its effectiveness. Evidence also supports the use of Salagen during XRT to reduce the degree of post-therapy dryness. Permanent facial hair loss also may result within high-dose regions.

10. What is the treatment for nonmetastatic esophagus cancer?

Total esophagectomy is the standard surgical approach to cancers of the esophagus. Concomitant chemoradiation (5 weeks of radiotherapy with 5-FU and cisplatin chemotherapy delivered during weeks 1, 5, 8, and 11) is the organ-preserving approach for this aggressive disease. Chemoradiation trials appear to have inferior results compared with esophagectomy series. On careful review, however, patients with locally advanced disease often are considered ineligible for surgical therapy, as are patients with alcohol- and tobacco-related medical problems. Such factors play a prominent role in patient outcome.

Although a randomized trial comparing these radically different approaches has never taken place, it is generally accepted that each is equally effective in similarly staged patients with squamous tumors. A randomized trial demonstrated that the addition of 5-FU/cisplatin to moderate doses of XRT significantly improved both local and distant tumor control as well as overall survival when compared with high-dose XRT alone. Current trials are determining if combining chemotherapy with higher XRT doses will improve outcome; median survival for esophagus cancer is only 11 months. Surgery is considered a more essential component of therapy for adenocarcinomas than squamous cell carcinomas. Current clinical trials are evaluating the role of coordinating surgery with chemoradiation in this subset of patients.

11. Does XRT have a role in resected or unresectable pancreatic cancer?

Yes. Although surgical resection of pancreatic cancer should be performed whenever techni- cally possible, adjuvant radiotherapy to the pancreatic bed is indicated in all patients unless metastatic disease is present. Numerous randomized trials have evaluated the role of RT with and without chemotherapy in patients with either resected or unresectable pancreas cancer. These studies uniformly demonstrate a survival improvement in treated patients and the superiority of combined chemoradiation to either modality alone. Despite aggressive therapy, median survival of patients with disease is poor: 22 months for patients with resected tumors and 8 months for pa- tients with unresectable disease.

12. Does radiation improve cure rates of colorectal cancer?

Rectal cancers located below the peritoneal reflection are anatomically confined within the pelvis. As a result, local failures of rectal cancers predictably occur within this isolated space. Pelvic radiation combined with 5-FU-based chemotherapy significantly improves both pelvic tumor control and long-term survival rates. The subgroups that benefit from this adjuvant com- bined modality therapy as determined in randomized trials include patients with T_{3-4} or node- positive tumors. The current NCI recommendations consist of two cycles of 5-FU–based chemotherapy followed by 5–6 weeks of concurrent chemoradiation therapy followed by chemotherapy alone for 7 more months. Side effects of pelvic XRT may include diarrhea, de- crease in WBC count, and fatigue.

The colon is not confined to a small anatomic space, traversing through both the retroperi- toneum and abdomen. Colon cancers therefore have a less predictable pattern of recurrence com- pared with rectal cancers. Adjuvant RT to the entire abdomen and retroperitoneum would be required to address all potential sites of "local failure," which is very morbid and has not been proved efficacious for colon cancer, regardless of stage. However, a current intergroup trial is evaluating the role of focal XRT for lesions at high risk for truly localized failure, defined as T_{3-4} lesions, or tumors associated with an abscess/perforation.

13. Do cancers of the anal canal require an abdominoperineal resection (APR)?

Decades ago, patients were treated with an APR for anal canal tumors, resulting in closure of the anus and placement of a permanent colostomy. Several series of preoperative chemoradiation demonstrated complete eradication of the tumor in two-thirds of patients. As a result, the stan- dard treatment has evolved to definitive chemotherapy (usually 5-FU/mitomycin or 5-FU/cis- platin) delivered concomitantly with RT. The RT is delivered to the anal tumor, including the regional lymph nodes (LNs) at risk (inguinal and pelvic). Doses range from 4500–5000 cGy in 5–6 weeks, depending on the primary tumor and nodal stages. Side effects of the RT include di- arrhea, dysuria, lowered blood counts, anal irritation, and desquamation of groin skin. The cur- rent role of surgery is diagnosis of the primary tumor and biopsy of suspicious palpable inguinal LNs. Overall 5-year survival for treated patients is 70–80%, which is an improvement over the older surgical approach to anal cancer.

14. What is the role of RT in the treatment of malignant brain tumors?

Gliomas comprise a spectrum of tumors of similar origin with varying degrees of aggressive- ness. Grade III–IV astrocytomas should be treated surgically whenever feasible, followed by de- finitive XRT. Standard treatment consists of 6 weeks of daily therapy (6000 cGy) to a field encompassing the tumor plus a margin or normal brain tissue. Chemotherapy is beneficial in many subsets of patients, and numerous trials are investigating optimal drug combinations and timing issues.

XRT is more controversial in the management of lower-grade astrocytomas, for which surgi- cal therapy alone is often adequate.

15. Are meningiomas "benign" brain tumors? How are they treated?

Meningiomas comprise 20% of all intracranial tumors and are more common in women and Caucasians. They arise from the arachnoid cells of the meninges and therefore develop along the brain convexities, sphenoid ridge, and parasagittal structures. The majority of meningiomas are slow-growing benign tumors, which do not have the ability to disseminate to other parts of the body or brain. Their designation as "benign," however, should not lead the clinician to underestimate the neurologic sequelae that a meningioma can cause when located adjacent to critical structures.

Standard therapy consists of surgical resection. When completely resected, recurrence rates are extremely low (4–10%). Radiotherapy is reserved for any patient in whom only a subtotal resection was achieved, and recurrence rates without further therapy range from 60–75%. XRT is delivered to the tumor plus margin to 5040 cGy in 28 fractions. Recurrence rates following adjuvant RT are 20–30% at 10 years.

There is a subset of **malignant** meningiomas that are locally aggressive tumors. Because of their much poorer prognosis, adjuvant RT to 6000 cGy is always delivered postoperatively, regardless of the extent of resection.

16. Should patients diagnosed with medulloblastoma be treated with radiotherapy even if they have had a complete resection?

Yes. Medulloblastomas are peripheral neuroectodermal tumors of the cerebellum, usually located at midline within the vermis, with a high predilection for dissemination throughout the neuraxis. Staging therefore always includes imaging of the entire brain and spine (MRI is preferred) as well as cytologic evaluation of cerebrospinal fluid. Even in the absence of documented dissemination, all medulloblastomas require postoperative radiotherapy to the entire neuraxis to minimize the incidence of diffuse CNS relapse. Standard treatment consists of 3600 cGy in 20 fractions to the entire brain and spine, with continued treatment to the posterior fossa to 5400 cGy. The role of chemotherapy in medulloblastoma is being investigated in pediatric national trials.

17. What are the advantages and disadvantages of curative XRT alone as treatment for early-stage Hodgkin's disease (HD)?

Patients with early-stage HD (stages I–II) are cured nearly 90% of the time, regardless of whether they are treated with definitive chemotherapy, radiotherapy, or a combination of the two. Treatment with definitive XRT avoids the leukemogenic potential of mechlorethamine, Oncovin, procarbazine, prednisone (MOPP) chemotherapy, and the cardiopulmonary toxicity associated with Adriamycin, bleomycin, vinblastine, dacarbazine (ABVD) chemotherapy. No diffuse hair loss or significantly lowered blood counts occur. Radiotherapy for patients with supradiaphragmatic disease results in preservation of fertility.

The acute side effects of XRT to the traditional fields for HD (mantle and para-aortic LNs) include temporary focal hair loss at the occiput, odynophagia, laryngitis, nausea, and mild suppression of white count and platelet count. Patients are generally pathologically staged before undergoing definitive XRT, which includes an exploratory laparotomy, para-aortic LN sampling, biopsies of both lobes of the liver, and a splenectomy. As a result, such patients are subject to the risk and discomfort associated with a laparotomy and general anesthesia. To avoid the risk of sepsis with gram-positive encapsulated organisms in a splenectomized patient, Pneumovax vaccines are necessary. Radiation does predispose patients to the risks of solid malignancies within irradiated areas. The risk of breast cancer is well documented, with increased risk of cancer development 7–20 years after XRT.

Current areas of research focus on combining shorter courses of chemotherapy with low doses of radiation to minimize the long-term risks of therapy in a young population of patients with a high probability of cure.

18. What is the role of XRT in the treatment of intermediate- and high-grade non-Hodgkin's lymphoma?

A randomized trial published in 1998 demonstrated that 3 cycles of cyclophosphamide, hydroxydaunomycin, Oncovin, and prednisone (CHOP) chemotherapy followed by involved field

XRT resulted in improved disease-free survival (DFS) and overall survival (OS), compared with 8 cycles of CHOP in patients with early-stage disease (stage I or II). This trial has set a new standard for treating such patients, resulting in 5-year DFS and OS rates of 77% and 82%, respectively. Radiotherapy is delivered only to known sites of disease to doses of 4000–5000 cGy in 4–5 weeks.

19. What are the benefits of treating localized prostate cancer with radiation rather than a radical prostatectomy?

Definitive XRT for prostate cancer is a noninvasive outpatient technique that generally requires 15 minutes per day over 7 weeks. Treatment outcome studies across the U.S. demonstrate that less than 25% of men who are sexually potent at the time of treatment become impotent as a result of XRT. In contrast, the traditional radical prostatectomy results in a nearly 100% impotency rate. The results of using the newer nerve-sparing surgical techniques highly depend on the experience of the surgeon, and only in the best of hands are comparable potency rates achieved. Furthermore, patients who have extracapsular extension, seminal vesicle involvement, and positive margins may require adjuvant XRT anyway. Urinary symptoms (dribbling and frank incontinence) also are less common following XRT than surgery. Conformal XRT technology has greatly enhanced the ability to treat prostate cancer and minimize toxicity to adjacent normal tissues, primarily the rectum and bladder. Combining definitive RT with androgen blockade agents has improved local control rates and is being studied in national trials.

Other radiotherapy treatment options include temporary or permanent implantation of radioactive seeds into the prostate gland with or without the addition of external beam RT. Such techniques are gaining popularity as treatment is completed in a much shorter time-span than conventional XRT. Less long-term data, however, are available on the results of these implant techniques, and methods have yet to be standardized.

20. How are early cervical cancers treated?

Patients with stage IA, IB1, and IIA cervical cancers can be treated equally well with either surgery (radical hysterectomy and lymph node dissection) or definitive radiotherapy. Cure rates range from 75–90% for these disease stages. XRT as curative treatment for cervical cancer always includes a combination of external beam radiotherapy to the pelvis followed by brachytherapy. The most common implantation technique uses a set of instruments called a tandem (inserted through the cervical os into the uterus) and 2 ovoids (placed in the lateral vaginal fornices on either side of the cervix). These instruments are later "loaded" with radioactive cesium or iridium to deliver further doses of radiation while minimizing dose to the rectum and bladder.

Surgery is preferred in young women when preservation of ovarian function is desirable. Definitive RT is generally reserved for women with multiple medical problems who are poor operative candidates and women with moderate-to-morbid obesity, which presents technical difficulties to the operating surgeon.

Side effects of definitive pelvic radiotherapy include short-term fatigue, diarrhea, and dysuria. Brachytherapy implants are associated with minimal-to-moderate discomfort. The entire treatment results in sterility in 100% of patients, but causes long-term bladder or rectal complications in less than 5% of women when standard dose guidelines are adhered to. To avoid development of vaginal adhesions in a patient who is not sexually active, instructions for use of a vaginal dilator are given. Without such precautions permanent vaginal scarring will prevent comfortable intercourse and the physician's ability to perform a pelvic exam and Papanicolaou smear of the cervix.

21. Is surgery a treatment option for locally advanced cervix cancers?

No. Patients with disease extension into the parametria (International Federation of Gynecology and Obstetrics [FIGO] stages IIB–IIIB) are not candidates for surgical resection because it is technically difficult to obtain satisfactory margins within the narrow confines of the lower pelvis. Radiotherapy is therefore the standard treatment for patients with advanced nonmetastatic cervical cancer, again using both external beam and brachytherapy techniques. Pelvic control rates for stages IIB and IIIB are 75% and 50%, respectively, with 5-year survival rates of

65% and 25–50%, respectively. The role of chemotherapy in locally advanced disease is currently being evaluated because standard therapy still results in poor control rates.

22. What role does radiotherapy play in the management of vulvar cancer?

The Gynecologic Oncology Group (GOG) has completed two randomized trials for vulvar cancer defining the situations in which radiotherapy is both effective and ineffective. Patients with positive inguinal lymph nodes following a groin dissection have both improved local control and survival when radiotherapy is delivered to the pelvis and groin postoperatively. On the other hand, radiotherapy as prophylactic treatment to clinically normal inguinal lymph nodes was inadequate, with an unacceptable local failure rate. Although radical vulvectomy is the standard surgical procedure for the primary tumor, elderly women who are inoperable candidates may be well served by definitive radiotherapy.

23. When is XRT used in the treatment of nonmelanomatous skin cancers?

As many skin cancers are diagnosed each year in the United States as all other cancers combined (approximately 1 million). Most squamous cell and basal cell carcinomas are treated equally well with surgery or radiation, with cure rates of approximately 95%. Radiotherapy is preferred when surgical intervention may result in a cosmetically or functionally unacceptable outcome. Lesions of the lip, eyelid, or infraorbital skin are therefore optimally treated with definitive XRT. Multiple large series demonstrate that multiple fractionation schemes are equally efficacious. Doses ranging from 2000 cGy in a single fraction to 6000 cGy over 6 weeks have equal control rates and cosmetic outcome. The short-term side effects of moist desquamation and epilation usually resolve within several weeks to months following treatment. Long-term side effects to treated skin include atrophy, hypopigmentation, and telangectasias. Lesions treated adjacent to the eye can cause ectropion or epiphora.

24. When is total body irradiation (TBI) used as part of a bone marrow transplant program?

Patients who are treated with a BMT for leukemia or genetic diseases are normally given bone marrow or cord blood cells from another individual, related or unrelated to the patient. In such cases, TBI plays an important role in both sterilizing residual tumor or affected marrow cells within the patient and enhancing immunosuppression to allow engraftment. When TBI is used, it is always combined with high-dose chemotherapy, which together form the "preparative" regimen for the transplant. The advantages of including TBI in the preparative regimen are that radiation respects no physical or blood–brain barriers, assuring adequate cell kill in all body regions. Unlike chemotherapy, in which tumor cells may have any one of several mechanisms to render the given drug ineffective (e.g., multidrug resistance genes, calcium channel pumps), TBI is effective because no anti-RT specific mechanism exists within tumor cells. However, TBI is extremely toxic and causes severe short-term mucositis and diarrhea. Long-term side effects in surviving patients are hormonal abnormalities, sterility, risk of secondary malignancies, cataracts, and subtle memory/cognitive deficits. The primary life-threatening toxicity associated with TBI is veno-occlusive disease of the lung or liver.

25. What are radiation oncology emergencies?

XRT is used on an emergent basis when tumors cause life-threatening organ obstruction or progressive neurologic compromise. The most common clinical examples include symptomatic cord compression, airway obstruction, and impending herniation due to an intracranial mass. Steroids are used initially to ameliorate the local swelling that tumors cause, and radiotherapy should be initiated as soon as it is feasible. In general, several days of treatment are required before symptomatic improvement is realized. Unfortunately, the longer a patient has had neurologic impairment as a result of cord compression, the less likely treatment will reverse the deficit.

26. What is the most common treatment for painful osseous metastases?

Irradiation of painful bone metastases is a simple and effective method for lessening pain. Palliative RT is delivered in an accelerated fractionation scheme that minimizes the number of treatment visits yet preserves treatment effectiveness. One large study of over 1000 patients demonstrated that 54% of patients achieve complete pain relief, and 90% experience some relief. Fractionation schemes considered equally effective include 3000 cGy in 2 weeks and 2000 cGy in 1 week. Patients with breast and prostate cancer are more likely to obtain complete pain relief than those with other primary tumor sites. In Europe, even shorter courses of radiation are used, delivering a single fraction of 800 cGy.

For patients with bone pain refractory to conventional XRT or who have painful sites too numerous to treat, strontium-89 chloride administration is another option.

27. Is RT ever used to treat nonmalignant conditions?

Yes. RT has proved effective in managing numerous benign conditions. Patients known to develop keloids following surgical incisions may undergo short-course radiotherapy postoperatively to prevent keloid formation. Infiltration of the extraoccular musculature in hyperthryoidism causes cosmetic deformity and often functional impairment with decreased ocular range of motion and even damage to the optic nerve. RT to the posterior orbits (2000 cGy in 10 treatments) is very effective in resolving the exophthalmos and preventing progressive visual dysfunction. Single fraction (700–800 cGy) treatment to joints known to be at high risk for heterotopic ossification essentially prevents this debilitating condition. In this setting RT can be delivered either pre- or postoperatively.

BIBLIOGRAPHY

1. Aalders J, Abeler V, Dolstad P, et al: Postoperative external irradiation and prognostic parameters in stage I endometrial carcinoma. Obstet Gynecol 56:419–426, 1980.
2. Fisher B, Costantino J, Redmond C, et al: Lumpectomy compared with lumpectomy and radiation therapy for the treatment of intraductal breast cancer. N Engl J Med 328:1581–1586, 1993.
3. Gastrointestinal Tumor Study Group: Prolongation of the disease-free interval in surgically treated rectal carcinoma. N Engl J Med 312:1465–1472, 1985.
4. Homesley H, Bundy B, Sedlis A, et al: Radiation therapy versus pelvic node resection for carcinoma of the vulva with positive groin nodes. Obstet Gynecol 68:733–740, 1986.
5. Miller TP, Dahlberg S, Cassady JR, et al: Chemotherapy alone compared with chemotherapy plus radiotherapy for localized intermediate- and high-grade non-Hodgkin's lymphoma. N Engl J Med 339:21–26, 1998.
6. Overgaard M, Hansen PS, Overgaard J, et al: Postoperative radiotherapy in high-risk premenopausal women with breast cancer who receive adjuvant chemotherapy. Danish Breast Cancer Cooperative Group 82b Trial. N Engl J Med 337:949–955, 1997.
7. The Department of Veterans Affairs Laryngeal Cancer Study Group: Induction chemotherapy plus radiation compared with surgery plus radiation in patients with advanced laryngeal cancer. N Engl J Med 324:1685–1690, 1991.

50. HYPERCALCEMIA OF MALIGNANCY

Andrew W. Steele, M.D., M.P.H., and Fred D. Hofeldt, M.D., FACP

1. What are the signs and symptoms of hypercalcemia?

They are frequently nonspecific but include irritability, confusion, weakness, fatigue, anorexia, nausea, vomiting, constipation, photophobia, and polyuria. The polyuria is caused by a hypercalcemia-induced nephrogenic diabetes insipidus. Severe hypercalcemia may be associated with central nervous system and cardiac depression with progressive stupor, coma, and shock. Hypercalcemia causes a shortening of the QT interval, a prolonged PR interval, T-wave changes on electrocardiography, and cardiac arrhythmias in some patients, especially if they are on digitalis. The hypercalcemic patient may manifest nephrolithiasis or nephrocalcinosis, peptic ulceration, or pancreatitis. As many as 1.5% of patients undergoing preventive care evaluations may be incidentally discovered to have a high serum calcium on routine chemistry panel. Among cancer patients the symptoms manifested can be influenced by age, sites of metastases, degree of hepatic or renal dysfunction, and the patient's performance status.

2. In a sick patient with a low albumin level, what is the correction for the serum calcium?
As a rule, approximately 45% of the measured serum calcium is protein-bound and 55% is diffusible. The protein-bound fraction is greatest for albumin compared with globulin. For a serum calcium of 10 mg/dl, approximately 0.8 mg/dl will be protein-bound to globulin and 3.7 mg/dl to albumin. For a low albumin state, the correction is that 1 gm of albumin will bind 0.8 mg of calcium.

For example: If the measured serum calcium is 7.6 mg/dl and albumin is 2.4 gm/dl, what is the corrected calcium? (Assume a normal serum albumin is 4.0 gm/dl.)

4.0	Normal albumin level
− 2.4	Patient albumin level
1.6	Difference
× 0.8	Amount calcium (mg) bound per gram of albumin
1.28	Add this to measured calcium to adjust for low albumin state
+ 7.6	
8.88	md/dl equals corrected calcium value

Hence, the calcium is adjusted into the normal range, 8.15–10.5 mg/dl (2.0–2.6 mmol/L), and is appropriately low for the level of hypoalbuminemia.

3. How is hypercalcemia evaluated when the serum albumin or total protein is elevated?

$$\text{Corrected serum calcium} = (\text{measured serum calcium}) \div \frac{(0.6 + \text{total serum protein})}{19.4}$$

4. What conditions cause hypercalcemia?
The following causes of hypercalcemia need to be considered in any patient with a bona fide elevation of serum calcium as documented on at least three repeat determinations:

Primary hyperparathyroidism
Sporadic (90–95% of all cases of hyperparathyroidism)
Familial syndromes (multiple endocrine neoplasia [MEN] types I and II)
MEN I (tumors of pituitary, pancreas, and parathyroid)
MEN IIa (medullary thyroid carcinoma, hyperparathyroidism, pheochromocytoma)
MEN IIb (medullary thyroid carcinoma, pheochromocytoma, mucosal neuromas, marfanoid habitus, and parathyroid hyperplasia)

Neoplastic diseases
Local osteolysis (breast and lung carcinoma metastatic to bone and myeloma)
Humoral hypercalcemia of malignancy

Endocrine disorders
Hyperthyroidism
Adrenal insufficiency
Benign familial hypocalciuric hypercalcemia (BFHH)

Medications
Thiazide diuretics
Vitamin D and rarely vitamin A intoxication
Mild-alkali syndrome
Lithium

Infectious diseases
Sarcoidosis
Berylliosis, tuberculosis, coccidioidomycosis, histoplasmosis
HIV infection

Miscellaneous
Immobilization (associated with high bone turnover rates, as in children or patients with Paget's disease)
Recovery phase of acute renal failure (rare)
Idiopathic hypercalcemia of infancy (rare)
Dehydration (due to hemoconcentration)

5. Which two medical conditions account for most cases of hypercalcemia?

Of the many causes of hypercalcemia listed above, the most common are malignancy (45%) and hyperparathyroidism (45%). The large differential diagnosis includes the other 10% of the causes of hypercalcemia. Hence, from a practical approach, the evaluation of hypercalcemic disorders can be broken down into two categories: parathyroid hormone (PTH)-mediated versus non–PTH-mediated hypercalcemia. Of note, hypercalcemia associated with malignancies is the most frequent cause of hypercalcemia among hospitalized patients.

6. What are the renal actions of PTH?

PTH has many actions on the renal proximal tubule. It causes increased renal loss of phosphate with phosphate wasting and hypophosphatemia. There is an increased tubular reabsorption of calcium. However, because the filtered load of calcium is high and the normal tubule reabsorption capacity of calcium is approximately 95% ± 2%, patients with hyperparathyroidism experience only mild hypercalciuria, whereas malignancy, in which PTH is suppressed, is associated with renal calcium wasting and urinary calciums as high as 400–600 mg/day.

Excessive PTH causes a type II renal tubular acidosis, which manifests as a hyperchloremic metabolic acidosis. PTH also stimulates renal gluconeogenesis and causes aminoaciduria. PTH acts as a trophic factor for renal 1α-hydroxylase regulation with generation of 1,25-dihydroxyvitamin D from its precursor 25-hydroxyvitamin D.

7. How does understanding these actions of PTH assist in distinguishing between hypercalcemia of malignancy and hyperparathyroidism?

Hypophosphatemia is seen in about 40–60% of patients with hyperparathyroidism, and its presentation varies considerably, depending on dietary phosphate intake. In patients with normal renal function, a chloride > 104 mmol/L suggests hyperparathyroidism, as does a serum bicarbonate in the mildly acidotic range. A chloride/phosphate ratio of > 33 suggests hyperparathyroidism. An elevated PTH is diagnostic. Today's generation of immunoradiometric (IRMA) and immunochemiluminometric PTH assays are highly specific for patients with primary hyperparathyroidism and in most cases enable differentiation from patients with non–PTH-mediated hypercalcemia, particularly those with malignancies. Three non-PTH causes of hypercalcemia can present with elevated PTH levels; lithium intake, BFHH, and, rarely, PTH-secreting ectopic tumors. The table below summarizes these differences.

PTH-mediated Hypercalcemia	*Non–PTH-mediated Hypercalcemia*
Laboratory values	
Low phosphate (< 2.4 mg/dl)	↓, normal, or ↑
High chloride (> 104 mEq/dl)	Chloride generally < 100 mEq/dl
Mild metabolic acidosis	Metabolic alkalosis
High Cl/PO$_4$ (> 33)	Low Cl/PO$_4$ (< 33)
High PTH	Low PTH
Specific disease	
Hyperparathyroidism*	Neoplasia with/without humoral hypercalcemia of malignancy
	Other non-PTH causes (see question 4)

• Remember BFHH.

8. Does a 24-hour urine calcium measurement help in evaluating a hypercalcemic patient?

Yes. Before establishing the diagnosis of hyperparathyroidism, it is important that BFHH be eliminated from consideration. This familial autosomal dominant condition has nearly complete penetrance and frequently affects family members with nonspecific symptoms, which may suggest a clinically significant disorder. However, when evaluated, they have a calcium/creatinine ratio of less than 0.01. These patients may have enlarged parathyroid glands due to increases in the amount of fat within the parathyroid glands. Parathyroidectomy does not cure the hypercalcemia. The calcium/creatinine ratio (Ca/Cr) is calculated as follows:

$$\text{Ca/Cr urine} = \frac{\text{Ca urine} \times \text{Cr plasma}}{\text{Cr urine} \times \text{Ca plasma*}}$$

* equals total calcium, not ionized fraction

A value > 0.1 is seen in other hypercalcemic disorders; a value < 0.01 is seen in BFHH.

9. Which malignancies are associated with hypercalcemia?

Hypercalcemia may occur in association with various malignancies with an incidence of 15–20 cases per 100,000 persons and life-long prevalence of 10–20% among cancer patients. It is highest in myeloma and breast cancer (40%) and slightly less common with other cancers such as squamous cell cancer of lung (25%) and adenocarcinomas of the kidney and pancreas. It also is seen with other hematologic malignancies such as lymphoma and adult T-cell acute leukemia. Other less commonly associated malignancies include islet cell carcinoma, pheochromocytoma, and squamous cell cancer of the esophagus, stomach, penis, parotid, and urothelium.

10. Discuss the mechanism for hypercalcemia in malignancy.

The malignant tumor may be primarily invasive in bone, which may locally activate bone reabsorption, or the tumor may be in a distal site from bone, with resorption stimulated by humoral substances that activate the osteoclast directly or indirectly. Immobilization may contribute to hypercalcemia. Many patients with cancer have bone involvement, but a minority develop hypercalcemia. Therefore, it is believed that the combination of bone invasion, humoral factors, and renal effects leads to hypercalcemia in such patients.

11. What are the mediators of humoral hypercalcemia of malignancy?

Tumors may produce cytokines (osteoclastic-activating factor), including interleukins, tumor necrosis factor, lymphotoxin, and colony-stimulating factor, or other humoral substances such as prostaglandins of the E series, 1,25-dihydroxyvitamin D, transforming growth factors, and the more recently described PTH-like or PTH-related peptide (PTHrP). 1,25-Dihydroxyvitamin D has been implicated in the hypercalcemia of melanoma, myeloma, and Hodgkin's and non-Hodgkin's lymphoma.

12. What is PTH-related peptide?

PTHrP was recently extracted and identified by complementary DNA probes and found to be produced by certain malignancies. PTHrP is encoded from genes that have been mapped to the short arms of chromosomes 11 and 12. PTHrP has been found in normal tissues such as brain, kidney, parathyroid, skin, atrium, uterus, and breast. These peptides are larger molecular species than PTH but retain homology to the PTH molecule, which allows it to imitate some of the actions of the parathyroid hormone, particularly activation of bone resorption, renal phosphate wasting, and generation of renal cyclic adenosine monophosphate. However, most often the Cl/PO_4 is < 33 in these malignancies.

13. What could be a mechanism of hypercalcemia in a patient with squamous cell carcinoma of the lung?

PTHrP has been identified and elevated serum values have been seen in hypercalcemic patients with squamous cell carcinoma of the lung. Similar PTHrP findings have been observed in patients with small-cell and anaplastic lung carcinoma, melanoma, prostate, and renal and breast carcinoma.

14. Is there a level of hypercalcemia that is considered critical?

Patients may manifest symptoms at variable levels of calcium. However, a serum calcium in excess of 14 mg/dl should be considered a critical value, and the patient should be treated under intensive monitoring. In this setting, hypercalcemic symptoms may include profound weakness, impaired mental function, nausea and vomiting, and central nervous system depression leading to stupor, lethargy, or coma.

15. What factors should be considered in deciding to treat on an inpatient vs. an outpatient basis?

In general, patients with serum calciums ≥ 12.0 mg/dl who have nausea or vomiting, dehydration, altered mental status, renal insufficiency, cardiac arrhythmias, ileus, or limited access to care or who live alone are best treated as inpatients.

16. What are the immediate therapeutic options to treat severe hypercalcemia?

Urgent Therapy of Hypercalcemia

Saline

Generally safe with 200–300 ml/hr but may need over 10 L/d with 20 mEq KCl/bottle (can follow NS:D5W); alternate 4:1 ratio with 20 mEq KCl bottle (can follow electrolytes and volume to document losses). May need 15 mg magnesium/hr.

Saline plus furosemide

Before using furosemide, be sure that the patient is adequately hydrated.

Aggressive management: 80–100 mg furosemide intravenously every 1–2 hr with close attention to fluid and electrolyte balance.

Less urgent management: 40 mg furosemide every 4–6 hr.

Intravenous biphosphonates

IV pamidronate (Aredia), 60–90 mg as single 4-hr (60 mg) or 24-hr (90 mg) infusion with adequate saline hydration. Allow minimum of 7 days to elapse before retreatment.

IV etidronate (Didronel) at dose of 7.5 mg/kg with 250 cc of saline over at least 2 hr and repeat daily for 3–7 days.

Calcitonin

4–8 IU subcutaneously every 6–12 hr.

Calcitonin plus glucocorticoids

4–8 IU/kg every 6–12 hr; prednisone, 40–60 mg/d for 3–5 days.

Gallium nitrate

Avoid use if creatinine > 2.5 mg/dl; give 100–200 mg/m^2 of body surface in 1,000 ml NS over 24 hr daily for 5 days.

Dialysis

Especially in patients with myeloma and marked renal insufficiency.

Intravenous phosphate

Caution: can cause hypertension. Avoid use if serum phosphate is elevated. Given as 1,000 mg elemental phosphate (0.16 mM/kg) over 8–12 hr during each 24-hr period.

Intravenous EDTA

Avoid use because of formation of insoluble calcium compounds that damage the kidney.

17. What are the options for management of chronic hypercalcemia of malignancy?

Chronic Therapy of Hypercalcemia*

Mobilization
Increased oral fluid intake
Oral phosphates

1,000–2,000 mg of elemental phosphate (start K-Phos, 3 tablets, 3 times daily).

Avoid use in patients with elevated serum phosphate or renal insufficiency.

Mithramycin

May also be used in semiacute situations, 25 µg/kg in 50 ml D5W given as infusion over 3 hr.

Glucocorticoids

Prednisone, 50–60 mg/day

Biphosphonates

Pamidronate (Aredia): 60–90 mg intravenously over 4–24 hr, once weekly to monthly.

Oral etidronate (Didronel): 5–20 mg/kg/day (not FDA-approved).

Oral alendronate (Fosamax): 10 mg/day (not FDA-approved).

Aspirin or indomethacin is probably ineffective.

• Adjust therapy in addition to treatment of primary cause.

18. Which patients may have a poor response to biphosphonates?

If the hypercalcemia is mediated by PTHrP, some of the biphosphonates (pamidronate and clodronate) do not seem to be as effective.

BIBLIOGRAPHY

1. Attie MF: Treatment of hypercalcemia. Endocrinol Metab Clin North Am 18:807, 1989.
2. Bilezician JP: Management of acute hypercalcemia. N Engl J Med 326:1196–1203, 1992.

3. Blind E, Schmidt-Gayk H, Scharla S, et al: Two-site assay of intact parathyroid hormone in the investigation of primary hyperparathyroidism and other disorders of calcium metabolism compared with a midregion assay. J Clin Endocrinol Metab 67:353, 1988.
4. Burtis WJ, Brady BS, Onloff JJ, et al: Immunochemical characterization of circulating parathyroid hormone-related peptide in patients with humoral hypercalcemia of cancer. N Engl J Med 322:1106–1112, 1990.
5. Chisholm MA, Mulloy AL, Taylor AT: Acute management of cancer-related hypercalcemia. Ann Pharmacother 30:507–513, 1996.
6. Danks JA, Ebeling PR, Hayman J, et al: Parathyroid hormone-related protein: Immunohistochemical localization in cancers and in normal skin. J Bone Miner Res 4:273, 1989.
7. DeVita VT, Hellman S, Rosenberg SA (eds): Cancer: Principles and Practice of Oncology, 5th ed. Philadelphia, J.B. Lippincott, 1997.
8. Henderson JE, Shustik C, Kremer R, et al: Circulating concentrations of parathyroid hormone-like peptide in malignancy and in hyperparathyroidism. J Bone Miner Res 5:105, 1990.
9. Licatta AA: Biphosphonate therapy. Am J Med Sci 313:17–22, 1997.
10. Nussbaum SR, Warrell RP, Rude R, et al: Dose-response study of alendronate sodium for the treatment of cancer-associated hypercalcemia. J Clin Oncol 11:1618–1623, 1993.

51. PARANEOPLASTIC NEUROLOGIC SYNDROMES

Bertrand C. Liang, M.D., and James P. Kelly, M.D.

1. What is the definition of paraneoplastic?

Paraneoplastic disturbances are remote effects of the neoplasm not related to direct invasion or compression from the tumor or to metastatic spread. Although paraneoplastic neurologic syndromes are the focus of this chapter, paraneoplasia may include hormonal, biochemical, or hematologic disturbances associated with malignancy.

2. What is the incidence of paraneoplastic syndromes?

In some reports, syndromes related to remote effects of cancer occur in as many as 10% of patients with tumors, but in other reports the incidence is 5–7%.

3. What type of cancer is most commonly associated with paraneoplastic syndromes?

Small-cell lung cancer accounts for the majority of cases, although breast and gynecologic cancers also are frequently capable of producing remote neurologic effects.

4. What are the typical neurologic features of paraneoplastic syndromes?

Virtually any level of the central and peripheral nervous systems can be affected, but cerebellar and neuropsychiatric features predominate. Common clinical presentations are agitation and confusion with memory dysfunction, ataxia, nystagmus or dysarthria, peripheral sensory loss, generalized weakness, and visual dysfunction. Neurologic paraneoplastic syndromes are frequently the most debilitating aspect of a cancer patient's disease process.

Clinical Presentations of Neurologic Syndromes

Limbic encephalitis	Peripheral neuropathy	Myasthenic syndromes
Brainstem encephalitis	• Sensory motor	Necrotizing myopathy
Cerebellar ataxia	• Motor	Visual loss/retinopathy
Myelitis	• Sensory neuropathy	Opsoclonus/myoclonus
	• Autonomic neuropathy	

5. What is the work-up for paraneoplastic syndromes?

Work-up includes a detailed history of what typically is a subacute onset of progressive dysfunction of the nervous system. Detailed examination of the affected central or peripheral nervous system offers information about the level of involvement. Neuroimaging, especially magnetic resonance imaging (MRI) scan, has been useful in detecting some evidence of inflammatory changes in the central nervous system. Analysis of spinal fluid by lumbar puncture is frequently useful and in most cases demonstrates a mononuclear pleocytosis, elevated immunoglobulin G (IgG) index, and oligoclonal bands. The diagnosis of paraneoplastic syndrome is *clinical*; thus a negative work-up does not rule out paraneoplastic syndrome. Serologic markers for cerebellar degeneration (anti-Purkinje cell or anti-Yo) and encephalopathy (anti-Hu or anti-Ri) are now commercially available; these markers are sensitive but not specific tests for paraneoplastic syndrome.

6. Does this syndrome ever precede other signs of cancer?

Yes. It is not uncommon for features of paraneoplastic syndrome to precede other symptoms of neoplasm by weeks to years. If paraneoplastic syndrome is suspected, a thorough work-up for any evidence of underlying cancer is warranted.

7. Can this problem be treated?

Most authors suggest that early detection and treatment of underlying cancer is the single best way to halt or even to reverse certain aspects of paraneoplastic syndrome. There have been reports of successful treatment with plasma exchange or immunosuppressive therapy, including cytotoxic agents or intravenous immunoglobulin. Unfortunately, in most cases, it is not possible to reverse the effects of paraneoplastic syndrome. All too often, the neurologic effects can be treated only symptomatically, despite association with relatively treatment-responsive tumors.

8. Is neuroimaging useful?

MRI scan is particularly useful in demonstrating abnormalities in the temporal lobes associated with limbic encephalitis. Otherwise, neuroimaging is of limited benefit.

9. Describe the difference between neurologic symptoms of a paraneoplastic syndrome and neurologic side effects of chemotherapy or radiation treatments.

This may be the most difficult clinical issue in any patient who already has been treated for cancer and exhibits cranial nerve damage, cerebellar ataxia, myelopathy, peripheral neuropathy, or even myopathy. Chemotherapy or radiation treatment is the more likely etiology if the agent or modality is known to cause the symptoms in question, because paraneoplastic syndrome is rare.

10. What other neurologic disorders must be considered in the differential diagnosis?

Other neurologic conditions associated with cancer include multiple cerebral infarctions, disseminated intravascular coagulation, nonbacterial thrombotic endocarditis that produces emboli, hemorrhage related to coagulopathy, and thrombocytopenia. On rare occasions, B-cell lymphoma produces encephalopathic changes through disseminated intravascular lymphomatosis.

11. Are there autonomic or endocrine features of paraneoplastic neurologic syndrome?

Yes. Various hypothalamic dysfunctions have been reported; the most common are orthostatic hypotension and syndrome of inappropriate secretion of antidiuretic hormone (SIADH).

12. What are the pathologic findings in paraneoplastic neurologic syndrome?

Neuronal loss
Perivascular mononuclear infiltrates
Demyelination and focal atrophy of the area of the nervous system involved.

CONTROVERSIES

13. Does the antibody marker cause paraneoplastic syndrome?

Although there is an association between the antibodies and the syndrome present, with the exception of the Lambert-Eaton syndrome, there is no direct evidence that the antibody produces the clinical syndrome.

14. Can paraneoplastic syndrome exist without associated malignancy?

For:

Virtually every type of neurologic paraneoplastic syndrome has been described in patients in whom no malignancy was detected on autopsy. Further studies may prove associations between other etiologic agents and so-called paraneoplastic findings, much as the true cause of progressive multifocal leukoencephalopathy (PML) was determined to be Jakob-Creutzfeldt (JC) virus rather than malignancy, as earlier thought.

Against:

The fact that no malignancy is detected at autopsy may reflect incomplete or flawed pathologic evaluation in these rare cases.

BIBLIOGRAPHY

1. Kalkman PH, Allen S, Birchall IWJ: Magnetic resonance imaging of limbic encephalitis. Can Assoc Radiol J 44:121–124, 1993.
2. Levin KH: Paraneoplastic neuromuscular syndromes. Neurol Clin 15:597–614, 1997.
3. Newman NJ, Bell IR, McKee AC: Paraneoplastic limbic encephalitis: Neuropsychiatric presentation. Soc Biol Psychiatry 27:529–542, 1990.
4. Peterson K, Rosenblum MK, Kotanides H, Posner JB: Paraneoplastic cerebellar degeneration. I. A clinical analysis of of 55 anti-Yo antibody-positive patients. Neurology 42:1931–1937, 1992.
5. Posner JB, Dalmau JO: Paraneoplastic syndromes affecting the central nervous system. Annu Rev Med 48:157–166, 1997.
6. Veilleux M, Bernier JP, Lamarche JB: Paraneoplastic encephalomyelitis subacute dysautonomia due to an occult atypical carcinoid tumor of the lung. Can J Neurol Sci 17:324–328, 1990.

52. ENDOCRINE PARANEOPLASTIC SYNDROMES

William J. Georgitis, M.D., FACP

1. Define endocrine paraneoplastic syndromes.

Syndromes are aggregates of signs and symptoms associated with any morbid process or disease. Endocrine paraneoplastic syndromes, also known as "ectopic" hormone syndromes, present with hormone-related manifestations, either remote or systemic, of a neoplasm not directly attributable to the physical effects of the primary tumor or its metastases. These manifestations may be systemic or affect an organ system not directly involved by the neoplasm.

2. Why is it important to recognize endocrine paraneoplastic syndromes?

Recognition may help direct the search for primary tumors. It could aid in the early detection of recurrence or even permit detection of an otherwise occult neoplasm.

3. What are some mechanisms for endocrine paraneoplastic syndromes?

Paraneoplastic syndromes usually result from circulating biologically active substances. Almost all of these substances are polypeptides. Tumor-associated peptides can be detected frequently in many types of malignancy, but clinical manifestations from those tumor products are relatively uncommon. This is in part due to the fact that not all immunoassayable peptides are biologically active. There are two major pathogenic paradigms for production of these substances by a tumor—random genetic "derepression" and "endocrine-cell" theory. The derepression model refers to genetic transformations occurring in neoplastic cells that release structural genes from normal inhibition. The resulting enhanced production of enzymes, intact hormones, or hormonally active polypeptides may then cause clinically evident paraneoplastic syndromes. The "endocrine-cell" theory explains the excess production of tumor products based on an abnormal proliferation of endocrine cells normally present in the tissue of origin. For example, diarrhea is seen with medullary carcinoma of the thyroid still confined to the thyroid.

4. Does a paraneoplastic syndrome always mean the tumor is malignant?

Not always. Oncogenic osteomalacia, a rare syndrome with bone pain, muscle weakness, and radiologic features of osteomalacia, has been cured by removal of benign mesenchymal tumors. On the other hand, oncogenic osteomalacia has been associated with prostate cancer and squamous cell lung cancer.

5. Does the resolution of paraneoplastic syndrome after tumor removal indicate cure?

Sometimes not. Paraneoplastic symptoms and signs may resolve when the concentrations of substances causing the paraneoplastic findings fall below a threshold level sufficient to create the syndrome. Recurrence of the tumor may cause hormone levels to rise again above the clinical detection threshold, causing the syndrome to reappear and indicating that a cure was not achieved.

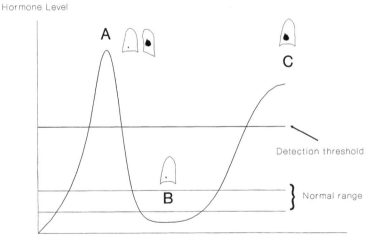

Time Course of Neoplasm

An endocrine paraneoplastic syndrome is evident when a tumor produces enough biologically active hormone to cause clinical signs and symptoms *(A)*. Resolution of the syndrome may occur when therapy for the malignancy reduces hormone levels below the detection threshold *(B)* but does not always indicate a cure. The paraneoplastic syndrome may reappear when hormone levels again rise with tumor recurrence *(C)*.

6. Are there effective treatments to palliate paraneoplastic syndromes?

Yes. Since the symptoms and signs result from excesses of biologically active substances, treatments directed at decreasing production, removal, or blocking the action of these humoral factors can benefit the patient in terms of improved quality of life. Effective treatment modalities sometimes include surgery, radiation therapy, medications, and plasmapheresis.

7. Which endocrine paraneoplastic syndrome was first reported?

In 1928, W.H. Brown reported Cushing's syndrome in a paper entitled "A case of pluriglandular syndrome: Diabetes of bearded women." The patient had a small-cell lung cancer and undoubtedly suffered from ectopic production of adrenocorticotropic hormone (ACTH). In addition to the proopiomelanocortin-derived ACTH molecule, small-cell carcinoma can also produce a variety of hormonally active peptides. For example, small-cell lung cancer can cause hyponatremia due to inappropriate antidiuretic hormone secretion or gynecomastia from chorionic gonadotropin. About half of ectopic ACTH cases result from small-cell lung cancers. Other tumors presenting with Cushing's syndrome include pheochromocytoma, thymoma, medullary thyroid carcinoma, and carcinoid tumors.

8. Can ectopically produced parathyroid hormone (PTH) cause hypercalcemia?

In contrast to what was believed several decades ago before assays and molecular biologic techniques became more refined, PTH is rarely produced ectopically. An elevated level of PTH is almost always diagnostic of primary hyperparathyroidism, a common outpatient diagnosis in middle-aged, asymptomatic hypercalcemic patients. With humoral hypercalcemia of malignancy a suppressed PTH level is expected. There are a few convincing case reports in the literature of hypercalcemia from ectopic PTH production by malignancies.

Hypercalcemia in patients with cancer without bony metastases is often due to humoral substances with parathyroidlike actions. These substances, designated as PTH-like, share sequence homology with PTH. Biologic effects, including hypercalcemia, hypophosphatemia, and phosphaturia, result from activation of PTH receptors. A variety of tumor types, including renal, bladder, adenocarcinomas, lymphomas, and squamous cell lung, head, and neck cancers, can impersonate hyperparathyroidism by producing PTH-like peptides.

9. Which tumors are associated with erythrocytosis?

Erythrocytosis is seen in approximately 50% of renal carcinomas, 20% of cerebellar hemangioblastomas, and 15% of benign renal cysts and adenomas. It has also been reported in association with a variety of other neoplasms, including hepatomas, uterine fibroids, virilizing ovarian tumors, lung cancers, thymomas, pheochromocytomas, paragangliomas, and parotid fibrous histiocytomas. Excess erythropoietin is often the cause. The kidney, in the adult, and the liver, in the fetus, make erythropoietin, thus explaining the major association of erythrocytosis with renal and hepatic neoplasms.

10. Can signs of an endocrine paraneoplastic syndrome be seen in the skin?

Yes. Hyperpigmentation can result from excess production of peptides with the melanocyte-stimulating hormone sequence, including ACTH and lipotropin. Hirsutism in women, usually severe with masculinization due to male-range testosterone levels, can result from excessive androgen production of adrenal or ovarian tumor origin. Excess glucagon from islet cell glucagonomas in the distal pancreas has been associated with a curious polymorphous, often evanescent rash termed necrolytic migratory erythema. Glossitis, dystrophic nails, anemia, diabetes, and weight loss are additional features of this often slowly developing syndrome.

11. Can hyperthyroidism result from a paraneoplastic mechanism?

Yes. Human chorionic gonadotropin (hCG) has sufficient sequence homology in its beta-chain with thyroid-stimulating hormone (TSH) to cause excess thyroid hormone production by stimulating the thyrotropin receptor—a form of cross-activation or "specificity spillover at the hormone receptor." Sensitive assays for TSH performed in women without thyroid disease have shown that hCG secreted by the placenta stimulates thyroid hormone production during pregnancy. Levels of hCG must be very high to cause overt thyrotoxicosis. Thyroxine levels correlate with the very high hCG levels from trophoblastic tumors, including choriocarcinoma and hydatiform moles in women. Rare cases of hyperthyroidism in men with testicular trophoblastic tumors or choriocarcinoma have been reported.

12. Does acromegaly often result from growth hormone-releasing hormone (GHRH)?

Very rarely. Nonpituitary tumors can produce acromegaly and pituitary somatrotroph hyperplasia by elaborating GHRH. As a rule, acromegaly is caused by growth hormone from large pituitary adenomas. Tumors reported to produce GHRH include carcinoids, pancreatic islet cell neoplasms, gastric, breast, and ovarian carcinomas. In fact, the 44-amino acid sequence of GHRH was characterized from extracts of tumors from patients with GHRH-dependent acromegalic syndrome. A study screening for excess serum GHRH levels in 177 asymptomatic patients failed to detect a single case, implying that ectopic GHRH production must be a rare cause of acromegaly.

13. Have other hypothalamic peptides been produced by tumors?

Yes. Corticotropin-releasing hormone (CRH), in association with ectopic ACTH, and somatostatin have been found in nonpituitary tumors. Thyroid-releasing hormone (TRH) and luteinizing hormone-releasing hormone (LHRH) have not yet been reported.

14. What is the most common ectopic hormone produced?

ACTH.

15. Is ectopic ACTH easily recognized?

Sometimes yes. A patient presenting with a pulmonary mass, hyperpigmentation, hypokalemia, weight loss, and muscle weakness should readily have the diagnosis of ectopic ACTH-induced Cushing's syndrome confirmed with appropriately elevated ACTH and cortisol levels.

Sometimes no. Ectopic ACTH can be notoriously difficult to distinguish from ACTH-producing pituitary adenomas causing Cushing's syndrome (Cushing's disease). Plasma ACTH levels can be normal or only mildly elevated in both. In cases of ectopic ACTH from carcinoid tumors and bronchial adenomas, cortisol may suppress with high-dose dexamethasone, the expected response for pituitary-dependent Cushing's syndrome. Simultaneous sampling for plasma ACTH from peripheral and petrosal veins draining the pituitary separates ectopic from eutopic ACTH but requires skillful specialists to perform the procedure and is not appropriate for every case.

16. What hormones and resulting signs and symptoms may be associated with pancreatic islet cell tumor?

There are five islet cell tumor types and etiologic hormones.

Islet Cell Tumor Syndromes

TUMOR	HORMONE	EPONYM	MANIFESTATIONS
Insulinoma	Insulin		Hypoglycemia
Gastrinoma	Gastrin	Zollinger-Ellison syndrome	Hyperacidity, peptic ulcers
VIPoma	Vasoactive intestinal polypeptide (VIP)	Werner-Morrison syndrome	Diarrhea
Glucagonoma	Glucagon		Rash, diarrhea, anemia, glucose intolerance
Somatostatinoma	Somatostatin		Abdominal pain, diarrhea, weight loss, hyperemia, gallbladder disease

BIBLIOGRAPHY

1. Doppman JL, Nieman LK, Cutler GB, et al: Adrenocorticotropic hormone-secreting islet cell tumors: Are they always malignant? Radiology 190:39, 1994.
2. Ezzat S, Asa SL, Stefaneanu L, et al: Somatotroph hyperplasia without pituitary adenoma associated with a long-standing growth hormone-releasing hormone-producing bronchial carcinoid. J Clin Endocrinol Metab 78:555, 1994.
3. Fradkin JE, Eastman RC, Lesniak MA, et al: Specificity spillover at the hormone receptor—Exploring its role in human disease. N Engl J Med 320:640, 1989.

4. Marino MT, Asp AA, Budayer AA, et al: Hypercalcemia and elevated levels of parathyroid hormone-related peptide in cutaneous squamous/basal cell carcinoma. J Intern Med 233:205, 1993.
5. Odell W, Wolfsen A, Yoshimoto Y, et al: Ectopic peptide synthesis: A universal concomitant of neoplasia. Trans Assoc Am Physicians 90:204, 1977.
6. Patel AM, Peters SG: Paraneoplastic syndromes associated with lung cancer. Mayo Clin Proc 6:278, 1993.
7. Raff H, Shaker JL, Seifert PE, et al: Intraoperative measurement of adrenocorticotropin (ACTH) during removal of ACTH-secreting bronchial carcinoid tumors. J Clin Endocrinol Metab 80:1036, 1995.
8. Wallace PM, Flannery MT, Stewart JM: Paraneoplastic syndromes for the primary care physician. Prim Care 19:727, 1992.
9. Wilkins GE, Granleese S, Hegele RC, et al: Oncogenic osteomalacia: Evidence for a humoral phosphaturic factor. J Clin Endocrinol Metab 80:1628, 1995.
10. Zieger MA, Pass HI, Doppman JD, et al: Surgical strategy in the management of non–small-cell ectopic adrenocorticotropic hormone syndrome. Surgery 112:994, 1992.

53. SPINAL CORD COMPRESSION

Alice M. Luknic, M.D.

1. Why is it important to recognize spinal cord compression?

Spinal cord compression is one of the true emergencies encountered in oncology. However, all physicians need to be aware of this emergency because 10–40% of patients who present with acute spinal cord compression have cancer but are not yet diagnosed. Without urgent evaluation, permanent paralysis and incontinence may occur. A delay of even one day may have devastating consequences.

2. What are the symptoms of spinal cord compression?

Back pain that gets worse with lying down is a hallmark symptom. Ninety-five percent of patients present with back pain first. It often is worse with a Valsalva maneuver or coughing. Pain may be localized to the back or be radicular in nature. Weakness or sensory loss generally follows the onset of back pain and may progress very rapidly to complete paralysis. Changes in bowel or bladder function are usually late findings and portend a poor prognosis.

3. Describe possible physical exam findings.

Pain is generally located directly over the vertebral body affected. Percussion in the area generally elicits tenderness. Careful neurologic evaluation to assess for weakness, sensory loss, loss of deep tendon reflexes, and loss of sphincter tone should be performed. If any such signs are found, evaluation and treatment should be pursued emergently.

4. Which studies should be ordered to confirm spinal cord compression?

Magnetic resonance imaging (MRI) is the imaging study of choice. It best images the spinal cord and assesses the extent of tumor, and should be ordered emergently with gadolinium contrast.

If MRI is not available, CT myelogram using contrast medium in the subarachnoid space can assess whether spinal cord compression is present. This study is more invasive and does not yield as much information as MRI scan.

Plain spine radiographs are abnormal in at least two-thirds of patients with spinal cord compression. They are 85% accurate in predicting the presence or absence of epidural metastases. However, normal films do not exclude the possibility of spinal cord compression. Bone scans are more sensitive than plain films in detecting spine metastases. However, they cannot confirm whether compression is present.

5. Which tumors are more likely to cause spinal cord compression?

More than 50% of all cases are accounted for by prostate cancer, breast cancer, and lung cancer. Other tumors associated with spinal cord compression include lymphoma, melanoma, renal cell cancer, sarcoma, and multiple myeloma. In children, sarcoma, neuroblastoma, and lymphoma are the most common.

6. What should be done before performing radiologic studies or beginning treatment?

Steroids should be prescribed. Steroids reduce surrounding edema, and dramatic improvement of symptoms may occur within hours. Dexamethasone is generally used, in doses of 10–100 mg IV initially, followed by 4–24 mg every 6 hours intravenously or orally. Whether the higher doses are better is unknown, and generally they are reserved for patients with severe or rapidly deteriorating symptoms. Steroids should be tapered once therapy begins. Long-term side effects are significant, and steroid-induced proximal myopathy may be particularly troublesome in patients who already have some weakness.

7. What are the treatment options for patients with spinal cord compression?

Emergent radiation therapy is the mainstay of therapy. It can provide rapid relief for most patients. Surgery with decompressive laminectomy has been shown to be no better in most instances than radiation, and the morbidity of surgery is sizeable. Surgery is usually reserved for patients who fail to respond to, or relapse after, radiotherapy. Chemotherapy is used occasionally in patients with drug-sensitive tumors, such as high-grade lymphomas. Children with Ewing's sarcoma or neuroblastoma also may be treated with chemotherapy.

8. Can the outcome following treatment for spinal cord compression be predicted?

The most valuable prognostic factor predicting outcome is the patient's neurologic status at the time he or she presents. Almost all patients who are ambulatory at presentation remain ambulatory. However, only 25% of patients who are nonambulatory regain the ability to walk. Fewer than 10% of paraplegic patients will walk again after therapy. Recognizing spinal cord compression while a patient is still ambulatory is very important.

9. What is the goal of treatment?

The goal of therapy in patients with spinal cord compression is to maintain ambulation and to prevent loss of bowel or bladder function. Treatment of an epidural metastasis will not treat the underlying malignancy, but should be pursued even if the tumor is incurable. Maintaining a patient's ambulatory status and freedom from dependence on Foley catheter, for example, is an important quality-of-life issue. In addition, radiation therapy can greatly alleviate pain. Treatment of the underlying malignancy may be tailored based on the patient and his or her tumor type.

BIBLIOGRAPHY

1. Byrne TN: Spinal cord compression from epidural metastases. N Engl J Med 327:614–619, 1992.
2. Grant R, Papadopoulos SM, Greenberg HS: Metastatic epidural spinal cord compression. Neurol Clin 9:825–841, 1991.
3. Loblaw D, Laperriere N: Emergency treatment of malignant extradural spinal cord compression: An evidence-based guideline. J Clin Oncol 16:1613–1624, 1998.

54. SUPERIOR VENA CAVA SYNDROME

Alice M. Luknic, M.D.

1. What is superior vena cava (SVC) syndrome?

Superior vena cava syndrome results when blood flow is obstructed in the superior vena cava, which may result from thrombosis within the vessel or from compression of the vein externally. External compression can lead to thrombosis within the vessel, so a combination of the two processes may occur. The superior vena cava runs through the middle mediastinum in a narrow space surrounded by the trachea, aorta, right main stem bronchus, pulmonary artery, sternum, and many lymph nodes. Enlargement of any of these structures can compress the vein and result in SVC syndrome.

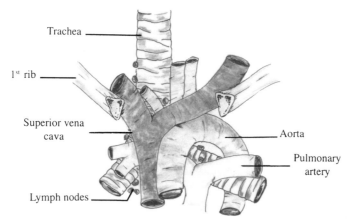

Diagram of superior vena cava anatomy.

2. What are the symptoms of SVC syndrome?

Patients usually complain of dyspnea, facial puffiness, a sense of fullness in the head, and often a cough. They may complain of edema in the arm or a dusky complexion. Symptoms often evolve slowly.

3. What are the usual physical findings in the patient with SVC syndrome?

The superior vena cava drains the head, neck, arms, and upper thorax. Two-thirds of patients with SVC syndrome have engorgement of the neck veins and of the veins over the chest wall, representing collateral circulation; half of patient have facial edema; and one-fourth have plethora and peripheral cyanosis. Upper extremity edema is not uncommon.

4. Is SVC syndrome truly an "oncologic emergency"?

SVC syndrome is rarely life-threatening. Although patients may present with impressive upper body edema, including the head, only rarely do such symptoms progress to laryngeal edema, seizures, coma, or death. Unless tracheal obstruction is impending, it is generally safe and prudent to establish the diagnosis before embarking on empiric treatment.

5. What are the chances that a patient with SVC syndrome has cancer? Which tumors are most common?

Approximately 80% of patients with SVC syndrome have an underlying malignancy, and 80% of these have lung cancer, most frequently small cell lung cancer. Non-Hodgkin's lymphoma comprises 13% of patients. Hodgkin's disease, germ cell tumors, and other mediastinal malignancies are less common.

6. Name some "benign" causes of SVC syndrome.

Currently, most benign causes are due to thrombosis as a sequela of central venous catheters or pacemakers. Mediastinal fibrosis from infection, sarcoidosis, benign tumors, and inflammatory diseases account for most of the remaining benign cases. In the 1950s tuberculosis and syphilitic aneurysms of the aorta were more common causes for SVC syndrome than they are today.

7. How should one proceed with establishing a diagnosis in a patient with SVC syndrome?

Evaluation should be pursued urgently. Chest x-ray can be obtained quickly and will show a mass in 80% of patients. Computed tomographic (CT) scanning better defines the anatomy of the region. Sputum cytology is noninvasive and often can yield the diagnosis of lung cancer. A thorough examination for lymphadenopathy should be performed before embarking on more invasive diagnostic procedures. Even in the presence of SVC syndrome, bronchoscopy and thoracotomy are generally safe.

8. How are patients with SVC syndrome managed?

Patients with small cell lung cancer, high-grade lymphoma, or germ cell tumors respond quickly to chemotherapy, making the knowledge of tumor type important. Emergency radiotherapy should be given only if symptoms are rapidly progressive and a tissue diagnosis cannot be made. In the setting of lymphoma, radiation may make it impossible to characterize the tumor, hindering definitive therapy. Non-small cell lung cancer patients generally are offered radiation therapy with or without chemotherapy. Patients with central venous catheters or pacemakers and thrombosis are treated with anticoagulation. Thrombolytic therapy should be reserved for patients without brain metastases.

BIBLIOGRAPHY

1. Abner A: Approach to the patient who presents with superior vena cava obstruction Chest 103:3945, 1993.
2. Adelstein DJ, Hinez JD, Carter SG, Sacco D: Thromboembolic events in patients with malignant superior vena cava syndrome and the role of anticoagulation. Cancer 62:2258, 1988.
3. Ahmamm FR: A reassessment of the clinical implications of the superior vena cava syndrome. J Clin Oncol 2:961, 1984.
4. Armstrong BA, Perez CA, Simpson JR, Hederman MA: Role of irradiation in the management of superior vena cava syndrome. Int J Radiat Oncol Biol Phys 13:531, 1987.

55. NEUTROPENIC FEVER

Miho Toi Scott, M.D., George R. Simon, M.D., and Madeleine A. Kane, M.D., Ph.D.

1. What is neutropenia?

Neutropenia is defined as a decrease in the absolute number of circulating terminally differentiated neutrophils. In Caucasians, the lower limit of normal for the absolute neutrophil count (ANC) is approximately 1800/μl; for African Americans, the lower limit for a normal ANC is approximately 1400/μl. Clinically significant neutropenia occurs with ANC < 1000 μl; with ANC < 500 μl, the risk of development of serious bacterial infection is very high.

2. What is neutropenic fever?

Neutropenic fever is defined as an oral temperature of 38° C twice or 38.5° C or more once in 24 hours in a person with an ANC < 1000/μl.

3. What is the clinical significance of neutropenic fever?

Neutropenic fever is considered a potentially life-threatening emergency. In the absence of sufficient neutrophils, overwhelming bacterial sepsis may develop rapidly. Unless diagnosed and treated immediately, a patient may die from systemic bacterial infection in less than 24 hours.

4. How should a patient who presents with neutropenic fever be evaluated?

The evaluating clinician must consider the possibility of neutropenia in all febrile patients because it poses a life-threatening emergency. A rapid but careful history to identify possible predisposing factors for neutropenia and symptoms suggesting an infectious source and thorough physical examination are essential. If suspicion of neutropenia is high on the basis of initial clinical impression, cultures should be obtained as part of the initial evaluation and empiric parenteral broad-spectrum antibiotics should be initiated. Historical clues include recent causative drugs such as chemotherapy, known diagnoses predisposing to neutropenia, toxic exposures to chemicals or radiation, or previous history of neutropenia. Physical examination should systematically address common sites of infection such as the pharynx, middle ears, lungs, abdomen, indwelling catheters, sinuses, periodontium, perineum, skin lesions, fingernails, and sites of recent procedures such as bone marrow biopsies. Multiple bacterial and fungal cultures must be obtained quickly before initiation of antibiotics.

Testing should include complete blood count, electrolytes, glucose, creatinine, liver function tests (including transaminases), alkaline phosphatase, lactate dehydrogenase, and total bilirubin. Imaging studies are essential and at minimum include chest radiograph. Depending on symptoms and clinical impression, sinus radiographs, head CT or MRI, abdominal or pelvic radiographs, ultrasound and/or CT may be indicated. In special situations, nuclear medicine studies such as gallium scan or bone scan may be useful. Echocardiography may be of use if endocarditis is suspected.

5. What cultures should be obtained from a patient with neutropenic fever?

At a minimum, blood, urine, throat, and sputum cultures should be obtained. At least two blood cultures must be obtained from separate sites, either two peripheral veins or one peripheral site and one culture from each lumen of an indwelling intravenous catheter. Sputum Gram stain and microscopic urinalysis may be helpful, but the lab must be alerted that a neutropenic patient may not exhibit the presence of the usual numbers of neutrophils even if these fluids are the site of infection. Throat swab and culture of the anterior nares, rectal area, and suspicious skin lesions should be performed; a lumbar puncture also should be done if the patient has altered mental status and/or meningismus. Cerebrospinal fluid must be Gram-stained, cultured for bacteria (including acid-fast bacilli), and assessed for glucose and protein. Pleocytosis may be absent in neutropenic patients with meningitis, but glucose level may be low and protein may be elevated. Diarrheal stools should be tested for *Clostridium difficile* toxin, enteric bacterial pathogens, protozoans, and possibly viruses. Fecal leukocytes may be absent in the presence of infection in neutropenic patients. Any other accessible suspicious sites of potential infection should be aspirated or biopsied and sent for stains and cultures.

6. What are the most likely causative organisms of neutropenic fever?

Most commonly, initial infections are caused by endogenous flora, but organisms are cultured in only about 50% of cases. Gram-negative and gram-positive bacteria are the most common isolates. Eighty-five percent of isolates are *Pseudomonas* spp., staphyloccoci, *Escherichia coli*, or *Klebsiella* spp. Other bacteria not infrequently cultured include group D streptococci (e.g., *S. faecalis*), alpha-hemolytic streptococci (e.g., *S. mutans* or *S. viridans*), anaerobic bacteria (e.g., *Bacteroides fragilis*, *Clostridium* spp.), and mycobacteria. *Candida* spp. are isolated in 5% of cases, and anaerobes and viruses are rarely identified. Subsequently, patients who require prolonged courses of broad-spectrum antibiotics may acquire antibiotic-resistant bacteria, filamentous fungi, and/or yeast. Cultures of the anterior nares may isolate *Staphylococcus aureus* or *Aspergillus* spp. Rectal cultures may isolate *Pseudomonas aeruginosa*, multiple drug-resistant gram-negative bacilli, *Candida* spp., or *Salmonella* spp.

7. **What are the disease-related causes of neutropenia?**

Both benign and malignant conditions may cause neutropenia:

Infections. Acute infections, such as gram-negative bacteria or viruses, can cause transient, sometimes severe, neutropenia. Persistent agranulocytosis may accompany some chronic infections, such as mycobacterial or fungal infections.

Autoimmune disorders. Neutropenia may be caused by immune destruction of neutrophils and sometimes myeloid precursors as well. Usually patients present with mild neutropenia, and no treatment is required. Examples of such disorders include polymyositis, systemic lupus erythematosus, and Felty's syndrome (rheumatoid arthritis, neutropenia, and splenomegaly).

Splenomegaly. Sequestration of neutrophils in an enlarged spleen from any cause may result in neutropenia. Examples include chronic liver disease causing congestive splenomegaly, Gaucher's disease, myeloid metaplasia, and idiopathic splenomegaly.

Chronic idiopathic neutropenia. Patients present with ANC 1000–2000/µl or less. Bone marrow biopsies often reveal many early myeloid precursors but reduced numbers of late metamyelocytes and mature granulocytes. The clinical course may be asymptomatic even with ANC approaching zero, or symptomatic with recurrent pyoderma (*S. aureus*, *E. coli*) and otitis media (pneumococci or *P. aeruginosa*) in children. This condition is more common in females. African Americans also may have a lower ANC than Caucasians, but the neutropenia is usually modest and not clinically significant.

Chronic cyclic neutropenia. Neutrophil counts oscillate, with nadirs at approximately 3-week intervals. At the nadir the ANC often drops to < 100/µl. Although life-threatening complications are rare, fevers, buccal, labial, or lingual ulcers, cervical adenopathy, carbuncles, cellulitis, infected cuts with lymphangitis, chronic gingivitis, and abscesses of the axillae or groin are common.

Nutritional deficiencies. Folic acid, vitamin B_{12}, and severe iron or copper deficiencies may cause suppressed or ineffective granulopoiesis. Neutropenia also may occur with starvation. Correction of the nutritional deficiency corrects the neutropenia.

Hematologic malignancies. Lymphomas, acute and chronic leukemias, multiple myeloma, hairy cell leukemia, myelodysplastic syndromes, and aplastic anemia may be accompanied by neutropenia. Granulopoiesis is suppressed by abnormal immune function or marrow infiltration with malignant cells.

Solid tumors. Neutropenia may occur secondary to marrow infiltration with metastatic solid tumors. Lung cancer, especially small-cell or oat cell lung cancer, prostate cancer, and breast cancer are the malignancies most commonly associated with neutropenia.

8. **What are the treatment-related causes of neutropenia?**

Medications may cause idiosyncratic or predictable neutropenia. Biologic response modifiers such as the interferons also cause predictable neutropenia, as does radiation therapy. Treatment with systemic radioactive isotopes, such as 89-strontium for bone metastases also may cause persistent neutropenia. Fatal cases of idiosyncratic agranulocytosis have been reported with various medications. Withdrawal of the causative agent usually results in normalization of granulocyte counts 7–14 days later. Common offending agents include:

Sulfonamides (trimethoprim-sulfamethoxazole)	Acetaminophen
Penicillins	Gold
Antithyroid drugs	Levamisole
Anticonvulsants (phenytoin, carbamazepine)	Penicillamine
Antipsychotics (clozapine)	Barbiturates
Procainamide	Benzodiazepines
Phenothiazines	Azidothymidine (AZT)
Aspirin	Ganciclovir

Most cancer chemotherapy drugs predictably cause neutropenia. For most chemotherapy drugs, the neutrophil nadir can be expected 7–10 days after treatment; counts should recover within 3–4 days. Examples include anthracyclines, such as adriamycin; alkylating agents, such as cyclophosphamide and nitrogen mustard; etoposide; taxol; and the vinca alkaloids, vinblastine and vinolrelbine. Nadirs may occur at 4–6 weeks after treatment with several other alkylating agents, including the nitrosoureas BCNU and CCNU, mitomycin-C, and melphalan. Prolonged and severe therapy-related neutropenia occurs in acute leukemias, in which the goal of treatment is to effect bone marrow hypoplasia to eradicate leukemia with the anticipation that normal stem cells will survive and eventually repopulate the marrow with normal cells. Nadirs may last several weeks after induction chemotherapy for acute leukemia. Hydroxyurea produces a much more rapid fall in neutrophils and malignant precursors, with count drops often observed in 12–24 hours with sufficient doses. Hydroxyurea is used for rapid lowering of extremely elevated WBCs in patients with leukemia.

Treatment with radiation therapy, especially together with chemotherapy, also may contribute to neutropenia. Biologic response modifiers, such as interferons and interleukins, also produce neutropenia in some patients.

9. How do you determine the cause of neutropenia?

Careful review of the current and recent medication history must be obtained. History and physical examination suggestive of infection or malignancy may help to determine the cause. Complete blood count, including platelets, and examination of the peripheral smear are mandatory. Bone marrow biopsy is likely to be helpful. Nutritional deficiency states can be evaluated by measuring folate, B_{12}, and iron in the blood, if suggested by the history and blood counts. Other potentially useful studies include antineutrophil antibodies, antinuclear antibodies with titer, quantitative immunoglobulins, and antiviral antibodies.

10. Discuss the potential complications of neutropenia.

Severe neutropenia ($< 500/\mu l$) predisposes to rapidly progressive, life-threatening bacterial infections. The clinical presentation may be misleading because the usual signs of inflammatory response may be blunted by the lack of neutrophils. Neutropenic patients form less pus, lack signs of pneumonic consolidation on physical exam and chest radiograph, and are less likely to present with exudate, swelling, heat, and regional adenopathy. Careful and frequent evaluations are needed for febrile neutropenic patients. The most likely routes of infection are the gastrointestinal tract and sites of invasive procedures (e.g., vascular access devices, bone marrow biopsy sites).

11. How should a patient with neutropenic fever be treated?

The key to successful life-saving therapy is immediate recognition of the clinical situation with rapid obtainment of appropriate cultures and immediate initiation of broad-spectrum empiric antibacterial therapy. Neutropenic precautions include a private room, scrupulous handwashing, and avoidance of fresh fruits, vegetables, and plants in the room until neutrophils recover. Persons with colds or other infections should avoid contact with neutropenic patients. The patient should wear a mask and possibly gown and gloves when leaving the hospital room.

Empiric antibiotic therapy usually includes more than one drug, but monotherapy with third-generation cephalosporins, carbapenam, or quinolones also has its advocates. The most common combination has been an aminoglycoside (gentamicin, tobramycin, or amikacin) with an antipseudomonal beta-lactam (e.g., ticarcillin, azlocillin, mezlocillin, piperacillin) or a third-generation cephalosporin (e.g., cefoperazone, ceftazidime). Quinolones may be substituted for aminoglycosides, especially in patients with tenuous renal function. If infection from an indwelling catheter is suspected, vancomycin should be added to cover methicillin-resistant staphylococci; usually the catheter can be preserved. In selected patients, outpatient antibiotic therapy is effective.

Antibiotic coverage should be adjusted based on the results of cultures and the sensitivities of identified culprit organisms. If new signs and symptoms of inflammation emerge during the initial course of antibiotics and/or fever persists, antibiotics should be changed and new ones possibly added. New abdominal pain or pulmonary abscess may prompt addition of anaerobe coverage. Changes are also necessary if unacceptable side effects such as drug rash or renal failure occur.

For patients with central venous catheters, indications for removal are tunnel infection, septic emboli, and nonpatent catheter. Removal also should be considered with certain types of infections, such as *Bacillus* spp., *Corynebacterium* spp. or the JK group, or *Candida* spp. because these microbes respond poorly to antibiotics.

In patients who become afebrile within the first three days of treatment, antibiotics should be continued (1) until cultures become negative, (2) until all sites of infection have resolved, (3) until all signs and symptoms of infection have resolved, (4) until neutrophils recover, and (5) for a minimum of 7 days if blood cultures are positive. If neutropenia is prolonged, discontinuation of antibiotics may be considered when (1) there is no fever for at least 7 days and antibiotics have been administered for 14 days; (2) all signs and symptoms of infection have resolved; and (3) mucositis is not present and skin remains intact. Such patients must be monitored closely for recurrence of signs and symptoms of infection, at which time new cultures should be rapidly obtained and empiric antibiotics restarted immediately.

Antiviral therapy should be started in patients with skin or mucous membrane lesions caused by herpes simplex or varicella zoster. Afebrile patients should be treated for positive viral cultures.

Prophylactic antibiotics are sometimes administered to patients who are expected to have a neutropenic nadir that will last only for a few days. Both sulfa combinations and quinolones have been used, but this is not standard practice. There is no role for granulocyte transfusions in the treatment of neutropenic fever.

12. What do you do if the fever persists despite appropriate broad-spectrum antibiotic coverage and the patient remains neutropenic?

Careful reassessment is needed when fever persists in neutropenic patients for 3 days despite empiric antibiotics. Occult sites of infection (e.g., sinuses, oral cavity and gums, perianal area) need to be reevaluated. Appropriate cultures need to be repeated, with identified causative organisms and their drug sensitivities reviewed. The possibility of inadequate serum or tissue antibiotic levels needs to be entertained. If the patient appears toxic and no new causative organism can be determined, empiric antifungal therapy needs to be initiated after 3–4 days, especially in patients in whom a prolonged nadir is expected, such as acute leukemics.

13. What should be done if the neutropenia resolves (ANC > 500/µl for 2 days) but the fever persists despite broad-spectrum antibiotics?

Discontinuation of antibiotics should be strongly considered unless the patient is clinically unstable or bacteremia was documented but antibiotics have been administered for less than 7 days. Cultures need to be repeated as part of a complete reevaluation, and antibiotics should be restarted based on culture results or clinical deterioration. Drug fever, which resolves with discontinuation of therapy, also needs to be considered.

14. What growth factors may be used to treat neutropenia?

Lineage-specific growth factors are now commercially available for use in neutropenia. Granulocyte colony-stimulating factor (G-CSF) specifically stimulates granulocyte production from stem cells, and granulocyte-macrophage colony-stimulating factor (GM-CSF) stimulates production of both lineages. Both are produced commercially by recombinant DNA technology.

G-CSF is an 18-kDa protein encoded by a gene on the long arm of chromosome 17. G-CSF both stimulates production of mature neutrophils and activates their function. It is normally produced by monocytes, macrophages, endothelial cells, and fibroblasts. Its production is stimulated by interleukin-1, tumor necrosis factor alpha, and/or endotoxin.

GM-CSF is a combination of 14–35-kDa glycoproteins encoded by a gene on the long arm of chromosome 5. GM-CSF stimulates clonal growth of multipotential colony-forming units, erythroid burst-forming units, megakaryocyte colony-forming units, granulocyte-macrophage progenitors, and eosinophil colony-forming cells. GM-CSF is produced by mast cells, T lymphocytes, endothelial cells, fibroblasts, and thymic epithelial cells. Its production is induced by interleukin-1, tumor necrosis factor, and phorbol esters.

15. What is the role of G-CSF and GM-CSF in the treatment of neutropenia with or without fever?

Both G-CSF and GM-CSF are effective in treating patients with cyclic neutropenia. They also have an important role in drug-induced neutropenia. In cancer treated with myelosuppressive chemotherapy, they may be administered prophylactically to patients who are likely to become neutropenic during the nadir, especially patients who have experienced complications of neutropenia from a previous cycle of chemotherapy and dose reduction is not desirable. G-CSF and GM-CSF also play a role in bone marrow transplantation; they are administered at the time of the grafted cells to stimulate bone marrow repopulation with neutrophils and to shorten the period of neutropenia. Neutropenia in patients with AIDS also has been successfully treated with G-CSF, whether HIV-related or drug-related. Neutropenic patients with myelodysplasia may respond to growth factors in about 25% of cases. Patients with granulocytic leukemia or refractory anemia with excessive blasts are usually not treated with growth factors because of the concern over potential stimulation of leukemic cell proliferation. Growth factors are not effective in patients who present with neutropenic fever and should not be used in this setting.

BIBLIOGRAPHY

1. American Society of Clinical Oncology: Recommendations for the use of hematopoietic colony-stimulating factors: Evidence-based, clinical practice guidelines. J Clin Oncol 12:2471–2508, 1994.
2. Bociek RG, Armitage JO: Hematopoietic growth factors. Cancer J Clin 46(3):165–184, 1996.
3. Chanock SJ, Pizzo PA: Fever in the neutropenic host. Infect Dis Clin North Am 10:777–796, 1996.
4. Coates T, Baehner R: Leukocytosis and leukopenia. In Hoffman R, Benz EJ Jr, Shattil SJ, et al (eds): Hematology: Basic Principles and Practice. New York, Churchill Livingstone, 1991, pp 553–566.
5. Dale DC: Hematopoietic growth factors for the treatment of severe chronic neutropenia. Stem Cells 13(2):94–100, 1995.
6. Coyle TE: Hematologic complications of human immunodeficiency virus infection and the acquired immunodeficiency syndrome. Med Clin North Am 81:449–470, 1997.
7. Hartmann LC, Tschetter LK, Habermann TM, et al: Granulocyte colony-stimulating factor in severe chemotherapy-induced afebrile neutropenia. N Engl J Med 336:1776–1780, 1997.
8. Jacobs P: Bone marrow failure: Pathophysiology and management. Dis Month 41(4)201–289, 1995.
9. Malik IA, Khan WA, Karim M, et al: Feasibility of outpatient management of fever in cancer patients with low-risk neutropenia: Results of a prospective randomized trial. Am J Med 98:224-231, 1995.
10. Ramphal R, Gucalp R, Rotstein C, et al: Clinical experience with single agent and combination regimens in the management of infection in the febrile neutropenic patient. Am J Med 100(6A):835–895, 1996.
11. Rusthoven JJ: Clinical needs for hematopoietic growth factors: Old and new. Cancer Invest 14:622–634, 1996.
12. Sugar AL: Empiric treatment of fungal infection in the neutropenic host. Arch Intern Med 150:2258–2264, 1990.

56. LEUKOSTASIS

Miho Toi Scott, M.D., and Madeleine A. Kane, M.D., Ph.D.

1. What is leukostasis?

Leukostasis is the plugging of capillaries with usually immature leukocytes; it results in organ dysfunction with possibly life-threatening consequences. Pulmonary and cerebral circulation are the most often affected symptomatically, but other circulations, such as renal, penile, and cardiac, also may be affected and lead to clinically significant complications.

2. Who gets leukostasis?

Patients with acute myelocytic leukemia (AML) or the accelerated or blast phases of chronic myelocytic leukemia (CML) with absolute myeloblast plus promyelocyte counts > 50,000/µl are at greatest risk for leukostasis. Patients with AML and leukostasis are also at increased risk for cerebral hemorrhage compared with patients with acute lymphocytic leukemia (ALL). Patients with ALL and chronic lymphocytic leukemia (CLL) are also at risk for leukostasis, but the absolute lymphoblast or lymphocyte count must exceed 150,000/μl, and leukostasis seldom is observed unless the count greatly exceeds 200,000/μl. Leukostasis has rarely been observed in patients with hairy cell leukemia and white blood cell count > 200,000/μl.

3. What causes leukostasis?

Excessive numbers of immature leukocytes seriously affect normal circulation by simply obstructing capillaries or by forming white cell thrombi in small vessels. The large size, rigidity, and stickiness of leukemic myeloblasts result in plugging of the microcirculation in the lungs, brain, and other, less critical organs. The leukemic blasts also compete for oxygen in the microcirculation, producing local tissue hypoxia and further organ dysfunction. As leukostasis progresses, endothelial injury occurs, vessels walls are damaged, and leukemic cells invade the surrounding tissue. In the pulmonary circulation, leukocyte thrombi and plugging of pulmonary microvascular channels lead to vascular rupture and infiltration of the lung parenchyma with resultant pulmonary edema and hypoxemia. In the brain, tumor nodules may form in the perivascular white matter, especially when circulating myeloblast counts are > 300,000/μl. Under these conditions, the risk for parenchymal cerebral hemorrhage increases substantially.

4. What are the clinical presentations of leukostasis?

Patients may present with serious but nonspecific systemic symptoms that initially suggest a broad differential diagnosis. Dyspnea, tachypnea, cough, chest discomfort, progressive hypoxemia, acidemia and bilateral infiltrates, pulmonary edema, and/or pleural effusions on chest radiograph typify pulmonary leukostasis. Physical exam reveals tachypnea and bilateral rales, possibly with wheezes and/or basilar dullness. Poor prognostic signs are hypercapnia, hypoxia, and progressive respiratory acidosis. Fever also may be present. Symptoms and signs of CNS leukostasis include headache, dizziness, tinnitus, ataxia, lethargy, disorientation, stupor, somnolence, visual changes, obtundation, seizures, and even coma. Physical exam may reveal papilledema and retinal vein distention. Imaging studies may show evidence of cerebral edema, intraparenchymal hemorrhage, or small tumors. Lumbar puncture is likely to reveal elevated protein and myeloblasts in the cerebral spinal fluid. Presentation also may include congestive heart failure, acute renal failure, hepatopathy, and priapism.

5. How is leukostasis diagnosed?

Leukostasis is diagnosed in a patient who presents with suggestive clinical symptoms and signs (see question 4) and has an absolute myeloblast count > 50,000/μl (AML, CML), lymphoblasts > 150,000/μl (ALL), or lymphocytes > 300,000/μl (CLL).

6. What can be done for the patient with leukostasis even before a definitive diagnosis is made and definitive treatment is begun?

A presumptive diagnosis of leukostasis must be considered an emergency, and immediate therapy must be instituted. During the history and physical exam, specific questions for leukostasis need to be addressed. Intensive monitoring of vital signs and EKG, supplemental oxygen, cautious but vigorous hydration, urine alkalinization, and allopurinol need to be initiated. Cytologic evaluation of cerebrospinal fluid may reveal CNS involvement. Blood transfusions should not be administered even for severe anemia until the myeloblast count is reduced to < 100,000/μl.

7. Can leukostasis be prevented?

Prevention of leukostasis requires the diagnosis of new or recurrent AML or CML before the absolute myeloblast count reaches > 50,000/μl or more. Although this is difficult, the risk of leukostasis can be reduced with appropriate treatment to lower the number of leukemic cells.

When leukemic patients present with a high blast count without signs or symptoms of leukostasis, they should be hydrated, urine should be alkalinized, and allopurinol should be started. When diagnosis is established, appropriate antileukemia treatment should be initiated.

8. Can patients with ALL develop leukostasis?

Unlike the leukemic blasts of AML, the lymphoblasts of ALL are quite deformable and are not sticky. Despite their large size, they do not predispose to capillary occlusion, endothelial injury, blast leakage, and growth of tumors in the involved tissues to anywhere near the same extent as myeloblasts. Although leukostasis occasionally occurs in ALL, the risk is much less than in AML because the absolute lymphoblast count must exceed 150,000/μl. Microvessel occlusion then occurs due to the sheer density of the large cells.

9. Can patients with CLL develop leukostasis?

Typical patients with CLL present with increased numbers of circulating mature lymphocytes. Thus they are at much less risk for leukostasis than patients with AML or CML or even ALL. A few cases of leukemic thrombi or aggregates have been reported in autopsy series of patients with CLL and leukocyte counts exceeding 300,000/μl. Although these postmortem histopathologic findings were not believed to be clinically significant, a recent case report illustrates the potential risk of leukostasis in patients with CLL. Prolymphocytic leukemia with leukostasis also has been reported.

10. What is likely to be found on a lung biopsy of a patient with AML and white blood cell count of 100,000/μl with 50% myeloblasts?

Vascular engorgement and accumulation of large aggregates of leukemic cells are found. Leukemic cells occupy most or all of the lumen of involved vessels. Fibrin strands are inconspicuous or absent. Degenerating leukemic blasts leaked into the pulmonary parenchyma may be seen. Leukemic infiltration and local hemorrhage into the pulmonary tissue also may be seen.

11. How can a practitioner determine whether a dyspneic patient with AML has pulmonary leukostasis, pneumonia, or an opportunistic infection due to immunocompromise?

The diagnosis of pulmonary leukostasis is a diagnosis of exclusion. However, leukostasis must be presumed to contribute to the clinical picture if the myeloblast count exceeds 50,000/μl. Infectious causes need to be pursued by vigorous diagnostic methods: blood cultures for bacteria and fungi, detailed history and physical exam, and urine, sputum, and skin lesion cultures. Suspicious skin lesions may require biopsy. Presumptive diagnosis of pneumonia also must be made in a neutropenic patient, and appropriate broad spectrum empiric antibiotics should be initiated. If opportunistic infection is suspected, lung biopsy may be necessary.

12. How is leukostasis treated?

Leukostasis is difficult to treat once it occurs. Chemotherapy, together with hydration, urine alkalinization, and allopurinol, must be initiated as soon as possible after the presumptive diagnosis is made. However, the effect of chemotherapy on the leukemic burden is relatively slow compared with leukapheresis or exchange transfusion, which also may be needed depending on clinical severity. Hydroxyurea (3 gm/m^2 of body surface area orally for 2 days) is often used because its impact may be seen within 12–48 hours. Anthracyclines and cytosine arabinoside also have been used successfully to reduce leukemic count in AML/CML. Vincristine, L-asparaginase, and prednisone may be successful in patients with ALL who present with high peripheral blast counts.

Leukapheresis can reduce the white blood cell count by 20–60% within a few hours. The risk of urate nephropathy and tumor lysis syndrome, which result from rapid lysis of leukemic cells after chemotherapy treatment, can be reduced by immediate initiation of leukapheresis even before allopurinol can take effect. The complications of hyperuricemia, hypocalcemia, hyperkalemia, and hyperphosphatemia are minimized in the initial treatment period, but the effects of leukapheresis are temporary. Chemotherapy must be started as well. In most cases, leukapheresis is a benign procedure that can be used safely, but fatal disseminated intravascular coagulation from fragmented leukemic cells has been reported. Leukapheresis has been used to control leukemia in pregnant women to avoid the toxic effects of chemotherapy on the first- or second-trimester fetus. Leukapheresis also may be used for rapid reduction of the white blood count in a patient who is clinically compromised by severe anemia (e.g., an elderly patient with symptomatic coronary artery disease) and needs to be transfused. Leukapheresis helps to avoid the increase in blood viscosity due to the transfused red blood cells.

Symptomatic leukostasis is the major clinical syndrome that accompanies peripheral myeloblast counts of 50,000–300,000/µl. At higher counts intracranial hemorrhage becomes the major complication. If the blast count exceeds 300,000/µl, tumor nodules in the brain are likely to be present. This situation increases the risk of intracranial hemorrhage. Although the reduction of blasts through leukapheresis has not been proved to reduce the risk of cerebral hemorrhage, it is reasonable to try it. Leukapheresis alone is not adequate therapy because it does not affect tumor nodules in the brain. Cranial radiation (600 cGy in a single fraction) has been effective in destroying intracerebral foci of leukemic cells, thus preventing or reducing risk of intracerebral leukostasis and intracranial hemorrhage.

Some clinicians advocate use of leukapheresis when myeloblast counts are 50,000–100,000/µl. Each case should be evaluated with consideration of the rate of increase in the blast count, if known, and the morphologic subtype of the leukemia. Leukapheresis is indicated when symptoms of leukostasis are present.

13. If a patient with evidence of leukostasis has severe anemia, which should be treated first? Why?

Leukostasis needs to be treated first before red blood cell transfusions are administered. Extreme leukocytosis is likely to raise blood viscosity. Increased viscosity results in impaired blood flow and worsening accumulation of cells in small vessels, particularly in the CNS, lungs, and kidneys, further contributing to tissue damage. The whole blood viscosity is lower in severely anemic patients than in patients with moderate anemia or normal hematocrit. Correction of anemia by transfusion before reduction in the leukocyte count worsens hyperviscosity with likely precipitation of neurologic and respiratory deterioration. Blood transfusion should not be administered until the peripheral myeloblast count is lowered to <100,000/µl.

14. Which patients are at greatest risk for leukostasis?

Leukostasis occurs much more frequently in myeloblastic than in lymphoblastic or lymphocytic leukemias. Highest-risk subtypes of AML or CML in blast crisis include the monocytic subtypes (French-American-British [FAB] classification M4 and M5) and the microgranular variant of acute promyelocytic leukemia (FAB M3). The increased risk of leukostasis with the monocytic subtypes is probably associated with the extreme leukocytosis often seen at presentation.

BIBLIOGRAPHY

1. Baer MR: Management of unusual presentations of acute leukemia. Hematol Oncol Clin North Am 7(1):275–292, 1993.
2. Bunin NJ, Kunkel K, Callihan TR: Cytoreductive procedures in the early management in cases of leukemia and hyperleukocytosis in children. Med Pediatr Oncol 15:232–235, 1987.
3. Dutcher JP, Schiffer CA, Wiernik PH: Hyperleukocytosis in adult acute nonlymphocytic leukemia: Impact on remission rate and duration, and survival. J Clin Oncol 5:1364–1372, 1987.
4. Grund FM, Armitage JO, Burns P: Hydroxyurea in the prevention of the effects of leukostasis in acute leukemia. Arch Intern Med 137:1246–1247, 1977.
5. Harris AL: Leukostasis associated with blood transfusion in acute myeloid leukaemia. BMJ 1:1169–1171, 1978.
6. Hild DH, Myers TJ: Hyperviscosity in chronic granulocytic leukemia.Cancer 46:1418–1421, 1980.
7. Lester TJ, Johnson JW, Cuttner J: Pulmonary leukostasis as the single worst prognostic factor in patients with acute myelocytic leukemia and hyperleukocytosis. Am J Med 79:43–48, 1985.
8. Maurer HS, Steinherz PG, Gaynon PS, et al: The effect of initial management of hyperleukocytosis on early complications and outcome of children with acute lymphoblastic leukemia. J Clin Oncol 6:1425 1432, 1988.

9. Megaludis AM, Winkelstein A, Zeigler ZR, Miller TR: Leukostasis: a phenomenon of prolymphocytic leukemia. Am J Hematol 32:146–147, 1989.
10. Sharma K, Rao S, Bhat SV: Effect of hydroxyurea on blood viscosity in chronic myelogenous leukemia with hyperleukocytosis. Physiol Chem Physics Med NMR 23:261–268, 1991.
11. van Buchem MA, Wondergem JH, Kool LJ, et al: Pulmonary leukostasis: Radiologic-pathologic study. Radiology 165:739–741, 1987.
12. Van Rybroek JJ, Olson JD, Burns CP: White cell fragmentation after therapeutic leukapheresis for acute leukemia. Transfusion 27:353–355, 1987.
13. Ventura GJ, Hester JP, Smith TL, Keating MJ: Acute myeloblastic leukemia with hyperleukocytosis: Risk factors for early mortality in induction. Am J Hematol 27:34–37, 1988.

57. PSYCHOSOCIAL ASPECTS OF CANCER CARE

Lari B. Wenzel, Ph.D., Ann D. Futterman-Collier, Ph.D., and Nathan A. Munn, M.D.

1. What are the most difficult cancer communication issues between the physician and patient/family?

People retain little just after hearing bad news. The acronym **FORM** serves as a reminder to form your messages carefully, particularly in the following circumstances:

First diagnosis is frightening. The initial diagnosis of cancer is often as difficult to say as it is to hear. With any first diagnosis, however, usually the hope of informed optimism accompanying first-line treatment quells the initial terror associated with cancer.

Oncologic care can be overwhelming for people who have never before had a serious illness. When conveying new treatment and future care information, limit the amount of information provided during the first appointment and schedule another, at which time the patient can bring a family member, friend, or even a tape recorder to be a "third ear."

Recurrence is not initially part of the cancer patient's vocabulary. This is a challenging issue, because hope for cure is typically removed. Informed optimism, if presented and understood realistically, includes holding the disease at bay and ameliorating symptoms as they occur.

Metastasis often signals the end of treatment. Depending on the location of the metastases, communication about end-of-life preferences should begin. This delicate subject is best addressed when feelings, values, and thoughts about death and dying have been examined.

2. How can cancer-related stress be buffered?

Recent literature suggests that positive, healthy adjustment and growth may result from the cancer experience. Positive growth is facilitated by a healthy range and expression of emotions, an optimistic attitude, social support, stress management through active coping, and spirituality.

3. When and how should patients/family be referred for psychosocial support?

When? If they ask your opinion about these services, they are looking for your endorsement and should be referred. If they call repeatedly with nonemergency questions, they are probably anxious and need to address their fears or concerns. If their mood (sad, angry, anxious, despondent) or symptoms (nausea/vomiting, pain, fatigue) interfere with their ability to enjoy and engage in aspects of daily life, individual care is needed. In addition, cognitive problems, sexual problems, or family communication difficulties may necessitate referral for counseling.

How? The physician wields considerable influence in steering the patient toward or away from assistance. Consequently, the delivery of your message should be clear and decisive. If you are clear that addressing emotional or social concerns related to cancer is important and beneficial, convey this attitude without hesitation. Some patients may feel singled out, feeling that you "think they are crazy." Begin with assurance that you view their cancer diagnosis and treatment as a highly stressful time. Some stressors can be reduced through emotional support.

4. What are the risks and benefits of individual counseling?

Individual counseling provided by a psychologist, psychiatrist, social worker, psychiatric nurse, or marriage and family counselor may be quickly beneficial because the counseling is tailored to the patient's unique concerns and circumstances. Within a hospital consultation setting, however, a patient may be offended by the concept of counseling related to cancer concerns. The physician can pave the way for the consultant by "normalizing" the consultation (i.e., "This is a service which we find valuable for our patients"). A more general risk involves therapy delivered by inexperienced and/or unqualified therapists, as well as paying for the cost of care, particularly as counseling is affected by managed care mandates.

5. What are the risks and benefits of support groups?

Support groups are seldom costly and have several known benefits. First, a skilled leader can deliver supportive expressive or psychoeducational strategies to suit the characteristics of the group (e.g., advanced disease vs. new diagnosis). Group strategies have repeatedly been shown to reduce distress and some physical symptoms (pain, fatigue, nausea) and to enhance social support, decision-making ability, and quality of life. Some research shows survival benefit associated with support group participation. A common risk occurs when a newly diagnosed patient attends a group in which some members are dying of the same disease (e.g., newly diagnosed, early-stage breast cancer vs. metastatic breast cancer). The newly diagnosed patient may be overwhelmed with fear that her disease, too, will advance, which overshadows any benefits from the group experience. A less dramatic risk involves having a blend of participants (e.g., breast and prostate, young and old adults), whose ability to relate with each other may be minimized by numerous differences in disease and life circumstances.

6. What symptoms of cancer or cancer treatment may affect mood and cognition?

The acronym **FOCUS** alerts practitioners to attend to the neuropsychological and physiologic components of the cancer disease course:

Fatigue. Cancer fatigue adversely affects significant aspects of patients' daily lives, including ability to work, meet family needs, and cope with the disease long after treatment completion.

Organic symptoms. Delirium may include symptoms of confusion, inattention, disorientation, gross misperceptions, memory disturbance, and sleep-wake cycle alterations.

Chemo brain. Chemotherapy together with antiemetic regimens may cause forgetfulness, memory lapses, somnolence, and altered orientation. Patients often refer to this phenomenon as "chemo brain."

Uncontrolled nervousness and agitation. Certain antiemetic regimens, reactions to steroids, or strong emotional reactions to new information may cause uncomfortable symptoms.

Severe pain. Poorly controlled pain exacerbates depression and anxiety.

7. Why do some patients with cancer feel nauseous or vomit before chemotherapy?

Despite recent advances in effective antiemetic medication, a small proportion of patients receiving chemotherapy develop anticipatory nausea or vomiting (ANV). ANV is thought to be an example of classic conditioning, a phenomenon in which cues associated with chemotherapy (e.g., smells of the hospital, appearance of the clinic, strong-tasting foods, the "thought" of chemotherapy) are conditioned to the unconditioned response of postchemotherapy nausea and vomiting. This phenomenon can be effectively treated through referral to a psychologist with expertise in behavior therapy.

8. What is delirium? What are the possible causes?

Delirium is characterized by a reduced ability to maintain attention, disorganized thinking, fluctuating level of consciousness, disorientation and disturbances in perceptions, and alterations in the sleep-wake cycle and memory. A helpful mnemonic for the numerous differential diagnoses is **I WATCH DEATH**.

I	= **I**nfection	(encephalitis, meningitis, syphilis)
W	= **W**ithdrawal	(alcohol, barbiturates, sedatives-hypnotics)
A	= **A**cute metabolic disturbances	(acidosis, alkalosis, electrolyte disturbance, hepatic failure, renal failure)
T	= **T**rauma	(heat stroke, postoperative state, severe burns)
C	= **C**NS pathology	(abscesses, hemorrhage, normal pressure hydrocephalus, seizures, stroke, tumors, vasculitis)
H	= **H**ypoxia	(anemia, carbon monoxide poisoning, hypotension, pulmonary/cardiac failure)
D	= **D**eficiencies	(vitamin B_{12}, hypovitaminosis, niacin, thiamine)
E	= **E**ndocrinopathies	(hyper- or hypoadrenalcorticism, hyper- or hypoglycemia)
A	= **A**cute vascular disorders	(hypertensive encephalopathy, shock)
T	= **T**oxins/drugs	(medications, pesticides, solvents)
H	= **H**eavy metals	(lead, manganese, mercury)

From Wise MG: Delirium. In Hales RE, Yudofsky SC (eds): Textbook of Neuropsychiatry. Washington, DC, American Psychiatric Press, 1987, with permission.

9. How does a physician determine whether a patient is competent to make medical decisions, including referral of care?

Competency is task-specific—for example, refusing chemotherapy or surgery—and should not be confused with general mental status. To determine competency, a physician must review the following:

- Ability to understand pertinent information about treatment
- Ability to communicate options concerning treatment (e.g., risks and benefits of treatment vs. no treatment)
- Presence of any psychiatric symptoms that may inhibit rational thinking (e.g., paranoia, suicidal ideation, or delirium)

10. How does psychiatric status interact with cancer pain?

Patients with a psychiatric diagnosis are more likely to report pain. However, psychological factors are too often used to explain the presence of pain when medical aspects have not been fully addressed.

11. What are some of the psychiatric treatment modalities for cancer pain?

Strategies include decreasing mood disturbance (with psychopharmacologic agents), providing psychosocial interventions (e.g., support, coping), and behavioral interventions (e.g., relaxation, hypnosis, cognitive therapy, communication, self-observation, documentations).

12. Does giving opiates to patients with cancer frequently turn them into opiate addicts?

No. The chance that patients with cancer will become addicted to opiates is very small.

13. What complicates the differential diagnosis of depression in patients with cancer?

Depressed mood may be caused by psychiatric illness (e.g., adjustment disorder, major depression, dysthymia), thyroid and other endocrine dysfunction, brain lesions (CNS tumor, stroke, encephalopathy), and medication side effects. It is difficult to diagnose major depression because the physical symptoms of depression—decreased energy, anorexia, sleep disturbance, and weight loss—also are characteristic of cancer per se. Thus, it is necessary to examine psychological symptoms—depressed mood, anhedonia, hopelessness, suicidal ideation—in diagnosing depression in patients with cancer or other medical illnesses.

14. Are antidepressants effective in depressed patients dying of cancer who are understandably depressed?

Yes. Although a major depression may seem understandable in a grave situation, antidepressants are still effective in relieving depressive symptoms and improving quality of life.

15. When is anxiety considered abnormal in patients with cancer?

If anxiety is so great that it disturbs the patient's functioning or ability to understand or cooperate, it is helpful either to prescribe anxiolytics or to have the patient learn a behavioral technique, such as relaxation and imagery.

16. What anxiety disorders may complicate cancer treatment?

First, the physical symptoms of panic disorder may complicate care because they can be interpreted, for example, as a myocardial infarction, pulmonary emboli, or neurologic disorders and possibly lead to unnecessary procedures. Second, agoraphobia (fear of being in places or situations from which escape may be difficult or help may be unavailable in the event of a panic attack) can lead to handicaps in seeking treatment or being able to comply with treatment. Third, obsessive compulsive disorder may cause severe anxiety in patients with cancer, especially in germ-free environmental situations.

17. What is a normal grief reaction to the death of a loved one? How is a normal reaction distinguished from a pathologic one?

Normal grief is characterized by decreased appetite, sleep disturbance, depressed mood, and crying. Pathologic grief is usually of a longer duration. It is characterized by negative self-evaluation (hopelessness, worthlessness, thoughts of suicide) and prolonged disruption of daily functioning.

18. How long after the death of a loved one should antidepressants be prescribed for people with pathologic grief?

The question is difficult, but most physicians would say 4–6 months.

19. Is there a link between major depression and development and/or progression of cancer?

The literature on the relationship between depression and cancer is contradictory at best. One possibility is that major depression poses a greater risk for patients with cancer because it directly interferes with immune processes. Clinically, many patients believe that their emotional states actually caused their cancer, and this belief leads them to feel guilty. Frequently, such patients are relieved when informed of the inconclusive data about this topic.

20. How does cancer genetic testing affect a patient's quality of life?

This new area of genetics has created both risks and benefits for the individual patient with cancer. For example, many patients who have undergone genetic counseling and testing feel empowered with information related to cancer risk factors, screening options, and potential prevention strategies. Yet cancer-specific distress may be heightened, and concerns related to first-degree relatives may be pronounced. Fears of job or insurance discrimination as a result of testing as well as concerns about how best to communicate genetic issues with the family remain unresolved. In addition, decision-making related to prophylactic surgeries may be a source of anxiety and conflict.

21. What concerns exist for long-term cancer survivors?

Recent survivorship research indicates that uncertainty and fear of recurrence, potential long-term cognitive changes, fatigue, and potential job or insurance discrimination challenge many long-term survivors. Of note, increased medical attention related to late effects of treatment is also needed.

BIBLIOGRAPHY

1. Breitbart W, Holland JC: Psychiatric complications of cancer. In Brian MC, Carbone PP (eds): Current Therapy in Hematology Oncology, vol. 3. Philadelphia, B.C. Decker, 1988, pp 268–274.
2. Fawzy FI, Cousins N, Kemeny ME, et al: A structured psychiatric intervention for cancer patients. I: Changes over time in methods of coping and affective disturbance. Arch Gen Psychiatry 47:726–732, 1993.
3. Heinrichs MA: Principles of psychosocial oncology. In Rubin P, McDonald S, Qazi R (eds): Clinical Oncology: A Multidisciplinary Approach for Physicians and Students, 7th ed. Philadelphia, W.B. Saunders, 1993.
4. Holland JC, Rowland JH (eds): Handbook of Psychooncology: Psychological Care of the Patient with Cancer. Oxford, Oxford University Press, 1990.
5. Lesko L: Psychologic issues. In DeVita VT, Hellman S, Rosenberg SA (eds): Cancer: Principles and Practice of Oncology, 5th ed. Philadelphia, Lippincott-Raven, 1997.
6. Seligman L: Promoting a Fighting Spirit: Psychotherapy for Cancer Patients, Survivors, and Their Families. San Francisco, Jossey-Bass, 1996.
7. Wise MG: Delirium. In Hales RE, Yudofsky SC (eds): Textbook of Neuropsychiatry. Washington, DC, American Psychiatric Press, 1987, pp 89–103.

58. PALLIATIVE CARE AND END-OF-LIFE DECISION MAKING

Lari B. Wenzel, Ph.D., Bradley J. Monk, M.D., and Daniel G. Petereit, M.D.

1. What is the most important point to remember in providing care to a person with advanced cancer?

Determining whether the disease is curable dictates the aggressiveness of therapy. Regardless of the intent of therapy, the most important aspect of patient care is to assess and provide adequately for the patient's needs. When caring for a patient with an advanced malignancy, the physician must concentrate on the quality as well as the quantity of remaining life. Therefore, the survival benefit of any treatment must be weighed against the potential impact on the quality of remaining life. Some cancer treatments (e.g., radiation therapy, certain chemotherapeutic agents) actually improve the quality of life as well as prolong survival.

2. How can quality of life be sustained for advanced cancer patients?

Quality of life should be the primary goal in treating patients with advanced cancers. Through a multidisciplinary team approach, many palliative care options are available to enhance quality of life or to minimize detrimental aspects of disease. In addition to physicians, team members may include rehabilitative services, psychosocial services, and home health/hospice services. Early assessment and treatment of problems, with regular monitoring, greatly enhance quality of life. Assessment should include an evaluation of such functions as eating, voiding, eliminating, hygiene, pain, and absence of significant dyspnea. Psychological and social factors are equally important in quality of life and should be assessed and, if disrupted, treated rigorously. Impairments may include mood or cognitive disturbance, problems interacting with significant others (or the reverse), or loss of esteem and purpose.

3. At what point in the care of a patient with cancer may you begin to understand the patient's end-of-life preferences? What questions should you ask to enhance your understanding?

Generally, patients are not prepared to discuss end-of-life decisions during the initial phases of diagnosis and treatment, regardless of the extent of disease. However, as the clinician develops a relationship with the patient, it is almost inevitable that such issues will be discussed. Asking questions in a manner that normalizes the situation allows the patient to discuss the topic without immediately vocalizing the personal threat. Examples include the following: (1) "Many people in a medical situation like yours have thoughts that they may not survive the disease. Have you experienced this?" (2) "Often when people have a potentially life-threatening diagnosis they think about things they have yet to do or want to do. What would you want to do with remaining time?" Such questions, without the immediate personal burden, may open a line of communication between physician and patient that can then extend from the patient to significant others. The patient often is grateful that someone helps him or her in courageously facing such difficult issues.

4. When may you find yourself in the dilemma of providing cardiopulmonary resuscitation (CPR) and prolonged mechanical ventilation for an advanced cancer patient?

Although patients with advanced cancer frequently succumb to their illness, many untreated patients with advanced cancer experience significant long-term survival. Therefore, the chance of long-term survival and/or cure must be weighed against the obvious pain and suffering from performing CPR and mechanical life support. If you are not aware of or if the patient has not completed a health care advance directive, living will, or durable power of attorney, you may be compelled to perform CPR or other immediate life-sustaining procedures.

5. How can a health care advance directive, living will, or health care durable power of attorney be useful?

The health care advance directive documents the patient's wishes about health care treatment plans, including but not limited to decisions about life-sustaining treatment, and selects an agent to make and communicate decisions for the patient. The living will is a legal document that states wishes about life-sustaining health care in the event of terminal illness. The durable power of attorney appoints someone to make health care decisions for the patient. These legal documents help to ensure that the patient's medical care choices are known ahead of time. Generally, the law respects any form of written directive about stated values and preferences regarding death and dying. Unfortunately, despite adequate documentation, many physicians and health care institutions have overlooked or disregarded such directives. Such oversights undermine the trust established in the physician-patient relationship and the physician-primary caregiver relationship and have potential negative legal implications.

6. How is it possible to differentiate terminating treatment from terminating care?

The comprehensive approach to oncologic care is the continuation of the physician-patient relationship, in which care of the patient does not cease. The type of treatment may change as illness progresses, but quality care should persist throughout the disease course. For example, as uncontrolled cancer progresses, the focus of the treatment changes from an emphasis on prolongation of life to an emphasis on palliation of symptoms and dying with dignity.

7. With what issues are you as a physician presented when a patient with metastatic or end-stage disease says, "Doctor, tell me honestly, how much time do I have?"

Although there is no correct answer, this question needs to be dealt with in a compassionate, sincere, and honest manner, respecting the needs of the patient. Your approach may differ depending on whether the patient is asymptomatic, has good performance status, and may survive 1–2 years or longer or has poor performance status and faces imminent death. If the patient likely has less than 1 year to live, it is helpful to say that "a 1–2-year life expectancy is probably not realistic" or to express the median survival of a patient's disease by stating, "Generally, half of my patients do not live beyond [a specified time]." It is also helpful to hear that no physician can predict when someone will die from cancer. In addition, the physician also may communicate that some patients survive well beyond their life expectancy. Although it may be argued that such broad, sweeping statements are ambiguous, it is important to offer hope. It is equally critical that patients know that you will care for them, regardless of treatment outcome. Patients are frequently worried about pain and suffering when cancer progresses. It is important to emphasize that numerous comfort and pain control options are available. To summarize, remember the following in counseling patients: (1) be honest; (2) be compassionate; (3) emphasize that no one can predict the future or the exact duration of life expectancy; (4) convey a sense of hope; and (5) assure patients that you will take care of their needs.

8. With what issues are you as a physician presented when a patient with metastatic or end-stage disease says, "Doctor, just do whatever it takes to get rid of this thing"?

Although this situation is rare, the occasional patient may deny the gravity of his or her illness. The physician may choose to reexplain the disease and the treatment options, with a realistic explanation of treatment risks and benefits. It is the physician's responsibility to educate the patient about the natural history of the disease and indications for therapeutic interventions. Particular attention should be given to the effect of therapy on the patient's quality of life. At this point, the physician's statements may shift toward a discussion of palliative care options.

9. How can a physician manage the potential controversy or conflict that evolves when a patient with advanced cancer receives active treatment and may simultaneously benefit from hospice care?

The goals of active (cytotoxic) treatment may be either to improve the quality of life or to prolong life. Fortunately, these goals are frequently not mutually exclusive. Thus, patients receiving cytotoxic therapy may experience significant palliation of symptoms related to cancer, such as airway obstruction, dyspnea due to a pleural effusion, or partial bowel obstruction due to intraperitoneal disease. The goals of hospice care and cytotoxic therapy do not necessarily conflict and, when properly conceptualized, may work closely together. The concept of hospice is to palliate symptoms, not to expedite death.

10. How should the concept of hope be communicated to a dying patient?

The physician should privately define his or her own meaning and attitude toward hope in care delivery, thus enabling optimal communication. A true sense of hopefulness departs from unrealistic goals to a sense of realistic and benevolent goals. As the clinician better understands a dying patient's wishes, the physician can help the patient generate hope in reaching these goals. For example, one may hope to see the birth of a grandchild or the graduation of a child from school. In addition, a dying patient may hope that he or she dies with dignity and does not suffer. All of these areas can generate significant hope within the dying patient, although there is no real hope for prolonging life or cure. This sense of hope can be communicated by encouraging patients to rely on family, close friends, religious beliefs (if applicable), and other sources of strength that a patient may possess.

11. How should the news of disease progression be communicated? Under what circumstances, if any, is it useful to inform family members first?

Frequently, the progression of cancer is manifested by the development of new symptoms. For example, a recurrent brain cancer may cause seizures or alteration in consciousness. Therefore, it is possible to communicate clearly the news of disease progression because it explains such symptoms. In the absence of symptoms, one can explain the findings, which suggest disease progression. For example, one may discuss an elevated level of prostate-specific antigen in a patient with prostate cancer or an abnormality detected on a chest radiograph in a patient with lung cancer. Speaking about these diagnostic tests cushions the news and perhaps makes it less devastating. News of disease progression, however, is difficult to communicate and should be shared with the patient in a sincere, sensitive, honest (but not brutally so) fashion. Of interest, patients often seem to be aware of bad news before communication. It is best to convey this message in person rather than by phone. It is initially useful to tell the patient what the studies revealed, followed by an expression of your sorrow. This latter statement is not superfluous, for it allows the patient to hear the compassion and sorrow conveyed by a trusted practitioner. Therefore, it is absolutely critical that words be chosen carefully and in a fashion that is honest but not brutally so. Like other issues addressed in this chapter, this discussion is highly individualized and depends on the physician-patient relationship. Typically within American culture, family members are informed first only if the patient is not mentally competent to grasp the information (e.g., dementia).

12. When should advice about discontinuing treatment be communicated?

Advising discontinuation of therapy is appropriate when the patient is deteriorating rapidly, the goals of treatment are unattainable, and/or the patient strongly desires discontinuation of therapy in the face of advancing cancer. In addition, cytotoxic therapy should be discontinued when the side effects outweigh any reasonable chance of improving survival or quality of life.

13. What physical aspects of dying require medical care to ensure comfort?

First, address the symptoms that affect a particular patient. Careful attention should be given to normal bodily functions such as eating, voiding, and normal elimination. In addition, every attempt should be made to relieve pain and dyspnea. Measures may include:

1. **Breathing:** sitting the patient in an upright position; home oxygen; thoracentesis, sclerosis, or pleurodesis for a malignant pleural effusion; tracheostomy for upper airway obstruction.

2. **Pain:** narcotic analgesia, nonsteroidal antiinflammatory drugs, antidepressants, nerve blocks, heat, and nerve stimulators.

3. **Hunger:** surprisingly, most patients dying of cancer who are unable to eat are not hungry; this phenomenon is poorly understood.

4. **Thirst:** patients who are unable to drink are frequently not thirsty; once again, this phenomenon is poorly understood.

5. **Elimination:** every attempt should be made to keep the patient dry; Foley catheters and anticathartics for diarrhea may be useful.

6. **Nausea and vomiting:** gastrostomy tubes may be useful in patients with high small bowel obstructions; antiemetic medications; sedation (useful in preventing nausea).

14. What are the advantages and disadvantages of caring for a dying person at home?

Frequently, patients prefer to die in their home environment, where they are most comfortable and which allows the family more input into the dying process. Dying at home is also less expensive than dying in an institution. However, it is not infrequent for the dying patient to create physical or emotional burdens on the primary caregiver and to disrupt the home environment. Thus, issues related to dying at home must be discussed carefully with the patient and the patient's family, with a realistic description of how the physical facility, resources, and, most importantly, primary caregiver's multiple roles should facilitate a comfortable environment.

15. How do psychological factors affect or interact with the experience of dying?

In general, the patient's affect, coping style, and coping resources are paramount in determining his or her interpretation of the dying process and how this interpretation unfolds behaviorally. One may predict how an individual patient will cope with advancing disease and death based on initial coping responses to diagnosis and treatment as well as responses to past stressful events. However, variability exists between younger and older patients, cultures, and reliance on social support and spirituality. In many circumstances, a dying family member may exacerbate long-standing family tensions or other dysfunctional family relationships that remain unresolved. In general, patients and their loved ones with good coping skills and resources will cope well through the course of the illness.

16. Under what circumstances is counseling indicated?

Ideally, all oncologic patients should have access to counseling to cope with the multiple levels of stress that arise from a diagnosis of cancer. Although some may advocate that all dying patients and family members can benefit from counseling, it is wise to define persons or situations in which counseling can be clearly beneficial. Examples may include patients requiring or desiring assistance in resolving issues, seeking emotional comfort, or reducing symptoms of depression or anxiety (for self and family). Counseling is most difficult when the patient denies the prognosis or severity of the illness. In this case, counseling may be experienced as threatening. Counseling may be offered in an individual, group, or family format and should be tailored to the needs of the patient.

17. How does spirituality and a sense of meaning and purpose in life interact with the experience of dying?

Once a taboo subject, the interplay of medicine and spirituality has recently become a vital topic. Most suggest that spirituality enhances the patient's ability to cope with disease and dying and provides a supportive buffer against the physical and psychological assaults that accompany advancing cancer. The sense of spirituality can provide significant meaning to end-of-life experiences. Once delegated only to clergy, health care professionals are now increasingly encouraged and willing to open a spiritual dialogue with patients with potential rewards to both.

BIBLIOGRAPHY

1. Brescia EJ, Kass F: Specialized care of the terminally ill. In DeVita VT, Hellman S, Rosenberg SA (eds): Cancer: Principles and Practices of Oncology, 5th ed. Philadelphia, Lippincott-Raven, 1997.
2. Cella DF: Quality of life as an outcome of cancer treatment. In Goenwald SL, Frogge MH, Goodman M, Yarbro CH (eds): Cancer Nursing: Principles and Practice, 3rd ed. Boston, Jones & Bartlett, 1993.
3. Emanuel EJ, Kass F: Ethical and legal aspects of caring for patients with cancer. In Holland JF, Frei E, Bast RC, et al (eds): Cancer Medicine, 3rd ed. Philadelphia, Lea & Febiger, 1993.
4. Holland JC, Rowland JH (eds): Handbook of Psychooncology: Psychological Care of the Patient with Cancer. Oxford, Oxford Press, 1990.

59. HOSPICE CARE

Jane M. McCabe, R.N., B.S.N., O.C.N.

1. Define hospice.

The term hospice has its origin in 19th century Europe. A hospice was a place where travelers or the homeless could seek food and shelter. Today the term hospice refers to a facility for supportive care of the terminally ill. However, in the United States 90% of hospice care is delivered in the home.

2. What is hospice care?

Hospice care is a coordinated, multidisciplinary patient/family-centered program of support with end-of-life care that maintains a primary focus on the integration of holistic palliative principles, including biopsychosocial, cultural, spiritual, and environmental quality of life.

3. What is palliative medicine?

Palliative medicine is the medical specialty that studies and manages patients with advanced disease and a limited prognosis by focusing on comfort and quality of life.

4. What is palliative care?

The World Health Organization defines palliative care as follows:

The active total care of patients whose disease is not responsive to curative treatment. Control of pain, of other symptoms, and of psychological, social, and spiritual problems, is paramount. The goal of palliative care is achievement of the best quality of life of patients and their families. Palliative care . . . affirms life and regards dying as a normal process . . . neither hastens nor postpones death . . . provides relief from pain and other distressing symptoms . . . integrates the psychological and the spiritual aspects of care . . . offers a support system to help patients live as actively as possible until death . . . offers a support system to help the family cope during the patient's illness and in their own bereavement.

5. What is the history of the hospice movement?

The early European pioneers of hospice recognized the need to provide comprehensive palliative care to people who were dying. In 1842 Jeanne Garnier opened several hospices in Lyons, France. In 1879 the Irish Sisters of Charity opened a hospice in Dublin, and in 1905 in east London the St. Joseph's Hospice was opened. The Calvary Hospital in New York City was opened in 1899. Modern hospice care in the United States began in the early 1970s with the opening of the New Haven hospice home care. Since that time thousands of programs have opened to offer hospice services across the United States.

6. How has hospice evolved over the past 10 years?

Palliative treatment interventions such as radiation, chemotherapy, hydration, and blood product support, which have been refused to hospice patients in the past, may be allowed today. Many hospice programs accept people who live alone, whereas in the past a 24-hour caregiver was required. Hospice programs of the past defined palliative care, whereas today the primary care physician and the hospice team define the palliative treatment plan together on an individual case basis. The hospice benefit has been extended to include terminal diseases other than cancer.

7. Are all hospice programs the same?

Although the basic hospice philosophy may be the foundation on which each program bases its services, organizational structure, affiliations, and aspects of services vary widely. Organizations offering services may be nonprofit or for-profit. The program may offer acute or skilled residential and/or respite facility hospice care with or without home care services. The organization may be new or well established in the community. It may be affiliated with other health care groups. It may be licensed to provide home health care services as well as hospice services. The services may be offered only to people who live within certain geographic boundaries. It may have limited insurance contracts or have contracts with most available plans in the area that it serves.

8. Where are hospice services delivered?

Hospice care may be offered in an acute care or skilled nursing care facility, nursing home, free-standing hospice residential center, or patient's home.

9. What criterion does the patient need to meet to be eligible for hospice care?

Any person of any age at any time during a life-limiting illness whose life expectancy is estimated to be days, weeks, or months may qualify for hospice care. The primary care physician and patient or guardian, along with the family, choose hospice care after the determination is made to seek palliative rather than curative medical interventions. The patient signs an agreement to enter a hospice program and may give up other types of insurance benefit coverage.

10. How is a hospice program chosen?

By law the patient is the decision maker. The primary care provider may recommend a program with which he or she is familiar or ask that the patient or family interview or visit several programs in their geographic area. Some patients/families may feel empowered by this activity and some overwhelmed. The choice may be limited by availability or insurance contracts.

11. What is unique about hospice care?

Hospice programs are a truly collaborative, case-managed, patient/family-centered delivery of palliative care. The care is delivered by a physician-directed interdisciplinary team of caring professionals and trained volunteers who have specialized expertise in palliative end-of-life pain and symptoms management. Most services are available on call 24 hours/day, 7 days/week. Individual and group bereavement follow-up support is extended to families in grief for at least 1 year after the death of the patient. Many services are available regardless of ability to pay.

12. Who makes a hospice referral?

The patient, family, or any health care provider may make initial contact with the hospice program. A physician must certify that the patient has been diagnosed with a terminal illness and has a limited life expectancy.

13. What happens after a hospice referral is made?

If the referral is made by anyone other than the patient's physician, the hospice contacts the physician for certification of hospice-appropriate care. Hospices may have medical staff available in the event that the patient has no physician. Next, the hospice contacts the patient/family to set up an initial visit. The program and services are explained and questions answered. The patient signs informed consent and insurance forms. An intake assessment of patient/family needs is made by a registered nurse. Equipment, supplies, and medication needs are determined and ordered. An initial plan of care is reviewed, and written physician orders are obtained. The plan of care is reviewed and revised as needed.

14. Once a hospice referral is made, can the patient change his or her mind?

Yes. The patient always has the right to leave a hospice program and return to traditional medical care. Occasionally the medical condition improves, or the disease goes into remission. When or if a discharged hospice patient wants to return to hospice care, Medicare, Medicaid, most HMOs, and most private insurance companies allow readmission.

15. What is covered under the hospice benefit plan?

Hospice benefits include physician services, nursing care, medical appliances, equipment, supplies, medications for symptom management and pain relief, home care, inpatient care, respite care, home health aide and homemaker services, physical therapy, occupational therapy, speech/language pathology services, medical social services, dietary and other support, and counseling.

16. How is hospice care reimbursed?

Hospice insurance coverage is widely available. It is reimbursed by Medicare nationwide, by Medicaid in some 38 states, and by most private health insurance policies. If stated policy coverage is not available, most insurance companies consider coverage on a case-by-case basis. Hospice providers are paid on a capitated daily rate set by Medicare for each provider, which is usually around $100–$150 per day for all services provided.

17. Does the patient have any out-of-pocket expenses for hospice services?

There may be a minimal out-of-pocket expense to the patient. Under Medicare the patient may be required to pay 5% or a $5 copayment for medications and a $5 copayment for inpatient respite care per day. Some insurance plans have a deductible or pay a percentage of fixed rates per patient per day.

18. Does signing onto the hospice program benefit the patient/family financially?

In most cases the patient/family out-of-pocket expenses decrease and the services increase. This alone may relieve pressure felt by patients and families about financial issues.

19. Is hospice care only for cancer patients?

The National Hospice Organization has developed guidelines to help health care professionals determine noncancer prognosis for end-stage renal disease, cardiac disease, liver disease, HIV/AIDS, dementia, pulmonary disease, stroke/cerebrovascular accident, and neuromuscular disease.

20. How does the cost of hospice care per day compare with hospital and home care?

In 1995 average charges per hospital day were estimated at $1,800 and for a skilled nursing facility at $325 per day compared with $100 per day for hospice care. In the last month of life, when most health care dollars are spent, Medicare's 1995 hospice program was estimated to save $1.65 for every dollar spent on Part A benefits.

21. Who are the members of the hospice team?

Medicare requires that the hospice core team members of the interdisciplinary group include at least a doctor of medicine or osteopathy, registered nurse, social worker, and pastor or other counselor. These team members may be volunteers or employees. The physician is the only member who may be contracted. In addition, noncore team members include physical, occupational, and speech therapists, home health aides, dieticians, volunteers, and bereavement counselors.

22. What if the patient has no money or insurance coverage?

Most hospices provide care for people who are unable to pay. Money is used from community fundraising and memorial and foundation gifts.

23. What is bereavement?

The term *bereavement* refers to the process experienced after a loved one dies. Bereavement counseling, provided as an important hospice benefit to help the family through this transitional process, attempts to minimize suffering from decline in physical and mental functioning associated with grief and loss. The hospice bereavement program offers services for at least 1 year after the death has occurred.

24. Explain advance directives.

Advance directives are written instructions concerning individual wishes about medical treatment. It is important to ask about advanced directives on initiation of your relationship with a patient as his or her care provider and to make an attempt to keep copies in the patient's medical record. Some patients may wear necklaces or bracelets with advance directive information. Fill-in-the-blank advance directive forms are available in health care institutions as well as retail office supply stores. (See chapters 38 and 58 for more information).

25. Explain the Patient Self-Determination Act.

The Patient Self-Determination Act was signed into law in December 1991. The law requires that a person who receives care from a Medicare- and Medicaid-funded agency be given written information about advance directives. The intention of the law is to allow people to begin the process of determining what care they would like to receive under what circumstances before they become too ill to communicate. Usually people are given information about living wills, medical durable power of attorney, medical proxies, guardians, and cardiopulmonary resuscitation (CPR).

26. Define living wills. When do they go into effect?

A living will is a written document giving the health care providers direction about artificial life support—the type of support that a person may want and how long he or she wants it to continue. This document usually goes into effect when two people have witnessed it and when at least two physicians agree in writing that the person has an irreversible condition. The living will may be cancelled or changed at any time by the individual.

27. What is meant by medical durable power of attorney?

A medical durable power of attorney is a document signed by the patient that names someone to act as the patient's agent immediately or only in the event that the patient is unable to make medical decisions for him- or herself. The agent may request copies of medical records to assist in decision making. The agent must be at least 18 years old.

28. What if the patient has a terminal illness and requires palliative symptom management and care but does not feel ready for a hospice program?

Many agencies who offer hospice care also offer prehospice home health care that uses the same staff members, who assist with the transitional process while delivering expert palliative care. Reimbursement is made under home care guidelines until the patient decides to enter the hospice program.

29. What parameters are used to determine when a patient is a hospice candidate?

Guidelines have been developed by the National Hospice Organization for the most common disease categories. In general, the patient indicators of terminal disease include an irreversible medical diagnosis or multiple diagnoses, patient choice of treatment goals directed toward comfort with relief of symptoms rather than cure, documented clinical progression due to the disease, multiple emergency department visits or hospitalizations over the past 6 months, unintentional weight loss greater than 10% over the past 6 months, Karnofsky performance status of 50% or less, and dependence in at least 3 of 6 activities of daily living.

30. Does a hospice referral mean giving up hope for the patient?

Many patients and families initially may dwell on their imminent loss of life when faced with a terminal illness rather than making the most of the remaining time. Hospice helps people to understand death as a life transition, which may lead to sadness, anger, and emotional pain as well as opportunities for reminiscence, laughter, reunion, and hope for living life to the fullest until death occurs.

31. What resources are available for more information about hospice?

Most hospice care agencies are listed in the yellow pages of the local telephone directory. For information in your area about Medicare-approved hospice care, contact the nearest Social Security Administration office. State and local health departments also have information, as do state hospice organizations. For free copies of the Medicare Handbook call 1-800-638-6833. The National Hospice Organization may be contacted at 1901 North Moore St., Suite 901, Arlington, VA 22209 (1-800-658-8898). The Internet has information for the general public as well as health care providers using the search words Hospice or Palliative Care. The Hospice Education Institute may be contacted at 5 Essex Square, P.O. Box 713, Essex, CT 06426. Hospice Link may be contacted at 1-800-331-1620.

ACKNOWLEDGMENT.   The author thanks the following people for their consultation on this chapter: Carolyn Jaffe, R.N.; Paula Nelson Marten, R.N., Ph.D., A.O.C.N.; Janelle McCallum Betley, R.N., B.S.N., M.S.M.; and Karen Saco, R.N., B.A.

BIBLIOGRAPHY

1. Banaszak-Holl J, Mor V: Differences in patient demographics and expenditures among Medicare hospice providers. Hospice J 11(3):1–19, 1996.
2. Donaldson MS, Field MJ: Measuring quality of care at the end of life. Arch Intern Med 158:121–128, 1998.
3. Doyle D, Hanks GWC, Macdonald N (eds): Oxford Textbook of Palliative Medicine, 2nd ed. Oxford, Oxford University Press, 1998.
4. Enck RE (ed): The Medical Care of Terminally Ill Patients. Baltimore, Johns Hopkins University Press, 1994.
5. Field MJ, Cassel CK (eds): Approaching Death: Improving Care at the End of Life. Washington, DC, National Academy Press, 1997.
6. Gordon AK: Hospice and minorities: A national study of organizational access and practice. Hospice J 11(1):49–70, 1996.
7. Groenwald SL: Cancer Nursing Principles and Practice, 4th ed. Sudbury, Jones & Bartlett, 1998.
8. Heaven CM, Maguire P: Disclosure of concerns by hospice patients and their identification by nurses. Palliat Med 11(4):283–290, 1997.
9. Hospice of Metro Denver: Hospice of Metro Denver Guide. Denver, Hospice of Metro Denver, 1996.
10. Jaffe C, Ehrlich CH: All Kinds of Love. Amityville, Baywood Publishing, 1997.
11. Merson M, Bradley EH: Enhancing awareness of hospice through physician assisted living: Public health perspectives. Conn Med 61(12):789–791, 1997.
12. National Hospice Organization: Medical Guidelines for Determining Prognosis in Selected Non-cancer Diseases. Arlington, VA, National Hospice Organization, 1995.
13. Sheehan DC, Forman WB (eds): Hospice and Palliative Care: Concepts and Practice. Boston, Jones & Bartlett, 1996.

V. Solid Tumors

60. HEAD AND NECK CANCER

Charles E. Leonard, B.A., M.D.

1. Explain the basic work-up for head and neck tumors.

A complete history and physical examination (thorough head and neck examination) are completed first. Diagnosis is confirmed by histologic examination of the lesion in question. Cervical lymphadenopathy can be evaluated with fine-needle aspiration. A chest radiograph is performed to rule out pulmonary metastasis. Bronchoscopy, direct laryngoscopy, and esophagoscopy (triple endoscopy) are done for staging purposes to rule out synchronous malignancies that may occur in 10% of patients. Other imaging studies that may prove useful include magnetic resonance imaging (MRI), computed tomography (CT) of the head and neck, panoramic evaluation of the mandible, angiography, and dental radiographs.

SINONASAL TUMORS

2. What is the most common malignancy of the sinonasal tract?

Squamous cell carcinoma accounts for more than 70% of the malignant lesions of the sinonasal tract. Minor salivary gland tumors comprise 10–15% of neoplasms of the sinonasal tract. Malignant melanoma occurs in 10–15% of nasal cavity tumors. Other histologic variants are lymphoma, esthesioneuroblastoma, sarcoma, and inverting papilloma. The most commonly involved site is the maxillary sinus, which is involved in about 70% of cases, followed by the nasal cavity in 20% and the ethmoid cavity in about 10%. Primary carcinomas of the frontal or sphenoid sinuses are rare.

3. List the most common signs and symptoms of patients with sinonasal tumors.

Unilateral nasal obstruction (48%)	Nasal discharge (37%)
Facial or palatal swelling (41%)	Epistaxis (35%)
Facial pain (41%)	

4. Do environmental factors play a role in sinonasal tract malignancies?

Nickel-refining processes have been implicated in squamous cell and anaplastic carcinomas, with a 250 times greater incidence than the general population and with a latent period of 18–36 years. Furniture workers exposed to hardwood dust have an increased incidence of adenocarcinoma of the ethmoid sinus. One of the better-known causative agents for maxillary sinus tumors is Thorotrast, a contrast agent that contains the radioactive metal thorium. It was used in the past to image the maxillary sinus. Workers involved in bookmaking or the production of isopropanol and mustard gas, as well as painters of luminous watch dials (use of radioactive paint), have been shown to be at a higher risk for sinonasal tract malignancies.

5. What are the most common metastatic tumors to the sinonasal tract?

The most common primary sources are kidney, breast, and lung, from which carcinomas metastasize to the maxillary, ethmoid, frontal, and sphenoid sinus in descending order. By far, renal cell carcinoma leads the list of neoplasms that metastasize to the sinonasal tract. Other sites in order of frequency are breast and lung. The most common sites of metastasis are the maxillary antrum and nasal cavity.

6. Discuss the treatment options for sinonasal carcinomas.

Surgery is the mainstay of treatment and is often combined with radiation therapy for positive margins, advanced disease, and perineural and perivascular invasion. Radiation alone may be used for unresectable lesions, lymphoreticular tumors, or poor surgical candidates. Chemotherapy currently is used mostly in palliation.

ORAL CAVITY

7. The oral cavity comprises which structures?

The oral cavity is the region from the vermilion border of the lips to the junction of the hard and soft palates superiorly and the circumvallate papillae inferiorly. The lips, buccal mucosa, alveolar ridges, retromolar trigone, anterior two-thirds of the tongue (oral tongue), floor of the mouth, and hard palate are also included.

8. What is the most common oral cancer? What risk factors are associated with oral cancer?

Squamous cell carcinoma represents over 95% of the oral malignancies. Others include minor salivary gland tumors, sarcomas, lymphomas, and melanomas. Other histologic types in descending order of frequency are lymphomas, minor salivary gland tumors, sarcomas, and melanomas. According to 1987 National Cancer Institute statistics, oral cancer comprises 4% of cancers in men and 2% in women. Smoking and alcohol ingestion are strongly linked to oral cancer, and concomitant use appears to have a synergistic effect. Patients who smoke more than 20 cigarettes a day have a sixfold increase in oral cancer. More than 6 ounces of hard liquor per day results in a tenfold increase of oral cancer. Excessive use of both tobacco and alcohol results in a 15-fold increased risk of oral cancer compared with abstinence from both substances. Patients cured of their original cancer who continue to smoke have about a 40% chance of developing a second head and neck primary. About 95% of the patients are over the age of 40, with an average age of 60 years.

9. Which areas of the oral cavity are most often associated with malignancy?

Excluding the lip, over 75% of the cases involving the oral cavity involve only 10% of the oral cavity—the anterior floor of the mouth along the gingivobuccal sulcus and lateral border of the tongue to the retromolar trigone and the anterior tonsillar pillar. This may be due to the flow and pooling of carcinogens in these areas. The most commonly involved site is the lip (45%), followed by the oral tongue (17%), floor of the mouth (12%), and lower gingiva (12%). Thirty-five percent of patients with oral tongue lesions present with evidence of adenopathy and 5% are bilateral. Thirty percent of patients without clinically positive nodes will develop neck disease if left untreated (either by neck dissection or radiotherapy).

10. What treatment modalities are available for oral cancer?

In general, radiation therapy and surgical therapy offer equal cure rates for small (T1 or T2) lesions. Radiation therapy can often result in superior speech and swallowing; however, this must be balanced with diminution of taste, xerostomia, and duration of treatment (usually 6 weeks). Radiation therapy is administered in two ways; either external beam radiotherapy or use of radioactive sources implanted into and around the tumor itself (brachytherapy). Radiotherapy also may result in complications involving the mandible, with complications occurring in approximately 6% of patients treated with external radiotherapy only and 10–20% treated with combinations of external radiotherapy and implants. Since surgical therapy is more rapid (not requiring a course as lengthy as radiotherapy) with equal cure rates, it is generally the most common treatment for smaller, early-stage lesions. Combined therapy (surgery and radiation) provides better cure rates for larger and more advanced (stages III and IV) cancers than either modality alone.

OROPHARYNGEAL CANCER

11. The oropharynx comprises what structures?

The base of the tongue (posterior to the circumvallate papillae), soft palate, uvula, tonsillar pillars, tonsillar fossa, tonsils, and posterior pharyngeal wall comprise the oropharynx. Waldeyer's ring is lymphatic tissue that lines the nasopharynx and oropharynx and is made up of the pharyngeal (adenoid), palatine, and lingual tonsils.

12. What are the most common malignancies of the oropharynx? Where are they located?

Squamous cell carcinoma accounts for 95% of the malignancies in the oropharynx. The tonsil and tonsillar fossa are the most common locations. Waldeyer's ring is a common site for head and neck lymphomas and accounts for about 16% of oropharyngeal malignancies. The remaining malignancies are the same as for oral carcinoma (see question 8).

13. Give the prognosis for base of tongue carcinoma.

The prognosis is often poor because of late diagnosis and regional metastasis to the cervical lymph nodes, which is about 70% due to the delay in diagnosis. Bilateral cervical metastasis is not unusual and occurs in about 30% of patients. Symptoms often include dysphagia, odynophagia, referred otalgia, "hot potato voice," and trismus. Approximately 50% of patients requiring a total glossectomy for treatment will require a laryngectomy to prevent aspiration.

14. Do oropharyngeal lesions in other sites have a high risk of lymph node involvement?

Approximately 40–50% and 70–80% of patients with anterior tonsillar pillar cancers and tonsillar fossa lesions have clinically evident disease. The risk of clinically occult disease at presentation is 10–15% and 50–60%, respectively. Patients with soft palate carcinoma have a 40–50% incidence of palpable neck disease (10% bilateral) at presentation, and another 20% have subclinical disease.

15. How is oropharyngeal cancer treated?

Early T1 or T2 lesions have equal cure rates with either radiotherapy or surgery; however, functional results may be slightly better with radiotherapy. More advanced lesions have usually been managed with a combination of radiotherapy and surgery. Some practitioners have argued that even advanced lesions should be treated with radiotherapy alone (reserving surgery for local-regional failures). The functional results after radical surgery may severely compromise quality of life without offering significant improvements in cure rates.

16. What is the main cause of treatment failure and death in patients who present with early-stage head and neck cancers?

Second primaries are the chief cause of failure in such patients. Daily treatment with isotretinoin is effective in preventing second primary tumors in patients previously treated for squamous cell carcinoma. Isotretinoin does not, however, prevent recurrences of the original tumor in local, regional, or distant sites.

NASOPHARYNX

17. Give the anatomic boundaries of the nasopharynx.

The nasopharynx extends from the base of the skull to the soft palate. The nasopharynx includes the eustachian tube, torus tubarus (the cartilaginous crescent-shaped posterior lip of the eustachian tube), and fossa of Rosenmüller (lateral nasopharyngeal recess), which is the most common site of nasopharyngeal carcinoma.

18. Which malignancies are found in the nasopharynx?

Malignancies of the nasopharynx can be divided into three main groups under light microscopy:

1. Squamous cell carcinomas (keratinizing, nonkeratinizing, and undifferentiated) (71%)
2. Lymphomas (18%)
3. Miscellaneous cancers consisting of adenocarcinomas, plasma cell myelomas, adenoid cystic carcinomas, melanomas, and fibrosarcomas (11%)

19. Describe the World Health Organization (WHO) classification system of nasopharyngeal carcinoma (NPC).

WHO divides the squamous cell carcinomas into three entities:
Squamous cell carcinomas (WHO type 1) (25%)
Nonkeratinizing carcinomas (WHO type 2) (12%)
Undifferentiated carcinomas (WHO type 3) (63%)

20. What are the clinical signs and symptoms of NPC?

Unilateral neck mass (60%) and aural fullness (41%) are the most common signs and symptoms. Other findings include hearing loss (37%), epistaxis (30%), nasal obstruction (29%), head pain (16%), and ear pain (14%). Adults with unilateral serous otitis media or a cranial nerve VI palsy should have a careful examination of the nasopharynx.

21. How often are cervical lymph nodes involved in patients with NPC?

Approximately 85–90% of patients have clinically evident lymph node metastases at presentation, and 50% of these are bilateral. Of note, some authors assert that the probability of neck metastasis does not correlate with T stage. Patients without clinical neck disease at presentation have a 30–50% risk of developing neck metastases if the neck is untreated.

22. What tests are helpful in the work-up of NPC?

A CT scan displays skull base invasion, which occurs in about 25% of cases. Immunologic and biochemical investigations have confirmed that the Epstein-Barr virus (EBV) is associated with NPC. Indirect immunofluorescence for immunoglobulins and antibodies to viral caspid antigen (VCA) and to the diffuse component of the early antigen (EA) are the most sensitive for diagnosis of NPC (the VCA [IgG] is the more specific test of the two). The antibody-dependent cell-mediated cytotoxicity (ADCC) is predictive of prognosis. The polymerase chain reaction (PCR) can be used to test for the presence of EBV genomes in metastatic squamous cell carcinoma of the neck obtained by fine-needle aspiration.

23. How is NPC treated?

Although the initial treatment of choice has been external-beam supravoltage radiotherapy (6500–7000 cGy), more recent evidence has suggested that the addition of chemotherapy may have a significant impact on increasing local control and survival.

LIP CANCER

24. How common is lip cancer?

Lip cancer is the most common malignant tumor of the oral cavity, accounting for approximately 40% of cases. About 90% of lip carcinomas are squamous cell, and about 90% of these occur on the lower lip.

25. What is a keratoacanthoma?

Keratoacanthoma is a benign, self-limiting epithelial lesion that can mimic squamous cell carcinoma. It appears as an ulcerated, circumscribed lesion with elevated or rolled margins, a keratinized central region, and an indurated base. It has a rapid initial growth phase and may be present for weeks or even months. Incisional biopsy is important for lesions that are present for several weeks to rule out squamous cell carcinoma.

26. What negative prognostic factors are important with respect to lip cancer?

Large primary tumor (> 3 cm)   Poorly differentiated histology
Cervical node metastasis   Mandibular invasion
Recurrent tumors   Commissure lesions
Perineural invasion

Primary lip cancers < 2 cm have a 5-year survival rate of about 90%. Larger tumors, such as those involving the mandible, have a 5-year survival rate of < 50%. The likelihood of recurrence correlates directly with the size of the primary tumor (e.g., a recurrence rate of 40% for lesions > 3 cm). Cervical nodal metastases decrease survival to between 25% and 50%. Well-differentiated squamous cell lesions have a higher survival rate (86–90%) than poorly differentiated lesions (38–62%). Recurrence reduces the 5-year survival rate to < 50%. Perineural invasion also is associated with a poor outcome.

27. Are other tumors associated with the lips?

Basal cell carcinoma is the second most common malignancy of the lips. It is actually more common in the upper lip than squamous cell carcinoma. These tumors are very slow-growing and rarely metastasize.

Minor salivary gland tumors are more commonly (85% of cases) associated with the upper lip. Only 17% of these minor salivary gland tumors are malignant, and the most common minor salivary gland neoplasm is a pleomorphic adenoma (a benign neoplasm). Other tumor types include melanoma, microcystic adenexal carcinoma, Merkel's cell carcinoma, malignant fibrous histiocytoma, and malignant granular cell tumors.

HYPOPHARYNGEAL CANCER

28. The hypopharynx comprises which structures?

The hypopharynx extends from the hyoid bone superiorly to the inferior border of the cricoid cartilage inferiorly. It is subdivided into three regions: piriform sinus (fossa), postcricoid region, and posterior hypopharyngeal wall.

29. Which areas of the hypopharynx are most commonly involved?

Piriform sinus (70%)
Postcricoid area (15%)
Posterior pharyngeal wall (< 15%)

30. What are some of the most common signs and symptoms of hypopharyngeal cancer?

Sore throat, odynophagia, dysphagia, unilateral ear pain, or enlarged neck nodes may be presenting signs associated with hypopharyngeal tumors.

31. Does hypopharyngeal cancer have unique pathologic characteristics?

As in other areas of the aerodigestive tract, epidermoid carcinoma accounts for 95% of the lesions. Most of the remaining 5% are adenocarcinomas. Submucosal spread is common and is more prevalent as the tumor approaches the cervical esophagus. Satellite tumors, or "skip areas," also are more common in this region. Cervical lymph node metastasis occurs in 75% of piriform sinus lesions, 40% of postcricoid lesions, and 60% of posterior hypopharyngeal wall lesions. Patients presenting without neck metastases will eventually manifest disease in 40–50% of cases if the neck is untreated.

32. How is hypopharyngeal cancer managed?

Radiation therapy alone may be used for small lesions (T1 and T2), and surgery is reserved for salvage if primary radiotherapy fails. Combined surgery and radiotherapy are used for larger lesions.

33. Does the addition of chemotherapy to surgery or radiotherapy improve local control or survival rates in advanced head and neck cancers?

Other than in the nasopharynx, no randomized trials have shown a significant benefit in local control or survival when chemotherapy is added to surgery or radiation alone or administered with/without radiation preoperatively. However, some recent evidence suggests that the combination of radiation and chemotherapy after surgical resection in some "high-risk" patients may result in significant survival and local control rates over radiation alone. This point is currently under study.

LARYNGEAL CARCINOMA

34. Is the larynx divided into separate structures?

The larynx is anatomically composed of the supraglottic, glottic, and subglottic regions. The supraglottic larynx contains the epiglottis, false vocal cords, ventricles, aryepiglottic folds, and arytenoids. The glottis consists of the true vocal cords and their commissures. The subglottic region is immediately beneath the vocal cords.

35. What is the most common benign neoplasm of the larynx?

Squamous papillomas are the most common benign laryngeal neoplasm and account for about 80% of benign laryngeal tumors. They are generally divided into juvenile- and adult-onset papillomas. Juvenile papillomas may have a viral etiology and commonly occur in infancy or childhood and present as hoarseness or stridor. Juvenile papillomatosis may be very aggressive, requiring multiple surgical procedures for control and protection of the airway. Adult-onset papillomas are commonly solitary and less aggressive than their juvenile counterpart. In many cases, a single surgical procedure may produce a cure.

36. Discuss the signs and symptoms associated with laryngeal neoplasms.

Hoarseness is the cardinal sign of laryngeal cancer. Dyspnea and stridor occur later when associated with airway obstruction. Pain may be confined to the throat or referred to the ipsilateral ear. Dysphagia and odynophagia are present with extralaryngeal involvement. Chronic cough and hemoptysis also are frequently present.

37. What are the important functions of the larynx?

Airway protection	Phonation
Respiration	Sphincteric action (Valsalva maneuver and lifting)

38. What is the most common laryngeal cancer? Where is it located?

Carcinoma of the glottic region (true vocal cords) is the most common type of laryngeal carcinoma (50–75%). Because it interferes with phonation, it is often diagnosed earlier than cancers in other areas of the aerodigestive tract. The most common malignant neoplasm of the larynx is squamous cell carcinoma. Other histopathologies are noninvasive squamous cell carcinoma (carcinoma in situ), small-cell carcinoma, and minor salivary carcinomas. Verrucous carcinoma also occurs in 1–2% of patients with carcinoma of the vocal cords.

39. Are there causes of vocal cord paralysis other than glottic cancer?

Vocal paralysis is a sign of disease and not a diagnosis. It may be due to a lesion anywhere from the cerebral cortex throughout the pathway of the vagus nerve to the muscles of the larynx. Surgical trauma is the most common cause of unilateral and bilateral vocal cord paralysis, most often occurring following thyroidectomy. Other surgical procedures associated with vocal cord paralysis include lung resection, carotid artery and cervical spine operations, mediastinoscopy, laryngectomy, radical neck dissection, and cardiac surgery. Other causes include malignancy (lung, esophageal, and thyroid), trauma, inflammation (pulmonary tuberculosis, jugular thrombophlebitis, thyroiditis, meningitis, and influenza), neurologic disease (cerebrovascular disease, Parkinson's disease, multiple sclerosis, poliomyelitis, amyotrophic lateral sclerosis, and epilepsy), and idiopathic causes.

40. How is carcinoma of the larynx managed?

For early stage (T1–T2) carcinoma of the larynx radiotherapy has generally been the treatment of choice, reserving surgery for salvage therapy. Although cordectomy and hemilaryngectomy result in similar high cure rates, resulting voice quality is not comparable to irradiation. There is even recent evidence that verrucous carcinoma of the glottic region (once thought incurable with radiation) can be managed successfully with radiation therapy alone, reserving surgery for salvage.

41. What is the best therapy for advanced laryngeal cancer?

Unfortunately, there is no clear answer to this question. Although surgery followed by radiation therapy has been the traditional management for advanced tumors (radiation alone for unresectable lesions), results have not been satisfactory. For unresectable tumors no consistent data support the use of chemotherapy (either alone or in addition to radiotherapy) to improve local control or survival; however, different radiation regimens utilizing multiple daily fractions (hyperfractionated radiotherapy) have been shown to have some success in improving local control and possibly survival rates. A number of trials currently under way will examine the role of all three treatment modalities for efficacy in cure as well as quality of life.

42. Since chemotherapy does not improve local control or survival, does it have a role in the management of head and neck tumors?

Substantial evidence suggests that when chemotherapy is added to radiotherapy, laryngeal function can be preserved in a large proportion of patients with more advanced laryngeal cancers that otherwise might have required laryngectomy. In addition, the survival of patients who have not undergone surgery is not compromised by this "organ preservation" management.

43. What is the risk of lymphatic spread in laryngeal cancer?

Fifty-five percent of patients with supraglottic cancer present with clinically positive nodes at diagnosis, and 16% are bilateral. Thirty-three percent of cases with clinically uninvolved neck lymph nodes will manifest clinically positive nodes if the neck is observed. Because the true vocal cords essentially have no or very little lymphatic drainage, the probability of cervical metastases in T1 and T2 cord lesions is 0–2% and 3–7%, respectively. However, the probability for cervical metastasis in T2–T3 or T2–T4 lesions is approximately 20–30%.

SALIVARY GLAND NEOPLASMS

44. Which salivary glands are responsible for most of the neoplasms?

Tumors of the parotid, submandibular, and sublingual salivary glands are termed major salivary gland tumors. Minor salivary gland tumors originate in the oral cavity, nasal cavity, nasopharynx, larynx, and trachea. About 80% of all salivary gland neoplasms arise in the parotid gland, 10–15% in the submandibular gland, and the remaining in the sublingual gland and minor salivary glands. The smaller the gland of origin, the more likely the tumor may be malignant. Approximately 80% of parotid tumors are benign, whereas 50% of submandibular and less than 40% of sublingual and minor salivary gland tumors are benign.

45. What is the most common salivary gland tumor in children?

Pleomorphic adenomas (mixed tumors), which are benign epithelial neoplasms, are the most common salivary gland tumors in children. Hemangiomas (benign nonepithelial vascular tumors) and mucoepidermoid carcinomas (malignant epithelial tumors) are the second most common salivary gland tumors in children. Other benign tumors include lymphangioma, lymphoepithelial tumor, and Warthin's tumor. Most of the malignant tumors arise in the parotid gland (85%), and approximately 50% of these are mucoepidermoid carcinoma. Acinic carcinoma is the second most frequently encountered malignant epithelial tumor, followed by adenoid cystic carcinoma, adenocarcinoma, and undifferentiated carcinoma.

46. What is the most common parotid gland tumor in adults?

Pleomorphic adenoma is the most common tumor of the parotid gland in adults (approximately 50%). In fact, this benign neoplasm is the most common tumor for each of the salivary glands and makes up about 65% of all salivary gland tumors. The second most common benign tumor of the parotid is Warthin's tumor (papillary cystadenoma lymphomatosum), which accounts for 6–10% of all parotid neoplasms. Other benign entities include oncocytoma, monomorphic adenoma, and benign lymphoepithelial lesions.

47. What is the most common malignancy of the parotid gland?

Mucoepidermoid carcinoma accounts for 6–9% of all major salivary gland neoplasms and 30% of malignant tumors of the parotid. Other malignancies include malignant mixed tumor, acinic cell carcinoma, adenocarcinoma, squamous cell carcinoma, undifferentiated carcinoma, and lymphoma.

48. What is the most common malignancy of the submandibular gland and minor salivary glands?

Adenoid cystic carcinoma accounts for 30–50% of malignant tumors of the submandibular and minor salivary glands. Perineural invasion, a typical feature of this neoplasm, makes eradication of this tumor difficult. Mucoepidermoid carcinoma is the next most common malignancy (20%), and the remainder of the malignant tumors include the same entities as the parotid gland.

49. Are some types of malignant salivary gland tumors more aggressive than others?

Salivary gland tumors have been divided into high-grade or more aggressive pathologies and low-grade types, which are not considered to be as aggressive. Malignant mixed tumors, adenoid cystic carcinoma, salivary duct carcinoma, lymphoepithelioma, and high-grade mucoepidermoid carcinoma are considered to be high-grade lesions. Acinic cell carcinoma and low-grade mucoepidermoid carcinoma are considered to be low-grade lesions.

50. How often do malignant parotid tumors involve cervical lymph nodes?

The probability of lymph node metastasis depends on the histologic type and size of the parotid tumor. High-grade tumors have clinically evident cervical lymph node metastases in 20–30% of patients. Forty percent to 50% of patients with high-grade lesions and 5% with low-grade lesions have been found to have clinically undetected lymph node involvement. Early stage (T1 and T2) tumors also have a 5% chance of subclinical lymph node involvement versus 50% for later-stage tumors.

51. How accurate is fine-needle aspiration in the diagnosis of head and neck and salivary gland neoplasms?

Although the results depend on the skill, expertise, and experience of the cytopathologist, fine-needle aspiration for squamous cell carcinoma of the head and neck has been reported to be > 90% accurate. The diagnostic accuracy for salivary gland neoplasms is somewhat less, between 60% and 80%. Use of fine-needle aspiration has not been associated with tumor seeding in the needle tract.

52. What is the treatment of choice for salivary gland neoplasms?

Surgical excision is the treatment of choice. Most parotid lesions are present in the region of the tail and are superficial to the facial nerve. Therefore, they are amenable to a superficial parotidectomy with identification and preservation of the facial nerve. Occasionally, the deep lobe may be involved, requiring a total parotidectomy. Submandibular gland lesions are usually limited to the gland, and gland excision is the treatment of choice. Malignant tumors of the submandibular gland may extend beyond the gland to important structures such as the marginal branch of the facial nerve, hypoglossal nerve, lingual nerve, mandible, tongue, and floor of the mouth. Radiation therapy is added postoperatively for malignant tumors with positive margins, nerve or deep lobe involvement, lymph node metastasis, extraglandular extension, rupture of the capsule, or very large lesions (> 5 cm). For benign lesions, postoperative radiation is added when there is tumor spillage, after two to three recurrences, or when questions of malignant transformation exist. Neutron therapy has been found to be more effective than supravoltage radiotherapy in a recent randomized trial. However, this study has been criticized because of the differences in patient characteristics between the two groups.

BIBLIOGRAPHY

1. Bailey JB, Calhoun KH, Coffey AR, Neely JG (eds): Head and Neck Surgery—Otolaryngology. Philadelphia, J.B. Lippincott, 1993.
2. Feinmesser R, Miyazaki I, et al: Diagnosis of the nasopharyngeal carcinoma by DNA amplification of tissue obtained by fine-needle aspiration. N Engl J Med 326:17–21, 1992.
3. Lee KJ: Essential Otolaryngology, 5th ed. New York, Medical Examination, 1991.
4. Lippman SM, Hong WK: Second malignant tumors in head and neck squamous cell carcinoma: The over-shadowing threat for patients with early-stage disease. Int J Radiat Oncol Biol Phys 17:691–694, 1989.
5. Moss WT, Cox JD (eds): Radiation Oncology: Rationale, Techniques, Results, 6th ed. St. Louis, Mosby, 1989.
6. Million RR, Cassisi NJ (eds): Management of Head and Neck Cancer: A Multidisciplinary Approach, 2nd ed. Philadelphia, J.B. Lippincott, 1993.
7. Perez CA, Brady LW (eds): Principles and Practice of Radiation Oncology, 3rd ed. Philadelphia, Lippincott-Raven, 1997.
8. Pfister DG, et al: Larynx preservation with combined chemotherapy and radiation therapy in advanced but resectable head and neck cancer. J Clin Oncol 9:850–859, 1991.
9. Stell PM: Adjuvant chemotherapy in head and neck cancer. Semin Radiat Oncol 2:195–205, 1992.
10. Thawley SE, Panje WR, Batsakis JG, Lindberg RD (eds): Comprehensive Management of Head and Neck Tumors, 2nd ed. Philadelphia, W.B. Saunders, 1998.

61. BREAST CANCER

Bronagh P. Murphy, M.D., and Scot M. Sedlacek, M.D.

1. What does lobular carcinoma in situ (LCIS) represent?

It is currently believed that LCIS does not represent malignancy (contrary to the "carcinoma" in its name), but rather a marker for a woman who is at increased risk for the development of breast cancer. Some pathologists are attempting to change the name to **lobular neoplasia**, which also includes atypical lobular neoplasia. In women with lobular neoplasia, the risk of breast cancer development is approximately 1% per year and persists indefinitely. Two-thirds of breast cancer cases occur in the ipsilateral breast and the remaining one-third occur in the contralateral breast. Nearly 50% of the invasive cancers that develop are invasive lobular carcinomas, which is a much higher figure than that seen in the general population of patients with breast cancer (7%).

2. After recognizing LCIS on a breast biopsy, what recommendations should be made concerning therapy?

Because LCIS is only a marker for the high risk of developing breast cancer, the woman should be placed on a close follow-up program consisting of monthly breast self-examination, yearly mammography, and a physician-conducted physical examination every 6 months. If other significant risk factors are present with a diagnosis of LCIS, such as a first-degree relative with breast cancer, and the patient is unwilling to accept this markedly increased risk, the other treatment option is bilateral prophylactic total mastectomy. Removing all of the breast tissue (including the nipple/areolerlomytex) should greatly reduce the probability of the subsequent development of breast cancer, but does not completely eliminate such a risk. Excision, radiation, and systemic therapy have no role in the treatment of LCIS. Women with LCIS have been included in the Breast Cancer Prevention Trial to determine whether tamoxifen can decrease the risk of breast cancer; however, results from the study will not be available for a few years.

3. How does ductal carcinoma in situ (DCIS) typically present and what is the appropriate treatment?

DCIS is a proliferation of malignant cells within the ductal system without evidence of stromal invasion and may potentially progress to invasive cancer. DCIS typically presents as abnormal calcifications seen on a mammogram. Before 1985, the standard of care was mastectomy with or without an axillary dissection, a modality that carried close to a 98% cure rate. The incidence of positive lymph node metastases in pure DCIS is <1%. Therefore, axillary dissections should not be routinely performed in women with DCIS; sadly, the most frequent procedure for such women in the United States remains the modified radical mastectomy. The National Surgical Adjuvant Breast Project (NSABP) protocol B-17 was published in 1993. Women with DCIS were treated with either a lumpectomy (with negative margins) or lumpectomy with radiation. Recurrence rates were 5.1% and 2.1% per year, respectively. Thus, breast conservation with radiation therapy offers a woman a high chance of retaining her breast and a minimal risk of ultimately dying from breast cancer. The Van Nuys Breast Center has developed a classification system for DCIS that uses histology size and margins to determine the appropriate treatment involving excision alone, excisions and radiation, or mastectomy. Confirming studies ultimately will prove the validity of the Center's classification system.

4. Do hormone receptors and/or DNA analysis currently have any role in DCIS?

No. the most important issue for the pathologist evaluating a case of suspected DCIS is whether there are any areas of invasive cancer. Therefore, all of the tissue is processed for histologic examination and none is preserved fresh for estrogen/progesterone receptor and/or DNA analysis. This information was of no value when the standard treatment for DCIS was total mastectomy, which provided a nearly 98% cure rate. Because breast conservation is presently being used more frequently for DCIS, hormone receptors and DNA analysis may play a role in determining the risk of local recurrence and possibly which cases are likely to recur locally as infiltrating ductal carcinoma.

5. Which surgical procedure is more aggressive and therefore offers a woman the best chance to live cancer-free after 10 years: modified radical mastectomy (MRM) or lumpectomy with radiation therapy (RT)?

For the woman with a breast cancer that is small enough (4–5 cm maximum diameter) to be excised with negative surgical margins and who is left with sufficient residual breast tissue for an acceptable cosmetic, postoperative RT to the breast offers her the *same* long-term prognosis for survival as a woman who has her entire breast removed via mastectomy. The two therapies obviously are quite different, with certain advantages and disadvantages that the patient and physician should discuss. The advantages and disadvantages of the two options are outlined below.

	Advantages	*Disadvantages*
Mastectomy	No need for RT	No breast
	No need for ipsilateral mammograms	May need breast reconstruction
Lumpectomy/RT	Have a breast	Need RT for 5–6 weeks
	No need for breast reconstruction	Risk of local recurrence
		Still needs mammograms of irradiated breast

6. What are the indications for RT in women treated with MRM?

1. Large T3 (>5 cm) primary tumors
2. Any T4 (skin or chest wall involvement) primary tumors
3. Inflammatory breast cancer (T4d)

4. ≥ 4 lymph nodes involved with cancer
5. Spread of the cancer outside of the lymph node capsule into the surrounding perinodal fat
6. Positive surgical margin

Any one of the above six clinicopathologic findings places a woman at significant (>20%) risk for local/regional recurrence on the chest wall after mastectomy and should prompt her physician to seriously consider RT.

7. In women treated with MRM but without postoperative RT who then develop a local recurrence on the chest wall, what therapeutic and diagnostic options should be considered?

1. To provide the best chance for local control, attempts should be made to excise the entire recurrence with negative surgical margins.

2. A metastatic work-up should be performed (bone scan, computed tomography [CT] scans of the chest and abdomen): one-fourth to one-third of women will have demonstrable deposits at the time of local recurrence.

3. RT should be administered not only to the site of recurrence but to the entire chest wall and draining lymph node chains, because they also are at risk of multifocal recurrence.

4. Adjuvant chemotherapy vs. hormonal therapy: approximately 20% of patients at risk following an isolated local recurrence will develop metastatic disease each year. Therefore, by 10 years 93% of the women have developed metastases and ultimately will die of their cancer; this statistic indicates that a local occurrence portends dissemination, even after preventive treatment with chemotherapy and/or hormonal therapy is attempted. Only one study published to date demonstrates that adjuvant tamoxifen delayed metastases by $4\frac{1}{2}$ years.

8. Is inflammatory breast cancer (redness and swelling of the overlying skin) a surgical emergency that warrants excision prior to rapid growth by this most aggressive malignancy?

On the contrary, attempts at complete surgical excision are fraught with complications and poor outcomes due to the cancer rapidly spreading through the skin and lymphatics. Initially, some form of biopsy should be performed to diagnose the process, including determinations of hormone receptors, followed by neoadjuvant or induction chemotherapy in an attempt to cytoreduce the tumor. A multimodality approach such as chemotherapy → surgery → chemotherapy → RT → hormonal therapy has improved outcome in a disease that in the past had a 1–2% 5-year survival rate to one with a 50–65% 5-year survival rate. In recent years, high-dose chemotherapy followed by stem cell rescue has been incorporated into the multimodality approach with promising early results.

9. How long should a patient be treated with adjuvant tamoxifen?

The answer to this question is not yet fully known. However, from extrapolation of current data, the standard of care in the United States is to treat patients with adjuvant tamoxifen for 5 years. The NSABP B-14 study of tamoxifen vs. placebo in node-negative, estrogen receptor (ER)-positive (+) women demonstrated no additional benefit for women treated with 10 years of tamoxifen vs. those treated with the 5-year regimen. The Scottish Adjuvant Trial, which included both ER+ and ER-negative (–) women, also was unable to show a benefit of 10 years of tamoxifen vs. 5 years. The Swedish Breast Cancer Co-operative Group showed a significant improvement in event-free and overall survival for women treated with 5 years of tamoxifen vs. 2 years.

10. Adjuvant tamoxifen has been shown to improve disease-free survival (DFS) and overall survival (OS). What other benefits are obtained from this hormonal agent?

- Decreased chest wall recurrences by 50%
- Decreased breast recurrences in lumpectomy/RT-treated patients by 50%
- Decreases new contralateral breast cancers by 50%
- Prevents calcium loss from the bone
- Improves lipid profile (decreases total cholesterol by lowering low-density lipoprotein [LDL] levels)
- Induces vaginal secretions in one-third of postmenopausal women

11. List the potential disadvantages of adjuvant tamoxifen.
- Exacerbation of preexisting hot flashes
- Menstrual irregularity in premenopausal women
- Vaginal discharge related to a resumption of vaginal secretions
- Increased incidence of endometrial cancer (~ 1 in 1500 chance/year)
- Cost of $85–$90/month
- Depression in 1–10% of patients
- Retinal effects (rare and usually reversible)
- Increased estrogen levels leading to PMSlike symptoms in young, premenopausal women
- Risk of thrombosis

12. Which patients should be considered for postoperative adjuvant chemotherapy and/or adjuvant hormonal therapy?

Because of the hundreds of randomized and nonrandomized trials performed throughout the world, this issue has always been a difficult challenge for the medical oncologist. To meet this challenge the Early Breast Cancer Trialists' Collaborative Group published the Oxford Review of all randomized trials worldwide that concern the treatment of primary breast cancer. Currently, 10 years of follow-up information is available. Key points from the overview are as follows:

1. In all patients <50 years of age and >50 years (<50 years was used as a surrogate for pre-menopausal status) tamoxifen produced a 25% reduction in odds of recurrence and a reduced odds of mortality by 16%. The benefit was similar for both node-negative and node-positive patients.

2. Patients who derived the most benefit from tamoxifen were those ≥50 years and those with ER+ tumors.

3. Women >50 years benefited from combined chemotherapy and tamoxifen than either alone, whereas women <50 clearly benefited from adjuvant chemotherapy; however, benefit from combined chemoendocrine therapy for this group was less convincing.

13. Is sequencing of chemotherapy important?

Much clinical research effort is now being channeled into sequences of combination chemotherapy in an attempt to improve overall outcomes in breast cancer. One trial in Milan, Italy studied patients with breast cancer with four or more positive lymph nodes. All patients received eight cycles of CMF (cyclophosphamide, methotrexate, and 5-fluorouracil [5-FU]) and four cycles of doxorubicin (Adriamycin) intravenously each 21 days over 33 weeks. Group 1 received (alternating therapy) two cycles of CMF followed by one cycle of doxorubicin to the above total, whereas group 2 received (sequential) four cycles of doxorubicin followed by eight cycles of CMF. A significant disease-free and overall survival advantage was observed in the sequential arm at 10-year follow-up. The sequential arm allows increased dose intensity of drug without increasing dose level. The concept of dose density (increasing dose intensity by shortening treatment time intervals) is evolving into a potentially important tool in the current development of chemotherapeutic regimens for breast cancer.

14. How should treatment of a patient with metastatic disease be approached?

Because the current treatment is not curative, the goal of the physician caring for women with metastatic disease is **palliation**! The average woman with metastatic breast cancer will live 18–24 months, a figure that has changed minimally over the last 50 years of advances in cancer therapy.

The first goal in such patients is to determine if they will respond to hormonal manipulations. Overall responses are much greater in ER+ tumors (up to 60%), but responses of up to 20% may be seen in ER– tumors. Responses tend to last approximately 6–12 months but may be longer. In general, patients who have a good initial response to hormonal therapy usually have a higher chance of responding to second- and third-line agents than do patients who are initially unresponsive. Hormonal therapy includes agents such as tamoxifen, megestrol acetate, anastrozole, amino-glutethimide, diethystilbestrol (DES), phioxymesterolone, goserelin, and leuprolide. Newer hormonal agents, especially antiestrogens such as toremifene, are being developed and investigated in the treatment of breast cancer. Chemotherapy is widely used to treat patients with metastatic breast cancer and may be the modality of choice in patients with immediate life-threatening disease, such as multiorgan involvement, significant liver involvement, and/or lymphatic spread in the lung.

Finally, radiation is an invaluable tool for the palliation of painful bony metastases, impending cord compression, and superior vena cava syndrome.

15. Describe the role of biophosphonates in the treatment of breast cancer.

Pamidronate and other related biophosphonates inhibit osteoclast function. In prospective randomized trials, pamidronate has been shown to decrease the incidence of skeletal complications of bone metastases in patients with breast cancer, such as pathologic fracture rate, the need for pain medication and palliative radiation, and hypercalcemia. Such agents are gaining widespread use clinically as adjunctive therapy to chemotherapy and hormonal therapy.

16. When is sentinel lymph node sampling appropriate?

Axillary lymph node sampling has been a mainstay of oncologic diagnosis, as well as a valuable therapeutic and prognostic tool in the management of breast cancer. This basic tenet is now being challenged. Seventy to 80% have a negative axillary dissection for metastases and 5–20% develop lymphadema from axillary lymph node sampling: many clinicians have investigated alternative methods to stage the cancer.

One approach has tried to develop other prognostic factors such as ER status, proliferative index, and tumor size as means of precisely defining risk enough to obviate the need for an axillary dissection. Unfortunately, a set of prognostic factors that can supplant axillary lymph node status as a more significant factor in predicting the rate of recurrence has not been defined yet.

Another approach is to limit the axillary sampling to the first set of lymph nodes that the breast cancer drains to; therefore, if the first set does not have malignant cell involvement, the search may stop. Sentinel lymph node sampling is fast becoming a more common procedure that American surgeons are using in an attempt to better define which patients truly need a more thorough axillary dissection, a procedure with attendant complications. With approximately a 97% negative predictive value in experienced hands, most clinicians would be willing to accept a 3% false-negative rate when faced with the choice of possible complications versus possible missed benefits of adjuvant therapy. It is a matter of time before all breast surgeons are trained in the limited axillary sampling technique.

CONTROVERSY

17. How effective is high-dose chemotherapy in the treatment of breast cancer?

Trials using high-dose chemotherapy and peripheral stem cell support have been mainly directed at two patient subgroups:

1. Patients with high-risk primary breast cancer (stage II or III breast cancer involving ≥10 axillary lymph nodes)

2. Patients with metastatic breast cancer.

In the first group of patients with high-risk breast cancer, Peters et al. reported a DFS rate of 72% at 3-year follow-up when the patients were treated with an intensive adjuvant chemotherapy, consisting of four cycles of cyclophosphamide, doxorubicin, and 5-FU (CAF) followed by one cycle of cisplatin, carmustine, and cyclophosphamide with autograft support. Large, randomized trials currently are being conducted on the basis of this trial and several other pilot studies comparing an intensive adjuvant approach to the conventional adjuvant approach. Until the results are published, high-dose chemotherapy in this setting remains investigational.

Conventionally dosed chemotherapy in metastatic breast cancer is given with palliative (not curative) intent. High-dose chemotherapy with peripheral stem cell support, on the other hand, was developed to improve patients' chance of survival. The results of many completed pilot studies reveal that although complete responses can be achieved in up to 70% of patients with metastatic breast cancer, the majority of patients relapse, resulting in a long-term remission rate of only 10–20%. One randomized study showed a statistically significant improvement in DFS vs. OS in patients treated with high-dose chemotherapy plus stem cell support compared to a group treated with conventional-dose chemotherapy. Large-scale randomized trials are needed to assess the efficacy of high-dose chemotherapy vs. conventional-dose chemotherapy in patients with metastatic breast cancer. Further developmental studies of the high-dose approach are needed to try to improve the overall long-term remission rate. Therefore, high-dose chemotherapy with peripheral stem cell support should still be considered an experimental approach.

BIBLIOGRAPHY

1. Banadonna G, Zambetti M, Valagussa P: Sequential or alternating doxorubicin and CMF in breast cancer with more than 3 positive nodes. Ten year results. JAMA 273:542, 1995.
2. Bezwoda WR, Seymour L, Dansey RD: High-dose chemotherapy with hematopoetic rescue vs. primary treatment for metastatic breast cancer: A randomized trial. J Clin Oncol 13:2483, 1995.
3. Early Breast Cancer Trialists' Collaborative Group: Systemic treatment of early breast cancer by hormonal, cytotoxic, or immune therapy. Lancet 1:71, 1992.
4. Fisher B, Anderson S, Redmond CK, et al: Reanalysis and results after 12 years of follow-up in a randomized clinical trial comparing total mastectomy with lumpectomy with or without irradiation in the treatment of breast cancer. N Engl J Med 333:1456, 1995.
5. Fisher B, Dignam J, Bryant J, et al: Five versus more than five years of tamoxifen therapy for breast cancer patients with negative lymph nodes and estrogen positive tumors. J NAH Cancer Ins 88:1529, 1996.
6. Fisher B, Digman J, Wolmark N, et al: Lumpectomy and radiation therapy for the treatment of intraductal breast cancer: Findings from National Surgical Adjuvant Breast and Bowel 1317. J Clin Oncol 16:441, 1998.
7. Giuliano AE, Jones RC, Brennan M and Statman R. Sentinel lymphadenectomy in breast cancer. J Clin Oncol 15:2345, 1997.
8. Harris J R, Lippman ME, Veronesi U, et al: Breast cancer. N Engl J Med 327:319, 1992.
9. Hortobagyi GN, Theriault RI, Porter L, et al: Efficacy of pamidronate in reducing skeletal complications in patients with breast cancer and lytic bone metastases. N Engl J Med 335:1785, 1996.
10. Krag D, Weaver D, Ashikaga T, et al: The sentinel node in breast cancer. A multicenter validation study. N Engl J Med 339:941, 1998.
11. Love RR, Mazess RB, Barden HS, et al: Effects of tamoxifen on bone mineral density in postmenopausal women with breast cancer. N Engl J Med 326:852, 1992.
12. Love RR, Newcomb PA, Wiebe DL, et al: Lipid and lipoprotein effects of tamoxifen therapy in postmenopausal women with node-negative breast cancer. J Natl Cancer Inst 82:1327, 1990.
13. Mansour EG, Gray R, Shatila AH, et al: Efficacy of adjuvant chemotherapy in high-risk node-negative breast cancer. An Intergroup Study. N Engl J Med 320:485, 1989.
14. Peter WP: High-dose chemotherapy and autologous bone marrow transplantation in the treatment of breast cancer. In DeVita VT Jr, Hellman S, Rosenberg SA (eds): Important Advances In Oncology, 5th ed. Philadelphia, Lippincott-Raven, pp 135–150, 1991.
15. Silverstein MJ, Paller DN, Waisman JR, et al: Prognostic classification of breast ductal carcinoma in situ. Lancet 345:1154, 1995.

62. LUNG CANCER

Karen Kelly, M.D.

1. What cancer is the leading cause of cancer deaths in both men and women in the United States?

Lung cancer. It is estimated that 171,000 Americans are diagnosed with lung cancer each year, and more than 85% die from the disease. Recently, lung cancer surpassed breast cancer as the leading cause of cancer deaths among women. This observation correlates with the increase in the number of women who smoke. In contrast, the number of men who smoke is decreasing. If a cigarette smoker quits smoking today, his or her risk of developing lung cancer declines, but even at 15 years the risk is still 4.0% (vs. 1.0% for a nonsmoker).

2. Besides smokers, who else gets lung cancer?

People exposed to asbestos (such as shipyard workers and insulators) and radon (from underground mining or previous radiation therapy) are at greater risk for lung cancer. Other substances associated with lung cancer include arsenic, nickel-cadmium, chromium, and chloromethyl ether. Underlying lung disease with scarring or chronic obstructive lung disease (COPD) predisposes patients to lung cancer. Passive smoking exposure accounts for 3–5% of all cases of lung cancer. These risks are dramatically increased in smokers vs. nonsmokers.

3. Patients with lung cancer often present with nonspecific pulmonary complaints such as cough, dyspnea, chest pain, hemoptysis, and/or weight loss. What test should raise your suspicion for lung cancer?

A mass on a chest radiograph. Although 85% of patients have symptoms, 15% are asymptomatic, and an incidental mass is discovered on a routine chest radiograph. Once a mass has been identified, the patient is presumed to have lung cancer until proved otherwise.

4. With what other symptoms may a patient with lung cancer present?

Various paraneoplastic syndromes are associated with lung cancer. Paraneoplastic syndromes are defined as signs and symptoms related to a peptide hormone secreted by the tumor. The most common are hypercalcemia associated with squamous cell lung cancer and hyponatremia associated with small-cell lung cancer. Treatment of the underlying tumor usually reverses the clinical manifestations of the paraneoplastic syndrome. In addition, return of the paraneoplastic syndrome may be the first sign of recurrence. Evidence of a paraneoplastic syndrome is not synonymous with metastatic disease. Documentation of metastatic disease is crucial to avoid subjecting a patient to palliative therapy when curative intervention is appropriate and vice versa.

5. Does the histologic type of lung cancer matter?

Yes. Management is based on whether the patient has small-cell lung cancer (SCLC) or non–small-cell lung cancer (NSCLC). Chemotherapy is the cornerstone of treatment for all patients with small-cell histology, whereas surgery, radiation, and/or chemotherapy may be recommended for patients with NSCLC. SCLC accounts for 20–25% of all lung cancers; therefore, most patients have NSCLC. NSCLC can be subdivided into adenocarcinoma (32%), squamous cell carcinoma (29%), large cell undifferentiated (9%), bronchoalveolar (3%), and unspecified (27%).

6. How does lung cancer spread?

NSCLC spreads to the peribronchial, hilar, then mediastinal lymph nodes. Distant sites of metastases include the opposite lung, liver, bone, brain, and adrenal glands. More than one-half of patients present with extrathoracic spread. Two-thirds of patients with SCLC present with extensive disease outside of the chest (liver, brain, bone, bone marrow).

7. Which tests can be used to identify areas of spread?

All patients require a complete history and physical examination, a routine complete blood count (CBC), and blood chemistries. For patients with NSCLC a staging work-up includes CT scan of the chest and abdomen, bone scan, and brain scan. If there is no evidence of metastatic disease and the patient is considered medically and surgically operable, a mediastinoscopy should be performed to stage the chest accurately. For patients diagnosed with SCLC the following additional tests are required: CT scan of the chest and abdomen, bone scan, brain scan, and bilateral bone marrow biopsies. Bone marrow biopsies are required only to prove that a patient has limited disease; otherwise, it is optional. Bone scans and brain scans are performed only if clinically indicated.

8. What are the stages of lung cancer?

The current staging schema for NSCLC uses the TNM classification to determine the extent of disease, which in turn determines treatment and prognosis. T describes the primary tumor, N identifies lymph node involvement, and M represents metastatic disease. The stages for NSCLC recently changed:

Stage I (T1N0M0, T2N0M0): tumor < 3cm (T1) or > 3 cm with or without extension to the visceral pleura (T2) and at least 2 cm from the carina; no lymph node or metastatic spread.

Stage II (T1N1M0, T2N1M0, T3N0M0): tumor as described in stage I but with extension into intrabronchial hilar lymph nodes (N1) or a tumor of any size that extends into the parietal pleura, chest wall, or mediastinal pleura (T3) but is not associated with lymph node involvement (N0).

Stage IIIa (T1–2N2M0, T3N1–2M0): tumor of any size (T1, T2) with ipsilateral mediastinal lymph node involvement (N2) or a T3 tumor with involvement of intrabronchial/hilar lymph nodes (N1) or ipsilateral mediastinal lymph node (N2).

Stage IIIb (T4 with any N or any T with N3): tumor of any size that invades mediastinal structures (heart, great vessels, esophagus, vertebrae) or is associated with a pleural effusion (T4) and/or involves contralateral hilar, mediastinal, or supraclavicular lymph nodes (N3).

Stage IV (any T or N with M1): tumor with evidence of distant metastasis.

Multiple tumor nodules: satellite tumors within the primary tumor lobe of the lung should be classified as T4. Intrapulmonary ipsilateral metastasis in a distant (separate) nonprimary tumor lobe(s) of the lung should be classsified as M1.

SCLC is staged as either limited or extensive disease. **Limited stage** is defined as disease confined to one hemithorax, mediastinal, hilar, or supraclavicular areas that can be encompassed within a single radiation therapy port. **Extensive stage** is any disease spread outside the previously stated areas.

9. What are the accepted treatment modalities for lung cancer?

For stage I and II NSCLC surgical resection of the lobe of the lung containing the tumor is the standard of care. Patients with stage IIIA disease represent a heterogenous population. Trials are under way to determine whether combined modality with chemotherapy plus radiation therapy with or without surgery is advantageous. For patients not eligible for trials the use of chemotherapy with radiation and/or surgery is a rational approach. Patients with stage IIIB disease are currently treated with chemotherapy plus radiation therapy given concurrently. Patients with metastatic disease are offered chemotherapy or best supportive care (which may include palliative radiation therapy). Concurrent radiation therapy and chemotherapy are the treatment of choice for patients with limited stage SCLC. Unlike NSCLC, all patients with extensive stage SCLC should receive chemotherapy because the majority will respond. Chemotherapy improves survival from 1 month without treatment to 9–12 months with treatment.

10. Does staging affect survival?

Yes. The following survival curve clearly demonstrates the impact of stage on 5-year survival in patients with NSCLC.

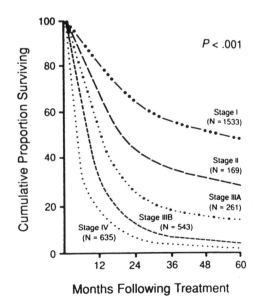

Survival of NSCLC patients by clinical stage. (From Mountain CF: Survival of NSCLC patients by clinical stage. Chest 89:225S–233S, 1986, with permission.)

The same holds true for patients with SCLC :

Limited SCLC	5–10% (5 yr), 15 months (median)
Extensive SCLC	0–1% (5 yr), 9 months (median)

11. How can we improve survival in lung cancer?

Because most patients die from distant metastases, the focus has been on developing more effective drugs. Several new chemotherapy agents (taxol, taxotere, gemcitabine, navelbine, topotecan, and CPT-11) that show increased activity with minimal toxicity have led to small advances in survival. For example, in patients with stage IV disease treated with newer agents, median survival has doubled from 6 to 12 months. The greatest impact, however, is expected to be in preventing tumor dissemination and/or killing micrometastatic disease associated with earlier stages of disease. Trials incorporating the new agents in the treatment of all stages of lung cancer are under way. Results are encouraging.

12. Do any tests detect lung cancer at an early, curative stage?

No. In the 1960s screening trials using chest radiograph and sputum cytology in a high-risk population of male smokers showed no survival benefit; this approach cannot be recommended. To date, no trial has evaluated chest radiographs alone, and a nationwide study is currently under way. Attempts to reevaluate sputum with more sensitive staining techniques are ongoing and show promising results.

CONTROVERSY

13. Should patients with stage IV NSCLC receive chemotherapy?

For:

1. Patients with NSCLC want therapy.

2. Patients who respond to chemotherapy live longer than patients who do not respond.

3. Patients who respond to therapy have a better quality of life.

4. Response can be predicted. Patients with good performance status, weight loss < 5%, female sex, and minimal tumor burden are more likely to respond to chemotherapy.

5. Four meta-analyses of randomized trials of chemotherapy vs. best supportive care concluded that chemotherapy offered a modest survival advantage over best supportive care.

6. The randomized trials of best supportive care vs. combination chemotherapy are flawed by small patient accruals, which do not allow detection of a small increase in survival.

7. Newer chemotherapy agents are more effective and less toxic.

Against:

1. Although some trials have shown a survival advantage, it is only in terms of weeks (7–17).

2. The response rate with the most active regimen is 20–30%; complete responders are rare (< 5%).

3. All drug regimens produce side effects.

BIBLIOGRAPHY

1. Bunn PA: Lung Cancer: Current Understanding of the Biology, Diagnosis, Staging, and Treatment [monograph]. 1992.
2. Bunn PA, Kelly K: New chemotherapeutic agents prolong survival and improve quality of life in non–small-cell lung cancer: Review of the literature and future directions. Clin Cancer Res In press, 1998.
3. Ihde DC: Chemotherapy of lung cancer. N Engl J Med 327:1434–1441, 1992.
4. Kelly K: Combined modality treatment for locally advanced non-small cell lung cancer. Semin Respir Crit Care Med 17:349–356, 1996.
5. Mountain CF: Revisions in the international system for staging of lung cancer. Chest 111:1710–1717, 1997.
6. Non-small Cell Lung Cancer Collaborative Group: Chemotherapy in non-small cell lung cancer: Meta-analysis using updated data on individual patients from 52 randomized clinical trials. BMJ 311:899–909, 1995.
7. Van Raemdonck DE, Schneider A, Ginsberg RJ: Surgical treatment for higher stage non-small cell lung cancer. Ann Thorac Surg 54:999–1013, 1992.

63. ESOPHAGEAL CANCER

Kathryn T. Howell, M.D.

1. What is the most common cell type in esophageal cancer?

The most common cell type in cancers found in the middle third of the esophagus is squamous cell carcinoma. Adenocarcinoma is more commonly seen in the lower third of the esophagus. Metastatic tumor, lymphomas, and sarcomas are very rare.

2. Does the incidence of esophageal cancer vary much geographically?

Esophageal carcinoma has the widest geographic variation of any malignancy with the highest rate in Hebi, China, and the lowest in Hunyuan, China. Although the rate of increase of squamous esophageal carcinoma has been steady since 1959, the rate of increase of adenocarcinoma has been on the rise. Esophageal carcinoma is more common in African Americans, although Caucasians have a greater incidence of adenocarcinoma. Men are more commonly affected than women.

3. What causes esophageal cancer in the United States?

Smoking has been proved to be associated with esophageal carcinoma, and alcohol also has been implicated as a causative factor in numerous studies. Worldwide, however, dietary and nutritional factors have been implicated as causative factors.

4. What other groups of people are at increased risk?

People with tylosis and achalasia have a high risk of esophageal carcinoma, with a much lower risk attributed to lye ingestion, Barrett's esophagus, esophageal diverticula, or webs.

5. How do most patients with esophageal cancer present?

The majority present with dysphagia and weight loss. Of interest, less than 50% present with odynophagia, despite the fact that symptoms do not generally appear until the diameter of the esophagus is less than 13 mm.

6. What are the best radiographic measures of resectability of esophageal cancer?

Resectability should be determined by the overall tumor burden, with consideration given to local factors in addition to ruling out distant metastatic disease. Barium swallow and endoscopic ultrasonography help to evaluate the length and circumferential involvement. Computed tomography (CT) is best at assessing local invasion as well as liver and adrenal metastases and celiac adenopathy, but it addresses poorly the length of the lesion. Magnetic resonance imaging (MRI) has many of the same qualities as CT but is better at defining the local vascular anatomy. The length of involvement of the esophagus is inversely related to curability. Tumors ≤ 5 cm have a 35% risk of metastatic disease, whereas 75% of tumors > 5 cm have metastases.

7. If surgery is considered for esophageal cancer, what other preoperative evaluations are useful?

A careful history and physical exam to evaluate patients for comorbid medical problems are essential. Routine chemistry screen (to evaluate nutritional status and metastatic disease to the liver and bone) and routine blood count as well the radiographic studies mentioned above should precede any consideration for surgery. Adequate cardiac evaluation (including electrocardiogram), pulmonary evaluation (including pulmonary function studies and, in the case of lesions of the upper two-thirds of the esophagus, bronchoscopy), and endoscopic evaluation with biopsy and brushings to confirm the histology are essential.

8. Are synchronous or metachronous second malignancies a significant problem in esophageal cancer?

Five percent to 12% of patients with esophageal carcinoma will have synchronous or metachronous malignancies of the aerodigestive tract, and about half of these are found in the head and neck. The oral cavity, pharynx, larynx, and lung are the most common sites.

9. Can esophageal cancer be surgically controlled?

It is estimated that only 20% of all esophageal cancers are truly localized to the esophagus. However, even though most patients are ultimately incurable, the only chance of local control as well as palliation should be aggressive attempts to control the primary tumor in the esophagus.

10. Is esophageal cancer ever considered cured?

Of patients resected for cure, only 20–25% will survive 5 years, regardless of the type of surgical resection. Unfortunately, 10-year survival continues to be less than 10% in some studies.

11. Does nutrition affect the surgical outcome of esophageal cancer?

Weight loss of greater than 10% preoperatively negatively influences subsequent survival; generally, patients with significant weight loss have more advanced disease. It has been shown that patients with optimal preoperative nutritional status have fewer complications; however, correcting nutritional status and/or weight loss before surgery does not change prognosis. Although nutritional status can be optimized with parenteral or intravenous alimentation, enteral feedings are preferred.

12. How large should surgical margins be in esophageal cancer?

Because the esophagus has no mesentery, segmental resection is not used as a curative surgical approach. Thus, the surgical approach includes removal of the tumor as well as the remaining distal esophagus and proximal stomach. Due to the lack of mesentery, esophageal cancer can spread a minimum of 5 cm in either direction. It is surprising that even in proximal esophageal lesions, 10% of patients have celiac lymph node metastases, and when the cancer is more distal, the number increases to as high as 50%.

13. What are advantages and disadvantages of surgery for esophageal cancer?

Although surgery alone can offer a 20% 5-year survival rate, operative mortality can range from 2–14%, with overall operative morbidity of 13–85%. Causes of morbidity include stricture, pneumonia, fistula, anastomotic and nonanastomotic leaks, adhesions, perforation, and bleeding. Surgical treatment is still difficult in the upper esophagus; irradiation tends to be used in this area.

14. What are advantages and disadvantages of radiation therapy in esophageal cancer?

Irradiation can be used for palliation with improvement in dysphagia in up to 75% of patients for 6–8 months. Cure can also be seen in 15–20% of selected patients. Treatment mortality is rare, but complications include perforation, hemorrhage, fistula, stricture, and pneumonitis. A course of treatment can take 5–7 weeks.

15. What are the contraindications to radiation therapy for esophageal cancer?

Established mediastinitis, hemorrhage, and tracheobronchial fistula.

16. Which drugs are effective against esophageal cancer?

Of the single agents tested, cisplatin and mitomycin appear to be the most active, with complete and partial responses between 14% and 40%. 5-Fluorouracil and bleomycin also have shown activity. Vindesine, vinorelbine, methylglyoxal-bis-guanylhydrazone (methyl-GAG), and paclitaxel (Taxol) appear promising. Multidrug regimens have had better total response rates.

17. How long do chemotherapy responses last in patients with esophageal cancers?

In general, patients receiving chemotherapy alone may tend to have advanced or inoperable disease. Responses in 25–35% of such patients are brief, lasting 1–2 months. Other patients may respond favorably for a median of 6–8 months with combination chemotherapy.

18. What is the best way to treat new esophageal cancers?

Currently, the most promising treatment for esophageal cancer appears to be chemotherapy combined with irradiation for inoperable disease and chemotherapy combined with irradiation followed by surgery for operable disease.

BIBLIOGRAPHY

1. Abeloff MO, Armitage JO, Lichter AS, Neiderhuber JE: Esophagus. In Clinical Oncology. New York, Churchill Livingstone, 1995, pp 1189–1208.
2. Bosset JF, Gignoux M, Triboulet JP, et al: Chemoradiotherapy followed by surgery compared with surgery alone in squamous-cell cancer of the esophagus. N Engl J Med 337:161–167, 1997.
3. Forastiere AA, Urba SG: Combined modality therapy for cancer of the esophagus. PPO Updates, Principles and Practice of Oncology 11:1–15, 1996.
4. Perez CA, Brady LW: Esophagus. In Perez CA, Brady LW (eds): Principles and Practice of Radiation Oncology. Philadelphia, J.B. Lippincott, 1992, pp 853–870.
5. Roth JA, Lichter AS, Putnam JB, Forastiere AA: Cancer of the esophagus. In DeVita VT Jr, Hellman S, Rosenberg SA (eds): Principles and Practice of Oncology, 4th ed. Philadelphia, J.B. Lippincott, 1993, pp 776–817.

64. GASTRIC CANCER

Dennis A. Sanders, M.D.

1. Is gastric cancer a common malignancy?

The incidence of gastric cancer is roughly 24,000 new cases per year since the late 1980s, which translates into a rate of 10:100,000 per year. For reasons that have not been fully understood, the incidence of gastric cancer in the United States has declined over the past seven decades, with a 60% decline in cancer mortality due to gastric cancer. However, of the new cases diagnosed each year, 60% eventually die from gastric cancer. In other countries, such as Japan, China, and Chile, the incidence of gastric cancer is roughly 75:100,000, making gastric cancer a major cause of mortality worldwide. Health care workers and scientists have been trying to discover why there is as much as a 7-fold difference in gastric cancer incidence worldwide, the answers to which may lead to unique strategies to prevent or treat gastric cancer.

2. Why are there differences in the incidence of gastric cancer around the world?

Epidemiologic studies suggest that environmental factors seem to be closely associated with the difference in gastric cancer incidence. Several population studies of migrants from high-incidence countries to low-incidence countries suggest that subsequent generations of the immigrant populations experience a significant decline in gastric cancer incidence, eventually mirroring that of the host country. Further studies have identified dietary factors, such as high intake of salted foods, smoked foods, and foods contaminated with aflatoxins, as causative factors for gastric cancer. Also noted is a two-fold higher incidence of gastric cancer in lower socioeconomic groups in the United States and Western Europe.

Potentially one of the most important risk factors identified since the late 1970s appears to be related to either exposure to or chronic infection by a bacterial pathogen known as *Helicobacter pylori*. *H. pylori* is unique in its ability not only to infect the human gastric mucosa under harsh conditions of low gastric pH but also to persist in the host for decades. It is speculated that the emergence of gastric cancer occurs decades after initial exposure to *H. pylori* through a series of several premalignant steps from gastric inflammation/ulceration to intestinal metaplasia and dysplasia and, finally, invasive cancer. Progression of these steps is thought to depend on the virulence of the bacterial strain, host genetic susceptibility to cancer, age at the time of *H. pylori* infection, and dietary influences.

Several studies have demonstrated *H. pylori* infection rates of 70–90% in high-incidence countries (developing world) versus rates of up to 30% in low-incidence countries, such as the United States. In the Andean region of Venezuela, gastric cancer is the leading cause of cancer mortality. Gastric biopsies obtained in a gastric cancer screening study revealed a prevalence rate of *H. pylori* infection in 95% of patients with atrophic gastritis or intestinal metaplasia, both known to be precancerous lesions.

3. Can gastric cancer be prevented?

Because gastric cancer is usually diagnosed in the more advanced stages, the long-term prognosis is poor. Therefore, strategies are being developed to take advantage of our expanding knowledge of causative factors for gastric cancer in an attempt to prevent this killer disease. With regard to *H. pylori*, Japanese researchers have reported that in patients with endoscopically detected early gastric carcinomas treated with surgery, no recurrences have been observed if patients were also successfully treated to eradicate *H. pylori* infection. From such studies, it is estimated that between 1 in 30 to 1 in 60 people infected with *H. pylori* will develop invasive gastric cancer. Therefore, it has been suggested that prophylactic treatment with antibiotics and acid-secretion blocking drugs may prevent gastric cancer in high-risk populations. In addition, *H. pylori* expresses various proteins on the bacterial coat that are immunogenic. Vaccines are currently being developed as another preventive approach. This approach may be especially appealing in developing countries such as southern China and Peru, where the prevalence of *H. pylori* infection ranges between 30% and 50% in children ages 1–5 and steadily rises to over 70% in the adult population.

Preventive dietary interventions also have been based on several epidemiologic observations that population deficiencies in nutrients such as beta-carotene, vitamin E, and selenium are associated with high gastric carcinoma incidence. The Henan Province in north-central China is such an area. Researchers supplemented the diets of 30,000 people at risk with selenium, vitamin E, and beta-carotene and found a significant decrease in gastric cancer incidence. These microurients are thought to act as antipromoting agents in the multistep process of carcinogenesis and to inhibit progressive damage of the gastric mucosa by *H. pylori*.

4. Is there a screening test for gastric cancer?

The incidence of gastric cancer in the United States is relatively small compared with other malignancies, and general population screening has not been deemed to be effective. However, in Japan, where gastric cancer causes 40% of all deaths from malignancy, an extensive screening program exists. Prior to screening strategies, only 4% of gastric carcinomas diagnosed in Japan were confined to the mucosa and submucosa. The Japanese use a combination of double-contrast radiography and endoscopy in the general population, and the rate of detection of these highly curable early gastric cancers increased to over 30%, which translates into a 90% survival rate for people diagnosed and treated in the early stages of gastric cancer.

5. How is gastric cancer diagnosed and treated?

In the United States, most patients present with relatively advanced stages of gastric cancer. The most common symptoms are weight loss, vague epigastric pain or fullness, early satiety, recurrent emesis, or anorexia. These symptoms usually lead to diagnostic procedures such as an upper GI contrast roentgenogram series and upper endoscopy. Once a biopsy-proven gastric cancer has been diagnosed, a metastatic evaluation is performed with computed tomography scans of the lungs and liver, which are the most common sites of distant metastatic disease.

Treatment of gastric cancer is dictated by how advanced the disease is at diagnosis. For patients without radiologic evidence of distant cancer, surgery is the most common treatment modality. Less than 20% of patients diagnosed in the United States have pathologically defined stage I disease, which has a 5-year survival rate of 50%. Roughly half of all patients diagnosed have locally advanced tumors that have metastasized to regional lymph nodes; thus their survival rate is between 10% and 30% at 5 years.

Patients with gross evidence of metastatic disease or locally advanced gastric cancer that cannot be technically resected are usually treated with palliative chemotherapy or radiation therapy, either alone or in combination. Either way, patients with stage IV gastric carcinoma have a dismal prognosis with a survival rate of less than 5% at 5 years.

Unfortunately, the survival rates for the various stages of gastric carcinoma have not improved markedly with standard approaches over the past three decades, and there have been attempts to improve survival outcomes with combined modality treatments in early stages of gastric cancer.

6. Are there any new treatment approaches for gastric cancer?

Initial approaches to the treatment of early-stage gastric carcinoma used adjuvant radiation therapy in an attempt to alter the local recurrence rate or systemic chemotherapy in an attempt to alter the rate of distant recurrence. Several clinical trials have randomized patients with stages II and III gastric tumors to surgery alone versus surgery plus adjuvant chemotherapy. At least 14 randomized trials have been reported, and no meaningful survival advantage has been observed with the use of adjuvant chemotherapy.

However, for patients with unresectable, locally advanced gastric carcinomas, several randomized clinical trials have demonstrated a significant survival advantage for patients treated with radiation therapy combined with chemotherapy compared with either modality alone. Current studies are under way to combine newer, radiosensitizing chemotherapeutic drugs with radiation. In addition, other trials are evaluating preoperative concurrent chemotherapy and radiation therapy in an attempt to improve total tumor resection rates.

In terms of metastatic gastric cancer, several trials have suggested that some of the newer antitumor drugs, such as paclitaxel, have significant single-agent activity against metastatic disease and will be combined with proven active drugs such as cisplatin and 5-fluorouracil in an attempt to improve survival and palliation rates.

BIBLIOGRAPHY

1. Anderson RL, Kelsen DP, Tepper JE: Cancer of the stomach. In DeVita VT Jr, Hellman S, Rosenberg SA (eds): Cancer: Principles and Practice of Oncology, 5th ed. Philadelphia, Lippincott-Raven, 1997, pp 1021–1049.
2. Blot WJ, Li J-Y, Taylor PR, et al: Nutritional intervention trials in Linxian, China: Supplementation with specific vitamin/mineral combinations, cancer incidence, and disease-specific mortality in the general population. J Natl Cancer Inst 85:1483–1492, 1993.
3. Cullinan SA, Moertel CG, Wieand HS, et al: Controlled evaluation of three drug combination regimens versus fluorouracil alone for the therapy of advanced gastric cancer. J Clin Oncol 12:412–416, 1994.
4. Dalton RR, Eisenberg BL: Rationale for the current surgical management of gastric adenocarcinoma. Oncology 8:99–106, 1994.
5. Hermans J, Bonenkamp JJ, Boon AMG, et al: Adjuvant therapy after curative resection for gastric cancer: Meta-analysis of randomized trials. J Clin Oncol 11:1441–1447, 1993.
6. Ilson DH, Kelsen DP: Adjuvant postoperative therapy of gastrointestinal malignancies. Oncology 8:75–90, 1994.
7. Kelsen D, Atiq OT, Saltz I, et al: FAMTX versus etoposide, doxorubicin and cisplatin: A random assignment trial in gastric cancer. J Clin Oncol 10:541–548, 1992.
8. Moertel CG, Gunderson LL, Mailliard JA, et al: Early evaluation of combined fluorouracil and leucovorin as a radiation enhancer for locally unresectable, residual, or recurrent gastrointestinal carcinoma. J Clin Oncol 12:21–27, 1994.
9. Munoz N, Kato I, Peraza S, et al: Prevalence of precancerous lesions of the stomach in Venezuela. Cancer Epidemiol Biomarkers Prev 5:41–46, 1996.
10. Pelayo C: *Helicobacter pylori* and gastric cancer: State of the art. Cancer Epidemiol Biomarkers Prev 5:477–481, 1996.

65. COLORECTAL CANCER

Allen L. Cohn, M.D.

1. What is the incidence of colorectal cancer in the United States?

Each year approximately 155,000 new cases of colorectal carcinoma are diagnosed in the United States, representing 15% of all cancers. Cancer of the large intestine affects approximately 1 in every 20 people in the United States.

2. What are some of the inherited syndromes associated with colorectal carcinoma?

Familial adenomatous polyposis (FAP) syndrome is an autosomal dominant trait with approximately 90% penetrance and affects approximately 1 person in 7000. Virtually 100% of patients affected by FAP syndrome will develop a colorectal cancer if no intervention takes place. Gardner's syndrome is an autosomal dominant trait that occurs at approximately one-half the frequency of FAP. Patients afflicted with this syndrome have many adenomas in the small and large intestines. Oldfield's syndrome is similar to Gardner's syndrome except patients also have multiple sebaceous cysts in addition to polyposis and adenocarcinoma of the colon. Turcot's syndrome is less common and is inherited as an autosomal recessive trait. Patients with Turcot's syndrome develop malignant tumors of the colon and central nervous system.

3. Are any familial cancer syndromes associated with colorectal cancer?

Yes. There are two hereditary nonpolyposis colorectal cancer syndromes. The first is inherited as an autosomal dominant trait with 90% penetrance. Patients present with multiple colon cancers at an early age. The second syndrome also is inherited as an autosomal dominant trait. Patients develop early onset of adenocarcinomas of the colon, ovary, pancreas, breast, bile duct, and ureters. First-degree relatives of patients afflicted with this syndrome have a seven-fold increase in cancer risk.

4. Is inflammatory bowel disease associated with an increased risk of colorectal carcinoma?

Yes. Patients with ulcerative colitis have about a 30-fold increase in the risk of colorectal cancer if no intervention takes place. Patients with Crohn's disease may have some increased risk of colorectal carcinoma but not to the degree associated with ulcerative colitis.

5. What preoperative evaluation should be done before surgery for suspected or confirmed colorectal carcinoma?

All patients should have a complete blood count, liver function tests, carcinoembryonic antigen (CEA) level, chest radiograph, and colonoscopy to rule out any synchronous primary tumors as well as polyps. In addition, a CT scan of the abdomen and pelvis should be done to rule out any metastatic disease.

6. What is the Astler-Collier modification of Duke's staging system for colorectal carcinoma?

Stage A is tumor penetration that is confined to the mucosa of the intestine. Duke's stage B1 is a tumor that penetrates into the muscularis layer. Duke's stage B2 is tumor penetration through the muscularis into the serosa or perirectal fat. Duke's stages C1 and C2 represent Duke's stages B1 and B2, respectively, with lymph node involvement. Duke's stage D represents metastatic disease.

7. What is the TNM staging system for colon carcinoma?

The TNM staging system looks at the size of the primary tumor (T), regional lymph node involvement (N), and metastatic disease (M). T1 represents invasion into the submucosa, T2 is invasion into the muscularis propria, T3 is invasion into the serosa or perirectal fat, and T4 is invasion into the free peritoneal cavity or into a contiguous organ. N0 represents no metastatic disease to regional lymph nodes, N1 represents 1–3 positive lymph nodes, and N2 represents 4 or more positive lymph nodes. M0 represents no metastatic disease, and M1 is the stage when distant metastases are present. Stage I cancer includes T1–T2 and N0 tumors, corresponding to Duke's stage A. Stage II corresponds to Duke's B cancers (T3–T4 and N0). Stage III is made up of any T stage and node-positive tumors (N1–N3), corresponding to Duke's stage C. Metastatic tumors are stage IV.

8. How are the patterns of metastatic spread different for rectal and colon carcinomas?

Colon cancer typically will metastasize to regional nodes and the liver because the venous drainage is through the portal system. Distal rectal cancers are more likely to have isolated lung metastasis, because the venous drainage of the distal rectum is through the inferior and medial hemorrhoidal veins and not the portal system.

9. What is the primary treatment for tumors of the colon and rectum?

Surgery is the primary treatment for most cases. Hemicolectomy is the surgery of choice for colon carcinomas. Low anterior resection or abdominal perineal resection is the surgery of choice for rectal carcinomas depending on the proximity of the tumor to the anal sphincter. For small rectal tumors near the sphincter, there are sphincter-sparing approaches such as a transanal resection, posterior proctectomy, or a coloanal pull-through.

10. Are any adjuvant treatments available for colon cancer after surgical resection?

Recent studies have shown a survival benefit for patients with Duke's stage C colon cancer treated with adjuvant 5-fluorouracil (5-FU) and levamisole for 1 year. New trials demonstrate that 5-FU and leucovorin chemotherapy for 6 months yields equivalent results as 5-FU and levamisole for 1 year. Both show a trend toward improved survival for Duke's stage B, but it is not statistically significant.

11. Are any adjuvant treatments available for rectal cancer?

Studies using the combination of postoperative radiation therapy and chemotherapy with 5-FU have shown improved survival rates as well as decreased local relapse rates for Duke's stages B2 and C rectal cancers.

12. Does surgery play any role in the treatment of isolated liver metastasis?

Patients with solitary liver metastasis or several metastases confined to one lobe of the liver are candidates for hepatic resection with intent to cure. Patients who are resected for cure have about a 20% 5-year survival rate.

13. Is chemotherapy effective for metastatic disease?

The combination of 5-FU and leucovorin is the standard chemotherapy for metastatic disease. Many different treatment regimens are available, yielding response rates between 25% and 35%, with little overall effect on survival.

14. Is any effective therapy available for metastatic disease in patients whose disease has progressed on 5-FU and leucovorin?

Recent studies have demonstrated a 15–20% response rate for irinotecan in patients whose disease has progressed on 5-FU and leucovorin or shortly after receiving 5-FU and leucovorin as surgical adjuvant treatment.

BIBLIOGRAPHY

1. Cunningham D: Current status of colorectal cancer: CPT-11 (irinotecan): A therapeutic innovation. Eur J Cancer 32A(Suppl 3):S1–S8, 1996.
2. DeVita VT, Hellman S, Rosenberg SA (eds): Cancer: Principles and Practice of Oncology, 5th ed. Philadelphia, Lippincott-Raven, 1997.

3. Erbe RW: Inherited gastrointestinal polyposis syndromes. N Engl J Med 294:1101–1104, 1976,

4. Fleming ID, Cooper JS, Henson DE, et al: Manual for Staging of Cancer, 5th ed. Philadelphia, Lippincott-Raven, 1997.

5. Huges KS, et al: Resection of the liver for colorectal carcinoma metastases: A multi-institutional study of patterns of recurrence. Surgery 100:778, 1986.

6. Lynch HT, Smyrk T, Watson P, et al: Hereditary colorectal cancer. Semin Oncol 18:337–366, 1991.

7. Moertel CG, Fleming TR, Macdonald JS, et al: Levamisole and fluorouracil for adjuvant therapy of resected colon carcinoma. N Engl J Med 322:352–356, 1990.

8. O'Connell M, Wieand H, Krook J, et al: Lack of value of methyl-CCNU (MeCCNU) as a component of effective rectal cancer surgical adjuvant therapy: Interim analysis of Intergroup Protocol 86-47-51. Proc Am Soc Clin Oncol 10:134, 1991 [abstract].

9. Olson RM, Perencevich NP, Malcom AW, et al: Patterns of recurrence following curative resection of adenocarcinoma of the colon and rectum. Cancer 45:2969–2974, 1980.

10. Poon MA, O'Connell MJ, Wieand HS, et al: Biochemical modulation of fluorouracil with leucovorin: Confirmatory evidence of improved therapeutic efficacy in advanced colorectal cancer. J Clin Oncol 9:1967–1972, 1991.

11. Roth MS: Hepatic resection for colorectal liver metastases. Hematol Oncol Clin North Am 3:171–184, 1989.

66. TUMORS OF THE LIVER AND BILIARY TREE

Marc S. Greenblatt, M.D.

1. What are the most common liver tumors?

The most common neoplasms found in the liver are metastases from extrahepatic primary cancers. Benign lesions account for approximately 10% of liver tumors. The most common benign tumors are hemangioma, focal nodular hyperplasia, bile duct adenoma, and hepatic adenoma. The most common primary liver cancer is hepatocellular carcinoma (HCC). The fibrolamellar variant of HCC is uncommon but appears to have a better survival rate than other types.

2. How common is primary hepatocellular carcinoma?

The worldwide incidence of HCC has a wide geographic variation. Its incidence is low in Western countries, but it is one of the most common malignancies in many areas of the world, such as Southeast Asia and sub-Saharan Africa. In the United States the incidence of primary HCC is 2–3 cases per 100,000, but rates up to 150/100,000 are found in high-incidence areas with multiple risk factors. Primary HCC is the ninth leading cause of cancer deaths in the United States.

3. What are the risk factors for hepatocellular carcinoma (HCC)?

The most common risk factor for HCC worldwide is chronic hepatitis B virus (HBV) infection. In high-risk areas such as China, Southeast Asia, and southern Africa, chronic HBV infection is endemic, affecting 15–20% of the population. Spread is mostly vertical, from mother to newborn; this population is at higher risk for HCC than people with horizontally acquired HBV infection. Recently, hepatitis C (HCV) virus appears to be increasing as a risk factor. The other environmental factor that predisposes to HCC in high-incidence areas is exposure to the chemical carcinogen aflatoxin B1 (AFB). AFB is produced by the fungus aspergillus flavus, which contaminates grain stores in some areas of China, African, and other areas of high HCC incidence. Epidemiologic studies demonstrate a synergistic effect of HBV infection and AFB exposure in risk of HCC. Basic science studies indicate that the mechanism of carcinogenesis involves both alterations to critical genes within the hepatocytes and increased cell proliferation due to viral infection.

Another risk factor for HCC is cirrhosis from any cause, including alcohol consumption, hereditary hemochromatosis, and alpha1-antitrypsin deficiency. Other less common risk factors are long-term treatment with steroid hormones, such as oral contraceptives and anabolic steroids, exposure to the radioactive contrast material thorium dioxide (Thorotrast) once used in radio-logic procedures, and exposure to the chemical carcinogen vinyl chloride.

4. What are the most common presenting symptoms and signs of HCC?

Abdominal pain is present in about 90% of patients in the United States. Abdominal swelling occurs in almost one-half of patients, and weight loss and anorexia in about one-third. Rapid worsening of a patient with known cirrhosis may signal the development of HCC. Uncommon but dramatic presentations of HCC include acute abdomen from massive intraperitoneal bleeding and Budd-Chiari syndrome from invasion of the inferior vena cava or hepatic vein. In Japan, where screening for HCC is common, more small asymptomatic tumors are found.

The most common sign on physical examination is hepatomegaly (90%); other common signs are ascites, jaundice, and splenomegaly. Fever occurs in up to one-half of cases, and hepatic bruits are detected in about 20%. Paraneoplastic hormonal syndromes include erythrocytosis, hypercalcemia, hypercholesterolemia, hypoglycemia, and sexual changes (i.e., gynecomastia, testicular atrophy).

5. How is HCC staged? What is the therapeutic significance of staging?

Stages I–IV are defined using the TNM system, which describes tumor features, lymph nodes, and metastases. The most important feature of HCC staging is defining which tumors are candidates for complete resection. Potentially curative resection is limited to patients with T1N0M0 or T2N0M0 tumors (stage I or II), which include solitary tumors < 2 cm, multiple tumors limited to one lobe and < 2 cm without vascular invasion, or a solitary tumor > 2 cm without vascular invasion. Although pathologic staging often detects more advanced disease than clinical staging, it is still appropriate to consider resection for all patients with clinical stage I or II disease. CT scan and intraoperative ultrasound are useful modalities in staging.

6. Which tumor marker is useful in the management of HCC?

Alpha fetoprotein (AFP) is a fetal antigen that is a tumor marker expressed in HCC, germ cell tumors, and occasionally other cancers, as well as in other liver diseases such as chronic hepatitis and cirrhosis. Serum AFP levels are elevated in 60–90% of HCC patients, often to extremely high levels. The clinical scenario of chronic liver disease with acute worsening, liver mass on imaging study, absence of testicular mass, and extremely high (> 400 ng/ml) AFP is virtually diagnostic of HCC. AFP may be used as a marker of disease recurrence or persistence after surgery. Its role as a screening test is debated.

7. What are the long-term survival rates following surgical resection of HCC? What factors limit resectability of primary HCC?

Survival is generally greater than 70% for resected stage I tumors. Unfortunately, such tumors are uncommon. Survival falls to 40–60% for stage II disease and is negligible if metastases are present in lymph nodes or distant organs. Other poor prognostic factors include more than 50% involvement of the liver, albumin < 3.0 mg/dl, and bilirubin > 3.0 mg/dl. Because most patients with HCC have severe underlying liver disease, the number of potentially curative resections is limited by the functional reserve of the remaining liver and general debility.

8. Is there a role for orthotopic liver transplantation (OLT) for HCC?

A small subset of patients may benefit from OLT for HCC. Patients with fewer than 4 tumors, none > 5 cm in size, and without vascular invasion have survival rates of 40–60% with OLT. Some of these tumors are discovered incidentally at the time of OLT for other diseases.

9. Are treatments other than resection effective against HCC?

Locoregional therapies to the liver can be effective in treating both primary and metastatic liver neoplasms. Such therapies include catheter insertion into the hepatic artery and infusion of chemotherapy or Lipiodol (lymphangiogram dye), transcatheter chemoembolization, percutaneous ethanol injection, or cryosurgery. Systemic chemotherapy and hormonal therapy are ineffective in prolonging survival or providing meaningful palliation.

10. How can HCC be prevented? Who should be screened for HCC?

Prevention of chronic HBV infection by vaccination against HBV at birth has reduced the incidence of childhood HCC in Taiwan. Treatment of HCV with interferon alpha may reduce the incidence of HCC. Screening with serum AFP and ultrasonography may identify asymptomatic tumors but have not been proved to improve survival rates. However, many authors recommend that high-risk patients, such as those with chronic active hepatitis and/or cirrhosis, undergo screening with serum AFP every 3–6 months and ultrasound every 4–12 months.

11. How common are tumors of the biliary tract?

In the United States carcinoma of the gallbladder represents two-thirds of biliary tree cancers and is the fifth most common malignancy of the gastrointestinal tract, with an incidence of 2.5–4.4 per 100,000 people. Cholangiocarcinoma, carcinoma of the intrahepatic and extrahepatic bile ducts, has an incidence of 1.0 per 100,000 in the United States. The most common histology in both sites is adenocarcinoma.

12. What are the risk factors for biliary tract tumors?

Seventy-five to 95% of patients with carcinoma of the gallbladder have chronic cholecystitis and cholelithiasis, although only 1–2% of gallbladders with chronic cholecystitis contain carcinoma. Large stones are more strongly associated with cancer. Precancerous dysplasia has been observed to be associated with chronic inflammation. Other risk factors implicated in gallbladder cancer include a diffusely calcified ("porcelain") gallbladder, gallbladder polyps, typhoid carriers, and working in the rubber and metal fabrication industries. Native American women of the southwestern United States have an incidence six times the general population.

Cholangiocarcinoma also has been strongly associated with sclerosing cholangitis, which often accompanies ulcerative colitis, and hepatolithiasis. Other etiologic agents include biliary parasites, Thorotrast, choledochal cysts, and ulcerative colitis, even in the absence of sclerosing cholangitis.

13. What are the clinical features of carcinoma of the gallbladder? How sensitive are imaging studies in its detection?

The most common symptoms reported in cases of gallbladder carcinoma, abdominal pain and nausea, mimic those of cholecystitis. About one-half of patients have right upper quadrant tenderness, one-half have a palpable mass, and one-half are jaundiced. Ultrasonography is usually abnormal but rarely diagnostic. If performed because of high clinical suspicion, CT usually demonstrates a mass and can help in determining resectability by assessing hepatic or vascular invasion and nodal metastases. However, no radiographic finding is diagnostic of gallbladder carcinoma. Historically, gallbladder cancer was not usually diagnosed preoperatively, but recent studies suggest that improved diagnostic methods have increased the number of preoperative diagnoses.

14. What is the natural history and response to therapy of gallbladder cancer?

Most gallbladder cancers have spread locally (invasion and/or lymph node metastases) and/or metastasized to the liver or other organs at the time of diagnosis; fewer than 25% are resectable. However, between 10 and 20% are discovered incidentally in gallbladders removed for symptomatic stones. The minority of tumors that are confined to the mucosa or muscularis (stage I or II) have a good prognosis after resection. Radical surgery including cholecystectomy, subsegmental liver resection, bile duct resection, and extensive node dissection appears to increase both survival and surgical mortality rates. Adjuvant therapy has not been adequately studied. Unresectable tumors cannot be cured by radiation or chemotherapy. Response rates to intravenous systemic chemotherapy are poor, but are reported to be greater than 30% with hepatic arterial infusion. Fewer than 5% of patients are alive at 5 years.

15. How does the location of a cholangiocarcinoma affect prognosis and treatment? What is a Klatskin tumor?

Bile duct tumors can be intrahepatic, at the bifurcation of the common hepatic duct, or in the mid and distal bile duct. Primary cholangiocarcinoma at the bifurcation of the hepatic duct in the hilum of the liver is known as a Klatskin tumor; a series of 13 was described by Klatskin in 1965. Intrahepatic and Klatskin tumors are rarely resectable and usually fatal, although long-term survivals of 10–35% have been reported if complete resection is possible. Most patients die from complications of locoregional disease. Tumors of the distal bile duct and of the ampulla of Vater can be difficult to distinguish clinically from pancreatic head cancers. However, they may be amenable to curative resection.

16. How common are biliary obstruction and cholangitis in cholangiocarcinoma? How do they affect management?

More than 90% of patients present with jaundice, but cholangitis is rare as a presenting symptom. The primary goals of initial management are to stage the tumor to determine whether or not it is resectable and to control symptoms of obstruction. If pruritus is not present, then immediate drainage may not be required while work-up for resectability proceeds. The risk of cholangitis increases dramatically after instrumentation of the biliary tract.

17. Which procedures should be performed in the initial evaluation of patients with biliary obstruction?

A multidisciplinary approach to biliary tract tumors is required. Tumor resectability often can be determined using some combination of CT, magnetic resonance imaging (MRI), cholangiography, and angiography to delineate involvement of bile ducts, liver, portal vessels, and distant metastases. A CT scan is often informative in documenting dilated bile ducts, lymphadenopathy, and distant metastases, although it identifies the primary tumor in only about 60% of cases. Cholangiography, either transhepatic or endoscopic, is important in establishing the most proximal extent of tumor, which determines resectability. Endoscopic retrograde cholangiopancreatography (ERCP) can provide visualization of bile duct anatomy, drainage of distal obstruction with a stent, and biopsy or cytologic specimens. However, cholangitis and pancreatitis are complications of ERCP that may complicate future surgery. Therefore, transhepatic drainage and imaging remain important modalities. Stents to drain the biliary tract may be placed by either method. Recent studies suggest that MRI can provide much of the desired information.

Tissue diagnosis is not necessary if resection is planned. Biliary tract cytology obtained at the time of percutaneous or endoscopic drainage is diagnostic in only one-half of cases. Percutaneous needle aspiration biopsy improves the diagnostic yield and is often the procedure of choice for diagnosis of unresectable lesions.

18. Is long-term survival common for any group of patients?

For distal bile duct tumors, long-term survival rates of 30–45% have been reported in multiple series if curative pancreatoduodenectomy (Whipple resection) can be performed. For proximal cholangiocarcinomas, survival rates after bile duct resection are lower, approximately 5–15%. Unfortunately, because of extensive local invasion or distant spread of disease at diagnosis, complete resection is possible only in about one-quarter of patients. Adjuvant therapy has not clearly been proved to improve survival. However, distal bile duct and ampullary cancers are usually treated with radiation plus chemotherapy with 5-fluorouracil because benefit has been demonstrated for this regimen in pancreatic adenocarcinoma.

19. What are the complications of progressive cholangiocarcinoma, and how are they treated or prevented?

The goals of palliative therapy are relief of pruritus from obstructive jaundice, prevention of hepatic failure from obstruction, and avoidance of cholangitis. Obstructive jaundice can be relieved by endoscopic or transhepatic stent placement or, in cases that are surgically explored, by surgical

Roux-en-Y resection with stent placement or cholangiojejunostomy. Obstructed stents causing cholangitis are a serious complication, although they can be replaced to reestablish drainage.

BIBLIOGRAPHY

1. Ahrendt SA, Cameron JL, Pitt HA: Current management of patients with cholangiocarcinoma. Adv Surg 30:427–452, 1997.
2. Campbell WL, Ferris JV, Holbert BL, et al: Biliary tract carcinoma complicating primary sclerosing cholangitis: Evaluation with CT, cholangiography, US, and MR imaging. Radiology 207:41–50, 1998.
3. Carr BI, Flickinger JC, Lotze MT: Hepatobiliary cancers. In DeVita VT, Hellman S, Rosenberg SA (eds): Cancer: Principles and Practice of Oncology, 5th ed. Philadelphia, Lippincott-Raven, 1997.
4. Chang MH, Chen CJ, Lai MS, et al: Universal hepatitis B vaccination in Taiwan and the incidence of hepatocellular carcinoma in children. N Engl J Med 336:1855–1859, 1997.
5. Choi J: Regional transcatheter therapy of hepatic neoplasms. Cancer Control 3:407–413, 1996.
6. Colombo M, De Franchis R, Del Ninno E, et al: Hepatocellular carcinoma in Italian patients with cirrhosis. N Engl J Med 325:675–680, 1991.
7. Izzo F, Cremona F, Ruffolo F, et al: Outcome of 67 patients with hepatocellular cancer detected during screening of 1125 patients with chronic hepatitis. Ann Surg 227:513–518, 1998.
8. Maibenco DC, Smith JL, Nava HR, et al: Carcinoma of the gallbladder. Cancer Invest 16:33–39, 1998.
9. Mazzaferro V, Regalia E, Doci R, et al: Liver transplantation for the treatment of small hepatocellular carcinomas in patients with cirrhosis. N Engl J Med 334:693–699, 1996.
10. Pitt HA, Grochow LB, Abrams RA: Cancer of the biliary tree. In DeVita VT, Hellman S, Rosenberg SA (eds): Cancer: Principles and Practice of Oncology, 5th ed. Philadelphia, Lippincott-Raven, 1997.
11. Venook AP: Treatment of hepatocellular carcinoma: Too many options? J Clin Oncol 12:1323–1334, 1994.

67. PANCREATIC CANCER

Marc S. Greenblatt, M.D.

1. How common is pancreatic cancer?

Pancreatic cancer is the 11th most common cancer in the United States, with a rate of approximately 9/100,000. However, it is the fifth most common cause of cancer deaths in the United States. Rates have remained stable for several decades. In 1997 there were over 27,000 cases and over 27,000 deaths. Few patients are cured of the disease, and the 5-year survival rate is only 3–4%. In the United States, African Americans are affected more frequently than Caucasians, and other racial and geographic variations in incidence occur worldwide. Risk rises with age, and the highest incidence rates are seen in persons aged 65–79 years.

2. What is the most common histologic type of pancreatic cancer? What other histologic types are seen frequently?

The pancreas consists of exocrine and endocrine cells. Approximately 90% of all primary pancreatic cancers are ductal adenocarcinomas of the exocrine pancreas; all discussions in this chapter refer to these tumors. The majority of the remaining tumors are islet cell tumors (neoplasms of the endocrine pancreas). Rare tumors in the pancreas include lymphomas, sarcomas, and cystadenocarcinomas (indolent mucin-filled tumors). Metastatic lesions from other primary sites are often seen at autopsy but are rarely clinically significant.

3. What risk factors and carcinogens have been linked with pancreatic cancer?

The best-established risk factor for pancreatic cancer is cigarette smoking; relative risks of 1.5–2.0% in smokers have been reported. A dose-response relationship has been observed, and the risk declines after smoking cessation. Approximately 25–30% of cases of pancreatic cancer are attributable to cigarette smoking. Other risk factors are less well established. High consumption of meat or fat has been associated with increased risk, and high consumption of fruits and vegetables has been associated with decreased risk. Partial gastrectomy for peptic ulcer disease has been associated with a 2- to 5-fold increased risk of pancreatic cancer. Caffeine consumption has been suggested but has not been consistently demonstrated to increase risk. Chronic pancreatitis may increase cancer risk. Type II diabetes is present in about 15% of patients with pancreatic cancer, but it appears to occur as a consequence of the disease and is not an independent risk factor. Prolonged exposure to solvents and DDT have been associated with increased risk.

4. Is pancreatic cancer hereditary?

The risk of pancreatic cancer is increased in close relatives of patients with pancreatic cancer. However, the genetic basis for this observation is not well understood. Pancreatic cancer is seen as an infrequent component of several hereditary syndromes in which other cancers are prominent, such as hereditary nonpolyposis colorectal cancer and hereditary breast cancer. Germline mutations in the p16 tumor suppressor gene are found in some families with inherited melanoma; these kindreds also have a high incidence of pancreatic cancer. Hereditary pancreatitis, an uncommon autosomal dominant syndrome, the genetics of which are unknown, is associated with a high incidence of pancreatic cancer. Much remains to be learned about the genetic basis of pancreatic cancer and interactions with environmental influences.

5. What are the most common presenting symptoms and signs of pancreatic cancer?

Most patients with pancreatic cancer are symptomatic at the time of diagnosis. Pain is the most common symptom. It is typically epigastric, radiating to the back, and is often described as gnawing. It may be steady or relieved by food or positional change. Presenting symptoms in addition to pain that occur in more than one-half of patients are anorexia, nausea, and weight loss. Other common constitutional or abdominal symptoms include fatigue, dyspepsia, bloating, constipation, and depression. Tumors in the head of the pancreas may cause jaundice early in the course, often accompanied by pruritus. Painless jaundice, however, is rare. Tumors of the body or tail of the pancreas rarely present with jaundice and almost always present with advanced, unresectable disease. Although metastases are usually present, only about one-fourth of all patients present with either palpable liver metastases or ascites due to peritoneal metastases. Courvoisier's sign—a nontender right upper quadrant mass—represents a distended gallbladder due to biliary obstruction. It occurs in fewer than one-third of patients.

6. Which tests are most useful for diagnosing pancreatic cancer? Can tumor markers such as CA 19-9 be used to diagnose pancreatic cancer?

The diagnosis of pancreatic cancer should be confirmed by identification of malignant adenocarcinoma cells by histology or cytology. Although the vast majority of pancreatic tumors identified clinically prove to be adenocarcinomas, prognosis and therapy may change dramatically in the rare cases in which alternative diagnoses are made. Various diagnostic tests are often used. In the nonjaundiced patient, both computed tomography (CT) and ultrasound (US) are used to evaluate abdominal masses; CT offers more advantages. Both tests may identify pancreatic masses 2 cm or larger, ductal dilation, and metastases to liver or other abdominal organs, but CT also shows extent of local invasion into surrounding vessels or retroperitoneal structures and peripancreatic, periportal, and retroperitoneal adenopathy. CT- or US-guided fine-needle aspiration and cytologic analysis of pancreatic or liver masses are a safe method of obtaining histologic diagnosis. Jaundiced patients are often evaluated by endoscopic retrograde cholangiopancreatography (ERCP). The pancreatogram can identify obstructed, stenotic, distorted, or sclerosed ducts. The double duct sign is dilation of both pancreatic and common bile ducts. Cytology of ductal brushings may be diagnostic and obviate the need for biopsy. Carcinomas of the ampulla of Vater or the distal common bile duct may or may not be distinguishable from pancreatic cancer. The procedure also may be therapeutic in relieving biliary obstruction. The CA 19-9 tumor marker, a mucinous glycoprotein initially identified on the surface of colon carcinoma cells, is often elevated but is not specific for pancreatic cancer. It may be elevated in other GI malignancies (colon, gastric, hepatic, biliary) as well as pancreatitis and nonmalignant hepatic disease. CA 19-9 generally cannot be used to confirm the diagnosis in the absence of tissue diagnosis. Mutations in the *ras* oncogene occur in most pancreatic cancers and can be detected in clinical specimens; theoretically they may be useful in differentiating malignant from benign lesions. However, this and other molecular abnormalities add little to the current management of pancreatic cancer.

7. How is pancreatic cancer staged? What is the value of staging? What proportion of patients present in each stage?

The tumor-node-metastasis (TNM) staging system evaluates tumor size and invasion, lymph node metastases, and distant metastases. T2 indicates limited and T3 indicates extensive direct extension into adjacent organs. Only T1–2 N0 M0 tumors are candidates for potentially curative resection. Almost one-half of patients have locally advanced unresectable disease, and 40–50% present with metastatic disease. Metastases are most common in the liver (40%) or peritoneum (35%), but widespread systemic metastases are also common.

8. How often is pancreatic cancer resectable? Which preoperative studies are helpful?

Only 5–20% of patients have potentially resectable tumors on presentation. Improvement in preoperative studies in recent years has meant that advanced disease usually can be identified before laparotomy. Thus, in recent years fewer attempts at major resections have been performed. Morbidity has been reduced at major centers where pancreatic resections are restricted to surgeons who are experienced in the procedure. Higher success rates have been reported in the fewer resected cases, but overall cure rate remains unchanged. In addition to ERCP, CT, and US, other useful procedures for evaluating resectability include laparoscopy, which allows biopsies of liver and omentum if potential metastatic deposits are seen, and occasionally angiography, which can identify vascular invasion.

9. What surgical procedures are of benefit?

The standard operation to resect pancreatic cancer is the Whipple procedure, the en bloc resection of the pancreatic head, duodenum, gallbladder, common bile duct, and distal stomach. Preservation of the distal stomach and pylorus, if possible, eliminates the morbidity of postgastrectomy syndrome but does not reduce survival. More extensive procedures (e.g., lymphatic dissection or total pancreatectomy) do not improve survival, and total pancreatectomy causes brittle diabetes mellitus.

10. Do patients benefit from adjuvant therapy after surgery?

Adjuvant therapy with a combination of radiation and 5-fluorouracil (5-FU) chemotherapy improves survival in patients who have undergone complete resection. In a small randomized trial (43 patients) of chemoradiotherapy vs. observation conducted by the Gastrointestinal Tumor Study Group (GITSG), treated patients had a median survival of 20 months vs. 11 months and 2- and 5-year survival rates of 43% and 14% vs. 18% and 4%, respectively. Another randomized trial demonstrated the superiority of radiation therapy plus chemotherapy to chemotherapy alone.

11. What are the therapeutic options for patients whose tumor is locally advanced and unresectable but not metastatic on presentation?

The GITSG studied patients with locally unresectable disease, comparing radiation therapy alone with radiation therapy plus 5-FU. Although not curative, radiation therapy plus 5-FU was superior to radiation alone for this group as well, with median survival of 10 vs. 5.5 months. Preoperative radiation therapy and specialized methods such as intraoperative radiation therapy and interstitial implants have been used at some centers but do not appear to improve survival.

12. Is chemotherapy effective for advanced or metastatic disease?

Although results remain disappointing, recently there have been advances in chemotherapy for pancreatic cancer. Historically, chemotherapy has not improved survival over patients treated with supportive care only. The most commonly used agent was 5-FU, with a response rate of less than 20%; other agents also had low response rates. Recently, a new chemotherapeutic agent, gemcitabine, has demonstrated clinically significant activity against pancreatic cancer. In a randomized trial comparing gemcitabine with 5-FU, efficacy was measured by survival and clinical benefit, defined as improvement in either pain, performance status, or weight. Clinical benefit was seen in 24% of patients treated with gemcitabine and only 5% of patients treated with 5-FU; objective response rates (reduction in tumor size) were 5% and 0%, respectively. The survival rates at 1 year were 18% for gemcitabine and 2% for 5-FU, with median survival times of 5.65 and 4.41 months, respectively. Clinical benefit was also seen in 27% of patients refractory to 5-FU. Further studies with gemcitabine and other agents are ongoing.

13. What are the common complications of pancreatic cancer? How are they managed?

Abdominal pain is an important problem for most patients and usually requires significant use of narcotic analgesics. Ablation of the celiac plexus with alcohol or phenol, either intraoperatively or percutaneously, can provide relief. Relief of obstructive jaundice is required for symptomatic pruritus or postobstructive infection. Jaundice is best relieved by placement of a stent during ERCP. In unresectable patients, surgical bypass can relieve biliary obstruction but is associated with a higher postoperative morbidity and mortality compared with ERCP and does not improve survival. Duodenal obstruction may require laparotomy. Trousseau's syndrome of migratory spontaneous venous thrombophlebitis may precede or follow the diagnosis of pancreatic cancer and is often difficult to manage. Treatment is long-term anticoagulation, but recurrent thrombosis is common despite warfarin or heparin therapy.

BIBLIOGRAPHY

1. Burris HA, Moore MJ, Andersen J, et al: Improvements in survival and clinical benefit with gemcitabine as first-line therapy for patients with advanced pancreatic cancer: A randomized trial. J Clin Oncol 15:2403–2413, 1997.
2. Dowsett JF, Russel RCG: Tumors of the pancreas. In Pechham M, Pinedo HM, Veronesi U (eds): Oxford Textbook of Oncology. Oxford, Oxford Medical Publishers, 1995.
3. Kalser MH, Ellenberg SS: Pancreatic cancer: Adjuvant combined radiation and chemotherapy following curative resection. Arch Surg 120:899–903, 1985.
4. Lynch HT, Smyrk T, Kern SE, et al: Familial pancreatic cancer: A review. Semin Oncol 23:251–275, 1996.
5. Moertel CG, Frytak S, Hahn RG, et al: Therapy of locally unresectable pancreatic carcinoma: A randomized comparison of high dose (6000 rads) radiation alone, moderate dose radiation (400 rads) + 5-fluorouracil, and high dose radiation + 5-fluorouracil. Cancer 48:1705–1710, 1981.
6. Parker SL, Tong T, Bolden S, Wingo PA: Cancer Statistics 1997. Cancer J Clin 47:5–27, 1997.
7. Silverman DT, Dunn JA, Hoover RN, et al: Cigarette smoking and pancreas cancer: A case-control study based on direct interviews. J Natl Cancer Inst 86:1510–1516, 1994.
8. Warshaw AL, Fernandez del Castillo C: Pancreatic carcinoma. N Engl J Med 326:455–465, 1992.

68. OVARIAN CANCER

Helen L. Frederickson, M.D.

1. What is the incidence of ovarian cancer? Which women are at an increased risk for developing the disease?

Ovarian cancer accounts for 5% of all cancers among women. Twelve of every 1000 women over 40 years of age in the United States will develop ovarian cancer. Epithelial cancers of the ovary are primarily seen in women older than 50 years of age. Incidence dramatically increases with age. Highest incidence rates are in the 65–85 year age group. The peak rate of ovarian cancer is 54 per 100,000 in the 75–79 year age group. Lifetime risk for the general population is 1 in 70.

Reproductive factors related to the risk of developing ovarian cancer include nulliparity, early menarche/late menopause, and infertility. Protective factors include prolonged oral contraceptive pill use, multiple pregnancies, tubal ligation, and hysterectomy. Thus the probability of developing ovarian cancer is related to the total number of ovulatory cycles.

The risk of ovarian cancer is increased twofold with a history of breast cancer. Risk increases from 1.4% to 5% with one first-degree relative and to 7% with two first-degree relatives. In the latter group, a 3% chance of having hereditary ovarian cancer syndrome is present. In such families, the lifetime risk of ovarian cancer is at least 40% (autosomal dominant inheritance with variable penetrance). See chapter 93 (Breast Cancer Genetics) for more information.

2. How does the typical patient with ovarian cancer present?

The majority of epithelial ovarian tumors are advanced-stage disease at diagnosis. Patients usually present with vague symptoms of nausea, dyspepsia, or lower abdominal discomfort. Eventually, most patients develop ascites that causes a sudden increase in abdominal girth. Many patients develop symptoms of partial small bowel obstruction.

Patients with early-stage disease often present with a very large pelvic mass and symptoms of pressure from the large mass. Up to 50% of patients with stage I disease have a negative CA125.

Seventy-five percent of ovarian cancer patients present with stage III disease. Eighty percent of patients with epithelial ovarian cancer have an elevated CA125.

3. Is there a screening test for ovarian cancer?

No. The true natural history of ovarian cancer is not known. To date no one has demonstrated that any screening technique significantly affects mortality, even when high-risk populations are screened. The use of vaginal probe ultrasound (often combined with color-flow Doppler) and CA125 drawn randomly has been investigated, but to date no evidence shows that such methods may be used to decrease mortality from ovarian cancer. In fact, their use may result in increased morbidity by leading to many unnecessary surgical procedures.

CA125 is not a good screening test, because the incidence of the disease in the general population is so low that the majority of positive tests are in fact false-positives. Many benign disease processes also may cause an elevated CA125.

4. How is ovarian cancer staged?

Surgical staging in the absence of obvious stage III disease includes (1) peritoneal washings; (2) multiple peritoneal biopsies in the pelvis and upper abdomen; (3) diaphragm assessment (may be by Pap smear); (4) pelvic and paraaortic node sampling; and (5) infracolic omentectomy.

Stages

I	Confined to the ovaries
IA	Confined to a single ovary
IB	Both ovaries involved
IC	No gross spread beyond the ovaries
	Malignant cells are present in cytologic washings or in ascites
	Tumor extends to the ovarian surface
	Tumor is ruptured at surgery
II	Tumor spread in the pelvis beyond the ovaries
IIA	Spread to the uterus or fallopian tubes
IIB	Spread to the other pelvic structures
IIC	Malignant cells present in cytologic washings or in ascites
	Tumor is ruptured at surgery
III	Extrapelvic spread confined to the abdominal cavity or inguinal nodes
IIIA	No gross spread beyond the pelvis, with microscopic implants to the upper abdomen
IIIB	Gross intraabdominal extrapelvic implants < 2 cm
IIIC	Gross intraabdominal extrapelvic implants > 2 cm
	Retroperitoneal spread to pelvic or aortic lymph nodes or the inguinal nodes
IV	Distant spread

5. What is the treatment for early-stage ovarian cancer?

Total abdominal hysterectomy and bilateral salpingo-oophorectomy with careful surgical staging is the best therapy for stage I lesions of the ovary. Adjuvant therapy postoperatively is reserved for high-grade tumors or stage IB and IC tumors. Combination chemotherapy with a platinum analog and paclitaxel (Taxol) is the most common combination used. No clear data show that combination chemotherapy is superior to single-agent therapy or no further therapy in early-stage disease.

In young women with stage IA disease who desire children a unilateral salpingo-oophorectomy and careful staging may be associated with minimal increased risk of recurrence.

6. What is the treatment for advanced-stage ovarian cancer?

Maximal tumor reductive surgery includes a total abdominal hysterectomy and omentectomy followed by adjuvant combination chemotherapy. Many retrospective studies suggest that survival is longer in advanced-stage patients with residual tumor size < 2 cm. Unless the patient can be debulked to a tumor volume < 2 cm, residual diameter does not influence survival. Interestingly, based on Gynecologic Oncology Group (GOG) studies, survival is greater in patients with small volume residual disease (< 1 cm) at the time of surgery than in patients who are debulked to a residual volume of < 1 cm.

The optimal time for debulking surgery has not been determined. Traditionally, surgery has been performed at the time of diagnosis and followed by chemotherapy. More recently, investigators have considered "interval" debulking. Such patients are treated with 1–3 cycles of multiagent chemotherapy followed by surgery and the remaining chemotherapy cycles.

7. Which chemotherapy regimens are used in ovarian cancer?

Presently, platinum-based chemotherapeutic regimens are first-line chemotherapy for ovarian cancer. Studies comparing single-agent chemotherapy with combination therapy demonstrate that combination therapy prolongs survival and progression-free interval. The cisplatin analog carboplatin has been shown to have significantly lower toxicity than cisplatin with no significant difference in progression-free interval or survival.

GOG did a large randomized study of cisplatin/cyclophosphamide vs. cisplatin/paclitaxel. The outcome was that overall response, pathologic response, progression-free interval, and median survival were all greater in the paclitaxel/cisplatin arm. The GOG trial was done with a 24-hour infusion of paclitaxel at a dosage of 135 mg/m^2. More recent studies have shown a benefit with 175 mg/m^2 of paclitaxel over 3 hours, both in response rate increase and toxicity decrease. More recently, the combination of paclitaxel (175 mg/m^2 over three hours) and carboplatin has become the most common first-line therapy in the United States, although this regimen has not been compared to the cisplatin/paclitaxel regimen of the GOG protocol.

The optimal length of therapy has not been established. A prospective randomized trial compared 5 cycles of paclitaxel with 10 cycles of platinum-based therapy and showed no statistical difference. Some early studies with paclitaxel have suggested that prolonged use of this drug may elicit further responses.

8. Is there a role for second-look laparotomy?

Yes. Second-look laparatomy is appropriate when a patient is part of a research protocol for either first-line or second-line therapy. In about one-half of patients with a complete clinical response (including a negative CA125), malignancy will be found during the second look. Surgical assessment of residual disease remains the only way to determine treatment effectiveness and, thus, the only way to determine the benefit of new treatment regimens.

The survival benefit of second-look laparotomy has not been proved. Patients with stage I and II disease have a high correlation between a negative second-look operation and subsequent survival, but the recurrence rate in higher-stage disease with a negative second-look laparotomy is at least 50%. This figure suggests that even with a negative second-look surgery, further adjuvant therapy should be considered. Unfortunately, no adjuvant therapy in this setting has been shown to effectively decrease the recurrence rate.

9. Is there a role for high-dose chemotherapy with autologous bone marrow support?

Approximately 50% of patients with refractory ovarian cancer who have undergone high-dose chemotherapy regimens with autologous bone marrow support salvage treatment have responded in various phase I trials. These trials are small and involve highly selected patients, but suggest that the earlier use of such treatment may improve complete response rates. GOG presently has an ongoing randomized prospective trial in patients with small-volume residual disease after first-line chemotherapy, comparing six more cycles of carboplatin and paclitaxel to high-dose chemotherapy with stem-cell rescue. Until the completion of prospective randomized trials, high-dose chemotherapy in ovarian cancer patients should be considered experimental therapy.

10. What is the prognosis of patients with ovarian cancer?

The 5-year survival for patients with Stage III or IV disease is only 25–30%. The most common cause of death is related to ascites, bowel obstruction, and essentially a slow starvation. Distant metastases, (including bone, lung, liver, and brain) are unusual.

International Federation of Gynecology and Obstetrics 5-year Survival Results by Stage

STAGE	% 5-YEAR SURVIVAL
IA	83.5
IB	79.3
IC	73.1
IIA	64.6
IIB	54.2
IIC	61.3
IIIA	51.7
IIIB	29.2
IIIC	17.7
IV	14.3

11. Is there a benefit to secondary debulking at second-look laparotomy or at recurrence after first-line therapy?

The benefit of secondary debulking is unproven. Patients who progress on therapy are unlikely to survive regardless of further therapy. Patients with bulky residual at second surgery also are unlikely to survive, but some studies suggest that if bulky disease can be converted to microscopic residual, patients may have a survival advantage with second-line treatments.

12. What second-line therapy is available for patients with ovarian cancer ?

Platinum-sensitivity determines the response rate to second-line therapy. Patients who have responded to first-line platinum-based chemotherapy and have had a $\geq$ 6-month disease-free interval are more likely to respond to both platinum-based and nonplatinum-based regimens.

Many drugs have been used as salvage therapy in ovarian cancer. Paclitaxel was initially approved for second-line therapy. Now that paclitaxel is used as first-line therapy, topotecan has been approved for second-line therapy. Other second-line drugs include VP-16, hexamethylenamine, 5-fluorouracil, gemcitabine, and Doxil.

13. What is the role of intraperitoneal chemotherapy for ovarian cancer?

Theoretically, intraperitoneal chemotherapy can provide a major pharmacokinetic advantage in treating ovarian cancer, which normally spreads on the surfaces of the intraperitoneal contents. To be advantageous, the tumor nodules must be very small to allow penetration by the drug. Thus only a subset of patients are good candidates for intraperitoneal therapy. Patients also cannot have extensive adhesive disease, which prevents thorough distribution of the drug.

Patients with persistent minimal residual ovarian cancer (microscopic disease or disease < 0.5 cm) following intravenous platinum-based chemotherapy are appropriate candidates for intraperitoneal chemotherapy. Recent studies suggest that first-line intraperitoneal chemotherapy may have an advantage over traditional combination intravenous therapy.

Drugs that have been used for intraperitoneal therapy include cisplatin, carboplatin, 5-fluorouracil, doxorubicin, and paclitaxel. Biologic agents, such as interleukin-2, tumor necrosis factor, and interferon are being used in clinical trials intraperitoneally.

14. Describe areas of current research in ovarian cancer.

Current research includes developing new agents to prevent, modify, or reverse drug resistance, clinical trials with tumor vaccines aimed at inducing antibody or T cell responses against ovarian cancer, and assessing the role of antiangiogenic agents in ovarian cancer.

15. What is the significance of an ovarian tumor of low malignant potential?

Tumors of low malignant potential are epithelial tumors of the ovary that have histologic and biologic features ranging between clearly benign and frankly malignant. Such tumors afflict younger women and have a survival rate of 95% 10-year survival. Conservative therapy in women who desire pregnancy is safe, especially if patients have stage IA disease.

Even lesions that behave in a malignant fashion have good long-term survival. Often spontaneous regression of peritoneal implants in advanced-stage disease occurs. Diagnosis is based on extensive sectioning of the neoplasm given or if the tumor has spread. Adjuvant therapy has not been shown to be effective in such tumors.

BIBLIOGRAPHY

1. Alberts DS et al: Phase III study of intraperitoneal cisplatin-intravenous cyclophosphamide versus intravenous cisplatin-intravenous cyclophosphamide in patients with optimal disease stage III ovarian cancer: A SWOG-GOG-ECOG Intergroup study. Int J Gynecol Cancer 1(suppl):28, 1996.
2. Bast RC, Klug TL, St John E, et al: A radioimmunoassay using a monoclonal antibody to monitor the course of epithelial ovarian cancer. N Engl J Med 309:883–887, 1983.
3. Boyd J: Molecular genetics of hereditary ovarian cancer. Oncology 12:399–406, 1998.
4. Dembo AJ: Epithelial ovarian cancer: The role of radiotherapy. Int J Radiat Oncol Biol Phys 22:835, 1985.
5. Griffiths CT, Parker LM, Fuller AF: Role of cytoreductive surgical treatment in the management of advanced ovarian cancer. Cancer Treat Rep 63:235–240, 1979.
6. Gross TP, Schlesslman JJ: The estimated effect of oral contraceptive use on the cumulative risk of epithelial ovarian cancer. Obstet Gynecol 83:419–424, 1994.
7. Hoskins WJ, Rubin SC, Dulaney E, et al: Influence of secondary cytoreduction at the time of second-look laparotomy on the survival of patients with epithelial ovarian carcinoma. Gynecol Oncol 34:365–371, 1989.
8. McGuire WP et al: A phase II trial comparing cisplatin/Cytoxan and cisplatin/paclitaxel in advanced ovarian cancer. Proc ASCO 12:255, 1993.
9. Potter ME, Hatch KD, Soong SJ, et al: Second-look laparotomy and salvage therapy: A research modality only? Gynecol Oncol 44:3–9, 1992.
10. Potter ME, Partridge EE, Hatch KD, et al: Primary surgical therapy of ovarian cancer: How much and when. Gynecol Oncol 40:195–200, 1991.
11. Vermorken JB, Pecorelli S: Clinical trials in patients with epithelial ovarian cancer: Past, present and future. Eur J Surg Oncol 22:455–466, 1996.

69. CARCINOMA OF THE UTERINE CERVIX AND ENDOMETRIUM

Helen L. Frederickson, M.D.

1. What are the presenting signs of cervical carcinoma?

The most frequent symptom is a bloody discharge presenting as postcoital bleeding, intermenstrual bleeding, or menorrhagia. Symptoms of more advanced disease include backache, leg pain, leg edema, or hematuria.

2. What are the risk factors for cervical carcinoma?

Established risk factors include: first coitus at a young age, multiple sexual partners, and lower socioeconomic status. Human papilloma virus probably acts as a cofactor in cervical carcinogenesis. Smoking also is a significant risk factor.

3. How is cervical cancer diagnosed?

A cervical biopsy is necessary to diagnose invasive cervical cancer; a Pap smear is **not** diagnostic. Unless a gross lesion is present, a cervical biopsy consistent with microinvasion requires a cone biopsy to evaluate for frankly invasive carcinoma,

4. What is the treatment for cervical cancer?

Patients with Stage I or IIA cervical cancer are candidates for primary surgical treatment. Primary radiation therapy is equally efficacious in early-stage disease, but in younger patients surgery is preferred to preserve ovarian function and prevent radiation changes to pelvic organs. Higher-stage disease is treated with primary radiation therapy.

5. Explain the theory that radiation therapy for cervical cancer is based on.

The cervix is accessible for application of radiation techniques and is surrounded by normal tissue (vaginal) that is highly radioresistant. The anatomy of the cervix allows delivery of intracavitary doses up to a total of 10,000 rads to the tumor. Because the dose of radiation decreases by the inverse square of the distance from the source, the bowel and bladder are protected by packing them away at the placement of the tandem and ovoids.

6. What is the most common location of recurrence after radical hysterectomy? After primary radiation therapy?

After radical hysterectomy, approximately one-third of recurrences are in the pelvic sidewall and approximately one-fourth are in the central pelvis. Recurrence after radiation therapy is in the parametrial area 43% of the time.

7. What is the prognosis for a patient with persistent or recurrent cervical carcinoma?

The 1-year survival rate is 10–15% for recurrent or persistent disease, which is compared to overall survival by stage:

Stage I	80–85%
Stage II	60–65%
Stage III	25–35%
Stage IV	8–14%

8. Which patients are candidates for pelvic exenteration?

Pelvic exenteration for recurrent carcinoma of the cervix is indicated only when the pelvic recurrence is centrally located and all metastatic evaluations are negative. The triad of unilateral leg edema, sciatic pain, and ureteral obstruction indicates unresectable disease.

9. Does chemotherapy have a role in the treatment of cervical cancer?

Chemotherapy traditionally has had a low response rate and short duration in cervical cancer. Cisplatin has been shown to be the most active single agent in squamous cell cancer. Concomitant radiation and chemotherapy in high-risk patients has recently shown an increased survival rate over radiation alone.

10. Is adenocarcinoma of the endocervix different than squamous carcinoma of the cervix?

Yes. A recent retrospective study found that 5-year survival rates for stages I, II, and III/IV were 75.9%, 62.9%, and 25.1% respectively. Adenosquamous adenocarcinoma had a better prognosis than endocervical columnar cell adenocarcinoma in early-stage disease. Survival also is shown to be better in early-stage disease if patients are treated with radical surgery instead of primary radiation therapy.

11. What is the incidence of endometrial adenocarcinoma? How does the incidence compare with other gynecologic malignancies?

The incidence of endometrial adenocarcinoma is about 72/100,000 women per year. It is the most common gynecologic malignancy and the fourth most common malignancy seen in women.

12. Describe the evidence that estrogens play a role in carcinogenesis in endometrial adenocarcinoma.

Endometrial adenocarcinoma is associated with disorders characterized by chronic production of endogenous estrogen in the absence of progesterone. Obesity increases a woman's risk of developing endometrial cancer threefold and late menopause increases risk by 2.4 fold. Amount of body fat has been associated with decreased levels of both progesterone and sex hormone-binding proteins.

Other studies demonstrate that the risk of developing endometrial cancer increases 3–7 times with the use of unopposed estrogen, but such studies are retrospective studies; relative risks vary with control groups. More recently, tamoxifen has been implicated as a risk factor for endometrial cancer. Although it is an antiestrogen, it is known to have some estrogenic properties.

13. Do women who develop endometrial adenocarcinoma on tamoxifen have a worse prognosis than women with non–tamoxifen-associated endometrial cancers?

No. Initially it was suggested that tamoxifen-associated endometrial cancers might be well-differentiated, superficially invasive cancers, similar to unopposed estrogen-associated endometrial cancers. Retrospective studies did not show an increase in poor prognostic histology, tumor differentiation, or stage compared to what may be expected in a similar group of patients with non–tamoxifen-associated endometrial cancer.

14. What is the most common presenting symptom of endometrial carcinoma?

Abnormal uterine bleeding is the most common presenting symptom. Any postmenopausal bleeding is considered abnormal. Any increase in menstrual bleeding (i.e., more frequent or heavier menses) or intermenstrual spotting should prompt an endometrial biopsy in the perimenopausal period.

15. How is endometrial cancer diagnosed?

An endometrial biopsy is used to diagnose endometrial carcinoma. The biopsy may be done with any of the multiple devices for office biopsies or with dilatation and curettage (D&C). Several studies indicate that the accuracy of the endometrial biopsy in detecting cancer is about 90%. The Pap smear is not useful for screening for endometrial cancer, but one-half to one-third of patients with endometrial cancers have abnormal smears on routine cervical screening. If endometrial cells are present on a Pap smear in a postmenopausal woman, she should have an endometrial biopsy.

16. Does ultrasound have a role in the diagnosis of endometrial cancer?

No. Ultrasound has been suggested as a diagnostic tool in evaluating women with irregular bleeding. The endometrial stripe seen with the transvaginal ultrasound relates to endometrial thickness. Some studies suggest that a thin endometrial stripe eliminates the need for histologic diagnosis. To date, no agreement exists on the cut-off measurement at which no endometrial sampling is necessary. Ultrasound evaluation of women on tamoxifen is unreliable, because endometrial thickness in the patient treated with tamoxifen is considerably thicker than in the patient not treated with tamoxifen.

Ultrasound also has been evaluated as a means for determining depth of myometrial invasion, which seems unreliable; depth of invasion should be determined at the time of surgery.

17. How does endometrial carcinoma spread?

Endometrial carcinoma arises from the glands of the endometrium; initial growth is slow. As the tumor grows, it eventually invades the underlying myometrium. Extrauterine spread occurs by lymphatics and blood. Lymphatic invasion results in metastasis to the parametrial, pelvic, aortic, or inguinal nodes. Hematogenous spread usually results in pulmonary metastasis but may involve bone and liver. Peritoneal implants may be caused by lymphatic spread or by transtubal or transmural penetration.

18. What is the incidence of pelvic node metastases in patients with disease limited to the uterus? What is the incidence of metastases to paraaortic nodes?

Overall, 9.6% of patients have positive pelvic nodes. Tumor grade is related to risk of positive nodes.

Grade	%Positive pelvic nodes	%Positive paraaortic nodes
G1	3	2
G2	9	5
G3	18	11

Nodal metastasis is also related to depth of myometrial invasion.

Maximal invasion	%Positive pelvic nodes	%Positive paraaortic nodes
Endometrium only	1	1
Superficial muscle	5	3
Intermediate muscle	6	1
Deep muscle	25	17

19. How is endometrial carcinoma staged?

Endometrial carcinoma is staged surgically as follows:

Stage		
Ia	G123	Tumor limited to endometrium
Ib	G123	Invasion of less than one-half of the myometrium
Ic	G123	Invasion of more than one-half of the myometrium
IIa	G123	Endocervical glandular involvement only
IIb	G123	Cervical stromal invasion
IIIa	G123	Tumor invades serosa and/or adnexae
IIIb	G123	Vaginal metastases
IIIc	G123	Metastases to pelvic and/or paraaortic lymph nodes
IVa	G123	Tumor invasion of bladder and/or bowel mucosa
IVb	G123	Distant metastases, including intraabdominal and/or inguinal lymph nodes

20. Which factors are of predictive prognostic value in endometrial adenocarcinoma?

Histologic type: Adenocarcinoma is the most common histologic subtype. Uterine papillary serous carcinoma and clear cell carcinomas have a worse prognosis than adenocarcinoma. Squamous differentiation does not affect survival.

Histologic differentiation: Grade 1 5-year survival is 96% and grade 3 5-year survival is 70%.

Five-year survival based on stage:

Stage	%5-year survival
I	86
II	66
III	44
IV	16

Myometrial invasion, lymph node metastasis, and adnexal metastasis also are prognostic factors.

21. How is endometrial carcinoma treated?

Endometrial carcinoma is treated with initial surgical staging, including peritoneal cytology, total abdominal hysterectomy, bilateral salpingo-oophorectomy, and pelvic and paraaortic node sampling. The results of staging determine the use of adjuvant radiation, chemotherapy, and hormonal therapy. Therapy after surgical staging in patients with disease limited to the uterus has not been evaluated in a prospective randomized study. Many clinicians recommend postoperative radiation therapy based on depth of invasion and grade of tumors regardless of nodal spread. Studies suggest that lymphadenectomy is therapeutic and that survival improves with lymphadenectomy alone without adjuvant whole pelvic radiation therapy.

The role of adjuvant chemotherapy has been evaluated by the Gynecologic Oncology Group. High-risk stage I and occult stage II patients were treated with surgery followed by external irradiation followed by randomization to doxorubicin for eight cycles vs. no further therapy. Twenty-three percent of the recurrences were found in the doxorubicin arm and 26% were present in the non-doxorubicin arm.

Treatment of advanced disease is limited and has a poor prognosis. Treatment with adjuvant chemotherapy has a response rate as high as 66%, but responses are of short duration (< 6 months). Consequently, because chemotherapy regimens are toxic and treatment-related deaths are not uncommon, treatment of stage III or IV disease must be individualized.

22. What are the most common sites of recurrence in patients treated with radiation therapy? In patients treated with surgery alone?

The most common sites of recurrence in patients treated with adjuvant radiation are the abdomen, liver, and bone. Patients treated with surgery alone may have recurrence at the vaginal apex, and a significant percentage of such patients can be salvaged with surgery and/or radiation therapy.

23. What is the role of hormonal therapy in endometrial carcinoma?

Patients with advanced or recurrent disease and positive progesterone or estrogen receptors may be treated with high doses of progestin therapy in addition to surgery and radiation. Responses may be slow and not apparent for 3 or more months. As long as disease remains stable, therapy is continued. The mean duration of response for progestin therapy in patients with recurrent or metastatic endometrial carcinoma is about 10–12 months. The level of progesterone receptors varies with degree of differentiation.

24. How effective are chemotherapeutic agents in advanced or recurrent adenocarcinoma of the endometrium?

The overall response rate with current agents for endometrial adenocarcinoma is about 20–30%. The duration of response is short, lasting on the average only 3–6 months. Combinations with doxorubicin and cisplatin or cyclophosphamide have shown similarly disappointing results.

25. What is uterine papillary serous adenocarcinoma? How does it commonly spread?

Papillary serous adenocarcinoma is a variant of endometrial carcinoma, characterized by histology resembling ovarian serous carcinoma. Papillary serous carcinomas tend to be very aggressive and up to 72% have extrauterine spread. Lymph node metastasis occurs in patients even with disease confined to the endometrium. Staging is critical in this disease, even though adjuvant therapy is difficult. Recently, combinations of paclitaxel and carboplatin have shown increased responses. Radiation of the pelvis is unsuccessful because most recurrences are outside the pelvis. Whole abdominal radiation may play a role in adjuvant therapy in this disease.

BIBLIOGRAPHY

1. Barakat RR, Wong G, Curtin JP, et al: Tamoxifen use in breast cancer patients who subsequently develop corpus cancer is not associated with a higher incidence of adverse histologic features. Gynecol Oncol 55:164–168, 1994.
2. Behbakht K, Jordan EL, Casey C, et al: Prognostic indicators of survival in advanced endometrial cancer. Gynecol Oncol 55:363–367, 1994.
3. Bokhman JV: Two pathogenetic types of endometrial carcinoma. Gynecol Oncol 15:10–17, 1983.
4. Boronow RC, et al: Surgical staging in endometrial cancer: Clinical pathological findings of a prospective study. Obstet Gynecol 63:825, 1985.
5. Creasman WT, Morrow CP, Bundy BN, et al: Surgical pathologic spread patterns of endometrial cancer: A Gynecologic Oncology Group study. Cancer 60:2035–2041, 1987.
6. Delgado G, Bundy B, Zairo R, et al: A prospective surgical pathological study of Stage I squamous carcinoma of the cervix: A Gynecologic Oncology Group study. Gynecol Oncol 35:314–320, 1989.
7. Goff BA, Kato D, Schmidt RA, et al: Uterine papillary serous carcinoma: Patterns of metastatic spread. Gynecol Oncol 54: 264–268, 1994.
8. Kilgore LC, Partridge EE, Alvarez RD, et al: Adenocarcinoma of the endometrium: Survival comparison of patients with and without pelvic node sampling. Gynecol Oncol 56:26, 1995.
9. Long JH, Langdon RM, Cha SS, et al: Phase II trial of methotrexate, vinblastine, doxorubicin and cisplatin in advanced/recurrent endometrial carcinomas. Gynecol Oncol 58:240, 1995.
10. Marrow CP, Panel Report: Is pelvic irradiation beneficial in the postoperative management of stage IB squamous cell carcinoma of the cervix with pelvic lymph node metastasis treated by radical hysterectomy and pelvic lymphadenectomy? Gynecol Oncol 23:127, 1986.
11. Moore TO, Phillips PH, Nerenstone SR, et al: Systemic treatment of advanced and recurrent endometrial carcinomas: current status and future direction. J Clin Oncol 9:1071, 1991.
12. Potter MD, Alvarez R, Shingleton HM, et al: Early invasive cervical cancer with pelvic lymph node involvement: To complete or not to complete radical hysterectomy? Gynecol Oncol 37:78, 1990.
13. Thigpen JT, Blessing JA, DiSaia, PJ, et al: A randomized comparison of doxorubicin alone versus doxorubicin plus cyclophosphamide in the management of advanced or recurrent endometrial carcinoma: A Gynecologic Oncology Group study. J Clin Oncol 12:1408–1414, 1994.
14. Thigpen JT, Blessing J, Homesley H, et al: Phase III trial of doxorubicin +/- cisplatin in advanced or recurrent endometrial carcinoma. Proc Am Soc Clin Oncol 12:26, 1993.
15. Weiss NS, Szekely DR, English DR, Schweid AI: Endometrial cancer in relation to patterns of menopausal estrogen use. JAMA 242:261–264, 1979.

70. TESTICULAR CANCER

Paul S. Unger, M.D.

1. What is included in the differential diagnosis of a new scrotal mass in a young man?

Epididymitis, spermatocele, hydrocele, orchitis, infarction, trauma, benign tumor of the testis, epididymis or tunica albuginea, and torsion.

2. What is the most common solid tumor in men aged 15–34?

A germ cell tumor.

3. How many new cases of testicular cancer occur in the United States every year?

7,200 or an incidence of 6 per 100,000.

4. What is the best-documented risk factor for testicular cancer?

Cryptorchidism is associated with 10% of all germ cell tumors with a 10- to 30-fold increase in risk.

5. Can the risk from cryptorchidism be eliminated as a risk factor?
Yes, partially. Orchiopexy performed before puberty reduces but does not completely eliminate the risk for both ipsilateral and contralateral testicles.

6. What is the etiology of germ cell tumors?
Unknown.

7. What percentage of solid testicular masses are malignant?
95%.

8. What percentage of testicular tumors are of germ cell origin?
95%.

9. Can the diagnosis of testicular cancer be made by blood test?
No. Although alpha fetoprotein (AFP) and/or beta human chorionic gonadotropin (β-hCG) levels are typically elevated in nonseminomatous germ cell tumors (NSGCTs), an orchiectomy must be performed for diagnosis.

10. Can the diagnosis of testicular cancer be made by biopsy, as with other cancers, thereby preserving the testis?
No. A radical inguinal exploration with ligation of the spermatic cord and orchiectomy is carried out. Vascular control should be achieved before manipulation of the tumor. Open biopsy is absolutely contraindicated, as is scrotal exploration.

11. Explain why transscrotal biopsy of the testis is contraindicated.
Transscrotal biopsy may contaminate the scrotum with malignant cells. Because the scrotum has a different lymphatic drainage from the testicle, transscrotal biopsy would compromise further surgical treatment by contaminating the inguinal and pelvic lymph node drainage basins.

12. How are malignant germ cell tumors classified?

Seminoma	Nonseminoma
Classic seminoma	Embryonal carcinoma
Spermatic seminoma	Teratoma
Anaplastic seminoma	Mature, immature, teratocarcinoma
	Choriocarcinoma
	Yolk sac tumor (endodermal sinus tumor)

13. Why is the distinction between seminoma and nonseminoma important?
The two tumors are treated differently. Seminomas tend to be less aggressive and also exquisitely radiosensitive. Both classes are equally chemosensitive. Seminomas are usually found at an earlier stage.

14. Which pure germ cell tumor is the most common?
Seminoma represents 40–50% of all germ cell tumors found in men.

15. Which is the most common type of germ cell tumor?
Mixed germ cell tumor, composed of a mixture of elements in any combination, accounts for approximately 50% of all testicular tumors.

16. What is the most common combination of NSGCT?
Embryonal carcinoma plus teratoma.

17. Which is the most aggressive type of germ cell carcinoma?
Pure choriocarcinoma.

18. How often is pure choriocarcinoma seen?
In less than 1% of all germ cell tumors.

19. Where else is choriocarcinoma seen?
It is most commonly seen in a small component of mixed tumors in which its presence has little bearing on clinical behavior and outcome. Choriocarcinoma also may be seen in the placenta in women, known as a molar pregnancy. It is easily cured with single-agent chemotherapy.

20. Why is staging of testicular cancer important?
To determine prognosis and treatment.

21. Describe the stages.

Stage 1	Tumor confined to the testis, epididymis, or spermatic cord
Stage 2A	Minimal nodal spread with nodes < 2 cm in size
Stage 2B	Nodes 2–5 cm in size
Stage 2C	Nodes > 5 cm in the retroperitoneum
Stage 3	Metastases above the diaphragm or involvement of solid visceral organs, such as brain or bone

22. What percentage of patients with NSGCTs present with stage 3 tumors?
Stage 3 tumors account for approximately 20% of all patients; 40% are stage 1 and 40% are stage 2.

23. Toward what end should the staging work-up be directed?
The staging work-up guides the treatment plan. Patients with stage 1 disease may be treated with retroperitoneal lymph node dissection (RPLND), observation, or adjuvant chemotherapy. Patients with stage 2 disease may be treated with chemotherapy and/or RPLND. Patients with stage 3 disease are usually treated with chemotherapy; RPLND is reserved for resection of residual masses.

24. Do any risk factors predict relapse when observation of clinical stage 1 disease is contemplated?
Vascular invasion, lymphatic invasion, tumors with mostly embryonal elements, and spermatic cord invasion portend a higher risk, along with lack of yolk sac elements.

25. What studies should be performed in the staging work-up?
Computed tomography (CT) scan of the chest, abdomen, and pelvis and assessment of AFP, β-hCG, and lactate dehydrogenase (LDH) levels should be performed.

26. Is a bipedal lymphangiogram useful?
No. It has low sensitivity (75–80%) and a high false-positive rate of 10–20%.

27. What percentage of patients with clinical stage 1 disease and high-risk features have lymph node involvement at the time of RPLND?
50%.

28. What percentage of patients with recurrent NSGCT have normal AFP and β-hCG levels?
10%.

29. What percentage of patients with clinical stage 1 NSGCT (normal CT scan and serum markers) have retroperitoneal lymph node involvement?
20%.

30. RPLND cures what percentage of patients with clinical stage 1 NSGCT and positive nodes (pathologic stage 2)?
Fifty percent will relapse after RPLND if no additional treatment is given; chemotherapy is given to patients who have positive nodes at the time of surgery.

31. What percentage of patients with NSGCT whose lymph nodes were negative by RPLND will develop recurrent disease?
10–20%.

32. If patients with stage 1 and resected stage 2 NSGCT are followed closely every month for 12 months and every 2 months for the second 12 months, virtually all who have recurrence will have minimal disease. What percentage of patients who have recurrences will be cured with cisplatin-based combination chemotherapy?
99%.

33. When do most malignant germ cell tumors recur after initial therapy?
In the first 24 months.

34. In what percentage of patients with clinical stage 1 NSGCT who undergo RPLND will no disease be found?
70%.

35. What percentage of men are sterile at the time of diagnosis?
About 80–90% of men are oligo- or azoospermic at the time of diagnosis before any therapy.

36. What is the main complication of RPLND?
Retrograde ejaculation.

37. What percentage of patients can maintain normal ejaculation with sympathetic nerve-sparing RPLND?
As many as 80–90%.

38. If patients with stage 1 disease are treated by RPLND and positive nodes are found, is it better to give two prophylactic (adjuvant) course of cisplatin, VP-16, and bleomycin after surgery or to follow them closely and treat if disease recurs?
It does not matter because the outcome is the same—very good.

39. How quickly should tumor markers return to normal after primary surgery?
The half-life of β-hCG is 24 hours, whereas the half-life of AFP is 5–7 days. If plots of decrease of tumor markers do not remain linear over time, recurrent or persistent disease should be suspected.

40. The prognosis of most germ cell tumors seems quite good. Is there any way to distinguish low-risk from high-risk patients?
Yes. Several risk factor systems have been well identified. The best study is from the University of Indiana.
Low risk
Minimal extent
  1. Elevated markers only
  2. Cervical nodes (with or without nonpalpable retroperitoneal nodes)
  3. Unresectable, nonpalpable retroperitoneal disease
  4. > 5 pulmonary metastases per lung field and largest metastasis < 2 cm (with or without nonpalpable retroperitoneal nodes)
Moderate extent
  1. Palpable abdominal mass only (no supradiaphragmatic disease)
  2. Moderate pulmonary metastases: 5–10 metastases per lung field and largest metastasis < 3 cm or solitary pulmonary metastasis of any size > 2 cm (with or without nonpalpable retroperitoneal disease)

High risk

Advanced extent

1. Advanced pulmonary metastases: primary mediastinal NSGCT *or* > 10 pulmonary metastases per lung field *or* multiple pulmonary metastases with largest > 3 cm (with or without nonpalpable retroperitoneal disease)
2. Palpable abdominal mass plus supradiaphragmatic disease
3. Liver, bone, or CNS metastases

41. For low-risk stage 3 disease, what is the most effective chemotherapy?

Three cycles of cisplatin, bleomycin, and etoposide (or four cycles of etoposide and cisplatin).

42. How many patients with stage 3 disease treated with cisplatin combination chemotherapy will relapse?

Less than 10% with low-risk disease and 15–20% with high-risk disease.

43. When should surgery be contemplated after chemotherapy?

When a residual retroperitoneal mass is seen by CT scan. It may represent residual tumor, benign teratoma, or scar tissue.

44. In what other setting is surgery to be considered?

A residual lung mass, especially if tumor markers have normalized, also may represent residual tumor, benign teratoma, or scar tissue.

45. What percentage of patients in complete remission will relapse?

10–20%.

46. What risk is associated with general anesthesia in patients who have received chemotherapy for germ cell tumors?

Postoperative respiratory failure is occasionally seen in patients who were treated with preoperative bleomycin, secondary to oxygen toxicity. Postoperative care, therefore, must be more careful than usual, and FiO$_2$ during surgery and postoperatively should be minimized.

47. Does bleomycin cause other long-term toxicity?

Bleomycin, especially with vinblastine and cisplatin, probably enhances the incidence of Raynaud's phenomenon and the risk of cardiovascular disease in the long term.

48. Can the use of bleomycin be avoided?

Four courses of cisplatin and VP-16 are equivalent to three courses of the same two drugs with bleomycin in patients with low-risk disease.

49. Radiation therapy is the treatment of choice for seminomas up to what stage?

Patients with clinical stage 1 disease are given 2500 rads (2500 cGy) to the infradiaphragmatic nodes, although surveillance is advocated by some. The same radiation therapy is used for nonbulky stage 2 disease.

50. Is it necessary to radiate the mediastinum prophylactically in patients with seminoma?

No.

51. What is the treatment for patients with a bulky stage 2 seminoma?

Chemotherapy with cisplatin, VP-16, and bleomycin (or cisplatin and etoposide).

52. What about stage 3 seminoma?

Use the same chemotherapy as for advanced extensive NSGCTs.

Treatment Recommendations

CLINICAL SETTING	STANDARD THERAPY	INVESTIGATIVE THERAPY
NSGCT		
Stage A	Retroperitoneal lymphadenopathy (modified or nerve-sparing) *or* Surveillance for 2 yr *First year:* CT scan of abdomen every 2 mo, chest radiograph and markers (AFP, β-hCG, LDH) every mo *Second year:* abdominal CT scan every 4 mo with chest radiograph and serum markers every 2 mo *or* 2 cycles of BEP (see below)	
Stage B1 or B2 (after RPLND)	Observation with PVP-16B on relapse or two cycles of PVP-16B as adjuvant	None
Stage B3 or C		
Minimal or moderate	PVP-16B × 3 cycles or cisplatin plus etoposide × 4 cycles plus resection of residual disease	Ongoing trials to minimize toxicity
Advanced	PVP-16B × 3 cycles plus resection of residual disease	Clinical trials ongoing, such as VIP (etoposide, ifosfamide + cisplatin) vs. PVP-16B; early integration of high-dose chemotherapy with autologous bone marrow transplant
Seminoma		
Stage A	Infradiaphragmatic radiotherapy (2,500 cGy)	Surveillance for 2 yr *First year:* CT scan of abdomen every 2 mo, chest radiograph and serum markers every mo *Second year:* abdominal CT scan every 4 mo with chest radiograph and serum markers every 2 mo
Stage B1 or B2	Infradiaphragmatic radiotherapy (2,500 cGy)	
Stage B3 (palpable or > 10 cm)	Infradiaphragmatic radiotherapy or cisplatin-based combination chemotherapy	Management of residual mass is controversial (observe, resect radiotherapy)
Stage C	PVP-16B × 4 cycles or other cisplatin-based combination therapy	Same as NSGCT clinical trials; based on tumor extent (good risk vs. poor risk)

53. Where else may germ cell tumors arise?

Most frequently in midline structures, such as the mediastinum and retroperitoneum.

54. What is the prognosis of extragonadal germ cell tumors in relation to their testicular counterparts?

Stage for stage, chemosensitivity may be the same, although patients with extragonadal germ cell tumors tend to present with more advanced disease that is more difficult to cure.

55. What is included in the differential diagnosis of extragonadal germ cell tumors?

They may be confused with adenocarcinomas, sarcomas, lymphomas, and melanomas. The germ cell tumors are much more curable and treated with different chemotherapy. The diagnosis is facilitated by testing for β-hCG and AFP.

56. What is the reproductive capacity of patients with germ cell tumors who are treated with chemotherapy?

Ninety-six percent of patients are azoospermic after 4 courses of cisplatin-based combination chemotherapy. However, one-half of patients eventually have normal sperm counts and motility.

57. Have congenital anomalies been seen in the offspring of patients who have had germ cell tumors treated with chemotherapy?

No.

58. Will patients resistant to first- and second-line chemotherapy inevitably die of their disease?

No. In some patients retroperitoneal and pulmonary metastases may be resected and never recur. Second-line therapy includes the use of ifosfamide in combination with vinblastine and cisplatin (approximate cure rate of 25%), whereas high-dose therapy with stem cell support rescues another 15–20%.

BIBLIOGRAPHY

1. Birch R, Williams S, et al: Prognostic factors for a favorable outcome in disseminated germ cell tumors. J Clin Oncol 4:400–407, 1986.
2. Bosl G, Bajorin D, et al: Cancer of the testis. In DeVita VT, Hellman S, Rosenberg SA (eds): Cancer: Principles and Practices of Oncology, 5th ed. Philadelphia, J.B. Lippincott, 1997, pp 1397–1425.
3. Bosl G, Motzer R: Testicular germ cell cancer. N Engl J Med 337:242–253, 1998.
4. Gospodarowicz MD, et al: Early stage and advanced seminoma: Role of radiation therapy, surgery and chemotherapy. Semin Oncol 25:160–173, 1998.
5. McCaffrey J, Bajorin D: Therapy for good risk germ cell tumors. Semin Oncol 25:186–193, 1998.

71. RENAL AND BLADDER CANCER

Mark K. Plante, M.D., FRCS

RENAL CANCER

1. What are the origins of renal tumors?

Eighty percent of renal tumors are of parenchymal origin; the remainder are of uroepithelial origin. The most common tumors of each origin are renal cell carcinoma and transitional carcinoma, respectively. Renal cell carcinoma is the most common solid renal tumor and arises from the cells of the proximal convoluted tubule.

2. What are the yearly incidence and mortality rate of renal cell carcinoma in the United States? What are the major patient demographics?

Approximate incidence: 27,000 new cases/year

Approximate mortality rate: 11,000 deaths/year

Men are affected twice as much as women. The median age is approximately 65 years, and the incidence rises from about age 40 onward.

3. How are most cases diagnosed? What is the classic triad?

Most cases ares now diagnosed incidentally as a result of the more routine use of abdominal ultrasonography and CT scanning in the work-up of a myriad of patient complaints. The classic triad refers to hematuria, flank pain, and a palpable flank mass. Fewer than 10% of patients now present with these findings; those that do more commonly harbor advanced disease.

4. What roles do ultrasonography, CT scanning, arteriography, and MRI play in the work-up of patients with a renal mass?

Ultrasonography	Best determination of solid vs. cystic masses
	Assessment of renal vein and inferior vena cava (IVC) for thrombus
CT scanning	Best anatomic detail
	Assessment of regional nodes
Arteriography	Reserved for arterial anatomy in difficult cases
MRI	Gold standard for assessing caval thrombus extension

5. List the more common associated paraneoplastic syndromes and their incidence.

Anemia	20–40%
Cachexia, fatigue, weight loss	33%
Fever	30%
Hypertension	24%
Hypercalcemia	10–15%

6. Define Stauffer's syndrome. What is its significance?

Stauffer's syndrome is elevation of hepatic transaminase levels in the absence of liver metastases. It may occur in up to 3–6% of patients. Failure of the transaminase levels to normalize after surgical tumor excision may signify persistent disease.

7. How is renal cell carcinoma staged? What are the stage groupings?

The most widely used system is the tumor-node-metastasis (TNM) system:

Tumor stage	T1	Tumor ≤ 2.5 cm and confined to kidney
	T2	Tumor > 2.5 cm and confined to kidney
	T3a	Tumor through renal capsule, confined to Gerota's fascia
	T3b	Extends into renal vein
	T3c	Extends into renal vein and IVC
	T4	Extends beyond Gerota's fascia
Nodal stage	Nx	Nodes not assessed
	N0	Nodes negative for metastasis
	N1	Single node < 2 cm involved
	N2	One or more nodes 2–5 cm
	N3	One or more nodes > 5 cm
Metastatic stage	Mx	Metastatic status not assessed
	M0	No evidence of distant metastasis
	M1	Distant metastases present

The stage groupings are as follows:

Stage I	T1	N0	M0
Stage II	T2	N0	M0
Stage III	T1–T2	N1	M0
	T3a–T3c	N0, N1	M0
Stage IV	T4	Any N	M0
	Any T	N2, N3	M0
	Any T	Any N	M1

8. Name the most common metastatic sites in decreasing order of frequency.

Lung, regional lymph nodes, liver, bone, adrenal gland, opposite kidney, and brain. The metastatic work-up of patients with no neurologic or bony complaints should include a chest radiograph, serum calcium levels, and liver function tests. A bone scan should be obtained if either the alkaline phosphatase or serum calcium level is abnormal.

9. What are the most important prognostic factors?

The most important prognostic factor is tumor stage. Five-year survival rates for patients with T1 disease are 88–100%; for T2 and T3a, approximately 60%. Patients with metastases at presentation, whether nodal or distant, have a much poorer prognosis with 5-year survival rates of 0–2%. Tumor size, grade, histologic type, and patient sex also correlate with outcome but are clearly secondary to the importance of stage.

10. Does renal venous and/or IVC extension affect the patient's ultimate prognosis?

In fact, if the thrombus is free-floating and can be removed intact, the prognosis is the same as that of an equally staged tumor with no thrombus. If the thrombus invades the wall of the renal vein and/or IVC, the prognosis is generally worse, even if surgical excision is possible. Tumor thrombi may extend to the level of the right atrium and in some cases require hypothermic circulatory arrest for removal.

11. What is the role of surgery? Chemotherapy? Radiotherapy?

Surgery is the single most effective treatment for renal cell carcinoma. Radical nephrectomy is the only curative treatment at present. For small lesions in patients with a solitary kidney or renal failure or any predisposition to form multiple tumors (e.g., von Hippel-Lindau disease), partial nephrectomy is an accepted treatment strategy. No chemotherapy regimen has yet been shown to be highly effective. Radiotherapy has a role only in the palliative control of metastatic and local disease symptoms.

12. Is there any role for the surgical removal of metastases?

Yes. In patients with solitary metastases, particularly to the lung, surgical excision of both primary tumor and metastatic deposit can achieve long disease-free intervals as well as the possibility of cure.

13. What other treatment modalities exist at present?

Immunotherapy is the only other accepted treatment modality. Interleukin-2 and interferon alone and in combination have shown response rates from 10–40% in numerous studies. Other investigational treatments include vaccine, cellular, and genetic therapies.

BLADDER CANCER

14. What are the yearly incidence and mortality rate of bladder cancer in the United States? What are the major patient demographics?

Approximate incidence: 40,000 new cases/year

Approximate mortality rate: 10,000 deaths/year

Men are affected 2–3 times more often than women; 80% of cases occur in persons older than 50 years.

15. Name the types of bladder cancer.

Ninety percent of cases are transitional cell carcinoma, 8% are squamous cell, and the remaining 2% are adenocarcinoma.

16. What are the risk factors for development of bladder cancer? Are there differences for each type of bladder cancer?

There are many proven and putative risk factors for the development of bladder cancer. Some risk factors are shared among the types of bladder cancer, and some are unique to one type.

Type	Risk Factors
Transitional (TCC)	Aromatic amines (b-naphthylamine, 4-aminobiphenyl, 4-nitrobiphenyl, 4,4-diaminobiphenyl)—exposure in dye, textile, rubber, cable, printing, and plastic industries
	Cigarette smoking

Type *(Cont.)*	Risk Factors *(Cont.)*
Squamous cell	Schistosomiasis (*Schistosoma haematobium*)
	Chronic indwelling catheters (5–10% of paraplegics)
	Urinary calculi
	Bladder diverticuli
Adenocarcinoma	Urachal origin
	Bladder exstrophy
	Endometriosis
Miscellaneous	Chronic urinary stasis and bladder inflammation
	Phenacetin abuse (analgesic)
	Cyclophosphamide (breakdown product—acrolein)
	Pelvic irradiation
	Genitourinary tuberculosis
	Saccharin ?, cyclamates ?

17. How do most patients present? What are the associated symptoms?

Most patients undergo work-up as a result of either gross or microscopic hematuria. Irritative voiding symptoms as well as flank pain (ureteral obstruction), pelvic pain (extension outside the bladder), and leg edema (lymphatic involvement) also may be present.

18. List the most widely used staging system. What are the stage groupings?

The tumor-node-metastasis (TNM) staging system is most widely used:

Tumor stage	Ta	Noninvasive papillary carcinoma
	Tis	Carcinoma in situ (CIS)
	T1	Invasion into lamina propria
	T2	Invasion into superficial muscle
	T3a	Invasion into deep muscle
	T3b	Invasion into perivesical fat
	T4	Invasion of adjacent organs
Nodal stage	Nx	Nodes not assessed
	N0	Nodes negative for metastasis
	N1	Single node < 2 cm
	N2	One or more nodes 2–5 cm
	N3	One or more nodes > 5 cm
Metastatic stage	Mx	Metastatic status not assessed
	M0	No evidence of distant metastasis
	M1	Distant metastases present

The stage groupings are as follows:

Stage 0a	Ta	N0	M0
Stage 0is	Tis	N0	M0
Stage I	T1	N0	M0
Stage II	T2–T3a	N0	M0
Stage III	T3b–T4	N0	M0
Stage IV	Any T	N1–3	M0
	Any T	Any N	M1

19. Discuss the pathophysiology of transitional cell carcinoma (TCC) of the bladder.

TCC of the bladder is often described as a field disease. Because the bladder serves a storage role, the urine comes in contact with the entire urothelium for extended periods. Tumors may arise anywhere in the bladder and may be solitary or multifocal. The base (or floor) of the bladder is the most commonly affected area.

20. Is TCC found anywhere else in the genitourinary tract?

Because the entire urinary collecting system, from the renal pelvis to the distal urethra, is lined by uroepithelium, TCC may arise at any level. The bladder is by far the most common site for the reason given above. Renal and ureteral lesions are much less frequently diagnosed and are associated with bladder lesions in up to 30% of cases. Conversely, renal/ureteral lesions are seen in only 3% of patients diagnosed with bladder TCC.

21. Discuss the diagnostic work-up for TCC of the bladder. What role does urinary cytology play? What new diagnostic modalities are under development?

Diagnosis is generally made during cytoscopy. However, larger lesions can be seen on ultrasound, intravenous pyelography, and CT scans. Bladder lesions require transurethral resection and, if too large, biopsy. The inclusion of bladder wall muscle in the pathologic specimen is necessary for staging. Intravenous urography is important to rule out concomitant upper collecting system pathology. Urinary cytology is used in the work-up of hematuria to detect tumor cells that are shed into the urine from abnormalities of the urothelium easily missed by the naked eye. It has an increased sensitivity for high-grade lesions and CIS. Newer rapid reagent strips for bladder tumor antigens are now available and may have better sensitivity than urinary cytology.

22. Why is a distinction made among superficial papillary tumors, CIS, and invasive tumors?

The natural history, treatment, and prognosis differ for each category. Most patients present with solitary superficial papillary tumor (Ta), which can be cured by complete resection alone. Up to 50%, however, may recur; therefore, patients must be closely surveyed by cytoscopy. Three percent progress to more invasive disease. CIS, on the other hand, recurs in up to 75% of cases and may progress in 25–50%. Invasive tumors are much more likely to recur and progress to distant metastases.

23. Why are tumors given a grade? What are some of the prognostic factors?

The grade refers to the histologic morphology determined by the degree of cellular atypia, nuclear abnormalities, and number of mitotic figures. Tumor grade and stage strongly correlate with tumor recurrence, progression, and survival. Overall, survival for patients with superficial tumors (Ta–T1) is excellent (80–90%). However, for patients with more invasive disease staged as T2, T3, or T4, survival declines sharply to approximately 50%, 40%, and 25%, respectively.

24. When is intravesical chemotherapy indicated?

The indications are (1) presence of CIS, (2) rapid tumor recurrence, (3) multicentricity, (4) progression to higher grade, and (5) lamina propria invasion.

25. List the commonly used intravesical chemotherapeutic agents and their significant toxicity. What are the contraindications to their use?

Agent	Toxicity
Bacille Calmette-Guérin (BCG)	Disseminated tuberculosis
Thiotepa	Myelosuppression
Mitomycin-C	Contact dermatitis
Interferon	Flulike symptoms

All agents may give irritative voiding symptoms. Contraindications, which increase the risk of systemic toxicity of intravesical therapy, include (1) traumatic catheterization, (2) hematuria, (3) bacterial cystitis, and (4) immunocompromised states.

26. What is the accepted treatment of clinically localized, muscle-invasive TCC of the bladder?

Radical cystectomy (with urinary diversion) is the present standard of therapy. Five-year disease-free survival rates of up to 75% have been reported; 50% is the more accepted figure.

27. Where are the most common metastatic sites in decreasing order of frequency?

Pelvic lymph nodes (obdurator chain—75%, external iliac chain—60%), liver, lung, and bone.

28. How is a patient with metastatic disease treated?

The most widely accepted treatment is systemic chemotherapy. The most studied and commonly used regimen is MVAC (methotrexate, vinblastine, Adriamycin, and cis-platinum). Although initial reports showed overall and complete response rates as high as 75% and 35%, respectively, the larger phase III trials have shown lower rates of 39% and 13%, respectively. Regardless of the response rate, the median survival is 12–13 months. For this reason, as well as the significant toxicity associated with MVAC, newer regimens with numerous other agents are under investigation. The most promising is paclitaxel (Taxol) combined with carboplatinum, which has demonstrated increased response rates and survival and decreased toxicity.

29. What role does radiotherapy have?

Radiotherapy is typically reserved for the palliation of local disease, commonly hematuria, and symptomatic distant metastases.

30. What combination treatments are available?

A large body of research is now directed at bladder preservation in invasive, localized disease by using a more radical transurethral resection combined with both chemotherapy and radiotherapy.

BIBLIOGRAPHY

1. Cohen SM: Urinary bladder carcinogenesis. Toxicol Pathol 26:121–127, 1998.
2. Gillenwater JY, Grayhack JT, Howards SS, Duckett JW: Adult and Pediatric Urology, 3rd ed. St. Louis, Mosby, 1996.
3. Lamm DL (ed): Superficial bladder cancer. Urol Clin North Am 19:421–620, 1993.
4. Novick AC (ed): Renal-sparing surgery for renal cell carcinoma. Urol Clin North Am 20:277–282, 1993.
5. Marshall FF, Stewart AK, Menk HR: The National Cancer Database: Report on kidney cancers. American College of Surgeons Committee on Cancer and the American Cancer Society. Cancer 80:2167–2174, 1997.
6. McCaffrey JA, Bajorin DF, Scher HI, Bosle GJ: Combined modality therapy for bladder cancer. Oncology 11 (9 Suppl 9):18–26, 1997.
7. Motzer RJ, Russo P, Nanus DM, Berg WJ: Renal cell carcinoma. Curr Probl Cancer 21(4):181–232, 1997.
8. Smith SJ, Bosniak MA, Megibow AJ, et al: Renal cell carcinoma: Earlier discovery and increased detection. Radiology 170:699–703, 1989.
9. Vogelzang NJ, Scardino PT, Shipley WU, Coffey DS: Comprehensive Textbook of Genitourinary Oncology. Baltimore, Williams & Wilkins, 1996.

72. PROSTATE CANCER

Michael R. Cooper, M.D.

1. What is the incidence of prostate cancer?

The incidence (number of new cases diagnosed) of prostate cancer in the United States in 1997 is estimated to be 209,900, with 41,800 deaths attributable to this disease. The incidence of the disease for 1997 had initially been projected to be slightly greater than 300,000. The apparently lower than anticipated incidence of the disease may reflect the result of PSA-directed screening for prostate cancer, which in previous years detected many cases that otherwise would not have been detected until the disease was more advanced. However, there is as yet no decrease in the death rate from prostate cancer. Apart from skin cancer, it is the most commonly diagnosed malignancy in men and second only to lung cancer as a cause of cancer-related death. The large difference between the incidence of prostate cancer and the death rate associated with the disease is a major source of the dilemma that surrounds screening for and treatment of early-stage prostate cancer.

2. What is the prevalence of prostate cancer?

The prevalence (number of cases existing at any one time) is difficult to obtain. However, in autopsy series, more than 30% of men over the age of 50 years had cancer in their prostate glands. Some autopsy studies have shown prostate cancer in greater than 10% of males between the ages of 20 and 40 years. The prevalence of low-grade or indolent prostate cancer appears to be similar in different races and geographic groups, but the development of clinically significant prostate cancer is highest in Western societies and is particularly high in African-American men. Dietary factors, particularly fat consumption, are thought to play a major role in these differences.

3. Describe the zones of the prostate.

The fetal prostate consists of the dorsal, ventral, and lateral lobes. In the adult, McNeal's description of the peripheral, anterior, and posterior zones with prostatic periurethral glands is generally accepted. The peripheral zone comprises 65% of total gland size, the central zone 25%, and the transition zone 5–10%. The majority of prostate cancers arise in the peripheral zone of the gland and hence may be detected by digital rectal examination.

4. Define PSA.

Prostate-specific antigen (PSA) is a kallikreinlike serine protease and is produced exclusively by the epithelial cells lining the acini and ducts of all types of prostatic tissue. It has recently been demonstrated that some PSA also is produced in the periurethral glands adjacent to the prostate. It is involved in the liquefaction of the seminal coagulum that is formed at the time of ejaculation. Although PSA is specific for the prostate or, more correctly, for prostatic epithelium, it is not specific for prostate cancer. Its concentration in serum can be elevated by a simple increase in the amount of prostatic epithelium (i.e., as the result of benign prostatic hyperplasia [BPH]), prostatic infection, infarction, and trauma. Although vigorous prostatic massage can increase the serum concentration of PSA, simple digital rectal examination and palpation of the prostate do not produce clinically significant increases.

5. What are normal values for PSA?

The normal value for the PSA is ≤ 4.0 ng/ml. The higher the PSA, the greater the probability that it is elevated as the result of prostate cancer. Some investigators have suggested the use of age-specific ranges for the PSA, since with increasing age the volume of prostatic epithelium and hence the PSA increase as the result of BPH. The use of age-specific PSA ranges would increase the number of younger men and decrease the number of older men subjected to prostatic biopsy, thereby potentially directing treatment of early-stage disease toward those more likely to benefit from it.

6. At what age should screening for prostate cancer be started?

Screening for prostate cancer is a controversial issue. Although clear evidence indicates that the use of PSA in screening for prostate cancer results in the detection of the disease at an earlier stage, it is not clear whether the therapies currently delivered with the intention of curing early-stage prostate cancer (e.g., radical prostatectomy or radiation therapy) make a significant difference in the natural history of the disease. Both techniques appear to be relatively effective against low-volume, low-grade prostate cancer, but it is not clear whether such slowly progressive prostate cancers would become clinically significant within patients' lifetimes. The American Cancer Society (ACS) recommends that both the PSA test and the digital rectal examination be offered annually beginning at age 50 to men who have a life expectancy of at least 10 years. In men who are at greater risk (e.g., African-American men or men with two or more affected first-degree relatives) screening may begin at 45 years. If either the PSA or the digital rectal examination is abnormal, referral to a urologist and subsequent ultrasound and biopsy are usually recommended.

7. Name the most likely areas of metastatic prostate cancer.

Following extension through the prostatic capsule, prostate cancer characteristically spreads to the seminal vesicles, pelvic lymph nodes, and occasionally to retroperitoneal lymph nodes. In addition to this route of spread, prostate cancer has a pronounced tendency to disseminate hematogenously, most often appearing as osteoblastic metastatic skeletal disease.

8. What are the clinical staging systems for prostate cancer commonly used today?

The two most commonly used systems are the Whitmore (ABCD) system and the TNM system. In dealing with early-stage (potentially organ-confined) prostate cancer, it is more common to use the TNM system, because it provides a greater degree of discrimination among different extents of early-stage disease. Now that prostate cancer is more often detected by transrectal sextant needle biopsies of the prostate gland (i.e., following the detection of an elevated PSA) rather than by transurethral prostatectomy for BPH, a new subclassification of T1 disease had to be created to describe prostate cancer detected by needle biopsy alone: T1c.

Prostate Cancer Staging

Clinical and Pathologic Staging of Prostate Cancer: TNM (ABCD) System		
STAGE	CLINICAL	PATHOLOGIC
T1 or A	cT1 (A): Tumor not palpable, incidental finding at surgery or on PSA test	pT1a (A1): < 5% of resected tissue involved (well differentiated; focal involvement) pT1b (A2): > 5% of resected tissue involved (moderately or poorly differentiated; multiple foci) pT1c (B0): identified by needle biopsy
T2 or B	cT2a (B1): tumor in ≤ ½ of one lobe on digital rectal exam cT2b (B2): tumor in > ½ of one lobe on digital rectal exam cT2c (B2): tumor in both lobes	pT2a (B1): tumor in ≤ ½ of single lobe pT2b (B1): tumor in > ½ of single lobe pT2c (B2): tumor in both lobes
T3 or C	cT3a (C1): unilateral prostatic capsular extension cT3b (C1): bilateral prostatic capsular extension cT3c: seminal vesicle involvement	pT3a (C1): unilateral prostatic capsular extension pT3b (C1): bilateral prostatic capsular extension pT3c: seminal vesicle invasion C2: bladder outlet or urethral obstruction
T4 or C2	C2: Bladder outlet or urethral obstruction	pT4a: tumor invasion of bladder neck, external sphincter, and/or rectum pT4b: tumor invasion of levator muscles
D0	Clinically local disease Elevated prostatic acid phosphatase	
N+ or D1	Regional lymph node involvement	N0: no regional lymph node involvement N1: single lymph node < 2 cm N2: single lymph node ≤ 5 cm N3: single lymph node > 5 cm D1: regional lymph nodes only
M+ or D2	Distant metastases Relapse of D2 after adequate endocrine therapy	M (D2): distant metastases (nonpelvic lymph nodes, bone, other sites)

Gleason Pattern Score	
SCORE	APPEARANCE
2–4	Well differentiated
5–7	Moderately differentiated
8–10	Poorly differentiated

Prostate Cancer Staging (Continued)

			American Joint Committee on Cancer Stage Groups	
STAGE	TUMOR	NODE	METASTASIS	HISTOLOGIC GRADE
0	T1a	N0	M0	G1 (well differentiated)
I	T1a	N0	M0	G2 (moderately differentiated) G3–4 (poorly differentiated or undifferentiated)
	T1b	N0	M0	Any G
	T1c	N0	M0	Any G
	T1	N0	M0	Any G
II	T2	N0	M0	Any G (well, moderately, poorly differentiated)
III	T3	N0	M0	Any G
IV	T4	N0	M0	Any G
	Any T	N1	M0	Any G
	Any T	N2	M0	Any G
	Any T	N3	M0	Any G
	Any T	Any N	M1	Any G

9. Name the methods of staging newly diagnosed prostate cancer.

Laboratory staging is essential in evaluating prostate cancer. However, the extent of laboratory studies varies according to the suspected extent of the disease. Before the advent of the PSA test, it was common to determine the serum concentration of acid phosphatase, elevation of which almost always portended the eventual development of metastatic disease. However, there is currently little point in determining acid phosphatase values. PSA is more sensitive for the detection of organ-confined prostate cancer and is less influenced by extraneous variables when monitoring the course of therapy. Anemia is common only in the setting of advanced (stage D2) disease. Bony metastatic disease often produces elevations in the alkaline phosphatase.

Radionuclide bone scanning may detect areas of bone metastasis. It is often used in the evaluation of patients with stage D2 disease to correlate symptoms with areas of increased activity on the scan, thereby suggesting appropriate targets for palliative external-beam radiation therapy. For many years radionuclide bone scans were also performed in the evaluation of patients thought to have early-stage disease that potentially could be cured by radical prostatectomy or radiation therapy. However, if the PSA level is less than 20 ng/ml, the chance of a positive bone scan is 0.3%. When the PSA is 15 ng/ml or lower, the chance of a negative bone scan is virtually 100%. The majority of patients considered for curative local therapy have PSA values less than or equal to 10 ng/ml.

CT scanning and MRI have little value in the evaluation of patients with early-stage prostate cancer. Pelvic lymph node involvement cannot be reliably detected with either technique and in the past has been assessed directly with pelvic lymph node dissection. A newer technique for the detection of pelvic lymph node metastases is a radiolabeled monoclonal murine antibody that recognizes a protein, prostate-specific membrane antigen, which is commonly expressed on the surface of prostate cancer cells. Extracapsular extension of prostate cancer may eventually be evaluable with newer MRI techniques, but these remain investigational.

10. What are the treatment options for prostate cancer believed to be confined to the gland (stages T1 and T2)?

There are several treatment options for patients with organ-confined prostate cancer, and current data do not allow one to discriminate readily among them in terms of their ability to alter the natural history of the disease. Patients and their physicians often choose different approaches to treatment (or refuse treatment altogether) based on their different side effects.

The time-honored approach to attempting cure of early-stage prostate cancer is the radical prostatectomy, a surgical procedure that removes the prostate gland, the seminal vesicles, and the more distal portions of the ejaculatory ducts. The nerve-sparing technique developed by Walsh, which preserves the capsular and periprostatic nerves, allows maintenance of potency in appropriately selected patients without compromising control over the tumor. A radical prostatectomy can be accomplished via a retropubic or perineal approach. The perineal prostatectomy has gained advocates recently with the advent of laparoscopic pelvic lymph node dissection. The perineal approach usually results in less blood loss, and recovery is more rapid than with the retropubic approach. This procedure, which gives limited exposure and does not allow pelvic lymph node sampling, is often chosen for removal of small tumors associated with a low PSA. The overall morbidity associated with this procedure includes impotence in 30–50% of men and incontinence in 1–5%.

Radiation therapy in the form of external irradiation is currently a popular treatment. Treatment includes the obturator, hypogastric, and iliac lymph nodes as well as the prostate gland. The incontinence and impotence rates are similar to radical prostatectomy but may take longer to develop. Other complications seen with radiation therapy include radiation cystitis and proctitis.

Brachytherapy, the placement of radioactive substances into the prostate gland, is an option in localized prostate cancer. Techniques include open implantation in combination with lymph node dissection and ultrasound-guided perineal placement. Substances most often used include iridium-192, gold-198, iodine-125, and palladium-103. Complications are similar to external beam radiotherapy and include the complications of a pelvic lymph node dissection.

11. What percentage of patients have rectal involvement?

Less than 1% of patients have local extension into the rectum because of Denonvilliers' fascia, a perineal vestige that lies between the prostate gland and the rectum and usually prevents extension from the gland to the rectum.

12. At what stage is prostate cancer most commonly detected?

It is estimated that some 60% of the new cases of prostate cancer are T3 (C), as determined clinically or after examination of pathologic material following radical prostatectomy. T3 or C disease indicates that the prostate cancer has extended through the capsule of the gland and may involve the seminal vesicles. T3 or C prostate cancer detected or suspected clinically is typically treated with external-beam radiation therapy. New information indicates that this group of patients also benefits from simultaneous therapy with a luteinizing hormone-releasing hormone (LHRH) agonist, which reduces serum testosterone concentrations to castrate levels.

13. Describe the hypothalamic-pituitary-testicular axis.

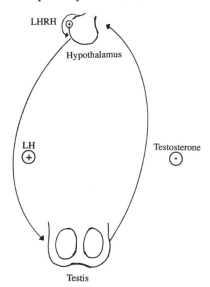

14. Who discovered the relationship between testosterone and prostate cancer?

Huggins and Hodges discovered that hormonal ablation caused regression of metastatic prostate cancer. The Nobel Prize was awarded to Huggins in 1953 for this discovery.

15. Which two methods are most commonly used to decrease circulating testosterone levels produced by the testicles?

Surgical removal of the testicles (bilateral orchiectomy) has been the mainstay of hormonal therapy for metastatic prostate cancer. The testosterone produced by the testicles accounts for 85–90% of circulating androgens, the remainder arising primarily from the adrenal glands. Bilateral orchiectomy produces objective and symptomatic improvement in 80–90% of men with metastatic (stage D2) disease.

Although the estrogen diethylstilbestrol (DES) was used for many years as an alternative to bilateral orchiectomy, it has been generally abandoned as a treatment for prostate cancer because its use is associated with excessive cardiovascular morbidity and mortality. Men taking DES are more likely to develop deep venous thrombosis, pulmonary embolism, myocardial infarction, and stroke. They also tend to develop peripheral edema, gynecomastia, and other signs of feminization.

Because of the problems associated with the use of DES, LHRH agonists were developed to suppress the testicular production of testosterone. The LHRH agonists currently available for use include leuprolide (Lupron) and goserelin acetate (Zoladex). Both are provided as depot formulations, which allow them to be given as once-monthly injections. The LHRH agonists bind to LHRH receptors normally present in the anterior pituitary gland. This binding of the LHRH agonist to the LHRH receptor initially stimulates the anterior pituitary gland to secrete luteinizing hormone (LH), which in turn stimulates the secretion of testosterone by the Leydig cells of the testis. However, because the concentration of LH agonist in the anterior pituitary gland is supraphysiologic and continuously maintained when patients are treated with either leuprolide or goserelin acetate, there is eventually a downregulation in the number of LHRH receptors in the pituitary and an ensuing shutdown in the secretion of LH.

16. Are there any contraindications to the use of an LHRH agonist?

Although there are no absolute contraindications to the use of leuprolide and goserelin acetate, there are situations in which these medications might not be the treatments of first choice. In men who have newly diagnosed metastatic prostate cancer and who present with life-threatening complications of the disease (e.g., spinal cord compression), an immediate decrease in serum testosterone concentrations is most desirable. The initial increase in serum concentrations of testosterone that follows LHRH agonist therapy could briefly accelerate the progression of the patient's disease, and castrate serum levels of testosterone would not be anticipated for some 2–4 weeks thereafter. Bilateral orchiectomy is a straightforward method for quickly reducing the serum testosterone concentration and avoids the potential "flare" in prostate cancer observed in approximately 10% of patients treated with an LHRH agonist.

17. Is it possible to avoid the "flare" in prostate cancer that may occur with LHRH agonist therapy?

A number of compounds (the nonsteroidal antiandrogens flutamide, bicalutamide,and nilutamide) have been developed that bind to the androgen receptor in the prostate cancer cell. Although these drugs bind to the androgen receptor, they do not result in stimulation of cellular proliferation, as do the natural ligands, testosterone and dihydrotestosterone. It is common practice to initiate therapy with a nonsteroidal antiandrogen for several days before the first injection of an LHRH agonist, thereby avoiding the potential worsening of the patient's disease, which could result from the transient increase in serum concentrations of testosterone.

18. For how long should therapy with a nonsteroidal antiandrogen be given?

Although it is rational to treat patients with a nonsteroidal antiandrogen for 5–7 days before and then during the month following the first injection of an LHRH agonist, it is not clear how long thereafter therapy with a nonsteroidal antiandrogen should be continued. It has been argued that, even after circulating concentrations of testosterone are within the castrate range, adrenal androgens continue to be a significant source of stimulation for the growth of the prostate cancer. Hence, it has been typical in the United States for patients to take a nonsteroidal antiandrogen indefinitely when given in combination with an LHRH agonist or as a supplement to orchiectomy. Support for this approach came from a large clinical trial performed cooperatively by several U.S. cancer groups, which demonstrated that in the treatment of men with stage D2 prostate cancer, the combination of leuprolide and flutamide produced an almost 7-month survival advantage compared with leuprolide alone. In this trial, flutamide was given until the time of disease progression.

However, more recently the Southwest Oncology Group (SWOG) reported the results of a large, randomized trial in the same patient population, in which all men were treated with orchiectomy and then received either flutamide or placebo. There was no difference in survival between the two groups, a result that argues against the importance of adrenal androgens in the progression of metastatic prostate cancer.

19. What are the potential sources of confusion about the use of nonsteroidal antiandrogens?

In the trial of leuprolide + flutamide versus leuprolide alone, the leuprolide injection was given as a daily subcutaneous injection. Depending on the degree of noncompliance with daily injections, it is possible that the flutamide provided some protection from intermittent increases in the serum concentration of testosterone. It is also possible that all of the benefit from flutamide therapy came from the first weeks of therapy when it may have prevented a worsening in the patient's disease resulting from the transient, LHRH-induced increase in serum concentrations of testosterone.

In addition, in patients who have taken flutamide for prolonged periods (greater than 1 year) and in whom the prostate cancer is progressing, cessation of therapy with flutamide can result in a decline in the serum concentration of PSA and in an improvement in disease-related signs and symptoms. This phenomenon is currently hypothesized to result from mutations in the androgen receptor of some prostate cancer cells, which cause the receptor to view flutamide no longer as an antagonist but rather as an agonist. In other words, prolonged therapy with flutamide may provide an advantage for the proliferation of a subset of prostate cancer cells with a mutated androgen receptor. A similar "withdrawal response" has been observed with other nonsteroidal antiandrogens.

20. What is hormone-refractory prostate cancer?

The term hormone-refractory prostate cancer refers to disease that is progressive in spite of castrate serum concentrations of testosterone (< 30 ng/ml). Although 80–90% of men with stage D2 prostate cancer respond to treatment with either bilateral orchiectomy or an LHRH agonist with a decline in PSA and an improvement in disease-related symptoms, disease progression, defined by an increase in the serum PSA concentration, occurs on average 18 months thereafter. PSA-defined progression antedates clinical evidence of progression by approximately 6 months. Median survival in patients with D2 prostate cancer, calculated from the time of initiation of androgen-deprivation therapy, is about 36 months.

21. How should hormone-refractory prostate cancer be treated?

Patients who exhibit evidence of disease progression in the face of castrate levels of serum testosterone should stop therapy with nonsteroidal antiandrogens (flutamide, casodex, nilutamide). Serial measurements of PSA taken over the following 4–6 weeks should identify a withdrawal response if it is to occur. Standard therapy otherwise is directed primarily at the relief of pain, which most often is related to skeletal metastases. Narcotic analgesics and external-beam radiation therapy directed to symptomatic or weight-bearing regions of bone are the mainstays of palliative treatment. Strontium-89 is a radioisotope that is chemically related to calcium and tends to accumulate in areas of bone metastasis. It is useful in treating patients with diffuse bone pain that cannot be easily treated with standard external-beam therapy.

22. Should chemotherapy be offered to patients with hormone-refractory prostate cancer?

No chemotherapeutic agent or combination of agents has been shown to alter survival in prostate cancer. However, mitoxantrone, a drug related structurally and mechanistically to doxorubicin (Adriamycin) when given in combination with low doses of prednisone, has been shown to help alleviate disease-related symptoms, particularly pain. Another promising approach in the field of cytotoxic chemotherapy is the combination of taxanes (paclitaxel and docetaxel) with estramustine phosphate. Estramustine phosphate is an estrogen molecule combined with nitrogen mustard. Although it has estrogenic side effects, its primary mechanism of action is to disrupt the function of tubulin, which is also the site of action of the taxanes.

BIBLIOGRAPHY

1. Bolla M, Gonzalez D, Warde P, et al: Improved survival in patients with locally advanced prostate cancer treated with radiotherapy and goserelin. N Engl J Med 337:295–300, 1997.
2. Crawford ED, et al: A controlled trial of leuprolide with and without flutamide in prostatic carcinoma. N Engl J Med 321:419–424, 1989.
3. Crawford ED: Changing paradigms in the treatment of advanced prostate cancer. Adv Oncol 12:14–21, 1996.
4. Crawford ED, DeAntoni EP, Hussain M, et al: Prostate cancer clinical trials of the Southwest Oncology Group. Oncology 11:1154–1163, 1997.
5. Hudes GR, Nathan F, Khater C, et al: Phase II trial of 96-hour paclitaxel plus oral estramustine phosphate in metastatic hormone-refractory prostate cancer. J Clin Oncol 15:3156–3163, 1997.
6. McNeal JE: Origin and development of carcinoma of the prostate. Cancer 23:24, 1969.
7. Sakr WA, Haas GP, Cassin BF, et al: The frequency of carcinoma and intraepithelial neoplasia of the prostate in young male patients. J Urol 150:370–385, 1993.
8. Scher HI, Kelly WK: Flutamide withdrawal syndrome: Its impact on clinical trials in hormone-refractory prostate cancer. J Clin Oncol 11:1566–1572, 1995.
9. Tannock IF, Osoba D, Stockler MR, et al: Chemotherapy with mitoxantrone plus prednisone or prednisone alone for symptomatic hormone-resistant prostate cancer: A Canadian randomized trial with palliative endpoints. J Clin Oncol 14:1756–1764, 1996.
10. von Eschenbach A, Ho R, Murphy GP, et al: American Cancer Society guideline for the early detection of prostate cancer: Update 1997. CA Cancer J Clin 47:261–264, 1997.
11. Wingo PA, Landis S, Ries LAG: An adjustment to the 1997 estimate for new prostate cancer cases. CA Cancer J Clin 47:239–242, 1997.

73. CUTANEOUS MELANOMA

Stephen J. Hoffman, M.D., Ph.D., and Lyndah K. Dreiling, M.D.

1. What is malignant melanoma?

Melanoma is a highly invasive and often fatal malignancy of the pigmented cells located at the base of the epidermis (melanocytes). During the early embryologic period, melanocytes migrate from the neuroectoderm to the skin, eye, respiratory tract, and gut. Nevi are thought to be nests of melanocytes at different levels of differentiation and represent the most common focus of primary cutaneous melanoma.

2. Is melanoma a tumor of more modern times?

John Hunter first reported a patient with a recurrent black "fungous excrescence" in 1787. An original specimen of the tumor was preserved in the Hunterian Museum of the Royal College of Surgeons of England. In 1968 examination of the specimen confirmed melanoma. René Laennec, however, was the first to describe melanoma as a disease in 1806.

3. How common is melanoma?

The incidence of melanoma is increasing dramatically in light-skinned people. The incidence rate for Caucasians in the United States ranges from 10–30 per 100,000 depending on geographic area. If present trends continue, this ratio may reach 1 in 75 by the year 2000.

4. What are the risk factors for melanoma?

In declining order of importance, risk factors are a changing mole, family history of melanoma, fair complexion, dysplastic nevi, history of nonmelanoma skin cancer, history of a severe blistering sunburn, large number of nevi and/or large size (5–10 mm) of nevi, and freckling tendency.

5. What is meant by a changing mole?

Generally, nevi become apparent on the skin beginning around puberty, complete development by adulthood, and involute during the geriatric years. Therefore, any new mole in an adult deserves evaluation. The warning signs of melanomas follow the **ABCD**s. They may show **a**symmetry of shape, color, or appearance. Their **b**orders may be irregular or notched, or they may **b**leed. The **c**olor of a mole may **c**hange from uniform brown to variable shades of blue, gray, pink, red, or white. The **d**iameter of most melanomas is > 6 mm, but small size is not uncommon and should not rule out malignancy.

6. How is melanoma diagnosed?

The diagnosis of melanoma is made histologically. Melanoma is evaluated on the basis of its depth of invasion into the skin and its thickness. **Clark's level of invasion** describes how deep into the skin the tumor has reached. The **Breslow thickness** measures in millimeters the tumor size from the granular layer of the epidermis to the deepest part of the tumor. In general, the deeper and thicker the primary tumor, the more likely it is to have metastasized.

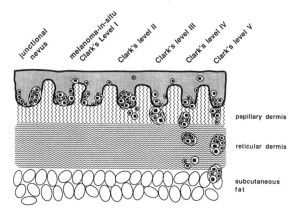

Determination of Clark's levels in primary melanoma.

7. What are the different types of melanoma?

Superficial spreading melanoma is the most common type and generally arises in preexisting nevi. It may grow slowly over years in a pattern that spreads over the superficial skin layer before penetrating into deeper layers. Nodular melanoma is the next most common type and, as implied by the name, is usually a nodule on the skin that often bleeds and is friable and ulcerated. Nodular melanomas grow deep rapidly and are known for early metastasis. Acral lentiginous melanoma occurs on the palms and soles and under the nails (non–hair-bearing skin). This type of melanoma is more common in nonwhites and generally carries a worse prognosis because its location delays diagnosis. Lentigo maligna melanoma is similar to the superficial spreading type and generally occurs on the face of elderly patients (Hutchinson's melanotic freckle).

8. Discuss several skin lesions that may simulate a cutaneous melanoma.

Seborrheic keratoses (greasy, "stuck-on"-appearing lesions on the trunk and face of older adults), benign nevi, pigmented basal cell carcinomas, and solar lentigo ("liver spots") are pigmented lesions that may mimic melanoma. Spitz nevi, previously known as juvenile melanoma, are pink-to-brown papules that occur in children, adolescents, and young adults and may simulate melanoma clinically and histologically. Pyogenic granulomas are friable, pink-to-red nodules that may simulate nodular melanoma.

9. How is a melanoma distinguished from mimic lesions?

Even experienced dermatologists can make diagnostic mistakes when evaluating a pigmented lesion by physical exam alone. Most changing lesions in an adult require a biopsy and histologic examination for accurate diagnosis before therapy.

10. What is the natural history of metastatic melanoma?

The most predictable factor about melanoma is its unpredictability. Unlike many malignancies, there is nothing magical about a 5-year disease-free survival. Probably in part because of the immune-related response to melanomas and possible waning of the same, melanoma may recur for long periods after excision of the primary tumor. The literature supports several cases of recurrence up to 40 years after primary diagnosis, although second unknown primaries may account for some cases.

11. Is there a genetic predisposition to development of melanoma?

Chromosome 1 and 6 rearrangements are the most frequent genetic abnormalities detected in melanoma. Chromosome 7 duplications are often found in late-stage metastatic tumors and suggest that melanoma oncogenes may be located on this chromosome. The germline mutations in people with either sporadic or familial melanoma involves one or more of the tumor suppressor genes in the p21 region of chromosome 9.

12. How should a patient with newly diagnosed melanoma be staged?

The hallmark of staging for melanoma is a complete history and physical examination. Because melanoma has a propensity to recur on the skin, all cutaneous areas must be fully examined, including the scalp, palms and soles, and genitals/perineum. Cutaneous lesions suspicious for second melanomas, atypical nevi, and/or subcutaneous metastases require biopsy. Palpable lymph nodes require histologic sampling by lymph node dissection or fine-needle aspiration. Minimal baseline staging procedures include chest radiographs (with computed tomography [CT]), if indicated, and evaluation of liver chemistries. Patients with histologic staging of Breslow depth > 4.00 mm thick or stage III disease also should undergo abdominal CT scanning. Patients complaining of central nervous system (CNS) symptoms or patients with deep primary lesions located in the head and neck region may require brain magnetic resonance imaging (MRI) to rule out intracranial metastases. A new procedure (radiolymphoscintigraphy) is used with more frequency to map the lymph node drainage of the primary tumor with blue dye, allowing biopsy of the sentinel node to assess for possible microscopic metastasis. If present, a regional lymph node dissection is completed. Based on the depth and thickness of the primary tumor, melanoma is staged by the American Joint Committee on Cancer Staging (AJCCS) criteria.

AJCCS Criteria for Staging of Cutaneous Melanoma

STAGE	CRITERIA
1a	Primary melanoma < 0.75 mm thick and/or Clark's level II (pT1); no nodal or systemic metastasis (N0, M0)
1b	Primary melanoma 0.76–1.50 mm thick and/or Clark's level III (pT2); N0, M0
IIa	Primary melanoma 1.51–4.00 mm thick and/or Clark's level IV (pT3); N0, M0
IIb	Primary melanoma > 4.00 mm thick and/or Clark's level V (pT4); N0, M0
III	Regional lymph node and/or in-transit metastasis (any pT, N1 or N2, M0)
IV	Systemic metastasis (any pT, any N, M1)

The AJCCS Melanoma Committee recommends that tumor thickness take precedence over Clark's level and should be used for pT (pathologic tumor) staging when differences arise or when Breslow's tumor thickness is unknown or cannot be measured.

13. Describe the treatment for stages I and II melanoma.

The appropriate treatment for stages I and II melanoma is surgical excision of the primary tumor with adequate margins. The current recommendations for surgical margins for excision of primary melanoma are as follows:

Thickness (mm)	Surgical Margins (cm)
In situ	0.5
≤ 1.0	1.0
≥ 1.0	2.0

14. What is the role of elective lymph node dissection in melanoma?

This area of melanoma treatment is controversial. Previously, elective removal of draining removal lymph nodes was performed based on the thought that melanoma metastasized via regional lymphatics and that removal of uninvolved nodes could prevent spread. Melanoma is now known also to metastasize via hematogenous routes. Adequate data from randomized studies show that elective lymph node dissection has no benefit for patients with primary melanomas of the extremities. For truncal and head/neck melanoma, the case is less clear, although any benefit is marginal and probably limited to patients with primary tumors at high risk to metastasize (e.g., thick or ulcerated tumors).

15. Is there any effective adjuvant therapy for resected melanoma?

Adjuvant therapy for resected melanomas with a moderate-to-high risk of recurrence should be considered within the setting of a clinical research protocol whenever possible. Emerging data from cooperative oncology groups indicate that certain types and schedules of immunotherapy may improve survival rates in this group of patients.

16. What is the prognosis for stage I or II melanoma?

In general, the prognosis is inversely proportional to the thickness and depth of the tumor. Total excision of a superficial melanoma, that is, malignant cells limited to the epidermis, is essentially curative. The 10-year survival rate for Clark's level II melanoma is 96%; for level III, 90%; for level IV, 67%; and for level V, 26%. Ten-year survival data by stage are 93% for stage I, 68% for stage II, 40% for stage III, and 0% for stage IV disease.

17. How often should patients with newly diagnosed melanoma be evaluated?

Patients with thin melanomas who have a lower risk for recurrence should be followed every 6 months for the first 2 years after diagnosis. Patients at a higher risk for recurrence (e.g., thick primary tumors, primary tumors of the head and neck region, ulcerated primary tumors) should be seen more often, such as every 3–4 months. Complete physical examination and review of systems should be performed with each evaluation. Follow-up radiologic and laboratory evaluations should be done every 6–12 months or as indicated.

18. What is the treatment for stage III melanoma?

Treatment for stage III disease (i.e., in-transit metastases or regional lymph node involvement) is surgical resection of tumor. Subsequent systemic or adjuvant therapies remain controversial and generally are offered in an experimental setting. Patients that advance from stage I/II disease to stage II need to be fully reevaluated to rule out both visceral and CNS metastases.

19. Discuss the therapeutic options for stage IV melanoma.

Surgery, radiation therapy, chemotherapy, immunotherapy, regional perfusion chemotherapy, and hyperthermia have been attempted and have some utility in treating the patient with advanced-stage disease. Radiation therapy is generally reserved for palliative treatment of certain tumors, because melanoma is highly radioresistant. Surgical excision of isolated visceral tumors is mostly palliative but in certain cases and in combination with chemotherapy may result in increased disease-free survival. The mainstay of treatment for advanced-stage disease is multi-agent chemotherapy, with immunotherapy (e.g., interferon alpha, interleukin-2) and hormonal therapy. Many other experimental therapies are currently under investigation, including other biologic response modifiers, monoclonal antibodies, and gene therapies. However, systemic therapy for metastatic melanoma remains a palliative intervention.

BIBLIOGRAPHY

1. Aapro MS: Advances in systemic treatment of malignant melanoma. Eur J Cancer 29A:613–617, 1993.
2. Balch CM, Houghton AN, Milton GW, et al (eds): Clinical Melanoma, 2nd ed. Philadelphia, J.B. Lippincott, 1992, p 223.
3. Friedman RJ, Heilman ER, Gottlieb GJ, et al: Malignant melanoma: Clinicopathologic correlations. In Friedman RJ, Rigel DS, Kopf AW, et al (eds): Cancer of the Skin. Philadelphia, W.B. Saunders, 1991, pp 148–176.
4. Friedman RJ, Rigel DS, Silverman MK, et al: Malignant melanoma in the 1990s: The continued importance of early detection and the role of physician examination and self-examination of the skin. CA 41:201–226, 1991.
5. Green RJ, Schuchter LM: Systemic treatment of metastatic melanoma with chemotherapy. Hematol Oncol Clin North Am 12:863–875, 1998.
6. Harris MN, Roses DF: Malignant melanoma: Treatment. In Friedman RJ, Rigel DS, Kopf AW, et al (eds): Cancer of the Skin. Philadelphia, W.B. Saunders, 1991, pp 177–197.
7. Hoffman SJ, Yohn JJ, Norris DA, et al: Cutaneous malignant melanoma. Curr Probl Dermatol V:1–44, 1993.
8. Kirkwood JM, Strawderman MH, Ernstoff MS, et al: Adjuvant therapy of high-risk resected cutaneous melanoma: The Eastern Cooperative Oncology Group Trial EST 1684. J Clin Oncol 14:7, 1996.
9. Koh HK: Cutaneous melanoma (see comments). N Engl J Med 325:171–182, 1991.
10. Legha SS, Ring S, Papadopoulos N, et al: A prospective evaluation of a triple-drug regimen containing cisplatin, vinblastine, and DTIC (CVD) for metastatic melanoma. Cancer 64:2024, 1989.
11. NIH Consensus Conference: Diagnosis and treatment of early melanoma. JAMA 268:1314–1319, 1992
12. Parmiani G: Future perspectives in specific immunotherapy of melanoma. Eur J Cancer 34(Suppl):S42–S47, 1998.
13. Pyrhonen S: The treatment of metastatic uveal melanoma. Eur J Cancer 34(Suppl)S27–S30, 1998.
14. Reintgen DS, Brobeil A: Lymphatic mapping and selective lymphadenopathy as an alternative to elective lymph node dissection in patients with malignant melanoma. Hematol Oncol Clin North Am 12:807–821, 1998.
15. Richards JM, Mehta N, Ramming K, Skosey P: Sequential chemoimmunotherapy in the treatment of metastatic melanoma. J Clin Oncol 10:1338–1343, 1992.
16. Shih IM, Herlyn M: Role of growth factors and their receptors in the development and progression of melanoma. J Invest Dermatol 100:196S–203S, 1993.
17. Stadelmann WK, Reintgen DS: Prognosis in malignant melanoma. Hematol Oncol Clin North Am 12:767–796, 1998.

74. NONMELANOMA SKIN CANCER

Patrick Walsh, M.D., and Timothy Egbert, B.S.

1. What is the most common cancer in humans?

Nonmelanoma skin cancer. An estimated 900,000–1.2 million new nonmelanoma skin cancers were diagnosed in 1998. Nonmelanoma skin cancer accounts for almost one-half of all cancers diagnosed in the U.S.

2. Are there different types of nonmelanoma skin cancer?

Yes. The most common type is basal cell carcinoma, accounting for approximately 75% of nonmelanoma skin cancer diagnosed in the U.S. Squamous cell carcinoma is the second most common form, accounting for slightly more than 20% of nonmelanoma skin cancer. Nonmelanoma skin cancers also include relatively rare adnexal tumors such as sebaceous carcinoma and eccrine porocarcinoma.

3. According to statistics from the National Cancer Institute, the incidence rate of all cancers declined an average of 0.7% per years between 1990 and 1995. Are skin cancer incidence rates also declining?

No. Melanoma and nonmelanoma skin cancers are the major exceptions to this national trend. Melanoma has the most rapidly increasing incidence rate of all solid tumors in the U.S., and the incidence of nonmelanoma skin cancer is increasing at a rate of about 2–4% each year.

4. What causes skin cancer?

Many factors predispose to the development of skin cancer and may be different for each type of skin cancer. The predominant cause of the development of nonmelanoma skin cancer is cumulative doses of ultraviolet radiation; approximately 40% of people who live to age 65 will develop at least one nonmelanoma skin cancer for this reason. Other causative factors include exposure to chemicals such as coal tar, polycyclic aromatic hydrocarbons, inorganic pentavalent arsenic, tobacco smoke tars, nitrogen mustard, and chromates. Exposure to ionizing radiation also predisposes to the development of skin cancer.

5. Do sunscreens cause skin cancer?

No. This misinterpretation of information by the lay press has received worldwide attention. Sunscreens that have a particular SPF (sun protective factor) are screens that block primarily ultraviolet radiation in the UVB range (290–320 nm wavelength), the wavelength that causes erythema and blistering (i.e., sunburn) of the skin most quickly. Cumulative doses of UVB are the most important etiologic factors in the development of nonmelanoma skin cancer. In contrast, brief, intense exposure to UVA (ultraviolet radiation in the range of 320–400 nm) also appears to predispose to the development of melanoma. It has been postulated (but not proved) that if people use UVB sunscreens to stay in the sun longer (because they are partially protected from the unpleasant sunburn range of ultraviolet radiation), they are increasing their exposure to UVA and therefore their chances of developing melanoma. This does not mean that sunscreens should not be used. The current recommendations for protection from the harmful effects of ultraviolet radiation include avoidance of exposure during peak periods of ultraviolet radiation (10 AM to 2 PM), use of sun-protective clothing, and use of broad-spectrum sunscreens that protect against both UVA and UVB radiation.

6. Define basal cell carcinoma (BCC) and describe the cellular layers of the epidermis.

BCC is a tumor of cells that have histologic and molecular characteristics similar to cells of the basal layer of the epidermis. The epidermis has several distinct cellular layers. The **basal layer** (stratum germativum) is the bottom layer overlying the basement membrane zone and the dermis, the only actively dividing layer (regenerative layer) of the epidermis. Above the basal layer is the **squamous layer** (stratum spinosum), then the **granular layer** (stratum granulosum), and then the **cornified cell layer** (stratum corneum).

7. Describe the appearance of BCC.

Each of the several forms of BCC looks slightly different. The most common form is the nodular BCC, which looks like a waxy or translucent bump that often has small dilated blood vessels on top. As the tumor grows, it often develops raised, rolled borders and a central indentation or ulceration. Pigmented BCC is similar to nodular BCC but has brown, blue, or black pigment distributed irregularly throughout the lesion. Other more uncommon variants include the superficial multifocal BCC, which appears as a well-demarcated red patch, and the morpheaform BCC, which is a poorly demarcated, firm, yellow, or waxy plaque.

8. Are there other lesions that look like BCC?

The differential diagnosis includes melanocytic nevus (e.g., an intradermal nevus, especially one that is not making much pigment), fibrous papule or angiofibroma, sebaceous hyperplasia, trichoepithelioma (a benign tumor of the skin), and other adnexal tumors.

9. How is BCC treated?

There are several effective treatments. Excision, electrodesiccation and curettage, and cryosurgery are each curative in > 90% of primary tumors. They are destructive to the tumor and its surrounding stroma.

10. What if BCC is not treated?

Left untreated, BCCs are usually only locally invasive. As they grow, they may invade and destroy underlying structures (e.g., muscle, nerve, bone), but usually do not travel through blood vessels or lymphatics.

11. What is Mohs' surgery?

Mohs' micrographic surgery is a surgical technique developed by Frederic Mohs. The fresh-tissue technique is a modification of the original technique first reported by Stegman and Tromovitch (two of Dr. Mohs' fellows). In this technique, the location and orientation of the tumor are mapped on excision, and the excised tumor is frozen and sectioned to allow microscopic analysis of all margins (including the deep margin). Any residual tumor can then be localized and removed. The procedure is curative in > 95% of cases. Mohs' surgery is indicated for recurrent skin cancers (which have only about a 50% cure rate using standard surgical techniques), skin cancers that occur in areas with a high rate of recurrence (e.g., pre- and posteroauricular areas, and the nasolabial sulcus), and for skin cancers that occur in cosmetically sensitive areas. Because only the involved tissue is excised, this tissue-sparing technique is ideal for lesions in such areas.

12. Define squamous cell carcinoma (SCC).

SCC, the second most common form of skin cancer, is a tumor composed of cells that have histologic and molecular characteristics similar to cells of the squamous layer of the epidermis.

13. Discuss the appearance of SCC.

Each form has a distinctive appearance. The earliest, most superficial form, SCC in situ, has three forms: Bowen's disease, erythroplasia of Queyrat, and bowenoid papulosis. Bowen's disease appears as a red, scaly patch or plaque with sharply defined borders. Erythroplasia of Queyrat is a bright red patch or plaque without scale that occurs on the glans penis. Bowenoid papulosis presents as multiple, flat-topped, red, brown, or flesh-colored bumps on the external genitalia. The more serious (and potentially metastatic) form of SCC is the invasive form. This tumor usually appears as an ill-defined, red, scaly bump that may ulcerate or bleed easily with trauma.

14. Are there other lesions that look like SCC?

Actinic keratoses, which may be precursors to SCC, appear as red, scaly patches on sun-exposed skin. Actinic keratoses may resemble Bowen's disease but usually have less well-defined borders. Inflammation of the glans penis, which may be caused by a variety of factors and conditions, may resemble erythroplasia of Queyrat. Inflammation can be distinguished by its usually transient character. Condyloma acuminata (venereal warts) may resemble bowenoid papulosis. Keratoacanthomas (KAs) are rapidly growing and frequently spontaneously involuting tumors that resemble invasive SCC. Some KAs are impossible to distinguish from well-differentiated SCC.

15. How is SCC treated?

Excision with dermatopathologic assessment of margins to ensure completeness of excision is the treatment of choice. Because of the chance of metastases, the destructive modalities used for BCCs, such as cryotherapy and electrodesiccation with curettage are usually not used unless a section of surrounding skin/mucosa is obtained with the procedure to allow assessment of completeness of destruction of the tumor. Mohs' surgery is recommended for recurrent SCC in any location, SCCs in cosmetically sensitive areas, and SCCs that demonstrate perineural or perivascular invasion.

16. What factors are associated with metastases of SCC?

Location, size, etiology, and tumor duration are factors strongly associated with metastases. SCC on the lower lip has an incidence of metastasis of 10–20%. SCCs that arise in burn scars, chronic ulcers, and sites exposed to high doses of ionizing radiation are usually less well differentiated and have up to a 20–30% incidence of metastasis. Tumors that have been present for long periods or are > 1.0 cm in diameter usually penetrate deeper into the skin, which may lead to penetration into lymphatics and superficial vasculature and increased potential to metastasize by these routes.

17. Who was Percival Pott?

Percival Pott was a London physician who accurately identified chemical carcinogenesis as the cause of SCC arising on the scrotum of chimney sweeps in 1775. He realized that the chimney sweeps' chronic occupational exposure to chimney soot led to the development of SCC. His analysis of the etiology of SCC of the scrotum is often cited as the beginning of cancer research and is probably the first accurate identification of a human carcinogen.

BIBLIOGRAPHY

1. Fitzpatrick TB, Eisen AZ, Wolff K, et al (eds): Dermatology in General Medicine, 4th ed. New York, McGraw-Hill, 1995.
2. http://www.cancer.org/cidSpecificCancers/non-melskin/stat.html
3. Miller SJ, Maloney ME (eds): Cutaneous Oncology: Pathophysiology, Diagnosis, and Treatment. Cambridge, MA, Blackwell Science, 1998.
4. Potter M: Percival Pott's contribution to cancer research. Bethesda, MD, National Cancer Institute, NCI Monograph 10:1–5, 1963.

75. PRIMARY BRAIN TUMORS

Bertrand C. Liang, M.D.

1. How common are brain tumors? At what ages do they occur?

Brain tumors are uncommon, representing only about 10% of all diagnosed cancers. However, they are the second most common cause of cancer-related death in children, the third most common cause of cancer-related death in the age group of 15–35 years, and the fourth leading cause of cancer-related death in the 36–45-year-old age group. Hence, although uncommon, they represent a high fraction of the number of cancer deaths and tend to occur in the younger age groups.

2. What are the most frequent types of primary brain tumors?

In adults, glioma and meningioma are the most common primary brain tumors; in children, glioma and medulloblastoma are most often diagnosed. Other tumors include oligodendroglioma, ependymoma, and primary central nervous system lymphoma, which are individually diagnosed in less than 10% of all patients with primary brain tumor neoplasms.

3. Is there a genetic predisposition to primary brain tumors?

In some instances. Various named syndromes (e.g., Li-Fraumeni, neurofibromatosis I/II, von Hippel-Lindau, tuberous sclerosis, Turcot, Gorlin, and mutliple endocrine neoplasia) and unnamed (uncharacterized) disorders are associated with a genetic predisposition to primary brain tumors. These are typically quite rare and are in general not associated with de novo tumors.

4. Have environmental factors been related to the development of brain tumors?

Little or no credible evidence suggests that brain tumors are derived from specific environmental factors. Although developmental *models* of brain tumors are associated with specific carcinogens, these have not been found to be etiologic in the development of such tumors in humans.

5. What are the clinical manifestations of persons with primary brain tumors?

The symptomatology is protean and reflects the area of the brain involved. Generalized symptoms are typical earlier in the course of the disease—focal signs and symptoms develop later. Signs and symptoms often reflect the grade of the tumor. For example, patients with lower-grade glioma often report neurologic symptoms for more than 1 year before diagnosis; patients with anaplastic astrocytoma may have symptoms 9–12 months before diagnosis; and patients with glioblastoma (the most malignant grade of glioma) may have symptoms for less than 6 (and often less than 3) months.

6. What grading system is used for gliomas?

Choice of grading system depends on the institution. Several grading systems are in use, which are either three- or four-tiered and are subtly different. Perhaps the one becoming most widely used is the three-level system, with astrocytoma as the lowest grade, anaplastic astrocytoma as the moderate (but malignant) grade, and glioblastoma multiforme as the most malignant grade. Glioblastoma is the most frequent glioma (and primary brain tumor), representing about 60% of all gliomas diagnosed.

7. What is the therapy for gliomas?

First, there is a paucity of double-blind studies that evaluate specific therapies for gliomas, especially those of lower grade. Astrocytoma tends to be treated with surgery, with or without radiotherapy. Currently, it is controversial whether radiation improves the outlook of patients with this lower-grade tumor. In general, chemotherapy is reserved for higher-grade tumors. Anaplastic astrocytoma and glioblastoma multiforme are typically treated with a multimodality approach that includes surgery, radiation, and chemotherapy. Only radiation therapy and chemotherapy have been shown to improve survival *prospectively* in astrocytomas and gliomas.

8. What is the prognosis of patients with astrocytomas or gliomas?

Patients with astrocytomas have an 80% 5-year survival rate. Retrospective analysis has shown good prognosis in patients who are young, have had gross total tumor resections, and have minimal or no postoperative neurologic or other deficits. Patients with anaplastic astrocytomas have a median survival of slightly more than 3 years; patients with glioblastoma multiforme have a median survival of 51 weeks. Better retrospective prognostic indicators in these tumors include an apoplectic presentation (e.g., seizure), longer history of symptoms, younger age, and good postoperative performance status. Of note, younger patients also have a higher incidence of responding to chemotherapy compared with patients older than 60 years.

9. What is the pattern of failure of gliomas?

In contrast to many systemic tumors, the failure of gliomas is local, within 2 cm of the original tumor margin, even with focal external beam radiation and systemic chemotherapy. The most likely cause is insufficient local control, since pathologic studies have shown tumor cells outside the 2-cm border zone.

10. Is there a glioma that actually responds to therapy?

The oligodendroglioma is thought to be a chemoresponsive primary brain tumor. Use of high-dose PCV chemotherapy (procarbazine, CCNU, and vincristine) results in a median survival greater than 5 years, with a 10-year survival rate of 24%. Good prognostic indicators from retrospective trials include more benign histology, inclusion of radiotherapy in the treatment regimen, gross total surgical resection, and good pre- and postsurgical performance status.

11. Is response on radiographic imaging (partial response [PR], stable disease [SD], progressive disease [PD]) prognostically predictive in patients with higher-grade gliomas?

This subject is extraordinarily controversial. The study by Macdonald et al. in 1990 defined a PR as greater than 50% decrease in contrast-enhancing cross-sectional area when evaluated by CT or MRI and suggested from empirical data that this was a reasonable approach to assess response and therefore prognosis. Recent data in patients with higher-grade gliomas suggest that there is no difference in overall outcome in patients who have had either a PR or SD when comparing adjuvant chemotherapy after radiation therapy (see Grant et al., 1997). A difference was noted only between PR/SD and PD, with the PD group having a significantly worse prognosis.

12. Are there any primary brain tumors associated with AIDS?

Despite some anecdotal associations of gliomas with AIDS, there has not been a confirmatory study. In contrast, primary CNS lymphomas (PCNSL) are common in the AIDS population, and AIDS is the number-one risk factor for developing PCNSL. PCNSL is the fourth leading cause of death in patients with AIDS.

13. Describe some "benign" primary brain tumors.

Meningiomas are considered benign primary brain tumors, although they are actually tumors of the meninges rather than the brain. Usually the sole therapy for these tumors is surgical resection. However, 10% of them recur after total surgical resection, and they have a 15% recurrence rate if a dural attachment is left after removal. Subtotal resection results in a 39% recurrence rate. Another glioma considered benign is pilocytic astrocytoma, primarily a tumor of children but occasionally seen in adults. This tumor usually requires only surgical resection, with no radiation or chemotherapy.

BIBLIOGRAPHY

1. Grant R, Liang BC, Page M, et al: Age influences chemotherapy response in glioma, irrespective of tumor grade. Neurology 45:929–933, 1995.
2. Grant R, Liang BC, Slattery J, et al: Chemotherapy response criteria in malignant glioma. Neurology 48:1336–1340, 1997.
3. Kimmelman AK, Liang BC: Familial brain tumor syndromes. Hosp Physician 32:17–26, 1996.
4. Liang BC, Thorton AF, Sandler H, Greenberg H: Malignant astrocytoma: Focal tumor recurrence after focal external beam radiation therapy. J Neurosurg 75:559–563, 1991.
5. Liang BC, Liang DM: Primary central nervous system neoplasms. In Biller J (ed): Practical Neurology. Philadelphia, Lippincott-Raven, 1997.
6. Macdonald DR, Cascino TL, Schold SC Jr, Cairncross JG: Response criteria for phase II studies of supratentorial malignant glioma. J Clin Oncol 8:1277–1280, 1990.

---

76. THYROID AND PARATHYROID CANCER

Bryan R. Haugen, M.D.

THYROID CANCER

1. A patient presents with an asymptomatic 3-cm thyroid nodule. What should I do?

Thyroid nodules are incredibly common. They are palpable in approximately 5% of the U.S. population, and most are asymptomatic. When ultrasound is performed for other reasons, a thyroid nodule is identified in close to 40% of patients. Fortunately, only 5–10% of palpable thyroid nodules are malignant. Many techniques are available for evaluating thyroid nodules (serum thyroid function tests, ultrasound, CT scan, radioiodine scan, fine-needle aspiration biopsy [FNAB]), but costs of multiple tests add up quickly. Currently, the most cost-effective work-up of a thyroid nodule is to perform an assay of serum thyroid stimulating hormone (TSH) and FNAB. Ultrasound and radioiodine scan do not add much to the initial work-up other than cost. If the serum TSH is low (5% of thyroid nodules), a radioiodine scan is helpful to determine whether the nodule is hot (rarely malignant) or cold (5–10% risk of cancer).

2. How is an FNAB performed?

The FNAB can be performed in many different ways. One needs to choose an approach that yields an adequate and representative specimen. I perform the FNAB with the patient in the supine position, using a 10-cc syringe and 23-gauge needle. After cleaning the skin and using local anesthesia, I immobilize the nodule between two fingers, insert the needle, and pull back the plunger to see whether fluid is present (hence no need for an ultrasound to determine whether it is cystic or solid). If no fluid is present or the fluid has been drained, I perform three more passes to get an adequate sample, which is at least six clusters of thyroid cells on two separate passes. The separate biopsies are performed in different areas of the nodule to ensure a representative sample.

3. What results can I expect from an FNAB? What should I do with them?

The results from an FNAB are four basic diagnoses, with four fairly simple treatment algorithms:

FNAB Diagnosis	% of Biopsies	% Malignant*	Next Step
Benign	60–70	1–2	Follow, with or without LT4 therapy
Malignant	5–10	98	Surgery
Inadequate	5–10	5–10	Repeat FNAB (ultrasound-guided?)
Suspicious	20	20–30	Surgery (in most cases)

LT4 = levothyroxine.
* Percentage found to be malignant at surgery.

4. The TSH level is normal, but the FNAB is malignant and suggestive of papillary carcinoma. Is anything other than surgery necessary?

Papillary thyroid cancer is the most common malignancy of the thyroid (60–70%), followed by follicular carcinoma (15–20%). These are called the differentiated thyroid cancers and are treated similarly with initial surgery (usually near-total thyroidectomy), followed by radioiodine (^{131}I) ablation of remaining thyroid tissue (30–100 mCi) or radioiodine treatment of residual cancer (> 100 mCi), depending on the stage of the cancer determined at surgery. A common staging system is the tumor-node-metastasis (TNM) classification, which relies heavily on age (> 45 years old), tumor size, and distant metastases. Lymph node involvement does not influence prognosis as heavily as with many other cancers. After the initial treatment with surgery and radioiodine, patients are placed on LT4 either to suppress the TSH mildly (0.1–0.5 mU/L) in low-risk disease (stage I/II) or to cause greater TSH suppression (< 0.1 mU/L) in high-risk disease (stage III/IV). Patients can be started on 2–2.5 μg/kg/day of LT4 to achieve mild-to-moderate TSH suppresson. Complications associated with long-term TSH suppression include osteoporosis and atrial fibrillation; thus careful monitoring is essential.

Young patients with tumors < 1–1.5 cm, no capsular or vascular invasion and no lymph node involvement can be followed after surgery on LT4 therapy alone and probably will not benefit from radioiodine ablation. Current recommendations are to use radioiodine for all other patients with differentiated thyroid cancer.

5. How do I follow this patient for disease recurrence?

Once a patient receives radioiodine ablation and is on LT4 therapy, follow-up occurs in two different forms: on LT4 therapy and off LT4 therapy. Patients are usually followed at 6-month intervals on LT4 therapy for the first few years until no disease recurrence is found. Low-risk patients may then be followed yearly, whereas high-risk patients are still followed every 6 months. Most often disease recurs in the first 5–10 years, but recurrence has been seen in some patients after 40 years of follow-up; thus continuous surveillance is required. Patients on LT4 therapy receive a physical examination, including a thorough exam of the neck. Serum thyroid function and serum thyroglobulin are also measured. Thyroglobulin is synthesized exclusively in thyroid cells (normal and malignant) and is an extremely sensitive and specific marker for thyroid cancer recurrence in patients who have received radioiodine ablation. In patients who have residual thyroid tissue, thyroglobulin is a less specific marker.

At 6–12 months after surgery and radioiodine ablation, patients are taken off LT4 therapy to raise endogenous levels of TSH and to stimulate any residual thyroid tissue or thyroid cancer to make thyroglobulin and concentrate radioiodine for a whole body scan. Serum TSH is measured 4–6 weeks off LT4 (cytomel [T3] may be used for the first 3–4 weeks) and is considered adequate at levels > 25 mU/L. Serum thyroglobulin is measured and whole body scan performed (2–5 mCi ^{131}I). If the scan is positive or serum thyroglobulin is elevated, therapy with ^{131}I (100–200 mCi) is considered. Serum thyroglobulin stimulated by an elevated TSH is the most sensitive marker of recurrent disease; if this test is negative, the likelihood of recurrent disease is minimal. This process is repeated again in 6–12 months, depending on the results and stage of disease. Patients with low-risk disease who have had 1–2 negative radioiodine scans may be followed on LT4 therapy, whereas patients with high-risk disease need intermittent withdrawal surveillance at 2–5-year intervals.

6. Do patients like to discontinue LT4 for scanning?

No. Withdrawal of LT4 causes all of the symptoms of hypothyroidism, some quite severe. Exogenous TSH (bovine and human pituitary extract) has been tried to raise serum TSH on LT4, but allergic/immune reactions to bovine TSH and concerns about slow viruses with human pituitary extracts have made such preparations difficult to use. Fortunately, recombinant human TSH (rhTSH), which is similar to recombinant human insulin and growth hormone, has been developed. It is safe and well-tolerated and avoids the symptoms of hypothyroidism because patients can remain on LT4 therapy. Use of rhTSH to stimulate serum thyroglobulin and radioiodine uptake for scanning is quite comparable to LT4 withdrawal and eventually may replace the more burdensome withdrawal technique.

7. Is there a downside to radioiodine therapy?

Radioiodine is a relatively safe and extremely effective therapy for differentiated thyroid cancer. Acute toxicity may occur with large doses, including sialadenitis, xerostomia, and bone marrow suppression. Bone marrow suppression is rare when less than 200 rad is delivered to the blood; this level is hard to get with doses < 200 mCi (unless a patient is very small or has renal insufficiency). Pulmonary fibrosis may occur in patients with widespread pulmonary metastases who receive large doses to the lungs. Long-term side effects, which may occur with cumulative doses of 600–800 mCi or more, include increased risk of secondary malignancies such as bladder cancer and certain types of leukemia.

8. Are alternative therapies available for patients with radioiodine-resistant cancer?

Fortunately, most patients with differentiated thyroid cancer respond to radioiodine therapy. Unfortunately, patients with cancer unresponsive to radioiodine have few other therapeutic options. Adriamycin appears to be the best studied single agent. Doses of > 60 mg/m^2 every 3 weeks produce a 30% partial response rate. No other single agent or combinations studied provide a superior response rate. External beam irradiation may be considered in patients with disease limited to the neck or solitary bone metastases. Retinoic acid derivatives are currently under study and may provide hope for redifferentiation of rare radioiodine-resistant tumors.

9. Are there other types of thyroid cancer?

Differentiated thyroid cancer accounts for > 90% of all thyroid cancers. Undifferentiated thyroid cancer (medullary and anaplastic) accounts for 5–10%, lymphoma for 2–5%, and metastatic cancer for the rest (about 1%).

Medullary thyroid cancer is the only inherited form of thyroid cancer (aside from the rare case of familial papillary cancer) and arises in the calcitonin-producing C cells. It is caused by an activating mutation in the RET oncogene. The only truly effective therapy is surgery, and the earlier the disease is caught, the more curative the surgery. Family members of patients with familial medullary thyroid cancer can be screened by sequencing the RET gene from DNA. This genetic test is commercially available. Surgery is recommended if they have the same mutation as the patient, even if no thyroid nodule is palpable. Surgery is usually curative if only C-cell hyperplasia is present, but it is rarely curative once a palpable nodule is present because lymph nodes are usually involved. Radioiodine is ineffective and not used. Medullary thyroid cancer is part of the multiple endocrine neoplasia (MEN) 2A (pheochromocytoma, hyperparathyroidism) and MEN 2B (pheochromocytoma, mucosal neuromas) syndromes; the possibility of these syndromes must be explored in all patients with medullary thyroid carcinoma.

Anaplastic thyroid cancer carries a 50% 6-month survival rate. Adriamycin in combination with external beam irradiation is used, but treatment is not very effective. A research protocol using paclitaxel as a single agent appears promising, and this agent in combination with others may improve survival.

Lymphoma often may be confused with anaplastic thyroid cancer on FNAB, but the therapy is quite different. Lymphoma generally responds to radiation therapy, and extensive surgery can be avoided if the disease is diagnosed early.

PARATHYROID CANCER

10. How does parathyroid cancer present?

Parathyroid cancer classically presents with marked hypercalcemia, increased parathyroid hormone (PTH) levels, and a neck mass. Parathyroid cancer probably accounts for < 1% of all cases of hyperparathyroidism. Parathyroid cancers are equally distributed between men and women and are often much larger at presentation than benign parathyroid adenomas. A palpable neck mass is present in up to 50% of cases when hyperparathyroidism is caused by parathyroid cancer. Mean serum calcium levels are > 14 mg/dl in 70% of patients with parathyroid cancer and may be as high as 24 mg/dl. PTH levels are often 5–10 times higher than the upper limits of normal in patients with parathyroid cancer compared with 2–3 times higher than normal in most patients with benign adenoma. Kidneys and bones are most often affected. In one series, 37 of 47 patients with parathyroid cancer had renal involvement and 34 of 62 had specific radiologic evidence of hyperparathyroid bone disease. In another large series, 84% had renal insufficiency and 91% had some evidence of bone involvement.

11. Discuss the treatment of parathyroid cancer.

Surgical resection is the only effective form of therapy. En bloc resection of the mass without biopsy is the initial procedure of choice. Intraoperative biopsy of the lesion is often associated with dissemination of malignant cells into the operative field, resulting in subsequent local recurrence. The average time between initial surgery and recurrence is 3 years, but intervals as long as 20 years have been reported. When tumor recurs, the most effective form of therapy is repeat surgery. Some patients have had as many as eight operations for recurrent disease. The possibility of surgical cure decreases markedly after the second operation, but subsequent surgery can provide long periods of reduced serum calcium levels and a significant improvement in quality of life. Radiation therapy, combination chemotherapy, calcitonin, mithramycin, and diphosphonates have been tried, and none has had any reliable effect on serum calcium or survival. Five-year survival is < 50%, and 10-year survival is approximately 35%.

BIBLIOGRAPHY

1. DeGroot LJ, Kaplan EL, McCormick M, Straus FH: Natural history, treatment and course of papillary thyroid carcinoma. J Clin Endocrinol Metab 71:414–424, 1990.

2. Dulgeroff AJ, Hershman JM: Medical therapy for differentiated thyroid carcinoma. Endocrine Rev 15:500–515, 1994.
3. Hay ID. Papillary thyroid carcinoma. Endocrinol Metab Clin North Am 19:545–575, 1990.
4. Ladenson PW, et al: Comparison of administration of recombinant human thyrotropin with withdrawal of thyroid hormone for radioactive iodine scanning in patients with thyroid carcinoma. N Engl J Med 337:888–896, 1997.
5. Mazzaferri EL, Jhiang SM: Long-term impact of initial surgical and medical therapy on papillary and follicular thyroid cancer. Am J Med 97:418–428, 1994.
6. Obara T, Fujimoto Y: Diagnosis and treatment of patients with parathyroid carcinoma: An update and review. World J Surg 15:738–744, 1991.
7. Pujol P, et al: Degree of thyrotropin suppression as a prognostic determinant in differentiated thyroid cancer. J Clin Endocrinol Metab 81:4318–4323, 1996.
8. Schlumberger MJ: Papillary and follicular thyroid carcinoma. N Engl J Med 338:297–306, 1998.
9. Shane E, Bilezikian JP: Parathyroid carcinoma: A review of 62 patients. Endocrine Rev 3:218–226, 1982.
10. Singer PA, et al: Treatment guidelines for patients with well-differentiated thyroid cancer. Arch Intern Med 156:2165–2172, 1996.
11. Solomon BL, Wartofsky L, Burman KD: Current trends in the management of well-differentiated thyroid carcinoma. J Clin Endocrinol Metab 81:333–339, 1996.
12. Sweeney DC, Johnston GS: Radioiodine therapy for thyroid cancer. Endocrinol Metab Clin North Am 24:803–840, 1995.
13. Wynne AG, Heerden JV, Carney JA, et al: Parathyroid carcinoma: Clinical and pathologic features in 43 patients. Medicine 71:197–205, 1992.

77. PITUITARY TUMORS AND ADRENAL CARCINOMA

Michael T. McDermott, M.D.

1. What kind of tumors occur in the pituitary gland?

Tumors of the pituitary gland may be nonfunctioning or functioning pituitary adenomas, craniopharyngiomas, carcinomas metastatic to the pituitary, and (rarely) pituitary carcinomas.

2. Which structures may be damaged by pituitary tumor growth?

Superiorly, pituitary tumors may compress the optic chiasm. Laterally, they can invade the cavernous sinuses and compress cranial nerves III, IV, V, and VI or the internal carotid arteries. Inferiorly, they may erode into the sphenoid sinus. These tumors also often compress or destroy the remaining normal pituitary tissue.

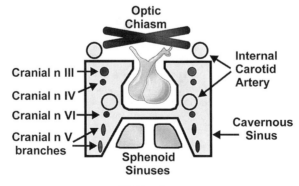

Pituitary fossa.

3. Discuss the clinical features of nonfunctioning pituitary tumors.

These tumors most often present as space-occupying masses, compressing nearby neurologic and/or vascular structures. Common clinical manifestations include headaches, visual field defects, visual loss, and extraocular nerve palsies. Pituitary compression may further result in adrenal insufficiency, hypothyroidism, hypogonadism, growth failure in children, and diabetes insipidus.

4. What is the treatment for a nonfunctioning pituitary tumor?

The treatment of choice is transsphenoidal surgery, in which access to the pituitary gland is gained through the sphenoid sinus. Because these tumors are usually quite large, surgical resection is often incomplete and postoperative radiation therapy may be advisable.

5. What are the clinical features of functioning pituitary tumors?

Prolactinomas produce galactorrhea and amenorrhea in women and impotence in men. Growth hormone–secreting tumors cause acromegaly in adults and gigantism in children. Corticotropin (ACTH)–secreting tumors produce Cushing's disease. Gonadotropin (LH, FSH)–producing tumors and thyrotropin (TSH)–producing tumors usually cause only mass effects but occasionally result in gonadal dysfunction or hyperthyroidism.

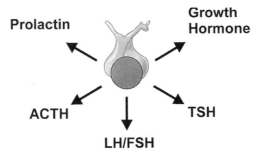

Functioning pituitary tumors.

6. How are functioning pituitary tumors treated?

Prolactinomas are treated with bromocriptine, pergolide, or cabergoline; surgery is performed if there is an inadequate response. Transsphenoidal surgery is the primary treatment for all other pituitary tumors. Growth hormone–secreting tumors also respond to octreotide, a somatostatin analogue. Radiation therapy may be used for any of these tumors, but its full effects are delayed for years.

7. Which cancers metastasize to the pituitary gland?

Metastatic disease to the pituitary gland occurs in approximately 3–5% of patients with widely disseminated carcinoma. The most commonly reported primary tumors are breast, lung, kidney, prostate, liver, pancreas, nasopharynx, plasmacytoma, sarcoma, and adenocarcinoma of unknown primary site.

8. Discuss the clinical features of pituitary carcinoma.

Pituitary carcinomas, which are extremely rare, expand rapidly and cause mass effects. Some secrete hormones causing endocrine syndromes similar to those seen with adenomas. Metastatic disease to the central nervous system, cervical lymph nodes, liver, and bone are commonly associated. Mean survival is approximately 4 years.

9. What is the treatment for pituitary carcinoma?

Transsphenoidal surgery is the primary therapy followed by postoperative radiation. Prolactin- and growth hormone–secreting carcinomas may partially respond to bromocriptine, pergolide, or cabergoline. There has been no significant reported use of chemotherapy for pituitary carcinomas.

10. What types of cancer occur in the adrenal glands?

Adrenal cortical carcinomas
Adrenal medullary carcinomas
Carcinomas metastatic from other sites

11. Discuss the clinical features of nonfunctioning adrenal cortical carcinomas.

Approximately 30–50% of adrenal cortical carcinomas do not produce hormones. They present clinically as abdominal or flank pain or as an incidentally discovered adrenal mass. They are locally invasive and metastasize most commonly to liver and lung. The mean survival is approximately 15 months, and the 5-year survival rate is about 20%.

12. Discuss the clinical features of functioning adrenal cortical carcinomas.

Adrenal cortical carcinomas may secrete aldosterone, cortisol, and androgens alone or in combination. Aldosterone excess, or Conn's syndrome, causes hypertension and hypokalemia. Cortisol overproduction results in the development of Cushing's syndrome. Androgen excess causes hirsutism and virilization in women and abnormal precocious puberty in children.

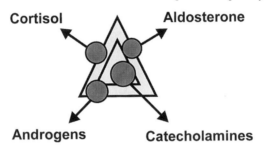

Functioning adrenal tumors.

13. What is the treatment for an adrenal cortical carcinoma?

The treatment of choice is surgery. Mitotane has produced partial or complete tumor regression, reduced adrenal hormone production and improved survival in nonrandomized, noncontrolled trials. Other chemotherapeutic agents and radiation therapy do not appear to be effective.

14. Discuss the clinical features of a malignant pheochromocytoma.

Pheochromocytomas cause hypertension, headaches, sweating, and palpitations. Approximately 10% of pheochromocytomas are malignant. In addition to elevated urinary excretion of vanillylmandelic acid (VMA), metanephrine, and catecholamines, malignant tumors often have a disproportionate increase in urinary dopamine and homovanillic acid. These tumors eventually metastasize to the liver, lung, and bone.

15. What is the treatment for a malignant pheochromocytoma?

Surgery is the treatment of choice. Alpha-adrenergic blocking agents such as phenoxybenzamine and prazosin are given preoperatively to control blood pressure and replete intravascular volume. These drugs and alpha-methyl tyrosine, a catecholamine synthesis inhibitor, also are effective long-term therapy for patients with unresectable tumors. Cyclophosphamide, vincristine, dacarbazine, and ^{131}I metaiodobenzylguanidine (MIBG) may cause partial regression of residual tumors.

16. What is the significance of metastases to the adrenal gland from other primary sites?

The vascular adrenal glands are a frequent site of bilateral metastatic spread from other tumors such as lung, breast, melanomas, stomach, pancreas, colon, kidney, and lymphomas. Acute adrenal crisis is rare. However, up to 33% of patients may have subtle adrenal insufficiency and experience improvement in their well-being when given physiologic corticosteroid replacement.

17. How should the incidentally discovered adrenal mass be managed?

Adrenal masses should be evaluated for oversecretion of cortisol, aldosterone, androgens, and catecholamines. Cancer is rare in tumors < 6 cm in size. All functioning tumors and nonfunctioning masses ≥ 6 cm should be removed surgically. Some experts recommend a size cutoff of 4.5 cm for surgery. Smaller masses should be reassessed in 3–6 months and then annually. They should be removed if there is growth or if hormone secretion develops.

BIBLIOGRAPHY

1. Branch CL Jr, Laws ER Jr: Metastatic tumors of the sella turcica masquerading as primary pituitary tumors. J Clin Endocrinol Metab 65:469–474, 1990.
2. Brennan MF: Adrenocortical carcinoma. CA 37:348–365, 1987.
3. Cheung AY, Sligh T, Bauserman S, Schultz G: Evaluation of modern pathologic nomenclature, tumor imaging and treatment of pituitary adenomas in a recent surgical series. J Neurooncol 37:145–153, 1998.
4. Copeland PM: The incidentally discovered adrenal mass. Ann Intern Med 98:940–945, 1983.
5. Katznelson L, Alexander JM, Klibanski A: Clinically non-functioning pituitary adenomas. J Clin Endocrinol Metab 76:1089–1094, 1993.
6. Klibanski A, Zervas NT: Diagnosis and management of hormone-secreting pituitary adenomas. N Engl J Med 324:822–831, 1991.
7. Luton J-P, Cerdas S, Billaud L, et al: Clinical features of adrenocortical carcinoma, prognostic factors, and the effect of mitotane therapy. N Engl J Med 322:1195–1201, 1990.
8. Molitch ME, Russell EJ: The pituitary "incidentaloma." Ann Intern Med 112:925–931, 1990.
9. Mountcastle RB, Roof BS, Mayfield RK, et al: Case report: Pituitary adenocarcinoma in an acromegalic patient: Response to bromocriptine and pituitary testing: A review of the literature on 36 cases of pituitary carcinoma. Am J Med Sci 298(2):109–118, 1989.
10. Schteingart DE: Treating adrenal cancer. Endocrinologist 2:149–157, 1992.

78. CARCINOID SYNDROME AND PANCREATIC ISLET CELL TUMORS

Michael T. McDermott, M.D.

1. What are carcinoid tumors?

Carcinoid tumors are neoplasms that arise from enterochromaffin cells. They are classified as coming from the foregut (bronchus, stomach, duodenum, bile ducts, pancreas), midgut (jejunum, ileum, appendix, ascending colon), or hindgut (transverse colon, descending and sigmoid colon, rectum). They occasionally occur in the gonads, prostate, kidney, breast, thymus, or skin.

2. What is the carcinoid syndrome?

The carcinoid syndrome is a humorally mediated syndrome. It consists of cutaneous flushing (90%), diarrhea (75%), wheezing (20%), endocardial fibrosis (33%), right heart valvular lesions, and occasionally pleural, peritoneal, or retroperitoneal fibrosis. Pellagra also may occur because of diversion of tryptophan from niacin to serotonin synthesis by the tumor.

3. Name the biochemical mediators of the carcinoid syndrome.

Carcinoid tumors produce a variety of humoral mediators, including serotonin, bradykinin, tachykinins, histamine, prostaglandins, neurotensin, and substance P. Diarrhea and fibrous tissue formation are probably caused by serotonin, whereas flushing and wheezing are likely due to kinins, histamine, or prostaglandins.

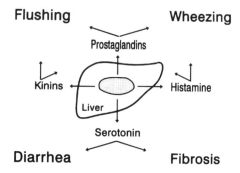

Carcinoid syndrome.

4. Under what circumstances does a carcinoid tumor cause the carcinoid syndrome?

Carcinoid syndrome results when humoral mediators reach the systemic circulation. Gastrointestinal carcinoids usually do not cause carcinoid syndrome unless there are hepatic metastases that impair metabolism of the mediators or secrete mediators directly into the hepatic vein. Extraintestinal carcinoids may cause carcinoid syndrome in the absence of metastases.

5. How is the diagnosis of carcinoid syndrome made?

The diagnosis is made by demonstrating increased serum concentrations of serotonin, neurotensin, or substance P, or increased urinary excretion of 5-hydroxyindoleacetic acid (5-HIAA), a breakdown product of serotonin.

6. Can patients with carcinoid syndrome be cured?

Benign extraintestinal tumors causing carcinoid syndrome may be cured by surgery. Malignant carcinoids with metastases are usually incurable but are slow growing, allowing prolonged survival. Extensive debulking is risky and rarely helpful. Chemotherapy and radiation are relatively ineffective.

7. How can the symptoms of carcinoid syndrome be controlled?

Niacin should be given to prevent pellagra. Flushing may decrease with histamine antagonists, phenoxybenzamine, phenothiazines, or glucocorticoids. Diarrhea may respond to methysergide, cyproheptadine, diphenoxylate, loperamide, or codeine. Octreotide, a somatostatin analogue, often controls both flushing and diarrhea.

8. What are pancreatic islet cell tumors?

These tumors, which arise from the islet cells of the pancreas, cause syndromes as a result of overproduction of hormones such as insulin, gastrin, glucagon, somatostatin, and vasoactive intestinal polypeptide (VIP). Insulinomas are benign in 80–90% of cases, but 40–60% of all other islet cell tumors are malignant.

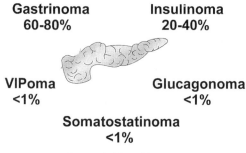

Pancreatic islet cell tumors.

9. Discuss the clinical manifestations of insulin-producing tumors.

Insulinomas produce excessive insulin causing hypoglycemia, which usually occurs in the fasting state or after exercise. The most common symptoms include confusion, slurred speech, blurred vision, seizures, and coma due to neuroglycopenia or reduced glucose delivery to the brain. Adrenergic symptoms of tremor, sweating, palpitations, headache, and nausea also occur occasionally.

10. How is the diagnosis of insulinoma made?

Hypoglycemia (glucose < 55 mg/dl in men, < 40 mg/dl in women) with hyperinsulinemia (insulin/glucose ratio > 0.33) during a 12–72-hour supervised fast is diagnostic. Measurement of C peptide, which is cosecreted with insulin, will help distinguish an insulinoma (high C peptide) from surreptitious insulin administration (low C peptide). The urine also should be screened for sulfonylureas.

11. Describe how to localize an insulinoma.

Imaging procedures such as computed tomographic (CT) scan, ultrasonography, transhepatic portal vein sampling, and splanchnic arteriography may all give the correct location, but some tumors cannot be found prior to surgery. Intraoperative palpation and/or ultrasonography usually provide correct localization in these cases.

12. What is the treatment for an insulinoma?

Solitary benign insulinomas should be removed surgically. Patients with unresectable malignant tumors should be treated with frequent feedings and inhibitors of insulin secretion such as diazoxide, verapamil, propranolol, phenytoin, and octreotide. Chemotherapy with streptozotocin and doxorubicin or 5-fluorouracil increases survival and improves symptoms.

13. Discuss the clinical manifestations of a gastrin-producing tumor.

Gastrinomas secrete excessive gastrin, which stimulates prolific gastric acid secretion. Patients develop severe peptic ulcer disease often associated with secretory diarrhea. Gastrinomas usually arise from the pancreatic islets but also may occur in the duodenum and stomach. This disorder also is known as the Zollinger-Ellison syndrome.

14. Explain how the diagnosis of gastrinoma is made.

The diagnosis is made by demonstrating the presence of high gastric acidity (pH < 3.0) in association with a fasting serum gastrin level > 1000 pg/ml or a moderately elevated gastrin that increases by more than 200 pg/ml within 15 minutes after the intravenous administration of secretin.

15. What is the best way to localize a gastrinoma?

Localization of the tumor may be pursued with a variety of techniques to include CT scan, magnetic resonance imaging (MRI), ultrasonography, endoscopic ultrasonography, transhepatic portal venous sampling, selective arterial secretin infusions, and radioactive octreotide scanning.

16. How is gastrinoma treated?

Most benign and some malignant gastrinomas can be cured by surgery. Otherwise, attention should be directed toward reduction of gastric acid overproduction. High-dose H_2 receptor antagonists, omeprazole, and octreotide effectively decrease acid secretion and symptoms in most patients. Refractory patients may require total gastrectomy for symptom relief.

17. Discuss the characteristics of glucagon-secreting tumors.

Glucagonomas cause diabetes mellitus, weight loss, anemia, and a skin rash known as necrolytic migratory erythema. The diagnosis depends on an elevated serum glucagon level (> 500 pg/ml). Treatment options include surgery for localized disease, octreotide to reduce glucagon secretion, and chemotherapy with streptozotocin, 5-fluorouracil, and dacarbazine.

18. Discuss the characteristics of somatostatin-secreting tumors.

Somatostatinomas cause diabetes mellitus, weight loss, steatorrhea, and cholelithiasis. The diagnosis is made by finding an elevated serum somatostatin level. Surgery is the treatment of choice. When surgery is not possible, streptozotocin may reduce somatostatin secretion and tumor size.

19. What are the characteristics of vasoactive intestinal polypeptide-secreting tumors (VIPomas)?

VIPomas cause watery diarrhea, hypokalemia, and achlorhydria (WDHA syndrome or pancreatic cholera). The diagnosis is made by finding an elevated serum VIP level. Surgery is the treatment of choice. Octreotide effectively reduces diarrhea in most patients. Radiation therapy, streptozotocin, and interferon alpha also may reduce diarrhea and tumor size.

BIBLIOGRAPHY

1. Feldman JM: The carcinoid syndrome. Endocrinologist 3:129–135, 1993.
2. Friesen SR: Tumors of the endocrine pancreas. N Engl J Med 306:580–590, 1982.
3. Godwin JD II: Carcinoid tumors: An analysis of 2837 cases. Cancer 36:560–569, 1975.
4. Jaffe BM: Current issues in the management of Zollinger-Ellison syndrome. Surgery 111:241–243, 1992.
5. Krejs GJ, Orci L, Conlon M, et al: Somatostatinoma syndrome: Biochemical, morphologic and clinical features. N Engl J Med 301:285–292, 1979.
6. Leichter SB: Clinical and metabolic aspects of glucagonoma. Medicine 59:100–113, 1980.
7. Moertel CG, Johnson CM, McKusick MA, et al: The management of patients with advanced carcinoid tumors and islet cell carcinomas. Ann Intern Med 120:302–309, 1994.
8. Perry RR, Vinik AI: Diagnosis and management of functioning islet cell tumors. J Clin Endocrinol Metab 80:2273–2278, 1995.
9. Service FJ, McMahon MM, O'Brien PC, Ballard DJ: Functioning insulinomas—Incidence, recurrence, and long-term survival of patients: A 60-year study. Mayo Clin Proc 66:711–719, 1991.
10. Wolfe MM, Jensen RT: Zollinger-Ellison syndrome: Current concepts in diagnosis and management. N Engl J Med 317:1200–1209, 1987.

79. OSTEOGENIC SARCOMA

Kyle M. Fink, M.D., Louis Bair, D.O., Victor Shada, D.O., and Ross M. Wilkins, M.D., M.S.

1. Who does osteosarcoma affect?

Osteosarcoma is the most common malignant primary bone tumor in childhood and adolescence and in all age groups with the exception of myeloma. Its highest prevalence is in males aged 10 to 22 years.

2. How common are malignant tumors of bone?

Only about 4,000 new cases are seen every year in the United States, which represents only about 0.2% of primary cancers.

3. In what bone(s) is osteosarcoma most commonly found?

In children and adolescents, osteosarcoma is usually found in the distal femur and proximal tibia. Those diagnosed in the elderly population are associated with Paget's disease and are found in the humerus, pelvis, and proximal femur.

4. How do patients with osteosarcoma present?

The typical symptoms are pain, tenderness, and enlargement of a localized area. Usually a decreased range of motion of an adjacent joint is found, and many patients have pain, particularly at night.

5. Do osteosarcomas frequently metastasize?

Yes. Over 80% of patients have micrometastatic disease secondary to hematogenous spread at diagnosis. The first recognizable site of metastases is the lungs. Regional lymph node spread is rare, although bone metastases may occur.

6. What are osteosarcomas composed of histologically?

They arise from primitive mesenchymal cells—usually malignant osteoblasts and spindle cells that produce immature fragments of trabecular bone often erratically located in the bone.

7. Which imaging studies of osteosarcoma are important?

The diagnosis of osteosarcoma is usually confirmed on plain roentgenographs. Computed tomography (CT) and magnetic resonance imaging (MRI) help in defining the osseous and soft tissue extent of the tumor and its involvement with adjacent joints and neurovascular structures. These images are particularly important with adjacent joints and neurovascular structures. These images are particularly important in comparison before and after chemotherapy. Imaging is vital in determining local recurrence and metastatic disease. Radionuclide bone scanning is helpful in locating bone metastases.

8. How are osteosarcomas staged?

Staging is based on grade, compartmentalization of the tumor, and metastases.

Surgical Staging of Bone Sarcomas

STAGE	GRADE	SITE
IA	Low	Intracompartmental
IB	Low	Extracompartmental
IIA	High	Intracompartmental
IIB	High	Extracompartmental
III	Low or high	Regional or distant metastasis

From Enneking WF, Spanier SS, Goodman MA: A system for the surgical staging of musculoskeletal sarcoma. Clin Orthop 153:106–120, 1980, with permission.

9. How are suspected osteosarcomas biopsied?

Open biopsy is preferred to sample these heterogenous tumors adequately. The biopsy should be done by the surgeon, who makes the ultimate decision regarding future operative procedures.

10. Is there a standard regimen for successful treatment of osteosarcomas?

Currently, patients undergo preoperative chemotherapy and in many protocols incorporate intra-arterial or intravenous chemotherapy using cisplatinum. After maximum response, the patient then undergoes limb-sparing surgery, if possible. Ninety percent of patients now retain their limb when the tumor involves the extremity, with only 10% having to undergo amputation. Based on the tumor kill at the time of resection, the patient then receives further postoperative adjuvant chemotherapy. If the tumor kill is > 90%, the same chemotherapy is used postoperatively, usually for three to four cycles. If there is < 90% tumor kill, different chemotherapeutic agents are used postoperatively versus those used preoperatively. Radiation therapy is generally only used for unresectable tumors.

11. What chemotherapeutic agents are commonly used?

The most effective agents are doxorubicin (Adriamycin), cisplatin, and high-dose methotrexate with leucovorin rescue. Recently, ifosfamide has also been shown to be a highly effective drug for osteosarcoma.

12. What is the overall survival for osteosarcomas?

With the advent of multidrug chemotherapy (used both pre- and postoperatively) in combination with surgical resection, the 5-year survival has risen from approximately 20% to over 80%. Unfortunately, if patients with osteosarcoma already have metastatic disease, particularly in the lung, long-term survival is poor. However, late pulmonary metastasis can be wedge resected for curative intent in about 20–25% of patients, which is the same as in soft tissue sarcomas.

BIBLIOGRAPHY

1. DeVita VT Jr, Hellman S, Rosenberg SA (eds): Principles and Practice of Oncology, 5th ed. Philadelphia, Lippincott-Raven, 1997.
2. Fink K, Wilkins R: Intra-arterial chemotherapy and limb preservation in osteosarcoma in children (abstract). American Society of Clinical Oncology, 1991, p 1126.
3. Fletcher BD: Response of osteosarcoma and Ewing sarcoma to chemotherapy: Imaging evaluation. Am J Roentgenol 157:825–833, 1991.
4. Holleb AI, et al (eds): Clinical Oncology, 2nd ed. Atlanta, American Cancer Society, 1991.
5. Jaffe N: Chemotherapy for malignant bone tumors. Orthop Clin North Am 30:487–499, 1989.
6. Klein MR, Kenan S, Lewis MM: Osteosarcoma: Clinical features and evolving surgical and chemotherapeutic strategies. Pediatr Clin North Am 38:317–348, 1991.
7. Meyer WH, Malawer MM: Osteosarcoma: Clinical features and evolving surgical and chemotherapeutic strategies. Pediatr Clin North Am 38:317–348, 1991.
8. Seeger LL, Gold RH, Chandnani VP: Diagnostic imaging of osteosarcoma. Clin Orthop Rel Res 270:254–263, 1991.
9. Sim FH, Bowman WE, Wilkins RM, Choa EYS: Limb salvage in primary malignant bone tumors. Orthopedics 8:574–581, 1985.
10. Wilkins RM, Sim FH: Evaluation of bone and soft tissue tumors. In D'Ambrosia (ed): Musculoskeletal Disorders: Regional Examination and Differential Diagnosis, 2nd ed. Philadelphia, J.B. Lippincott, 1986.

80. SOFT TISSUE SARCOMAS

Kyle M. Fink, M.D., Louis Bair, D.O., Victor Shada, D.O.,
and Ross M. Wilkins, M.D., M.S.

1. What is a soft tissue sarcoma?

This refers to a large group of malignant tumors arising embryonically from the primitive mesoderm. The primitive mesenchyme within the mesoderm differentiates into the various connective tissues of the body—tendon, ligament, muscle, and bone. Tumors of these tissues are referred to as soft tissue sarcomas. Because of imprecise differentiation, some sarcomas have ectodermal and epithelial origins.

2. How common are soft tissue sarcomas?

They account for an estimated 5,700 cases a year, with an incidence similar to testicular cancer and slightly less frequent than Hodgkin's disease. Approximately 3,100 people die of the disease annually.

3. Where do soft tissue sarcomas arise?

The most common site is the lower extremities, but they also are found in various other body sites.

Anatomic Sites of Soft Tissue Sarcomas

SITE	INCIDENCE (%)
Lower extremity	38.9
Retroperitoneal/intra-abdominal	15.2
Trunk	12.9
Upper extremity	10.9
Genitourinary	7.2
Visceral	5.4
Head and neck	4.8
Other	4.6

From Posnar MC, Brennan MF: Soft tissue sarcomas. In Holleb AI, et al (eds): Clinical Oncology, 2nd ed. Atlanta, American Cancer Society, 1991, with permission.

4. What is the clinical presentation of sarcoma?

Sarcomas in the extremities are usually painless, slow-growing masses. Retroperitoneal sarcomas are typically asymptomatic until late in their course when patients generally complain of an abdominal mass with associated abdominal fullness, vague abdominal pain, or early satiety. They also may have initial symptoms of diffuse retroperiteoneumlike low back pain. This is a constant boring pain even at rest, particularly at night, which is relieved by sitting up or even motion. Occasionally, pain is associated with signs of peripheral or nerve root compression.

5. What predilections do soft tissue sarcomas have?

Soft tissue sarcomas show no predilection for any group or sex. A database study done by memorial Sloan-Kettering Cancer Center from July 1982 to December 1987 of 1,091 patients with soft tissue carcinomas showed a median age of 50 years, 54% to 46% male to female ratio; 90% of patients were Caucasian.

6. Are there risk factors for soft tissue sarcomas?

No clear etiologic factor has been defined. Patients with neurofibromatosis (von Recklinghausen's disease) have a 10–15% risk of developing neurofibrosarcomas. Chronic lymphedema, particularly in the arms after radical mastectomy and radiotherapy (Steward-Treves syndrome), has resulted in cases of lymphangiosarcomas. Radiation injury and chemical carcinogen exposure also appear to be responsible for a small number of sarcomas. The *majority* of soft tissue sarcomas arise spontaneously.

7. Where do sarcomas metastasize?

The lung is the most frequent site of metastatic involvement. A few histopathologic types have regional lymph node involvement.

8. Which imaging studies are useful in the diagnosis and work-up of a patient with a soft tissue sarcoma?

Recently, when compared with computed tomography (CT) and angiography, magnetic resonance imaging (MRI) has proved to be superior in assessing soft tissue tumors because of better resolution and enhanced distinction between normal and abnormal tissue.

9. Describe how soft tissue sarcomas are staged.

Staging is based on histologic grade, tumor size, regional lymph node involvement, and presence of metastases. However, tumor *grade* is the best prognostic indicator. Grading criteria to type a sarcoma high-grade or low-grade are listed below.

Guidelines to Histologic Grading of Sarcomas

LOW GRADE	HIGH GRADE
Well differentiated	Poorly differentiated
Hypocellular	Hypercellular
Much stroma	Minimal stroma
Hypovascular	Hypervascular
Minimal necrosis	Much necrosis
< 5 mitosis/10 hpf	> 5 mitosis/10 hpf

hpf = high-power field.

10. How are soft tissue sarcomas biopsied for diagnosis?

The procedure of choice is an open biopsy or core-needle biopsy for extremity lesions. The biopsy must be done with an awareness of the subsequent treatment plan if the tissue is malignant. Incisional biopsy should be oriented longitudinally in the extremity for a possible subsequent limb preservation surgical procedure.

11. What is the definitive treatment of soft tissue sarcomas?

Surgery is the primary treatment of all soft tissue sarcomas. In extremity lesions, the goal is limb-sparing surgery if the tumor can be removed and a functional extremity remains. If the surgeon cannot remove the entire tumor, the tumor, in general, cannot be cured with irradiation or chemotherapy alone. If there is already metastatic disease present, particularly in the lungs at the time of presentation of a primary soft tissue sarcoma, cure is almost always impossible.

12. Explain the roles that chemotherapy and radiation play in the treatment of soft tissue sarcoma.

Irradiation may allow less aggressive surgery in selected cases when used as a local adjuvant. The role of systemic chemotherapy for soft tissue sarcomas has not been well defined, particularly in the adjuvant setting. Chemotherapy is currently reserved for palliation of metastatic disease. Generally, if the surgeon does not adequately resect the disease in soft tissue sarcomas, the disease then recurs and treatment becomes palliative with chemotherapy and radiation therapy.

13. Which chemotherapeutic agents are used in the treatment of soft tissue sarcomas?

The most common agent used is doxorubicin (Adriamycin). Other agents used are cyclophosphamide, DTIC, and most recently, ifosfamide.

14. Are patients with pulmonary metastases potentially curable?

If the primary site has been deemed disease free, up to 20–25% of patients with resected pulmonary metastases have been alive and disease free at 5 years in numerous trials. The major factors for their prognosis include tumor doubling time > 20 days, disease-free interval > 12 months, and the presence of less than four nodules. The two surgical procedures being used are lateral thoracotomy and, more recently, median sternotomy.

15. What is the risk of local recurrence following treatment of soft tissue sarcomas?

Local recurrence remains a problem, with rates as high as 40–50% for head, neck, and truncal sarcomas and 75% for retroperitoneal sarcomas. Extremity sarcomas, however, have shown more favorable results of 25% or less owing to multimodality therapy.

16. List the factors predictive of the likelihood of a local recurrence.

Age > 50 years	Certain specific histopathologies
Presentation with recurrent disease	Inadequate margins in resection
High-grade tumor	Size (particularly ≥ 10 cm)

17. What factors are predictive of likelihood to metastasize?

Size of the tumor appears to be a major predictor, with the greater size the more likely to metastasize. Other predictors include high-grade tumors and proximal site on an extremity.

18. List the factors predictive of decreased survival.

Age > 50 years	Size ≥ 10 cm
High tumor grade	Regional lymph node involvement
Painful mass a presentation	Inadequate margins
Proximal site	Amputation

BIBLIOGRAPHY

1. DeVita VT Jr, Hellman S, Rosenberg SA (eds): Principles and Practice of Oncology, 5th ed. Philadelphia, Lippincott-Raven, 1997.
2. Eilber FR, et al (eds): The Soft Tissue Sarcomas. Orlando, FL, Grune & Stratton, 1987.
3. Geer RJ, Woodruff J, Casper ES, et al: Management of small soft-tissue sarcoma of the extremity in adults. Arch Surg 127:1285–1289, 1992.
4. Hoekstra HJ, Schraffordt KH, Molenaar WM, et al: A combination of intraarterial chemotherapy, preoperative and postoperative radiotherapy, and surgery as limb-saving treatment of primarily unresectable high-grade soft tissue sarcomas of the extremities. Cancer 63:59–62, 1989.
5. Holleb AI, et al (eds): Clinical Oncology, 2nd ed. Atlanta, American Cancer Society, 1991.
6. Jaffe KA, Morris SG: Resection and reconstruction for soft-tissue sarcomas of the extremity. Orthop Clin North Am 22:151–176, 1991.
7. Sondak VK, Economou JS, Eilber FR: Soft tissue sarcomas of the extremity and retroperitoneum: Advance in management. Adv Surg 24:333–359, 1991.
8. Springfield DS: Introduction to limb-salvage surgery for sarcomas. Orthop Clin North Am 22:1–5, 1991.
9. Wilkins RM, Sim FH: Evaluation of bone and soft tissue tumors. In D'ambrosia R (ed): Musculoskeletal Disorders: Regional Examination and Differential Diagnosis, 2nd ed. Philadelphia, J.B. Lippincott, 1986, pp 189–217.

81. CANCER OF UNKNOWN PRIMARY SITE

Kerry Scott Fisher, M.D.

1. What is cancer of unknown primary site?

When a histologically confirmed cancer is identified in a site not consistent with a primary tumor in that organ and no primary site is apparent after a reasonable search, the diagnosis is cancer of unknown primary site (CUP).

2. IS CUP a common problem?

Yes. It accounts for 4–15% of histologies in all patients with solid tumors and is the eighth most common form of cancer. It usually affects older individuals, with an average age at diagnosis of 60 years.

3. How does the biology of CUP differ from cancer in which the primary site is known?

When the primary site is established during the patient's life or at autopsy in a patient with an unknown primary site, the tumor is often found in an organ not expected from the common patterns of spread in known primary tumors (their usual natural history). If the primary site is identified, the pattern of metastasis is often unexpected for that cancer. Aside from lung cancer, cancers that occur commonly in the general population make up a small percentage of unknown primary tumors.

4. Discuss the most common histology and the usual sites of presentation of CUP.

Adenocarcinoma and undifferentiated carcinoma account for > 75% of cases. Most present below the diaphragm. Squamous carcinoma in the cervical area and undifferentiated neoplasms in midline locations are important and potentially curable subsets.

5. When a primary site is eventually found, which sites are most common?

Even at autopsy fewer than 50% of patients have an identifiable primary tumor. A primary tumor in the pancreas accounts for about 25% of cases, and lung cancer is diagnosed in 20%. Stomach, colorectal, and kidney primary tumors account for a smaller but significant percentage.

6. Which diagnostic studies are most helpful in CUP?

The shotgun approach is out. Extensive, expensive, and uncomfortable evaluations are diagnostic of the primary site in only 5–30% of patients. Even if the primary site is suspected, the antemortem diagnosis is found at autopsy to be wrong in 25% of cases. Most diagnoses are made on follow-up when specific symptoms direct diagnostic evaluations. The goal in evaluating such patients is to identify treatable tumors, anticipate complications, and avoid low-yield, invasive, or costly procedures. The most productive evaluation consists of a thorough history and physical examination, routine laboratory evaluation, and chest radiograph.

7. How can the pathologist help in the diagnosis of CUP?

The importance of direct communication with the pathologist cannot be overemphasized; precise histologic diagnosis is essential in evaluating such patients. Morphologic clues may suggest certain anatomic sites. The distinction among adenocarcinoma, squamous carcinoma, and undifferentiated carcinoma also narrows the diagnostic possibilities. Providing the pathologist with clinical clues can direct the optimal use of special stains, immunohistochemistry, flow cytometry, and electron microscopy.

8. Is electron microscopy useful in finding a CUP?

A small percentage of patients with poorly differentiated carcinoma and an unknown primary site are found with electron microscopy to have neuroendocrine features. The pathognomonic finding is the dense-core granule. This subset of patients is especially important to recognize, because they tend to respond well to cisplatin-based chemotherapy regimens and a small number (10–20%) are actually cured.

9. Are any clues from the history and physical examination helpful in finding the primary site of a tumor?

Yes—and it is a cost-effective approach. Findings from a detailed history and physical examination can direct subsequent diagnostic and staging evaluation. More than 50% of patients have more than one metastatic site. The review of systems may identify locations that deserve further diagnostic evaluation. Careful examination of the thyroid, breasts, prostate, testis, and skin may yield a primary diagnosis. Rectal and pelvic examinations are often wrongly overlooked.

10. If the tumor presents in the cervical nodes, what should you do?

Biopsy of suspicious nodes should not be done until a complete diagnostic examination is performed. A careful endoscopic examination of the upper respiratory tract and computed tomographic (CT) scans of the neck are required. Of patients with squamous carcinoma in cervical nodes, 30–40% have potentially curable cancers. Treatment is often a combination of surgery and radiation therapy.

11. Which laboratory studies are indicated in diagnosing a primary tumor?

Routine laboratory tests may help in diagnosing a primary tumor (e.g., red cells in the urine suggest renal cell carcinoma) and determining the extent of metastatic spread (e.g., liver enzymes and alkaline phosphatase).

12. Are tumor markers helpful in CUP?

Although assays for a number of tumor-associated markers are available, lack of specificity limits their usefulness. Many patients with CUP express multiple serum tumor markers. A few specific markers do exist, however. Prostate-specific antigen can suggest prostate cancer in a man with carcinoma of unknown primary site. Young men with unknown primary sites, especially those with mediastinal masses, should be screened for germ cell tumors with beta human chorionic gonadotropin and alpha-fetoprotein. In women with adenocarcinomas CA-125, which may suggest an ovarian cancer, should be determined, and material should be submitted for hormone receptor analysis, which may correctly identify breast cancer. These studies may have diagnostic and therapeutic implications.

13. What is the prognosis of a patient with CUP?

The prognosis of patients with CUP is not improved by correctly identifying the primary tumor. Patients who present with upper cervical nodes have a 5-year survival rate of 30–50%. Metastasis at any other site is associated with a median survival rate of 3–5 months and a 5-year survival rate of < 5%.

14. If a young man is found to have a poorly differentiated neoplasm in a midline location, how should he be treated?

The patient should be assumed to have a germ cell tumor and should be treated with cisplatin-based combination chemotherapy. Germ cell tumors account for about 20% of most series and are potentially curable.

15. What is the best treatment for patients with CUP?

Most patients who present with CUP have tumors that are not curable with chemotherapy. The evaluation should be directed at diagnosing treatable malignancies such as breast, ovarian, germ cell, or prostate cancer. About 20% of patients with adenocarcinoma of unknown primary site respond to fluorouracil, but survival is not affected. Newer treatment regimens using combinations of drugs such as paclitaxel, carboplatin, and etoposide have response rates as high as 47%. Patients with the highest performance status should be chosen because they benefit the most from the palliative effects of treatment and have the least toxicity. The patient's performance status remains the best predictor of response to therapy and prognosis.

BIBLIOGRAPHY

1. Abbruzzese JL, Abbruzzese MC, Hess KR, et al: Unknown primary carcinoma: Natural history and prognostic factors in 657 consecutive patients. J Clin Oncol 12:1272–1280, 1994.
2. Briasoulis E, Pavlidis N: Cancer of unknown primary origin. Oncologist 2:142–152, 1997.
3. Gaber AO, Rice P, Eaton C, et al: Metastatic malignant disease of unknown origin. Am J Surg 145:493–497, 1983.
4. Greco FA, Vaugn WK, Hainsworth JD: Advanced poorly differentiated carcinoma of unknown primary site: Recognition of a treatable syndrome. Ann Intern Med 104:547–553, 1986.
5. Hainsworth JD, Erland JB, Thomas M, et al: Treatment of carcinoma of unknown primary site (CUP) with paclitaxel, carboplatin and etoposide: A Minnie Pearl Cancer Research Network phase 11 trial. Proc Am Soc Clin Oncol 16:275a[abstract 975], 1997.
6. Hainsworth JD, Greco FA: Treatment of patients with cancer of unknown primary site. N Engl J Med 329:257–263, 1993.
7. Hainsworth JD, Johnson DH, Greco FA: Poorly differentiated neuroendocrine carcinoma of unknown primary site. Ann Intern Med 109:364–371, 1988.
8. Nystrom JS, Weiner JM, Wolf RM, et al: Identifying the primary site in metastatic cancer of unknown origin: Inadequacy of roentgenographic procedures. JAMA 241:381–383, 1979.
9. Osteen RT, Kopf G, Wilson RE: In pursuit of the unknown primary. Am J Surg 135:494–498, 1978.
10. Pasterz R, Savaaj N, Burgess M: Prognostic factors in metastatic carcinoma of unknown primary. J Clin Oncol 4:1562–1565, 1986.
11. Schildt RR, Kennedy PS, Chen TT, et al: Management of patients with metastatic adenocarcinoma of unknown origin: A southwest Oncology Group Study. Cancer Treat Rep 67:77–79, 1983.

VI. Pediatric Oncology

82. WILMS TUMOR

Sharon L. Space, M.D., and Edythe A. Albano, M.D.

1. Define Wilms tumor.

Wilms tumor, also known as nephroblastoma, is a malignancy arising from the kidney. It is the third most common solid tumor in childhood.

2. Estimate the frequency of occurrence of Wilms tumor in the U.S.

Wilms tumor occurs at a rate of 8.1 cases per million Caucasian children and 7.8 cases per million African-American children each year (in children < 15 years of age) in the U.S. Approximately 460 new cases are diagnosed annually in the U.S., accounting for 5–6% of cancers in children < 15 years of age.

3. What is the National Wilms Tumor Study (NWTS)?

The NWTS is a cooperative clinical trial carried out in the U.S., Canada, and several other countries to study Wilms tumor. Clinical trials began in 1969 with NWTS 1. NWTS 5 opened in 1997. Much of the treatment progress has resulted from these large, multinational, randomized studies. Such progress could not have been made in single- or small-group studies. As a result of cooperative trials, the 2-year survival rate of children with Wilms tumor has risen from 20% 2 years after diagnosis to 90% in the 1990s. With these excellent survival rates, NWTS is focusing on decreasing therapy and associated adverse effects, evaluation of tumor biology, and evaluation of cost-effectiveness.

4. At what age is a child typically diagnosed with Wilms tumor?

The average age at diagnosis is 3–4 years. Eighty percent of cases are diagnosed in children < 5 years of age. It is extremely rare after 15 years of age. Males tend to present at a younger age. Bilateral tumors also are more common in younger children.

	Unilateral tumor (months)	Bilateral tumor (months)
Female	43	30
Male	36	23

5. What congenital anomalies are associated with Wilms tumor?

Associated congenital anomalies are found in 7.6% of children diagnosed with Wilms tumor. They include aniridia, hemihypertrophy, and genitourinary anomalies (including hypospadias, cryptorchidism, duplication of renal collecting system, gonadal dysgenesis, pseudohermaphroditism, and horseshoe kidney). Additionally, syndromes such as Beckwith-Wiedemann syndrome (BWS) (visceromegaly, macroglossia, omphalocele, hemihypertrophy, mental retardation), WAGR (**W**ilms tumor, **A**niridia, **G**enitourinary malformations, Mental **R**etardation), Denys-Drash syndrome (nephropathy, ambiguous genitalia), Perlman syndrome (macrocephaly, characteristic facies, macrosomia, organomegaly), and cerebral gigantism (cerebral overgrowth, macrocephaly, developmental delay) are associated with an increased incidence of Wilms tumor. Children with BWS have a 3–5% risk of Wilms tumor, and those with WAGR have a > 30% risk.

Congenital Anomalies Associated with Wilms Tumor

CONGENITAL ANOMALY	PREVALENCE IN GENERAL POPULATION (per 1000)	PREVALENCE IN PATIENTS WITH WILMS TUMOR (per 1000)
Aniridia	0.02	7.6
Hemihypertrophy	0.03	32.6
Genitourinary malformations	10	62.5

6. What screening is recommended in children predisposed to Wilms tumor?

Abdominal ultrasound and urinalysis for microscopic hematuria at 4–month intervals through age 7 years is recommended for children with aniridia, hemihypertrophy, BWS, WAGR syndrome, and Denys-Drash syndrome.

7. How does a patient with Wilms tumor usually present?

An asymptomatic abdominal mass or abdominal swelling noted by a parent brings most children to medical attention (83%). Occasionally this is detected on routine physical exam by the child's primary care provider. Less common presenting complaints include fever (23%), abdominal pain (most often due to hemorrhage into the tumor or tumor rupture), and constitutional symptoms (weight loss, anemia, malaise). Approximately 25% of children with Wilms tumor are hypertensive at presentation. Microscopic hematuria is found in 21% of patients, but gross hematuria is rare. The three clinical scenarios in which patients with Wilms tumor present are (1) sporadic cases who present most commonly with an asymptomatic abdominal mass, (2) children with a predisposition to Wilms tumor due to an underlying congenital anomaly (2%), and (3) those with a familial predisposition believed to be autosomally transmitted with low and variable expressivity (1–2%).

8. What is the differential diagnosis of congestive heart failure (CHF) in a patient being evaluated for Wilms tumor?

Severe hypertension secondary to hyperreninemia, tumor thrombi in the pulmonary arteries, or tumor extension into the right atrium causing tamponade may cause CHF.

9. What is the differential diagnosis for an abdominal mass in a child?

The differential diagnosis for an abdominal mass includes renal masses such as Wilms tumor, mesoblastic nephroma (a benign lesion typically seen in neonates), renal cell carcinoma, polycystic kidney disease, and hydronephrosis; liver masses such as hepatoblastoma or hepatocellular carcinoma; other malignancies such as neuroblastoma (a malignancy arising from the adrenal gland or parasympathetic ganglia), or lymphoma; and splenomegaly.

Neuroblastoma, the most common retroperitoneal malignancy in childhood, also is the most common misdiagnosis in the preoperative assessment. In a recent study, neuroblastoma was the incorrect preoperative diagnosis one-third of the time. With the increased use of abdominal computed tomography (CT) in evaluating children with abdominal masses, this is less likely but still occurs.

10. How is Wilms tumor distinguished from abdominal neuroblastoma?

Neuroblastoma arises from extrarenal sites and displaces the kidney. In contrast, Wilms tumor is intrarenal and distorts the kidney, which can be detected on abdominal ultrasound, CT, or intravenous pyelography. On plain films calcifications are frequently seen with neuroblastoma (> 50%) but are uncommon in Wilms tumor (10–15%). Clinically, children with advanced stage neuroblastoma appear much more ill than children with Wilms tumor with weight loss, fever, and irritability.

11. To which sites does Wilms tumor metastasize?

Wilms tumor metastasizes to regional lymph nodes, lung, and liver. Eighty percent of patients with stage IV tumors have lung metastases and 15% have liver metastases.

12. Which diagnostic imaging studies are used to evaluate the child with a suspected Wilms tumor?

Abdominal ultrasonography or CT is most commonly used. The radiographic examination should identify an intrarenal mass. Additionally, it is essential to evaluate the contralateral kidney for its presence and function, as well as synchronous Wilms tumor. The inferior vena cava (IVC) needs to be evaluated for the presence and extent of tumor thrombus. The liver also should be imaged for metastatic disease. Phase-contrast magnetic resonance angiography may be useful in defining intrarenal vasculature if renal-sparing surgery is indicated. A plain radiograph of the chest (4-view) should be obtained to check for pulmonary metastases. The use of chest CT is controversial because it may be overly sensitive in detecting abnormalities. Its role is currently being investigated in a clinical trial.

13. What are the histologic features of a classic Wilms tumor?

A Wilms tumor is composed of three elements (triphasic pattern) that mimic normal kidney: blastema (cellular component), epithelium (tubules), and stroma. The ratio of the components varies among tumors. Multiple tissues of neonatal types, including skeletal muscle, squamous epithelium, cartilage, and neuroglia, also may be seen in Wilms tumor.

14. Is the histologic subtype of Wilms tumor of prognostic significance?

Analysis of the clinical trial NWTS-4 shows that epithelial-predominant tumors are more likely to present at a lower stage (81.3% at stage I) and at a younger age (mean age at diagnosis = 17 months). In contrast, diffuse blastemal tumors are more aggressive: 76.3% of patients have stage III or IV disease at diagnosis. Such patients also tend to be older at diagnosis (mean age = 57 months). With the current therapies all subtypes are associated with high survival rates.

15. What does the term *unfavorable histology* refer to?

The term *unfavorable histology* refers to the presence of anaplasia (extreme nuclear atypia), clear cell sarcoma of the kidney (CCSK), and rhabdoid tumor of the kidney (RTK). In early Wilms tumor studies these three unique histologies were associated with markedly worse outcome when compared with favorable histology Wilms tumor. Five percent of Wilms tumors are of unfavorable histology. Anaplasia is believed to be a marker of resistance to chemotherapeutic agents and not a marker of more aggressive disease. It is rare in children diagnosed with Wilms tumor before 2 years of age and more common (10% of cases) in children diagnosed after 5 years of age.

CCSK and RTK are no longer considered to be Wilms tumor variants, but rather separate renal malignancies. CCSK, sometimes referred to as "bone-metastasizing renal tumor of childhood," is a much more aggressive disease than Wilms tumor and more likely to present with metastases to lung, brain, and bone. RTK, more commonly seen in male infants, also is a more aggressive neoplasm that metastasizes to the brain.

16. What is the significance of focal vs. diffuse anaplasia?

The extent of anaplasia was based originally on the proportion of microscopic fields that contained anaplasia without regard to the distribution of anaplastic elements (< 10% of fields with focal anaplasia). Although patients with diffuse anaplasia tended to have a poorer prognosis, this trend was not significant. More recently, focal anaplasia has been redefined as anaplastic changes confined to one or more clearly defined regions within the primary tumor and absent from extrarenal extension and metastatic lesions. This revised definition has significant prognostic implications. Focal anaplasia with complete surgical resection of the anaplastic, or chemotherapy-resistant, cells is not associated with a worse prognosis and does not require more aggressive treatment, whereas diffuse anaplasia is associated with a worse prognosis and requires more aggressive treatment for cure. In the current trials a diagnosis of focal anaplasia in stage I Wilms tumor does not receive intensified therapy. However, focal anaplasia in stage II, III, or IV or diffuse anaplasia at any stage is associated with higher rates of relapse and death and therefore is treated more intensively.

17. Define the term *nephrogenic rest*.

Nephrogenic rests are islands of cells resembling metanephric blastema (persistent embryonal remnants) and are believed to be precursors to Wilms tumor. Perilobar nephrogenic rests (PLNR) are often numerous and found in the periphery of the renal lobe. They are found in 25% of cases of Wilms tumor and 60% of Wilms tumor cases associated with BWS or hemihypertrophy. Intralobar nephrogenic rests (ILNR) are solitary lesions found anywhere in the deep renal cortex or renal medulla. ILNR are found in 15% of cases with underlying WAGR or Denys-Drash syndrome. Patients with an underlying predisposition to Wilms tumor and the presence of nephrogenic rests have an increased incidence of a second Wilms tumor in the contralateral kidney. Such patients receive more frequent follow-up for a longer duration.

18. Which constitutional chromosomal abnormalities have been linked to predisposition to Wilms tumor?

Three distinct chromosomal abnormalities are associated with the development of Wilms tumor.

WT1 gene: Patients with Wilms tumor and underlying WAGR syndrome have a constitutional deletion at the 11p13 locus, which includes the genes WT1 and PAX6. The gene product for WT1 is a transcriptional factor vital for normal kidney and gonadal development. WT1 is a tumor suppressor gene, which means that loss of both alleles is required for tumorogenesis. Loss of one allele of WT1 is associated with genitourinary defects. PAX6, the gene for aniridia, is contiguous with the WT1 gene. Loss of one allele of PAX6 is associated with aniridia, but not with the predisposition to Wilms tumor. All patients with Denys-Drash syndrome also have constitutional mutations of WT1. Abnormalities of WT1 are found in only 5–10% of sporadic cases of Wilms tumor.

WT2 gene: The BWS locus maps to 11p15. Additionally, some sporadic cases of Wilms tumor have loss of heterozygosity (LOH) of 11p15, prompting the identification of 11p15 as the locus for WT2, a second tumor suppressor gene associated with Wilms tumor. The WT2 gene has not been identified. The insulinlike growth factor II gene (IGF2), which encodes an embryonal growth factor, and H19, a gene adjacent to IGF2 on chromosome 11p15 that functions as a regulatory RNA molecule, are under investigation as being WT2.

Familial Wilms tumor: The chromosomal abnormality associated with this rare form of Wilms tumor (1–2% of cases) has not been identified. Abnormalities of WT1, WT2, and other chromosomal abnormalities associated with Wilms tumor have been ruled out, implicating a third and not yet identified gene.

19. What other chromosomal abnormalities have been identified in Wilms tumor?

Several tumor-specific chromosomal abnormalities are associated with more aggressive Wilms tumors, including LOH at 16q (15–20% of Wilms tumors) and LOH at 1p (10%). Abnormalities of p53, a tumor suppressor gene located at 17p13, although common in many adult cancers, are rare in Wilms tumor and have been identified only in the presence of anaplasia.

Ploidy, or DNA content of the tumor, is being investigated as a prognostic variable in Wilms tumor. Aneuploidy is identified more often in anaplastic tumors. Tetraploidy also has been associated with worse outcomes in some studies. Several studies have found that a higher DNA index is associated with a worse prognosis (DNA index < 1.5 = 2-year survival rate of 97.1%; DNA index > 1.5 = 2-year survival rate of 66.7%).

20. How is Wilms tumor staged?

The clinical stage is determined after surgical evaluation and confirmed by the pathologist.

Stage I: Tumor limited to the kidney and completely excised
Stage II: Tumor extends beyond the kidney but is completely excised. There is no residual tumor beyond the margins of excision.
Stage III: Residual nonhematogenous tumor confined to the abdomen
Stage IIIa: Lymph node involvement
Stage IIIb: Diffuse peritoneal contamination by tumor

Stage IIIc: Peritoneal implants are found
Stage IIId: Tumor beyond surgical margins (microscopic or gross)
Stage IIIe: Unresectable tumor infiltrating into vital structures
Stage IV: Hematogenous metastases (lung or liver)
Stage V: Bilateral renal involvement

21. Name four factors that independently predict the likelihood of relapse-free survival in Wilms tumor.

1. Favorable histology
2. Lymph nodes negative for tumor
3. Age < 24 months at diagnosis
4. Tumor weight < 250 gm

22. How is Wilms tumor treated in the U.S.?

Wilms tumor is treated with multimodal therapy based on staging. Treatment begins with surgical exploration of the abdomen. A transabdominal approach allows the following:

1. Inspection and palpation of the contralateral kidney for tumor involvement (7% of patients have bilateral disease at diagnosis, but in one-third of these patients there is no evidence of this on preoperative imaging studies).

2. Inspection and biopsy of suspicious liver and periaortic nodes.

3. En bloc resection of tumor and involved kidney.

These cannot be accomplished with a flank incision. Following surgical excision and pathologic examination, the patient is assigned a stage that defines further therapy with chemotherapy with or without radiation therapy.

The U.S. approach differs from the European one, in which chemotherapy is given before surgical resection. However, important histologic staging parameters are lost with this approach, and all patients are treated more intensively.

23. What is the role of radiotherapy in the treatment of Wilms tumor?

The current treatment recommendations are against radiotherapy for children with stage I or II disease. Children with stage III and IV Wilms tumor receive 1080 cGy to the abdomen. Whole-lung irradiation is indicated when lung metastases are identified on chest x-ray. With the use of prophylactic trimethoprim/sulfamethoxazole and reduced chemotherapy dosing immediately after completion of radiotherapy, no deaths due to interstitial pneumonitis occurred in NWTS 4.

24. When should radiotherapy begin?

Radiotherapy should begin within 10 days of nephrectomy. Higher rates of relapse occur if radiotherapy is delayed.

25. Which chemotherapeutic agents are used in the treatment of Wilms tumor?

Vincristine and actinomycin D are used in the treatment of all patients with Wilms tumor; doxorubicin (Adriamycin) is administered to patients with stage III and IV tumors. Early information suggests that pulse-intensive (single-dose) actinomycin D versus actinomycin D daily over 5 days is less hematologically toxic and more cost-effective with comparable event-free survival.

26. When is chemotherapy begun after nephrectomy?

Chemotherapy is begun by postoperative day 5 (surgery = day 0). As with radiotherapy, higher relapse rates are reported if chemotherapy is delayed.

27. What is the duration of chemotherapy?

Preliminary data suggest no survival advantage with longer courses of chemotherapy (54–60 weeks) compared with shorter courses (18–24 weeks). The following are current treatment recommendations in NWTS 5:

Stage/Histology	Treatment
I FH or anaplasia (focal or diffuse) and II FH	18 weeks (actinomycin D and vincristine)
III or IV FH and II–IV focal anaplasia	24 weeks (actinomycin D, vincristine, and doxorubicin)
II–IV diffuse anaplasia	24 weeks (actinomycin D, vincristine, doxorubicin, and Cytoxan)

28. What is the 4-year event-free survival (EFS) and survival of patients with tumor by stage and histology?

Four-Year Survival of Patients with Wilms Tumor (Based on NWTS 3)

STAGE/HISTOLOGY	EVENT-FREE SURVIVAL (%)	SURVIVAL (%)
I/FH	90.4	96.5
II/FH	88	92.2
III/FH	79	86.9
IV/FH	74	82.5
I–III/UH	64.7	68
IV/UH	55.6	55.7
Overall	**83.3**	**89.1**

FH, favorable histology; UH, unfavorable histology (including diffuse anaplasia, CCSK, and rhabdoid tumor)

29. What are the current recommendations for treatment of relapsed Wilms tumor?

The NWTS 5 protocol for treatment of relapsed Wilms tumor is investigating the role of autologous bone marrow transplantation, as well as less nephrotoxic chemotherapies, such as etoposide and carboplatin. The prognosis in relapsed Wilms tumor depends on previous therapy; patients who did not receive radiation therapy or doxorubicin as part of their initial treatment have improved survival.

30. What long-term complications of Wilms tumor therapy do survivors face?

Long-term toxicity of Wilms tumor therapy includes musculoskeletal abnormalities (e.g., scoliosis, atrophy) in patients treated with radiation (60% develop scoliosis after abdominal radiotherapy > 3000 cGy), cardiovascular abnormalities in patients who receive doxorubicin (< 2%), renal insufficiency (< 1%), and second malignancies (including leukemia, lymphoma, and sarcomas, with a cumulative incidence of 1.6%).

BIBLIOGRAPHY

1. Beckwith JB, Zuppan CE, Browning NG, et al: Histological analysis of aggressiveness and responsiveness in Wilms' tumor. Med Pediatr Oncol 27:422–428, 1996.
2. Birch JM, Breslow N: Epidemiology features of Wilms' tumor. Hematol Oncol Clin North Am 9:1157–1177, 1995.
3. Breslow NE, Takashima JR, Whitton JA, et al: Second malignant neoplasms following treatment for Wilms tumor: A report from the National Wilms' Tumor Study Group. J Clin Oncol 13:1851–1859, 1995.
4. Clericusio CL, Johnson C: Screening for Wilms' tumor in high-risk individuals. Hematol Oncol Clin North Am 9:1253–1265, 1995.
5. Coppes MJ, Haber DA, Grundy PE: Genetic events in the development of Wilms' tumor. N Engl J Med 331:586–590, 1994.
6. Green DM, Coppes MJ: Future directions in clinical research of Wilms' tumor. Hematol Oncol Clin North Am 9:1157–1177, 1995.
7. Green DM, Coppes MJ, Breslow NE, et al: Wilms tumor. In Pizzo PA, Poplack DG (eds): Principles and Practice of Pediatric Oncology, 3rd ed. Philadelphia, Lippincott-Raven, 1997.
8. Green DM, Thomas PRM, Shochat S: The treatment of Wilms' tumor. Hematol Oncol Clin North Am 9:1267–1274, 1995.

9. Grundy PE, Coppes MJ: An overview of the clinical and molecular genetics of Wilms' tumor. Med Pediatr Oncol 27:394–397, 1996.
10. Haase GM: Current surgical management of Wilms' tumor. Curr Opin Pediatr 8:268–275, 1996.
11. Miser JM, Tournade MF: The management of relapsed Wilms' tumor. Hematol Oncol Clin North Am 9:1287–1302, 1995.
12. Ritchey ML, Azizhan RG, Beckwith JB, et al: Neonatal Wilms' tumor. J Pediatr Surg 30:856–859, 1995.

83. CHILDHOOD ACUTE LYMPHOBLASTIC LEUKEMIA

Linda C. Stork, M.D.

1. What is acute leukemia?

Acute leukemia is defined as the presence of > 25% hematopoietic blasts in a bone marrow smear. It is an uncontrolled proliferation of white blood cells at an early stage of maturation.

2. Name the types of acute leukemia that occur in childhood.

Acute lymphoblastic leukemia (ALL) is the most common acute childhood leukemia, representing about 80% of cases. Acute nonlymphocytic (ANLL), or acute myelogenous leukemia (AML), accounts for the remaining 20%. ALL is treated very differently from ANLL (AML), and thus the distinction between the two is very important.

3. Give the incidence of acute leukemia in childhood.

Acute leukemia is the most common malignancy of childhood. New cases are diagnosed in about 2,500 children each year in the United States, with an incidence of about 1 in 25,000 children per year (< 15 years of age).

4. How is ALL distinguished from ANLL (AML)?

The clinical presentations of ALL and ANLL (AML) are generally similar. The morphology of blasts on a bone marrow aspirate stained with Wright/Giemsa distinguishes the majority of cases of ALL from ANLL (AML). Lymphoblasts are typically small, with cell diameters equal to that of approximately two red blood cell (RBC) diameters. They have a scant amount of cytoplasm, usually without granules. The nucleus usually contains none or one small indistinct nucleolus. Blasts of the myeloid leukemias are usually much larger than two RBC diameters and have more cytoplasm surrounding the nucleus than do lymphoblasts. RBC diameters have more cytoplasm surrounding the nucleus than do lymphoblasts. Granules are often present in the cytoplasm of an ANLL blast, and the nucleus usually contains one or more distinct nucleoli. Cytochemical stains also distinguish ALL from ANLL blasts. The latter cells stain with myeloperoxidase and/or nonspecific esterase, whereas the former cells do not (see chapter 27 for more details).

5. What cell type is the blast of ALL?

Immunophenotyping of ALL blasts, using monoclonal antibodies and flow cytometry, has helped us understand the heterogeneity of ALL. About 80% of cases are of B-cell lineage and 20% T-cell lineage. Lymphoblasts of B-cell lineage are found at various stages of B-cell development, but the majority are at an early stage of B-cell maturation before the synthesis of immunoglobulins. However, some B-lineage lymphoblasts have immunoglobulin chains within their cytoplasm and, very rarely, immunoglobulins on their surface. In general, the lymphoblasts of T-cell lineage are found at a stage before helper or suppressor T-cell functions are expressed (see chapter 27 for more details).

6. Discuss the usual presenting clinical findings in ALL.

Signs and symptoms of patients presenting with ALL include those related to decreased bone marrow production of RBCs, white blood cells (WBCs), and platelets. Pallor and easy bruisability with purpura or petechiae are seen in over 50% of cases. Intermittent fevers are common owing to the leukemia itself or to infections secondary to a decreased number of functioning WBCs. About 25% of patients experience bone pain, especially of the pelvis, vertebral bodies, and legs. Signs and symptoms may also be related to leukemic infiltration of extramedullary (outside the bone marrow) sites. Generalized lymphadenopathy, hepatomegaly, and splenomegaly occur in over 50% of cases. Some patients, particularly those with T-cell leukemia, present with a mediastinal mass that may cause respiratory distress, orthopnea, and airway compromise.

The differential diagnosis of ALL initially includes juvenile rheumatoid arthritis, infectious mononucleosis, idiopathic thrombocytopenic purpura (ITP), and aplastic anemia.

7. What are the laboratory abnormalities found at diagnosis in ALL?

The complete blood cell count (CBC) with differential is the most useful initial laboratory test for determining if a patient has ALL. Ninety-nine percent of patients have decreased numbers of at least one cell type (leukopenia, neutropenia, thrombocytopenia, or anemia), and the majority of patients have decreased numbers of two blood cell types. The WBCs are low or normal (WBCs < 10,000/μl) in about 50% of patients, but a differential often shows neutropenia (absolute neutrophil count < 1000/μl) along with a small percentage of blasts amid normal lymphocytes. In 30% of patients, the WBC is > 10,000/μl and in 20% of cases it is > 50,000/μl, occasionally > 300,000/μl. Blasts are usually readily identifiable on peripheral smears of patients with elevated WBCs. Blasts on peripheral blood smears may not look identical to those in bone marrow aspirates, but the lymphoid versus myeloid nature of these blasts usually can be recognized.

The majority of patients with ALL have decreased platelet counts (< 150,000/μl) and decreased hemoglobin (< 11 gm/dl) at diagnosis, although cases with normal platelet counts and hemoglobin do occur.

Several serum chemistries, particularly uric acid and lactate dehydrogenase (LDH), are often elevated at diagnosis in patients with ALL. Uric acid and LDH are intracellular products released after cell breakdown. Liver function tests may be mildly abnormal as well because of leukemic infiltration.

8. Define tumor lysis syndrome (TLS). How is it managed?

TLS results from rapid cell breakdown once chemotherapy has been initiated for ALL or T-cell and B-cell lymphomas. Chemotherapy causes lymphoblasts to release cellular contents into the blood stream. Uric acid, a purine metabolite, can precipitate in the kidneys as chemotherapy is initiated and cause acute renal failure.

Patients are always treated with oral allopurinol prior to and during initial chemotherapy. Allopurinol inhibits the synthesis of uric acid from xanthine and hypoxanthine and helps to prevent uric acid nephropathy. Patients are always treated with hydration to maintain high urine output (approximately 1.5 × the hourly maintenance rate) along with sodium bicarbonate alkalinization, because uric acid is more soluble in alkaline than acidic urine. Intracellular phosphates also are released following initiation of chemotherapy, potentially resulting in phosphate deposition in kidneys. Hyperphosphatemia may be accompanied by hypocalcemia and tetany. To prevent hyperphosphatemia, oral phosphate binders like Amphojel (aluminum hydroxide) may be helpful. Once hyperphosphatemia is present, urine should no longer be alkalinized, because phosphates are poorly soluble in alkaline urine. Intracellular potassium also is released from the blasts and hyperkalemia can result, requiring dialysis to prevent a fatal arrhythmia. Intravenous fluids during initial chemotherapy should not contain K+ unless the serum level is less than 2.5 mg/dl. Dialysis may also be required for hyperphosphatemia with tetany or fluid overload. TLS usually is at its worst 3 days into chemotherapy and diminishes thereafter.

9. What is the current treatment for ALL?

A number of chemotherapeutic agents in combination are used to treat ALL. Treatment is generally divided into a number of phases. The first month of therapy consists of induction, at the end of which over 95% of patients exhibit remission bone marrows. Consolidation is the second phase of treatment, during which intrathecal chemotherapy and sometimes cranial irradiation is given to treat lymphoblasts that may be present in the meninges of the central nervous system (CNS). Maintenance therapy is the third phase of treatment and usually has fewer acute side effects than the other two phases. In the Children's Cancer Group protocols, one or two short courses of intensive chemotherapy are interspersed among the maintenance chemotherapy treatment.

Chemotherapeutic agents commonly used in induction include oral prednisone, intravenous vincristine, intramuscular L-asparaginase, intrathecal methotrexate, and intravenous daunorubicin. For T-cell ALL, intravenous cyclophosphamide may be given in induction as well. Maintenance treatment of ALL generally includes oral daily 6-mercaptopurine (6MP), weekly oral or intramuscular methotrexate, and monthly pulses of intravenous vincristine and oral prednisone. Intrathecal chemotherapy, either with methotrexate alone or combined with cytarabine and hydrocortisone, is usually administered every 2–3 months. In the Children's Cancer Group protocols, girls are currently treated for about 2 years and boys for about 3 years, because previous statistical analyses found that boys required longer treatment than girls for an equivalent cure rate.

10. Can ALL be cured?

The chance of cure depends to some degree on specific prognostic features that are present at diagnosis of ALL. The two most important prognostic features include WBC count and age. In the 1970s, it became clear that children with WBCs < 50,000/µl had a much better chance of cure than did children with WBCs > 50,000/µl receiving the same chemotherapy. Children from ages 1 to 9 years have a better chance of cure than do younger or older patients. Certain chromosome abnormalities present in the leukemic blasts at diagnosis also have prognostic significance. Patients with a translocation between chromosomes 9 and 22: t(9;22) have a very poor chance of cure even with intensive therapy. Patients with translocation between chromosomes 4 and 11: t(4;11) generally have a poorer chance of cure than do other patients with ALL. On the other hand, patients whose blasts are hyperdiploid (contain > 50 chromosomes instead of the normal 46) have a better chance of cure than do patients without hyperdiploidy, particularly if the extra chromosomes include 4 and 10. A recently identified gene rearrangement called TEL-AML1 occurs in blasts of about 25% of children with ALL and is associated with an excellent prognosis. This rearrangement of genetic material involves chromosomes 12 and 21 and is detected by molecular but not by cytogenetic techniques.

Treatment for ALL currently is tailored to prognostic groups. A child between the ages of 1 and 9 years with WBCs at diagnosis of < 50,000/µl and without t(9;22) or t(4;11) would be treated with less intensive therapy than a patient with WBCs ≥ 50,000/µl or a patient > 10 years old. This treatment approach has significantly increased the cure rate among patients with the less favorable prognostic features while minimizing treatment-related toxicities in those with favorable prognostic features. The overall chance of cure for childhood ALL is now at least 70%.

11. What is meant by "extramedullary relapse"?

The CNS and the testes are considered sanctuary sites of extramedullary leukemia. Systemic chemotherapy does not penetrate these tissues as well as it penetrates most organs. "Presymptomatic" intrathecal chemotherapy is a critical part of all ALL treatment protocols to prevent leukemic relapse in the CNS. Before the institution of such therapy in the 1970s, the CNS was a major site of initial leukemic relapse. Lymphoblasts are presumed to be present in the CNS at diagnosis in all patients with ALL even if not detected in spinal fluid samples. Lymphoblasts probably reach the CNS via hematogenous spread by migrating out of blood vessels into meninges or by direct extension from cranial bone marrow into the arachnoid. Now about 10% of patients with ALL have leukemic relapse in the CNS. Symptoms suggestive of CNS disease include headache, nausea and vomiting, irritability, nuchal rigidity, and cranial nerve palsies.

Boys may experience leukemic relapse in their testes during or after completion of chemotherapy, usually presenting with unilateral painless testicular enlargement. The incidence of testicular relapse has decreased significantly as treatment for ALL has intensified, suggesting that more chemotherapy may be penetrating the "blood-testes" barrier. Routine follow-up of boys on treatment and off treatment includes examination of the testes.

12. Is there a role for bone marrow transplant in ALL?

Bone marrow transplant is rarely used as initial treatment following induction of remission for ALL because the majority of patients are cured without it. However, patients with certain chromosome abnormalities in their leukemic blasts, like t(9;22), appear to have a much better cure rate with early bone marrow transplantation from an HLA-DR-matched donor than with intensive chemotherapy. Infants with t(4;11) or rearrangements of chromosome 11 at the 11q23 region (detected by cytogenetics or molecular genetics) also appear to have a better cure rate with bone marrow transplantation in first remission than with chemotherapy alone. Bone marrow transplant does play a role for patients who have relapsed with ALL, particularly if the relapse is during the course of treatment or within several months of completion. For these patients, bone marrow transplant may provide a cure, provided a second remission is first achieved with chemotherapy.

13. What medical problems may develop in long-term survivors of ALL?

The majority of patients treated for ALL will have normal gonadal function and fertility. Boys who received testicular radiation for testicular relapse will be infertile and some may need testosterone replacement. Patients, especially those < 10 years old, who received cranial irradiation as "presymptomatic" treatment of CNS leukemia may develop learning disabilities as a result. Patients who received spinal radiation for CNS leukemia may lose several centimeters of expected height. CNS radiation also may cause endocrinopathies, including hypothyroidism and growth hormone deficiencies, both of which can be corrected with hormone replacement. Cardiac failure has been reported in patients who received high cumulative doses of anthracyclines (daunorubicin, doxorubicin) as treatment for ALL. Aside from brain tumors after cranial irradiation, second malignancies have been reported infrequently in long-term survivors of ALL. As these children are followed into their fourth and fifth decades, more medical problems secondary to the treatment of ALL may surface.

BIBLIOGRAPHY

1. Bennett JM, Catorsky D, Daniel MT, et al: Proposal for the classification of acute leukemia. Br J Haematol 33:451, 1976.
2. Beyer WA, Poplack DG: Prophylaxis and treatment of leukemia in central nervous system and other sanctuaries. Semin Oncol 12:121, 1985.
3. Borowitz MJ: Immunologic markers in childhood acute lymphoblastic leukemia. Hematol Oncol Clin North Am 4:743–765, 1990.
4. Cohen LF, Balow JE, Magrath IT: Acute tumor lysis syndrome: A review of 37 patients with Burkitt's lymphoma. Am J Med 68:486, 1980.
5. Meadows AT, Silber J: Delayed consequences of therapy of childhood cancer. Cancer 35:271, 1985.
6. Poplack DG: Acute lymphoblastic leukemia. In Pizzo PA, Poplack DG (eds): Principles and Practice of Pediatric Oncology, 2nd ed. Philadelphia, J.B. Lippincott, 1993.
7. Pui CH: Childhood leukemia. N Engl J Med 332:1618, 1995.
8. Ribeiro RC, Abromowitch M, Raimondi SC, et al: Clinical and biologic hallmarks of the Philadelphia chromosome in childhood acute lymphoblastic leukemia. Blood 70:948, 1987.
9. Sanders JE, Thomas ED, Buckner D, et al: Marrow transplantation for children with acute lymphoblastic leukemia in second remission. Blood 70:324, 1987.
10. Smith M, Arthur D, Camitta B, et al: Uniform approach to risk classification and treatment assignment for children with ALL. J Clin Oncol 14:18, 1996.

84. OSTEOGENIC SARCOMA AND EWING'S SARCOMA IN CHILDREN

Brian S. Greffe, M.D., C.M.

1. When does the peak incidence of osteogenic sarcoma and Ewing's sarcoma occur in childhood?

The second decade of life is usually the peak incidence for **osteogenic sarcoma** (OS). This is the time of the adolescent growth spurt. Of interest, there may be a relationship between this period of growth and the development of OS. The disease occurs at an earlier age in girls than in boys, corresponding to their more advanced skeletal age and earlier adolescent growth spurt. OS also has a predilection for the metaphyseal portions of the most rapidly growing bones in adolescents. People diagnosed with bilateral retinoblastoma (inherited form) are at significant risk of developing OS as a second malignancy later in life. OS is also seen as a second malignancy in the field of previous tumor irradiation.

Ewing's sarcoma (ES) is seen most commonly in the early to midportion of the second decade of life and rarely occurs in children less than 5 years old or in adults older than 30 years. It is extremely uncommon in African Americans and Chinese.

2. What are the most common sites of presentation for OS and ES?

OS usually involves the long bones. These tumors can be found most commonly in the distal femur and proximal tibia. The proximal humerus and mid and proximal femur also are frequently involved. Involvement of the axial skeleton (such as the pelvis) accounts for only 10% of cases in the pediatric age group.

ES, on the other hand, is seen most commonly in the pelvis and frequently involves the axial skeleton. It also commonly occurs in the humerus and femur.

3. What are the clinical manifestations of OS and ES?

The most common symptoms for both tumors at the time of presentation include pain and swelling of the involved bone and surrounding tissue. In newly diagnosed cases of OS, 10–20% of patients have gross metastatic disease at the time of presentation. Up to 30% of patients with ES have macrometastatic disease at diagnosis. The most common sites of metastatic disease include lung (OS, ES) and bone marrow (ES). Multifocal bone disease is present in 1–3% of patients with OS at presentation. Patients with metastatic disease may present with fever, respiratory distress, and, in the case of bone marrow involvement, pancytopenia.

4. What radiographic studies are important in the diagnosis of ES and OS?

Plain films of the involved area are usually the first radiographic studies obtained. In ES, the area of the tumor usually shows a moth-eaten pattern of bony destruction. An onionskin appearance secondary to elevation of the periosteum also may be present. In OS, the bony destruction seen on radiography is usually accompanied by periosteal new bone formation and lifting of the cortex with formation of Codman's triangle.

A radionuclide bone scan is helpful in defining the extent of the primary tumor and, in the case of OS, can also be useful in identifying "skip lesions" that are seen infrequently in these patients. Computed tomography (CT) scanning can be helpful in defining the extent of the primary tumor in the medullary cavity and soft tissues. Magnetic resonance imaging (MRI) may be more sensitive in this regard and in some centers is replacing CT. CT scan of the chest and chest radiography are necessary to identify pulmonary lesions.

5. Which laboratory tests should be considered in patients with newly diagnosed bone malignancies?

There are no specific tumor markers identified as yet for OS and ES. Serum levels of lactate dehydrogenase (LDH) and alkaline phosphatase, however, may be of prognostic value in patients with OS. Patients in whom either of these markers is elevated at the time of diagnosis appear to have a worse outcome. Erythrocyte sedimentation rate (ESR) may be elevated at the time of diagnosis in patients with ES and may be of value in following response to therapy and monitoring for recurrence. Bone marrow examination (bilateral aspirates and biopsies) is essential in patients with ES before initiation of therapy.

6. What are the histologic considerations in evaluation of a biopsy specimen in patients with OS or ES?

The presence of osteoid formation on biopsy combined with a connective tissue stroma containing large, atypical, spindle-shaped cells that are highly malignant with irregular nuclei and abnormal mitotic figures usually confirms the diagnosis of OS.

In ES, electron microscopy is essential in confirming the diagnosis. ES must be differentiated from other tumors containing small, round blue cells, including lymphoma, neuroblastoma, rhabdomyosarcoma, and peripheral neuroepithelioma.

7. What are the tumor cytogenetic abnormalities seen in OS and ES?

In the majority of patients with ES, a translocation of chromosomes 11 and 22 is seen in the tumor cells. This translocation also is seen in peripheral neuroepithelioma, another small, round blue cell tumor. This chromosomal abnormality is characterized by translocation of the c-*sis*-oncogene from chromosome 22 to chromosome 11. C-*sis* appears not to be expressed; however, the oncogene c-*ets*, located near the breakpoint on chromosome 11, is variably expressed.

In OS, analysis of the DNA content of the tumor cells has shown that patients whose tumors contain a low percentage of diploid cells and an aneuploid peak are more likely to develop metastatic disease. Furthermore, the tumor suppressor gene p53 located on chromosome region 17(p13-1) may play an important role in malignant transformation of OS.

8. What prognostic factors are important in patients with bone malignancies?

The site of primary disease without metastases is an important prognostic variable in patients presenting with ES. Pelvic and sacral sites appear to have the least favorable outcome.

In both OS and ES, the presence of metastatic disease at the time of diagnosis portends a poor outcome. In OS, patients who present with pulmonary metastatic disease can expect to have a disease-free survival of only 11–40% at 5 years. Ten to twenty percent of patients with metastatic ES will be cured of their disease. OS presenting with multifocal bony metastases is uniformly fatal.

In patients with OS, the levels of LDH and alkaline phosphatase at the time of diagnosis appear to have prognostic implications. Patients presenting with high LDH or alkaline phosphate levels have a worse outcome. Patients with primaries of the axial skeleton and poor tumor kill (< 90%) with preoperative chemotherapy also have a less favorable prognosis.

9. What role does surgery play in the treatment of OS and ES?

Surgery plays a very important role in both of these bone malignancies. To prevent local recurrence, it is essential to remove all gross and microscopic tumors. Surgery is usually performed after several courses of preoperative chemotherapy have been given. The chemotherapeutic agents are useful in making the primary tumor more amenable to resection as well as controlling micrometastatic disease. Micrometastatic disease, principally in the lung, is usually present at the time of diagnosis.

Surgery for primary bone tumors can be accomplished either with an amputation or a limb-salvage procedure. Amputation provides removal of all gross and microscopic tumor with clean margins and good local control. Limb-salvage procedures are reserved for tumors that can be removed en bloc with a margin of normal tissue and do not have a large extramedullary component.

Once the tumor has been removed, restoration of the structural integrity of the involved extremity is obtained using biologic materials such as cadaveric allografts or autologous grafts and metallic endoprosthetic devices. Patients who have not yet achieved their full growth potential may not be ideal candidates for a limb-salvage procedure, because they may develop a leg length discrepancy later in life.

10. What chemotherapeutic agents are useful in patients with OS or ES?

Chemotherapy plays a role in the preoperative and postoperative phases of therapy. Response to preoperative chemotherapy (as measured by the percentage of tumor kill in the resected specimen) is in fact an important prognostic factor particularly in OS. Patients whose tumors demonstrate greater than 90% tumor kill with preoperative therapy are more likely to survive disease-free.

Chemotherapeutic agents effective in OS include cisplatin, doxorubicin (Adriamycin), methotrexate, vincristine, and ifosfamide. Selected pediatric oncology centers are currently using intraarterial cisplatin in preoperative patients to deliver intense chemotherapy directly into the tumor, potentially maximizing tumor kill. A new biologic agent, MTP-PE (muramyl tripeptide phosphatidylethanolamine), which is a macrophage stimulator, is currently being investigated in the new Pediatric Intergroup Osteosarcoma Study.

ES responds to a variety of agents such as cyclophosphamide, Adriamycin, vincristine, actinomycin, etoposide, and ifosfamide, all of which are given by the standard intravenous route. The most recently completed Pediatric Intergroup ES Study reported a superior outcome in patients with localized disease using the above six agents in combination compared with cyclophosphamide, doxorubicin, actinomycin, and vincristine alone. The present ES study will investigate the role of dose intensification of alkylating agents in the treatment of local disease.

11. What is the indication for radiation therapy in the treatment of OS and ES?

Radiation therapy plays an important role in the local control phase of treatment in patients with ES. Although the tumor is sensitive to radiation, high doses (> 5000 cGy) are usually needed to achieve adequate control. It is important to realize that radiation therapy can interfere with growth potential in young children, and surgery in fact may be the local control measure of choice in these patients. Patients with ES metastatic to the lungs may achieve limited benefit from radiation therapy. The maximum amount of total radiation to the lungs, however, cannot exceed 2000 cGy, which is below the amount of radiation needed to achieve adequate control (usually between 4000 and 5000 cGy).

Radiation therapy plays a small role in the treatment of OS, because the tumor is not particularly radiosensitive.

12. Does bone marrow transplant play a role in the treatment of bone malignancies?

Patients with poor prognosis ES at the time of diagnosis (pelvic primaries, metastatic disease) have been treated with intensive chemotherapy ± total body irradiation and autologous bone marrow transplant. Bone marrow transplant is currently limited to certain pediatric oncology centers. The majority of institutions use a multimodality approach (chemotherapy, surgery, radiation therapy).

13. What is the therapy for patients who develop pulmonary metastases after treatment for OS?

Patients who develop pulmonary nodules more than 1 year after initial surgery for OS still have a chance for cure compared with those who develop pulmonary nodules within 6 months of the surgery. Once metastatic disease is diagnosed, a thorough search for other metastatic sites should be undertaken using CT scan and radionuclide bone scans. The primary tumor site also should be evaluated radiologically for evidence of local recurrence if a limb-salvage procedure has been performed. In patients with resectable disease, a surgical procedure such as a thoracotomy or median sternotomy should be performed to remove all evidence of disease. Patients with three nodules or less may have long-term survival with surgery alone. Adjuvant chemotherapy should be considered for patients with more than three nodules, incompletely resected metastatic disease, or evidence of disruption of the pleura by tumor.

BIBLIOGRAPHY

1. Gehan EA, Nesbit ME, Burget EO, et al: Prognostic factors in children with Ewing's sarcoma. Natl Cancer Inst Monogr 56:273–278, 1981.
2. Glass AG, Fraumeni JF: Epidemiology of bone cancer in children. J Natl Cancer Inst 44:187, 199, 1970.
3. Grier H, Krailo M, Link M, et al: Improved outcome in nonmetastatic Ewing's sarcoma (EWS) and PNET of bone with the addition of ifosfamide (I) and etoposide (E) to vincristine (V), Adriamycin (Ad), cyclophosphamide (C), and actinomycin (A): A Children's Cancer Group (CCG) and Pediatric Oncology Group (POG) report. Proc Annu Meet Am Soc Clin Oncol 13:A1443, 1994.
4. Huvos AG: Bone Tumors: Diagnosis, Treatment, and Prognosis, 2nd ed. Philadelphia, W.B. Saunders, 1991.
5. Knudson AG: Hereditary cancer, oncogenes, and antioncogenes. Cancer Res 45:1437–1443, 1985.
6. Mankin H, Conner J, Schiller A, et al: Grading of bone tumors by analysis of nuclear DNA content using flow cytometry. J Bone Joint Surg 67:404–413, 1985.
7. Meyers PA: Malignant bone tumors in children: Osteosarcoma. Hematol Oncol Clin North Am 4:655–665, 1987.
8. Meyers PA: Malignant bone tumors in children: Ewing's sarcoma. Hematol Oncol Clin North Am 4:667–673, 1987.
9. Meyers PA, Heller G, Healey J, et al: Chemotherapy for nonmetastatic osteosarcoma: The Memorial Sloan-Kettering experience. J Clin Oncol 10:5–15, 1992.
10. Miser JS, Steis R, Longo DL, et al: Treatment of newly diagnosed high risk sarcomas and primitive neuroectodermal tumors (PNET) in children and young adults. Proc ASCO 4:C-935, 1985.
11. Murray JL, Kleinerman ES, Cunningham JE, et al: Phase I trial of liposomal muramyl tripeptide phosphatidylethanolamine in cancer patients. J Clin Oncol 7:1915–1925, 1989.
12. Pizzo PA, Poplack DG (eds): Principles and Practice of Pediatric Oncology, 3rd ed. Philadelphia, Lippincott-Raven, 1997.
13. Price C: Primary bone-forming tumours and their relationship to skeletal growth. J Bone Joint Surg 40:574–593, 1958.
14. Young JL, Miller RW: Incidence of malignant tumors in U.S. children. J Pediatr 86:245–258, 1975.

85. CHILDHOOD BRAIN TUMORS

Nicholas K. Foreman, M.B., B. Chir., Lorrie F. Odom, M.D.

1. How common are brain tumors in children?

Brain tumors are the second most common type of childhood cancer and the most common solid tumor of childhood, next in frequency only to acute leukemia. Brain tumors account for about 25% of all pediatric malignancies. In the United States, they are the leading cause of death from cancer in children under 16 years of age. About 1700 new malignant central nervous system tumors occur in children under 15 years of age each year, an incidence of 2.5–3.5 per 100,000 children.

2. Where do most childhood brain tumors commonly arise and what symptoms are usually present at diagnosis?

Over one-half of brain tumors in children arise in the posterior fossa and include medulloblastomas, cerebellar astrocytomas, brain stem gliomas, and fourth ventricle ependymomas. The most common symptoms at diagnosis are usually related to increased intracranial pressure and include headaches, morning vomiting, and lethargy. Such symptoms also may be associated with unsteadiness of gait and diplopia. Persistent head tilt is a common but often missed sign of a posterior fossa tumor. Supratentorial tumors, especially in teenagers, may present with personality changes and academic failure.

3. What are the most common types of childhood brain tumors?

Almost 60% of childhood central nervous system (CNS) tumors are of astrocytic origin. Seventy-five percent of them are low-grade astrocytomas (LGA). Thus, LGA are a heterogenous group of tumors varying in incidence, biologic behavior, and microscopic features, representing the largest group of CNS tumors. The group includes juvenile pilocytic, fibrillary and protoplasmic astrocytomas, oligodendrogliomas, gangliogliomas, and low-grade mixed gliomas. In the currently favored classification system the two other subgroups of childhood astrocytomas are anaplastic astrocytoma and glioblastoma multiforme.

4. In what locations do axial LGA commonly occur?

Such tumors commonly occur in optic pathways, the suprasellar region, and the brain stem. Degeneration into a malignant neoplasm may occur in approximately 5–6% of patients.

5. How common is neuraxis dissemination at the time of diagnosis of malignant tumors in children?

Reports of neuraxis dissemination at diagnosis range between 10 and 46% of children with primary CNS tumors. Such spread is most common in children with medulloblastoma, other malignant embryonal tumors (cerebral primitive neuroectodermal tumor [PNET] and pineoblastoma), and malignant gliomas (such as anaplastic astrocytoma or glioblastoma multiforme), as well as in children under 5 years of age at diagnosis. Recently, neuraxis spread of low-grade gliomas has been increasingly documented. Leptomeningeal involvement may be determined by obtaining cerebrospinal fluid (CSF) cytology (cytocentrifuge examination of the spinal fluid). Neuraxis "drop metastases" may be diagnosed by gadolinium-enhanced magnetic resonance imaging (MRI) of the neuraxis to include sagittal and axial views and/or myelography.

6. What is the most common malignant brain tumor in children and at what age does it usually occur?

Medulloblastoma (considered to be synonymous with PNET) is the most common malignant brain tumor in children. Medulloblastoma (MB) or PNET usually occurs within the first decade of life, with a peak incidence between 5 and 10 years of age and a 1.7 to 2.2 male to female ratio. Such tumors commonly arise in the posterior fossa in the midline cerebellar vermis with variable extension into the fourth ventricle. MB or PNET, therefore, usually causes brain stem or cerebellar dysfunction and is often associated with blockage of the fourth ventricle and hydrocephalus. Affected children typically present with symptoms of increased intracranial pressure, including vomiting, lethargy, and morning headaches. They also may have unsteadiness of gait and diplopia. If the tumor occurs under the age of 1 year, the clinical presentation may be different and consist of increasing lethargy and head size.

7. What outcome of treatment for children with MB or PNET can currently be expected?

"Favorable" MB or PNET is considered grossly resected tumor without neuraxis dissemination. Standard radiation therapy (5400 cGy to the posterior fossa tumor bed and 3600 cGy to the remaining neuraxis) yields a greater than 70% 5-year disease-free survival (DFS).

"Unfavorable" tumors have neuraxis dissemination at the time of diagnosis. Other adverse factors, although probably less important, are residual tumor size > 1.5 cm^2 after resection and age < 4 years.

Prognostic Factors in Children with MB or PNET

	FAVORABLE	UNFAVORABLE
Extent of disease	Nondisseminated	Disseminated
Residual tumor (radiographic)	< 1.5 cm^2	> 1.5 cm^2
Age	> 4 years	< 4 years

It is clear that patients with metastatic disease at diagnosis have an improved outcome with the addition of chemotherapy. Treatment that incorporates radiotherapy, however, especially in a young child, often results in significant neurologic, endocrinologic, and intellectual sequelae.

8. What other posterior fossa/brain stem tumors occur in childhood?

Brain stem gliomas represent the third most common posterior fossa tumor of childhood and occur most frequently between the ages of 5 and 10 years. Most are diffuse pontine in type. Although more aggressive approaches to treatment are being investigated, mean survival for diffuse pontine remains < 1 year, with < 5% 3-year survival. Children with brain stem gliomas that are exophytic, midbrain, or medullary have a better prognosis.

Ependymomas are the least common posterior fossa neoplasm and represent 8–10% of CNS tumors of childhood. Over one-half of such tumors occur in children < 3 years of age. About 70% of them arise from ependyma of the fourth ventricle and grow to fill that ventricle. Using microsurgical techniques, gross total resection can be accomplished in 30–40% of children. Good prognostic factors correlating with an 80–85% 5-year relapse-free survival (RFS) are gross total resection, no evidence of leptomeningeal dissemination, and age > 2–3 years. Less favorable prognostic factors associated with < 40% 5-year RFS are subtotal surgical resection, leptomeningeal dissemination, and age < 2–3 years.

Choroid plexus tumors are amongst the most common posterior fossa tumors in the first year of life.

9. Do the clinical presentations of the various childhood posterior fossa/ brain stem tumors vary?

Children with MB usually have symptoms of relatively short duration; the majority of patients are symptomatic for less than 4 months prior to diagnosis. Ependymomas of the posterior fossa are most likely to mimic MB in their clinical presentation. However, symptoms caused by ependymomas tend to be present for a longer period of time (6–12 months), and cranial nerve palsies tend to be more frequent with ependymomas. Cerebellar astrocytomas tend to present with limb ataxia and nonspecific unsteadiness. Symptoms may be present for up to 2 years before diagnosis, although they are more commonly present 6–12 months.

10. What imaging studies are useful in diagnosing brain tumors in children?

In infants whose fontanelle has not closed, head sonography through the fontanelle is a useful screening study. Supratentorial tumors are usually well visualized by computed tomography (CT) scan of the head with and without contrast, but MRI may be preferred by the neurosurgeon for surgical planning. Posterior fossa tumors are best imaged by a gadolinium-enhanced MRI scan. Consideration should be given to imaging the spine preoperatively if MB is suspected; CT scanning may miss pineal and brain stem tumors. Neuraxis "drop metastases" may be diagnosed by gadolinium-enhanced MRI scan. Increasingly widely available imaging techniques are position emission tomography (PET) and single position emission computed tomography (SPECT) scanning. PET scanning may help distinguish necrosis due to radiation or chemotherapy (hypometabolic) from recurrent tumor (hypermetabolic). Thallium SPECT scanning has been helpful in the evaluation of recurrent neoplasm in adults. MR spectroscopy shows potential and is currently undergoing clinical trials.

11. Describe the new approaches available for the management of LGA of childhood.

In the past, LGAs of childhood were treated with excision of as much tumor as possible and irradiation of visible residual tumor. More recently, it became apparent that children with cerebellar astrocytomas may do very well even with incomplete excision of their tumors and no irradiation. The growth of certain infiltrative LGA may arrest, in some cases spontaneously, and in other cases after subtotal excision. Management of axial LGA presents a particular challenge, and for many decades, extreme conservatism dominated the neurosurgical attitude toward these tumors. In recent years, many technologic advances have greatly increased the safety of an open surgical approach to such midline tumors. Long-term follow-up has confirmed the efficacy of vincristine and carboplatin in LGA. The use of these agents may prove to be of particular value in the treatment of young children, in whom it is advisable to delay irradiation to the brain as long as possible or omit it altogether. Follow-up studies with extensive morbidity data are needed to assess the relative places of chemotherapy, radiotherapy, and aggressive surgery in LGA.

12. When should radiotherapy be used to treat residual LGA in children?

Radiotherapy should be restricted to patients with LGA who are > 5 years of age, who can be treated only by biopsy, who have tumors that show evidence of progressive growth despite resection or tumors that are significantly interfering with either visual or neurologic function. As evidence of the efficacy of certain chemotherapeutic agents for such tumors mounts, it may become advisable to offer an initial trial of chemotherapy in an effort to further delay or omit radiotherapy.

13. What is the current approach to the management of high-grade gliomas in children?

If a child is suspected of having a high-grade glioma, high-dose dexamethasone (Decadron) should be given preoperatively. It is vital to restrict intravenous fluids before the operation. Complete surgical resection combined with other therapies may mean possible long-term survival to a minority of children. The prognosis of incompletely resected high-grade astrocytomas is so poor that second-look surgery should be considered. Postoperative radiation is indicated. The use of chemotherapy, including high-dose therapy with rescue, is currently being explored in national trials.

14. Does the dose of dexamethasone affect the symptomatic management of patients with brain tumors?

Clinical experience with dexamethasone indicates that dose dependency exists in patients with brain tumors. Occasionally, patients deteriorate neurologically or functionally while steroid dose is being tapered. A temporary boost in dosage followed by a slower taper usually reverses this pattern. The side-effects of prolonged dexamethasone are both mentally and physically severe: all efforts must be made to wean the child from steroids.

15. Discuss the specific neurosurgical technologic advances that have occurred in recent years.

Advances include the magnification and illumination of the operating microscope, the gentleness of the ultrasonic tissue aspirator and CO_2 laser, and the accuracy of computerized stereotactic resection. Various computerized intraoperative guidance systems, such as the Viewing Wand (ISG Technologies, Toronto) and a jointed robotic position-sensing arm, are now available. These systems enable precise resection of a radiographically identified abnormality with sparing of normal brain.

16. What new techniques are available for more precise delivery of local treatment to children with brain tumors?

With advances in computer technology and treatment planning, it is now possible to treat the tumor and surrounding brain while sparing distant brain from unnecessary radiotherapy (RT). Three-dimensional conformal RT, a new method for delivering RT precisely to gliomas and other tumors, is currently undergoing trials. The technique involves shaping the isodose surface of an RT plane to conform to the tumor's three-dimensional anatomic boundaries. Its advantages include the following:

1. Minimizing RT exposure of surrounding healthy tissue (i.e., 30–50% reduction in amount of surrounding tissue irradiated).

2. Safely delivering higher-dose RT to the tumor than was previously possible.

3. Ability to reirradiate a tumor at recurrence.

Following standard RT, stereotactic radiosurgery (SRS), stereotactic fractionated radiotherapy (SFR), or brachytherapy (BT) may be used to boost the total tumor dose. The roles of SRS, SFR, and BT in the therapy of children still have to be defined.

BIBLIOGRAPHY

1. Ater JL, Moore BD 3rd, Francis DJ, et al: Correlation of medical and neurosurgical events with neuropsychological status in children at diagnosis of astrocytoma: Utilization of a neurological severity score. J Child Neurol 11:462–469, 1996.
2. Bouffet E, Perilongo G, Canete A, et al: Intracranial ependymomas in children: A critical review of prognostic factors and a plea for cooperation. Med Pediatr Oncol 30:319–329, 1998.
3. Comi AM, Backstrom JW, Burger PC, et al: Clinical and neuroradiologic findings in infants with intracranial ependymomas. Pediatric Oncology Group. Pediatr Neurol 18:23–29, 1998.
4. Duffner PK, Krischer JP, Burger PC, et al: Treatment of infants with malignant gliomas: The Pediatric Oncology Group experience. J Neurooncol 28:245–256, 1996.
5. Duffner PK, Horowitz ME, Krischer JP, et al: Postoperative chemotherapy and delayed radiation in children less than three years of age with malignant brain tumors. N Engl J Med 328:1725–1731, 1993.
6. Dunkel IJ, Garvin JH Jr, Goldman S, et al: High dose chemotherapy with autologous bone marrow rescue for children with diffuse pontine brain stem tumors: A report of the Children's Cancer Group. J Neurooncol 37:67–73, 1998.
7. Finlay JL, Boyett JM, Yates AJ, et al: Randomized phase III trial in childhood high-grade astrocytoma comparing vincristine, lomustine, and prednisone with the eight-drugs-in-1-day regimen: A report of the Children's Cancer Group. J Clin Oncol 13:112–123, 1995.
8. Foreman NK, Love S, Thorne R: Intracranial ependymomas: Analysis of prognostic factors in a population-based series. Pediatr Neurosurg 24:119–125, 1996.
9. Gajjar A, Sanford RA, Heideman R, et al: Low-grade astrocytoma: A decade of experience at St. Jude Children's Research Hospital. J Clin Oncol 15:2792–2799, 1997.
10. Kaplan AM, Albright AL, Zimmerman RA, et al: Brain stem gliomas in children: A Children's Cancer Group review of 119 cases. Pediatr Neurosurg 24:185–192, 1996.
11. Mulhern RK, Kepner JL, Thomas PR, et al: Neuropsychologic functioning of survivors of childhood medulloblastoma randomized to receive conventional or reduced-dose craniospinal radiation: A Pediatric Oncology Group study. J Clin Oncol 16:1723–1728, 1998.
12. Packer RJ, Ater J, Allen J, et al: Carboplatin and vincristine chemotherapy for children with newly diagnosed progressive low-grade gliomas. J Neurooncol 6:747–754, 1997.
13. Reddy AT, Packer RJ: Pediatric central nervous system tumors. Curr Opin Oncol: 10:186–193, 1998.
14. Robertson PL, Zeltzer PM, Boyett JM, et al: Survival and prognostic factors following radiation therapy and chemotherapy for ependymomas in children: A report of the Children's Cancer Group. J Neurosurg 88:695–703, 1998.
15. Wisoff JH, Boyett JM, Berger MS, et al: Current neurosurgical management of the extent of resection in the treatment of malignant gliomas of childhood: A report of the Children's Cancer Group trial no. CCG-945. J Neurosurg 89:52–59, 1998.

VII. HIV-Related Diseases

86. AIDS-ASSOCIATED NON-HODGKIN'S LYMPHOMAS

Jill Lacy, M.D.

1. What is the incidence of non-Hodgkin's lymphoma (NHL) in patients with acquired immunodeficiency syndrome (AIDS)?

The exact incidence of NHL in human immunodeficiency virus (HIV)-infected patients is uncertain. Among a cohort of 55 patients followed at the National Cancer Institute since 1985, 14.5% have developed lymphoma. Other studies place the incidence at 2–5%. The incidence of NHL in HIV-infected patients is apparently increasing in part because of longer survival made possible by antiretroviral agents and improved treatment and prophylaxis of opportunistic infections.

2. Which patients with HIV infection are at risk for developing NHL?

In contrast to Kaposi's sarcoma, which is seen almost exclusively in homosexual males, AIDS-associated NHL is encountered in all HIV risk groups. Virtually any patient with HIV infection is at risk for the development of NHL, including asymptomatic patients as well as those with overt AIDS. However, the risk increases sharply as the CD4 count falls below 50/mm^3, indicating that the severity of immunodeficiency is a key risk factor.

3. Describe the clinical features of AIDS-associated NHL.

It is a biologically aggressive tumor, and patients typically present with advanced-stage disease. Involvement of extranodal sites is common (> 75% of patients). Although the most frequent extranodal sites of involvement are bone marrow, liver, brain, leptomeninges, and gastrointestinal (GI) tract, virtually any site can be involved (e.g., myocardium, urethra, common bile duct). "B" symptoms (fevers, night sweats, weight loss) occur in about 50% of patients.

4. Are AIDS-associated lymphomas usually T- or B-cell lymphomas?

Virtually all are B-cell tumors.

5. Describe the pathologic subtypes of NHL associated with AIDS.

AIDS-associated NHLs are invariably intermediate- or high-grade lesions and fall into one of three diffuse aggressive histologic subtypes in the NCI Working Formulation:

1. Burkitt-like small noncleaved cell (high grade)
2. Immunoblastic sarcoma (high grade)
3. Diffuse large cell (intermediate grade)

6. Which human herpesvirus is implicated in the etiology of AIDS-associated NHL?

Epstein-Barr virus (EBV). EBV is present in at least one-half of AIDS-associated NHLs; tumor cells carry EBV DNA and express viral proteins. Of interest, all of the primary central nervous system (CNS) lymphomas encountered in patients with AIDS are EBV-positive. Recently, the Kaposi's sarcoma-associated herpesvirus (KSHV) has been identified in AIDS-associated lymphomas that involve serosal surfaces (so-called body cavity-based lymphomas).

7. What characteristic cytogenetic abnormality occurs in about one-half of AIDS-associated NHLs?

The t(8;14) chromosomal translocation that juxtaposes the heavy chain immunoglobulin locus with the *c-myc* oncogene.

8. What is the overall prognosis of patients with AIDS-associated NHL?

Most patients with AIDS-associated NHL have a poor prognosis, with an overall median survival in the range of 4–7 months. The two major causes of death are opportunistic infection (50–70%) and progressive lymphoma (30–50%).

9. What is the single most important prognostic factor for survival in AIDS-associated NHL?

CD4 count. Patients with CD4 counts > 100 have a median survival of 24 months vs. 2–4 months for CD4 counts < 100. Of importance, about one-half of patients with AIDS-associated NHL have a CD4 count > 100 at presentation. Additional poor prognostic factors include prior AIDS-defining illness, prior opportunistic infections, and poor performance status.

10. Describe the appropriate staging evaluation in patients diagnosed with AIDS-associated NHL.

The staging evaluation in patients with AIDS-associated NHL is similar to the evaluation performed in immunocompetent patients with lymphoma and includes the following: careful history and physical examination with special attention to GI and CNS signs and symptoms; chest radiograph or chest computed tomographic (CT) scan; abdominal and pelvic CT scan; and bone marrow biopsy. In addition, because of the high incidence of leptomeningeal disease, a lumbar puncture should be performed routinely. The presence of GI symptoms or heme-positive stools may indicate lymphomatous involvement of the GI tract, necessitating an upper GI series or endoscopy. A CT scan or MRI of the brain should be performed in any patient with cognitive changes or focal neurologic signs. In addition to the staging evaluation, patients with fever should be thoroughly evaluated for concurrent opportunistic infections. If identified, such infections should be treated before initiation of chemotherapy.

11. Multidrug chemotherapy is highly effective treatment for intermediate- and high-grade NHLs in immunocompetent patients. What is the role of chemotherapy in AIDS-associated NHL?

If untreated, AIDS-associated NHLs are rapidly fatal. Thus, most patients should be treated with cytotoxic drugs. The standard multidrug chemotherapy regimens that are effective in the treatment of intermediate- and high-grade NHL in immunocompetent patients (e.g., cyclophosphamide, doxorubicin, vincristine, and prednisone [CHOP] or methotrexate, bleomycin, doxorubicin, cyclophosphamide, vincristine, and dexamethasone [M-BACOD]) are also highly effective in the treatment of AIDS-associated NHL. Of importance, most patients derive significant palliation from the administration of multidrug chemotherapy. Response rates are about 50–70%, and 30–50% of patients achieve complete remission. However, relapses are common and occur early (25–50% of complete responders relapse within 6 months of completing therapy), and overall median survival is short (4–7 months). About 15% of patients have a durable remission (> 2 years).

12. What are some of the reasons for the poor outcome of chemotherapy in the treatment of AIDS-associated NHL compared with NHL in immunocompetent patients?

1. Death due to nonneoplastic complications of AIDS (e.g., opportunistic infections, wasting syndrome)

2. Inability to administer full doses of chemotherapy drugs on schedule because of impaired hematologic reserve and intercurrent opportunistic infections

3. Advanced stage of disease at presentation

13. Explain the role of colony-stimulating factors in the management of AIDS-associated NHLs.

Severe and prolonged neutropenia is a frequent complication of chemotherapy in patients with AIDS. The use of colony-stimulating factors (granulocyte CSF or granulocyte-macrophage CSF) reduces both severity and duration of neutropenia and its associated infectious sequelae. In addition, the administration of full doses of chemotherapy is often possible when the CSFs are used.

14. Should patients with AIDS-associated NHL receive standard or reduced doses of cytotoxic drugs used in the treatment of NHL in immunocompetent patients?

A recent cooperative group study demonstrated that the response rate and overall survival with a dose-reduced chemotherapy regimen (low-dose M-BACOD) were equivalent to the standard full-dose regimen with less toxicity. This study suggests that reductions in doses of the marrow-suppressive drugs do not appear to affect outcome adversely in patients with AIDS-related lymphomas.

15. Should patients continue antiretroviral therapy while receiving chemotherapy?

The widely used antiretroviral agent azidothymidine (AZT) is marrow-suppressive and markedly enhances the marrow toxicity of cytotoxic drugs. Thus, AZT should not be administered routinely to patients who are receiving chemotherapy. Non–marrow-suppressive antiretrovirals can be administered with chemotherapy, although careful attention to additive toxicities (e.g., peripheral neuropathy from ddI and vincristine) is important.

16. Should patients routinely receive *Pneumocystis carinii* prophylaxis while on systemic chemotherapy?

Yes. Patients should receive *P. carinii* prophylaxis regardless of CD4 counts because standard cytotoxic agents and prednisone are likely to cause further immunosuppression.

17. What is the role of intrathecal chemotherapy in the management of AIDS-associated NHL?

Given the propensity for AIDS-associated NHL to involve the leptomeninges, it is common practice to administer prophylactic intrathecal chemotherapy with either cytosine arabinoside (ara-C) or methotrexate weekly or biweekly for 4–6 doses. Patients with overt involvement of the leptomeninges at presentation (i.e., positive CSF cytology) should receive a more prolonged course of intrathecal chemotherapy as well as whole-brain irradiation.

18. Describe the clinical features of primary CNS lymphoma in patients with AIDS.

Patients present with lymphomatous involvement of the brain with or without leptomeningeal involvement and without overt systemic lymphoma. They are usually profoundly immunocompromised with low CD4 counts, and their prognosis is extremely poor (median survival: < 2 months). The most common presentation is cognitive changes that can be confused with AIDS-related dementia. Other presenting signs and symptoms include focal neurologic signs, seizures, and cranial nerve palsies.

19. What difficulties are encountered in the diagnosis of AIDS-associated primary CNS lymphoma?

The diagnosis of AIDS-associated NHL is often problematic because standard radiographic evaluation (brain CT scan or MRI) cannot reliably distinguish the mass lesion(s) of lymphoma from toxoplasmosis or, on occasion, progressive multifocal leukoencephalopathy. A reasonable approach to the patient with a mass lesion and HIV infection is to check toxoplasmosis titers. If the titers are positive, the patient is treated for toxoplasmosis; if there is no improvement clinically and radiographically after 1 week of therapy, a brain biopsy is performed. If toxoplasmosis titers are negative, a stereotactic brain biopsy should be performed immediately. Recently, thallium-210 single-photon emission CT imaging of the brain and polymerase chain reaction-based analysis of cerebrospinal fluid for the presence of EBV have proved helpful in the noninvasive diagnosis of primary CNS lymphoma in patients with AIDS.

20. How is AIDS-associated primary CNS lymphoma treated?

Whole-brain radiation therapy with dexamethasone (Decadron). Most patients experience improvement in symptoms with radiation therapy, and about one-half achieve complete radiographic remission. Nonetheless, survival remains poor; opportunistic infections are a major cause of death. Systemic chemotherapy is not routinely recommended.

BIBLIOGRAPHY

 1. Antinori A, Ammassari A, DeLuca A, et al: Diagnosis of AIDS-related focal brain lesions: A decision-making analysis based on clinical and neuroradiologic characteristics combined with polymerase chain reaction assays in CSF. Neurology 48:687–694, 1997.
 2. Ballerini P, Gaidano C, Gong JZ, et al: Multiple genetic lesions in acquired immunodeficiency syndrome-related non-Hodgkin's lymphoma. Blood 81:166–167, 1993.
 3. Baumgartner JE, Rachlin JR, Beckstead JH, et al: Primary central nervous system lymphomas: Natural history and response to radiation therapy in 55 patients with acquired immunodeficiency syndrome. J Neurosurg 73:206–211, 1990.
 4. Beral V, Peterman T, Berkelman R, Jaffe H: AIDS-associated non-Hodgkin's lymphoma. Lancet 337:805–809, 1991.
 5. Cesarman E, Chang Y, Moore PS, et al: Kaposi's sarcoma-associated herpesvirus-like DNA sequences in AIDS-related body-cavity-based lymphomas. N Engl J Med 332:1186–1191, 1995.
 6. Gill PS, Levine AM, Meyer PR, et al: Primary central nervous system lymphoma in homosexual men: Clinical, immunologic, and pathologic features. Am J Med 78:742–748, 1985.
 7. Hamilton-Dutoit SJ, Raphael M, Audouin J, et al: In situ demonstration of Epstein-Barr virus small RNAs (EBER 1) in acquired immunodeficiency syndrome-related lymphomas: Correlation with tumor morphology and primary site. Blood 82:619–624, 1993.
 8. Kaplan LD, Abrams DI, Feigal E, et al: AIDS-associated non-Hodgkin's lymphoma in San Francisco. JAMA 261:719–724, 1989.
 9. Kaplan LD, Kahn JO, Crowe S, et al: Clinical and virologic effects of recombinant human granulocyte-macrophage colony stimulating factor in patients receiving chemotherapy for human immunodeficiency virus-associated non-Hodgkin's lymphoma. Results of a randomized trial. J Clin Oncol 9:929–940, 1991.
10. Kaplan LD, Straus DJ, Testa MA, et al: Low dose compared with standard-dose m-BACOD chemotherapy for non-Hodgkin's lymphoma associated with human immunodeficiency virus infection. National Institute of Allergy and infectious Diseases AIDS Clinical Trials Group. N Engl J Med 336:1641–1648, 1997.
11. Levine AM: Acquired immunodeficiency syndrome-related lymphoma. Blood 80:8–20, 1992.
12. Levine AM, Wernz JC, Kaplan L, et al: Low-dose chemotherapy with central nervous system prophylaxis and zidovudine maintenance in AIDS-related lymphoma. JAMA 266:84–88, 1991.
13. MacMahon EME, Glass JD, Hayward SD, et al: Epstein-Barr virus in AIDS-related primary central nervous system lymphoma. Lancet 338:969–973, 1991.
14. Pluda JM, Venzon DJ, Tosata G, et al: Parameters affecting the development of non-Hodgkin's lymphoma in patients with severe human immunodeficiency virus infection receiving antiretroviral therapy. J Clin Oncol 11:1099–1107, 1993.
15. Sandler AS, Kaplan DL: Diagnosis and management of systemic non-Hodgkin's lymphoma in HIV disease. Hematol Oncol Clin North Am 10:1111–1124, 1996.

87. KAPOSI'S SARCOMA

George R. Simon, M.D., Madeleine A. Kane, M.D., Ph.D., and Adam M. Myers, M.D., FACP

1. What is Kaposi's sarcoma (KS)?

KS is a dermal malignancy that is multifocal in origin. Lesions may be flat or raised and are typically of purplish color. Histopathologically, lesions are composed of spindle cells and vascular structures with lymphocyte, macrophage and plasma cell infiltration. Fibrosis is variably present.

2. Who gets KS?

The following populations are at risk for KS:

1. Elderly men of eastern European or Mediterranean descent (classic KS)
2. Equatorial Africa (endemic KS)
3. Organ transplant recipients (400–500 fold increased risk)
4. People with HIV infection (epidemic KS). This variety of KS has been seen since the AIDS epidemic began, and its biologic activity is significantly more aggressive. It remains the most common malignancy associated with HIV infection, occurring in approximately 9% of gay or bisexual men. The incidence of KS is declining, perhaps in part as a result of adherence to safe sex practices and the diminished risk for contracting sexually transmitted diseases (i.e., herpes virus infection).

3. Is KS seen in all people with AIDS?

KS is rarely seen in people who contract AIDS as a result of blood product transfusion (e.g., hemophiliacs). It is also significantly less common in women who have AIDS as a result of heterosexual contact or intravenous drug use (IDU). Ninety percent of cases of KS occur in homosexual or bisexual men.

4. What is the cause of KS?

Recent epidemiologic data suggest that a novel human herpes virus (KSHV or HHV-8), a member of the gamma herpes family of viruses, may be etiologically linked to the development of KS. Genomic DNA from KSHV is found in KS tissues and in the peripheral blood and semen of patients with KS. KSHV DNA was also detected in the peripheral blood of HIV-infected high-risk gay or bisexual men without KS as well as in classical and endemic cases.

5. What is the pathogenesis of KS?

Although experimental details remain to be worked out, a model of KS pathogenesis is emerging. This model involves infection with KSHV, leading to alterations in levels of cytokines (e.g., interleukin [IL]-1, tumor necrosis factor-α [TNF], IL-6, oncostatin-M) and abnormal modulation of growth by HIV Tat. These factors predispose to malignant transformation and development of KS. If KSHV is cotransmitted with HIV via certain routes (such as oral-genital and anal sex) but not others (such as blood transfusions), this cotransmission may explain why HIV-infected homosexual and bisexual men are specifically affected.

6. How is KS diagnosed?

Traditionally, cancer lesions should be confirmed by biopsy. However, biopsy of lesions for KS is not uniformly necessary, although it is sometimes done to confirm the clinical impression. Kaposi's lesions, when characteristic and multiple, are hard to confuse with other processes. For example, an experienced bronchoscopist can note typical KS lesions in the endobronchial tree without biopsy. The vascular nature of lesions may result in significant hemorrhage if the lesions are biopsied. Single cutaneous lesions may be misidentified and should be biopsied. In one case, for example, *Pneumocystis carinii* involvement of the skin was mistaken for KS.

7. How is the response of treatment for KS evaluated?

It is important to document the extent of KS carefully before initiation of therapy. Standard body diagrams are useful for recording lesions. Lesions should be described in terms of color, whether they are raised or ulcerated, and whether they are associated with edema and halos. A yellow halo around a lesion is the result of heme products leaking from lesions and may indicate active growth. Usually 3–5 lesions are chosen to monitor as target lesions with bidimensional measurements. Polaroid photographs also can be taken to document the appearance of lesions before therapy.

8. How does KS behave? Does it truly metastasize?

KS is thought to be a multicentric disease. However, metastases do occur, especially to visceral organs. Epidemic KS has been reported to involve, at one time or the other, almost every organ site, but skin, oral mucosa, gastrointestinal tract, and lungs are most commonly involved. The central nervous system is generally spared.

9. How do you determine the extent of KS involvement?

It is important to document the extent of KS so that responses to treatment can be assessed. It is reasonable to estimate the number of KS lesions as none, 1–10, >10 but < 50, or > 50 rather than to attempt an exact count that would be hard to duplicate on subsequent visits. A thorough physical examination is essential, including examination of the gingiva and mouth. The presence of gingival and palatal lesion is associated with a greater risk for mucosal lesions at sites such as the GI tract and respiratory tree. Aside from a chest radiograph and routine laboratory tests, including determination of the CD4+ cell count and viral loads, more extensive and invasive studies are not routinely justified. An evaluation of the patient's immune status by performing a CD4+ cell count and assessing viral burden at time of diagnosis of KS is generally recommended because it can influence therapeutic decisions.

10. How should information be organized to make it more meaningful?

Several staging systems have been proposed. The following system helps to characterize a patient's disease and to guide decisions about therapy. Tumor extent and location, immune status (CD4 cell count and viral burden), and presence or absence of symptoms have therapeutic implications.

	Good Risk (All of the Following)	Poor Risk (Any of the Following)
Tumor (T)	Confined to skin and/or nodes Minimal oral disease (nonnodular) KS confined to palate	Tumor-associated edema or ulceration Extensive oral KS (nodular) KS in visceral sites
Immune system (I)	CD4 cells > 200/ml	CD4 cells < 200/ml
Systemic factors	No history of opportunistic infections or thrush No "B" symptoms* Karnofsky Performance Status > 70	History of opportunistic infections and/or thrush "B" symptoms present Karnofsky Performance Status < 70 Other HIV-related illnesses (e.g., neurologic disease, lymphoma)

* "B" symptoms are unexplained fever, night sweats, more than 10% involuntary weight loss, or diarrhea persisting more than 2 weeks.

11. What are the complications of KS?

KS is commonly asymptomatic. However, cutaneous lesions may be associated with mild-to-moderately severe edema, especially if the lesions are confluent or located in the lower extremities or periorbitally. Patients with marked edema often are found to have lymph node involvement by KS. Lesions that are protuberant or ulcerative in the mouth or gingiva can severely compromise oral intake and worsen the patient's nutritional status. Visceral KS is associated with the greatest morbidity. Diffuse involvement of the gastrointestinal tract or lungs may cause significant pain, dysphagia, and diarrhea or dyspnea and hypoxemia, respectively. Although a morbid complication of AIDS, KS is not commonly the primary cause of death.

12. How is KS treated?

It is best to categorize treatment as either local or systemic. Isolated asymptomatic lesions need not be treated. Lesions may be observed after triple antiretroviral therapy is initiated. No known therapies are considered to be curative. Treatment is palliative. It is difficult to palliate an asymptomatic patient, especially when therapies have potentially significant toxicities. In addition, regression of cutaneous or mucosal KS lesions may be seen after the initiation of highly active antiretroviral therapy (HAART) with three-drug combinations that contain a protease inhibitor.

13. What local treatments are available for KS?

Local therapies used to treat KS include radiation therapy, cryotherapy (with liquid nitrogen), injection of lesions with a dilute solution of an antineoplastic agent (i.e., vinblastine), or painting with dinitrochlorbenzene (DNCB) in sensitized patients. Topical retinoids and intralesional injections of interferon alpha (IFNα) are also options. Except for radiotherapy, these treatments should not be used on facial lesions or lesions on the soles of the feet. With topical therapies, lesions are treated weekly until an appropriate inflammatory reaction develops; then the patient is observed to assess the status of the lesions when the inflammation resolves. This approach should be used only for light-skinned people. Intralesional injections are done every 2 weeks for up to a total of 3 injections. Painful gingival lesions may be injected with 3% sodium tetradecyl sulfate solution.

Probably the most effective local treatment is radiotherapy. Typically, radiotherapy is used to treat confluent areas of disease, painful single geographic sites, and severely ulcerated or edematous lesions or to facilitate effective cosmetic control. Radiotherapy usually results in reduction of pain and/or swelling and often leads to flattening and fading of lesions. Lesions rarely disappear completely.

14. Discuss systemic therapies for KS.

Systemic therapies include IFNα and various chemotherapeutic agents. Asymptomatic patients with CD4+ cells ≥ 200 cells/μl are good candidates for INFα, usually in conjunction with HAART. Patients who have had AIDS-related opportunistic infections or KS-related "B" symptoms are generally not candidates for therapy with INFα.

Poor-risk patients (CD4+ cells < 200 cells/μl) should be considered for systemic therapy with antineoplastic agents. The single most effective systemic agent against KS is the antimicrotubule agent paclitaxel (Taxol). Partial responses of 65% are seen when paclitaxel is used in a dose of 135 mg/m^2 over 3 hours every 3 weeks. Similar results with paclitaxel were reported with lower doses of 100 mg/m^2 or less over 3 hours every 2 weeks. Liposomal preparations of anthracyclines, such as doxorubicin or daunorubicin, are other effective modalities. These drugs are nearly as effective as paclitaxel and, like paclitaxel, can be used as first-line systemic therapy. Other antineoplastic agents, such as vincristine, vinblastine, bleomycin, doxorubicin, and VP-16, may be used singly or in combination. VP-16 has the added advantage of oral administration. Combination chemotherapy with doxorubicin, bleomycin, and vincristine (ABV) was considered the most effective systemic therapy until the advent of paclitaxel and the liposomal formulated anthracyclines. ABV is quite toxic and often poorly tolerated. Therapy with less toxic single agents, such as bleomycin with or without vincristine, affords reasonable palliation. Patients' quality of life is improved by liposomal anthracycline therapy compared with ABV. Nausea, vomiting, alopecia, and treatment-related neuropathy are reduced.

Whether or not to treat with systemic therapy is often a difficult decision. Patients may have asymptomatic KS lesions and yet have other clinical conditions associated with AIDS that cause significant morbidity. In this situation, antineoplastic chemotherapy may actually increase the risk for opportunistic infections or worsen coexistent conditions by further depressing immunity. Most effective antineoplastic agents are marrow-suppressive; thus, they complicate the use of other myelosuppressive agents such as azidothymidine (AZT), sulfamethoxazole-trimethoprim, or ganciclovir. Close observation without therapy may be appropriate; therapy should be initiated if KS-related symptoms develop and/or a more aggressive tumor biology ensues (e.g., rapid increase in size and/or number of lesions and/or development of visceral KS).

15. Do KS lesions sometimes regress spontaneously?

KS may wax and wane in its appearance, particularly in patients whose immune function is relatively preserved (CD4 count > 400 cells/μl). This clearly supports the contention that KS behaves like an opportunistic malignancy in immunocompromised patients. Perhaps the most dramatic example of KS regression is seen in patients who are given immunosuppressive therapy to enable engraftment of a transplanted organ. In this situation, if immunosuppressive therapy is discontinued or reduced, KS often spontaneously regresses.

16. What newer and innovative anti-KS therapies are under development?

Angiogenesis is critical for KS development. Various antiangiogenic agents are undergoing clinical evaluation (e.g., thalidomide, TNP 470, flavoperidol, endoglin). The prototypic antiangiogenic agent is IFNα. Other cytokines such as INFδ and IL-12 are also under evaluation.

Several lines of evidence support the contention that both viral and host cytokines play pivotal roles in the emergence and perpetuation of AIDS-KS. Tat, the protein product of the HIV transactivating gene *tat*, promotes the growth of AIDS-KS from normal vascular cells, especially if the normal vascular cells have been primed by inflammatory cytokines such as fibroblast growth factors (FGFs). Novel gene therapy strategies against these molecules are under evaluation. Antisense oligonucleotides directed against tat mRNA and FGFs are in preclinical phases of development.

Intralesional injection of human chorionic gonadotropin (HCG) has also led to the regression of lesions. This treatment is based on the observation that pregnant mice are resistant to the establishment and dissemination of KS lesions, an effect postulated to be due to the high levels of CG associated with pregnancy. Studies are currently under way to evaluate the systemic use of HCG.

BIBLIOGRAPHY

1. Chang Y, Cesarman E, Pessin MS, et al: Identification of herpesvirus-like DNA sequences in AIDS-associated Kaposi's sarcoma. Science 266:1865, 1994.
2. Gallo RC: Some aspects of the pathogenesis of HIV-1-associated Kaposi's sarcoma. J Natl Cancer Inst (23):55–57, 1998.
3. Gill PS, Espina BM, Muggia F, et al: Phase I/II clinical and pharmacokinetic evaluation of liposomal daunorubicin. J Clin Oncol 13:996–1003, 1995.
4. Karp JE, Pluda JM, Yarchoan R: AIDS-related Kaposi's sarcoma. A template for the translation of molecular pathogenesis into targeted therapeutic approaches. Hematol Oncol Clin North Am 10:1031–1049, 1996.
5. Krown SE: Interferon-alpha: Evolving therapy for AIDS-associated Kaposi's sarcoma. J Interferon Cytokine Res 18:209–214, 1998.
6. Krown SE, Metroka C, Weinz JC: Kaposi's sarcoma in the acquired immune deficiency syndrome: A proposal for uniform evaluation response and staging criteria. AIDS Clinical Trials Group Oncology Committee. J Clin Oncol 7: 1201–1207, 1989.
7. Paredes J, Kahn JO, Tong WP, et al: Weekly oral etoposide in patients with Kaposi's sarcoma associated with human immunodeficiency virus infection: A phase I multicenter trial of the AIDS Clinical Trials Group. J Acquir Immune Defic Syndr Hum Retrovirol 9:138–144, 1995.
8. Saville MW, Leitzau J Pluda JM, et al: Treatment of HIV-associated Kaposi's sarcoma with paclitaxel. Lancet 346:26–28, 1995.
9. Stribling J, Weitzner S, Smith GV: Kaposi's sarcoma in renal allograft recipients. Cancer 42:442–446, 1978.

88. HEMATOLOGIC ABNORMALITIES IN HIV INFECTION

George R. Simon, M.D., Miho Toi Scott, M.D.,
Madeleine A. Kane, M.D., Ph.D., and Adam M. Myers, M.D., FACP

ANEMIA

1. How common is anemia in human immunodeficiency virus (HIV) infection?

Anemia is common in HIV infection, and the incidence increases with disease progression. Anemia is seen in 10–20% of patients with asymptomatic HIV infection and in 70–90% of patients with full-blown acquired immunodeficiency syndrome (AIDS), with or without opportunistic infections.

2. What are the causes of anemia in HIV infection?

In HIV infection, all three of the basic mechanisms of anemia may contribute to the development of anemia: (1) decreased production of red cells by bone marrow, (2) increased peripheral destruction of red cells, and (3) blood loss. By direct and indirect mechanisms, HIV induces dysplastic changes in the bone marrow, leading to ineffective hematopoiesis. In HIV-infected people, up to 40% of primitive hematopoietic cells may be eliminated because of the presence of cell surface CD4 and fusin receptors, which are the receptors necessary for a cell to be infectable by HIV. Secondary complications of AIDS, such as malignancies and opportunistic infections, and their treatments also may suppress the bone marrow. Dysregulation of the host immune system with increased autoimmune peripheral destruction of red cells also may be a contributing factor. Splenomegaly may decrease circulating erythrocyte counts by sequestration. Acute and chronic gastrointestinal (GI) blood loss secondary to GI infections and malignancies may contribute to anemia in HIV infection.

3. What peripheral blood smear abnormalities are seen in HIV-associated anemias?

Normocytic normochromic anemia is the predominant type of anemia seen in HIV infection. Macrocytosis may result from treatment with thymidine analogs, such as ziduvidine (AZT) or stavudine (D4T). Protease inhibitors, such as ritonavir, indinavir or nelfinavir, dapsone, and sulfamethoxazole-trimethoprim (used for prophylaxis and treatment of opportunistic infection with *Pneumocystis carinii)*, and chemotherapeutic drugs may contribute to macrocytosis. The reticulocyte count is usually inappropriately normal or low, suggesting depressed erythropoiesis. Frequently, there is evidence of early erythrocyte release from the bone marrow in the form of polychromasia. Enlarged, left-shifted, hyposegmented neutrophils, large vacuolated monocytes, and large granular lymphocytes also may be seen. Thrombocytopenia is common.

4. What are the characteristic bone marrow findings in patients with AIDS?

Even in the presence of peripheral cytopenias the marrow cellularity is characteristically normocellular or hypercellular. Dysplastic changes are common. Erythroid precursors are decreased and frequently dysplastic, and the myeloid-to-erythroid ratio varies from 2:1 to 5:1 (normal ratio = 1:2). Megakaryocytes are either adequate or increased and show dysplastic changes in the form of multiple, small nuclei. Paratrabecular benign atypical lymphoid aggregates are often present. Increased reticulin formation, granulomas, plasma cells, and increased eosinophils are also common. The increased reticulin formation may account for the many "dry taps" when marrow aspirations are performed in patients with AIDS.

5. What do iron studies show in patients with HIV-associated anemia?

The iron profile of HIV-related anemia resembles that of anemia of chronic disease. Hypoferremia with decreased iron reutilization but increased iron stores is typical. Therefore, one sees low serum iron and total iron-binding capacity and an elevated serum ferritin. Iron stores may be especially increased when the patient is transfusion-dependent.

6. What happens to serum B_{12} levels in patients with symptomatic HIV infection?

B_{12} levels are lower than normal in as many as 25% of patients with symptomatic HIV infection. Characteristically, the low B_{12} levels occur in the absence of neutrophilic hypersegmentation, erythrocytosis, macrocytosis, and megaloblastic changes in bone marrow. Treatment with B_{12} usually fails to produce a response. Although this reduction is not usually clinically significant or associated with complications, it may increase the hematologic toxicity of AZT. Conversely, in a subset of profoundly anemic patients, macrocytosis with moderate anisopoikilocytosis may be seen, but such patients do not have low B_{12} or folate levels. Marrow examination shows a hypocellular and dysplastic marrow. Again, B_{12} or folate supplementation does not reverse abnormalities.

7. How often does hemolysis occur in patients with HIV infection?

Although hemolytic anemia is rarely seen, a direct Coombs' test may be positive in up to 20% of patients with advanced HIV infection. The positive test is due to the nonspecific adsorption of immune complexes and polyclonal antibodies to the red cell and, not surprisingly, is often associated with hypergammaglobulinemia. An increase in autoantibodies specific to the red cell is also seen in HIV infection, but it is rarely associated with hemolysis. Hemolysis, when present, is characteristically without an appropriate reticulocyte response, despite the presence of erythroid hyperplasia in the marrow. Up to 30% of HIV-infected patients with autoimmune hemolysis have an associated autoimmune thrombocytopenia (Evan's syndrome).

8. What should you suspect if you see significantly depressed red cell count in the presence of normal or near normal white cell and platelet counts in a patient with AIDS?

Mycobacterium avium complex (MAC) needs to be excluded. This infection is seen in AIDS patients when the CD4 cell counts fall below 100/μl. Parvovirus also may induce anemia or occasionally pancytopenia; it is associated with increased giant pronormoblasts in the bone marrow. Anemia in association with other cytopenias is seen with many conditions that affect the bone marrow, including systemic *pneumocystis carinii* infection, fungal infections, cytomegalovirus (CMV) infection, and non-Hodgkin's lymphoma.

9. How is anemia in HIV infection treated?

Treatment is aimed at the underlying cause and may include antiretroviral agents, treatment of opportunistic infections and malignancies, replacement of deficient nutrients, discontinuance of myelosuppressive medications, and treatment of hemolysis or blood loss. Occasionally, repeated transfusions may be necessary to maintain hematocrit.

10. What is the role of erythropoietin in the treatment of anemia associated with HIV infection?

Erythropoietin (EPO) is a glycoprotein hormone produced by the kidney. EPO levels in blood increase in response to decreasing red cell mass. The increase in EPO in response to anemia may be blunted in HIV infection, particularly in patients taking AZT. Treatment with EPO has been found to be especially useful in patients with endogenous EPO levels less than 500 IU/L. In such patients an increase in red cell mass, a decrease in transfusion requirement, and an improvement in quality of life have been noted. Treatment with EPO is not recommended if the endogenous EPO level is higher than 500 IU/L. In HIV-infected patients with anemia and endogenous EPO levels of less than 500 IU/L, treatment with EPO may be an alternative to blood transfusions or AZT dose reduction. Use of EPO increases the cost of treatment, and the decision to use it must be made after careful consideration. Monitoring of iron levels is recommended during therapy with EPO; iron supplementation may also be needed.

THROMBOCYTOPENIA

11. Define thrombocytopenia (TCP).

TCP is defined as a platelet count of less than 150,000/μl. HIV-infected persons with TCP usually have a moderate presentation with platelet counts ranging between 40,000 and 60,000/μl. Occasionally platelet counts less than 10,000/μl are seen.

12. How common is TCP in HIV infection?

TCP is often seen as an isolated finding in HIV-infected people with a 3–8% incidence. Thirty to 40% of patients with AIDS will have TCP sometime during the course of their illness, often in association with anemia and/or neutropenia. TCP is often seen early in HIV infection, but its occurrence has no prognostic significance and does not predict the onset of AIDS. TCP may occur in any risk group (e.g., homosexual men, intravenous drug users, hemophiliacs). In any person, TCP without apparent cause should raise the suspicion of possible underlying HIV infection. Immune thrombocytopenia (ITP) is the most frequently observed HIV-related condition seen in HIV-positive hemophiliacs. The cumulative 10-year incidence of TCP in HIV-positive hemophiliacs was found to be 43% in adults and 27% in children.

13. What are the mechanisms of TCP in HIV infection?

TCP may result from increased peripheral destruction of platelets, decreased production as a result of depressed bone marrow function, or both.

Increased peripheral destruction of platelets may be mediated by immune mechanisms (ITP), increased splenic sequestration of platelets, or increased peripheral consumption of platelets as in disseminated intravascular coagulation (DIC) and thrombotic thrombocytopenic purpura (TTP).

Decreased production as a result of depressed bone marrow function. Bone marrow function in HIV infection is depressed by various factors, including use of myelotoxic drugs (e.g., sufamethoxazole-trimethoprim, AZT, chemotherapy) and involvement of bone marrow by opportunistic infections and malignancies.

Even in the absence of identifiable secondary causes of marrow suppression, bone marrow function may be perturbed by HIV. Some of these mechanisms are still under investigation, including inhibition of hematopoiesis by gp120/anti-gp120 complexes, infection of CD34+ hematopoietic stem cells, which express CD4+ receptor, and alteration in the cytokine milieu of the bone marrow induced by infection of the stromal cells by HIV. Most commonly, however, isolated TCP occurs in HIV infection through immune mechanisms.

14. How do HIV-infected patients with ITP usually present?

The clinical profile resembles that of ITP in HIV-seronegative patients with the important exception of the common presence of splenomegaly. One-third of HIV-infected patients with ITP present with easy bruising or petechiae. Spontaneous, clinically significant bleeding usually does not occur. Other hematologic abnormalities, such as anemia or neutropenia, are found in up to 60%.

15. When should a bone marrow aspiration and biopsy be performed in the evaluation of a patient with HIV-associated TCP?

A bone marrow aspiration and biopsy may be performed when the cause of TCP is not clear from a detailed history and physical examination, complete blood count, and peripheral smear examination. Often this procedure is performed when a more severe diagnosis than ITP is suspected. Megakaryocytes in the bone marrow may be increased in number and appear dysplastic. Although the bone marrow looks hypercellular in HIV infection, which may suggest increased peripheral destruction, decreased production of peripheral cells is likely because of the ineffective hematopoiesis in such patients. Drug toxicity may be evidenced by increased vacuolation of erythroid precursors and/or marrow hypoplasia.

16. Why is clinically significant bleeding not present in patients with ITP?

ITP is well tolerated in HIV-infected persons. Two factors contribute to the low incidence of significant bleeding. One is the better quality of the platelets in ITP. The circulating platelets are relatively young because of increased production and early release, and young platelets function more efficiently. The relatively larger size of the younger platelets gives rise to the increased mean platelet volume in the peripheral smear. In addition, peripheral destruction of platelets induces the release of platelet factor 3 (PF-3). Increased presence of PF-3 in the plasma induces the intrinsic clotting pathway, which in turn offsets the risk of significant bleeding. In TCP, which is caused by underproduction as a result of suppressed bone marrow (e.g., hypoplasia due to AZT toxicity), more severe bleeding is likely to occur at higher platelet counts.

17. When should ITP be treated in HIV infection?

ITP in HIV infection should be treated if platelet counts are less than 20,000/µl or at any level of platelet count if clinically significant bleeding occurs. In addition, treatment may be indicated if a patient has a low platelet count, especially less than 50,000/µl, if elective or emergency surgery is required. A patient is more likely to bleed if low platelet counts are associated with anemia or fever; if the rate of decrease of platelets was fairly rapid; or if the patient is taking antiplatelet drugs (e.g., aspirin), which render the residual platelets dysfunctional.

18. What drug therapies should be considered in HIV-infected patients with ITP?

Highly active antiretroviral therapy (HAART) should be initiated. HAART consists of three antiretroviral drugs, including a protease inhibitor. Even AZT alone has been found to increase platelet levels within 2 weeks of initiation of therapy.

Intravenous immunoglobulin G (IVIG) is transiently effective in most patients. IVIG can be used when a more immediate response is clinically indicated (i.e., acute hemorrhage), if the platelet counts are critically low, or if elective surgery is planned. The doses commonly used are either 1 gm/kg/day for 1 or 2 days or 400 mg/kg/day for 5 days. The use of IVIG is limited by its transient effects and high cost.

Adrenal glucocorticoids demonstrate a 70–90% response rate. Prednisone, 80 mg/day in divided doses, should begin to raise platelet counts in 3–5 days, but few patients maintain the response when steroids are discontinued. Continuous high-dose steroids should be used cautiously in HIV-infected patients because of the added immunosuppression and increased risk of opportunistic infections.

Danazol is an attenuated androgen with mild virilizing effects and can spare or reduce the use of corticosteroids. Better response rates are seen with the use of danazol in HIV-negative patients with ITP than in HIV-positive patients with ITP, although long-term remissions on danazol are rare even in the HIV-seronegative population. The commonly used dose is 300–800 mg/day. Response is usually seen within 2 months, but it may take up to 6 months if lower doses are used. Although danazol is generally well tolerated, common side effects include fluid retention, persistent nausea, and hepatitis.

Splenectomy induces a response in 75% of cases. This intervention can either convert previously steroid-resistant ITP to steroid-responsive ITP or even permit discontinuation of steroids in previously steroid-responsive patients. Antipneumococcal vaccine should be administered at least 10–14 days before splenectomy.

Alpha-interferon (α-IFN) in low doses (3 million units 3 times weekly) has been tried in a few cases and found to be effective. Because of its antiretroviral action, α-IFN may be of particular use in HIV-infected patients with ITP.

In one study, injected **anti-rhesus antibodies** (anti-Rho(D) immunoglobulin, WinRho SDF) were found to be effective in 9 of 14 RH+(D+) patients. The advantage of this therapy is that it may be administered every 3–4 weeks and is less expensive than IVIG. However, treatment usually must be continued indefinitely.

19. When should patients with ITP be transfused?

An acutely bleeding patient with ITP should be transfused quickly. If the urgency of the situation permits, the platelet transfusion may be given after a dose of IVIG. Prophylactic transfusions are generally not recommended unless the patient has critically low platelet counts ($< 5,000/\mu l$) or has bled previously at a higher platelet count.

20. Does the presence of ITP predict the clinical course of HIV infection?

The presence of ITP is not a prognostic factor in HIV-seropositive people and does not predict the onset of AIDS. However, earlier studies reported that the frequency of ITP was inversely correlated with the CD4 lymphocyte counts. The incidence of ITP was found to be 2.9% with CD4 cells $> 700/\mu l$ and 10.8% with CD4 cells $< 250/\mu l$.

NEUTROPENIA

21. How common is neutropenia in HIV infection?

Up to 50% of patients with AIDS experience neutropenia at some time during the course of their illness.

22. What causes neutropenia in HIV infection?

Of primary importance in evaluating neutropenia in HIV infection is the exclusion of secondary causes. Drugs are implicated, some of the common culprits being ganciclovir, trimethoprim/sulfamethoxazole, pyrimethamine/sulfadiazine, and anticancer chemotherapy. Opportunistic infections and neoplasms that involve the bone marrow usually cause neutropenia in conjunction with other cytopenias (pancytopenia) and rarely cause neutropenia alone.

23. What are the consequences of neutropenia in HIV infection?

It is not clear how neutropenia contributes to the alteration in host defenses. Preliminary studies suggest that the risk of documented bacterial infection increased approximately 2-fold and 8-fold if the neutrophil counts dropped below 1000 cells per mm^3 and 500 cells per mm^3, respectively. However, the frequency of such infections is low (3–5 infections per 100 patient years).

24. How do you treat neutropenia in HIV infection?

If the decrease in neutrophil count is modest and the patient is afebrile, no active intervention may be required other than close observation. If the patient is taking a myelosuppressive medication, discontinuation should be considered. Growth factors may be used when the clinical situation requires the continued use of myelosuppressive medications (e.g., intravenous ganciclovir for CMV infection or chemotherapy for non-Hodgkin's lymphoma). In addition, growth factors also may be used for primary bone marrow failure. In phase I and II studies the combined use of granulocyte colony-stimulating factor (G-CSF) and erythropoietin abrogated the neutropenia and anemia due to primary bone marrow failure, allowing the continued use of AZT. A large phase III trial is currently under way to better define the use of growth factors in neutropenia.

25. What are the negative consequences of using growth factors in HIV infection?

The common side effects of growth factors in HIV infection are bone pain and flulike symptoms, which include myalgias, arthralgias, malaise, lethargy, and occasionally fever. Pulmonary capillary leak syndrome is rare with currently used growth factors (G-CSF, granulocyte macrophage colony-stimulating factor [GM-CSF], erythropoietin) but may be a problem with some of the newer cytokines, such as interleukin-2 (IL-2). In initial studies, concern was raised over whether growth factors would increase viral loads. More recent studies did not find this to be the case. Currently, the use of growth factors is considered safe in HIV infection.

BIBLIOGRAPHY

1. Ballem PJ, Belzberg A, Devine DV, et al: Kinetic studies of the mechanisms of thrombocytopenia in patients with human immunodeficiency virus infection. N Engl J Med 327:1779, 1992.
2. Costella A, Croxson TS, Mildvan D, et al: The bone marrow in AIDS: A histologic, hematologic and microbiologic study. Am J Clin Pathol 84:425, 1985.
3. Glatt AE, Anand A: Thrombocytopenia in patients infected with human immunodeficiency virus: Treatment update. Clin Infect Dis 21:415–423, 1995.
4. Harbol AW, Liesveld JL, Simpson-Haidaris PJ, Abbound CN: Mechanisms of cytopenia in human immunodeficiency virus infection. Blood Rev 8:241, 1994.
5. Henry DH, Beall GN, Benson CA, et al: Recombinant human erythropoietin in the treatment of anemia associated with human immunodeficiency virus (HIV) infection and zidovudine therapy: Overview of four clinical trials. Ann Intern Med 117:739, 1992.
6. Kreuzer KA, Rockstroh JK: Pathogenesis and pathophysiology of anemia in HIV infection. Ann Hematol 75:179–187, 1997.
7. Leaf AN, Laubenstein IJ, Raphael B, et al: Thrombotic thrombocytopenic purpura associated with human immunodeficiency virus type 1 (HIV-1) infection. Ann Intern Med 109:194, 1988.
8. Nigro G, Gattinara GC, Mattia S, et al: Parvovirus–B19-related pancytopenia in children with HIV infection. Lancet 340:115, 1992.
9. Oksenhendler E, Bierling P, Brossard Y, et al: Anti-rh immunoglobin therapy for human immunodeficiency virus-related immune thrombocytopenic purpura. Blood 7195:1499, 1988.
10. Oksenhendler E, Bierling P, Farcet JP, et al: Response to therapy in 37 patients with HIV-related thrombocytopenic purpura. Br J Haematol 66:491, 1987.
11. Pelteir J-Y, Lambin P, Doinel C, et al: Frequency and prognostic importance of thrombocytopenia in symptom-free HIV-infected individuals: A 5-year prospective study. AIDS 5:381, 1991.
12. Scadden DT, Zon LI, Groopman JE, et al: Pathophysiology and management of HIV-associated hematologic disorders. Blood 74:1455, 1989.
13. Spada C, Treitinger A, Hoshikawa-Fujimura AY: HIV influence on hematopoiesis at the initial stage of infection. Eur J Haematol 61:255–260, 1998.

VIII. Cancer Genetics

89. THE USE OF MOLECULAR DIAGNOSTICS IN MALIGNANCY

David W. Yandell, Sc.D.

1. What exactly does the term *molecular diagnostics* mean, and how does it differ from traditional laboratory diagnostic methods?

Molecular diagnostics is a relatively new term that refers to an array of diagnostic technologies that are very different from traditional clinical laboratory tests based on biochemical analysis or those based on imaging of cells or tissues using stains or immune reagents. Molecular diagnostic methods usually examine the information coded in genes or the structure or arrangement of genes or aberrations in genes. These methods are typical of molecular genetics research and are often recently translated from the research laboratory setting. Interpretation of such tests may require a detailed knowledge of gene structure and function. It is not unusual for molecular diagnostic tests to be very new to direct clinical application; the sensitivity and specificity may not be well characterized and the test itself—as well as the reagents required—may not be FDA approved.

2. What types of tests are in the field of molecular diagnostics?

Molecular diagnostic technology is impacting many areas, including forensics, paternity, microbiology and infectious disease, medical genetics, organ transplantation, and oncology. The molecular diagnostic tests relevant to malignancy detect the presence of the following:

- **Carrier status for inherited genetic diseases** (e.g., inherited cancer predisposition syndromes, such as familial breast and ovarian cancer (FBOC), hereditary nonpolyposis colorectal cancer (HNPCC), familial adenomatomous polyposis (FAP), Li-Fraumeni syndrome (LFS), Wilms tumor (WT), retinoblastoma [RB])
- **Infectious pathogens** (e.g., the subtyping of cancer-causing viruses, such as human papilloma viruses (HPV), in cervical cancers or pap smears)
- **Gene amplification or overexpression** (e.g., HER2/*neu* in breast tumors or N-*myc* amplification in neuroblastoma)
- **Somatic (nonheritable) alterations of oncogenes, tumor suppressor genes, or other loci** (e.g., analysis of the p53 gene or microsatellite instability in tumors)
- **Specific gene translocations** (e.g., translocations involving the EWS [Ewing sarcoma] gene in the Ewing family of malignancies)
- **Clonality,** which needs to be differentiated from nonclonal or inflammatory proliferation (e.g., analysis of clonality of immunoglobulin gene rearrangements for diagnosis of lymphoma, or microsatellite instability [MIN])
- **Highly accurate identity typing** (e.g., analysis of outgrowth of donor cells or host-versus-donor tumor origin in a transplant recipient, or high-resolution HLA-typing for matching donor and recipient)

3. Are molecular diagnostic tests superior to or more accurate than other forms of clinical laboratory testing?

Not necessarily. The information provided is often different, however, and it may be performed in an entirely different setting because of the technology used and the requirement for isolation of some aspects of molecular diagnostic testing. In some cases, such as presymptomatic testing for cancer predisposition syndromes, molecular diagnostic technology offers definitive information that cannot be obtained any other way and creates new opportunities for disease surveillance and prevention. **The molecular diagnostic test result may be the final and determinative piece of information that leads to a diagnosis.** In other cases, such as tissue typing for transplantation, molecular techniques may provide a higher resolution HLA-type and very robust information, but the usefulness of this information is dependent on many other considerations: simple practical concerns limit the value of the molecular diagnostic result. Monitoring of minimal residual disease after therapeutic treatment for leukemia is an excellent example of a third category, in which the extraordinarily high sensitivity of molecular techniques creates a threshold for detection of remaining leukemic cells several orders of magnitude lower than other available technologies. However, the usefulness of this information is qualified and the interpretation difficult, because the presence of small numbers of cancer cells systemically is not necessarily predictive of the recurrence of clinical disease.

4. What is the difference between a genetic marker and a gene?

A genetic marker has no biologic function, and physical variability in the genetic marker (alterations in DNA sequence or structure) is not pathogenic. A gene has a function, and alterations of the gene sequence or structure usually change the function of the gene and may cause disease. Genetic markers are commonly used in molecular diagnostics to flag a region of the genome near an important cancer gene to follow inheritance of the cancer gene in families, or loss of the cancer gene in tumor cells. Genetic markers are extremely abundant in the normal human genome; their usefulness is high and the cost and difficulty of assaying these markers is minimal. Gene alterations, and particularly mutations in cancer genes in tumors, are usually unique to one individual or one tumor (often to a clone or subclone of the tumor) and can be difficult and expensive to identify. Although direct analysis of a gene sequence or structure is often necessary, a testing laboratory sometimes may be able to offer alternative approaches to direct gene sequencing or analysis that are less expensive, faster, and based on nearby genetic markers.

5. When is a genetic error a germline mutation?

Genetic variation is part of the evolutionary process and occurs regularly in the gametes. When a deleterious genetic error occurs in a reproductive gamete, it becomes a **germline mutation** and may result in a genetic disease that is transmitted to future generations. Somatic mutations, which occur in cells other than gametes or their precursors, are not transmissible to future generations and the primary pathogenic result (if any) of somatic mutation may be a lack of organization or growth control leading to cancer. It is important to understand that, although hereditary disease may be present for many generations in a family, new germline mutations occur in all genes: thus, it is not necessary for a person to have a prior family history of disease for him or her to be affected by a hereditary disease. For the familial form of retinoblastoma, for example, three out of four cases are due to new germline mutations, whereas only one in four has a prior family history of the disease. The ratio of new germline mutations to preexisting inherited mutations differs for different inherited syndromes. Molecular diagnostic analysis of the patient's blood determines whether a germline mutation is present; analysis of the parents' blood is required to determine whether the mutation is a new germline mutation or a preexisting familial mutation.

6. Describe the term *loss of heterozygosity;* how is it relevant to malignancy?

Tumor suppressor genes on the autosomes function in pairs (one derived from the mother, one from the father) in normal cells. These genes function to control and regulate growth; in most cases, even a single copy of the functional tumor suppressor gene is sufficient to limit growth and prevent the cell from replicating in a "malignant" way. Loss of heterozygosity (LOH) is a term describing a common occurrence in tumor formation in which one of two copies of an autosomal gene—usually a tumor suppressor gene—appears to have been lost in the process of malignant progression. LOH occurs in a cell in which mutation or inactivation of one copy of the tumor suppressor gene has already occurred, so that the only remaining functional copy of the gene is lost. LOH often occurs by loss of a whole chromosome, or by loss of a chromosome followed by endoreduplication of the remaining chromosome so that two copies of the nonfunctional gene (either paternal or maternal) remain. After no functional copy of the tumor suppressor gene remains, the cell is no longer responsive to normal growth regulatory signals and begins the process of uncontrolled division. No molecular diagnostic tests are based solely on LOH of a gene or markers tagging a gene, although LOH analysis in certain tumor types may occasionally provide useful prognostic information.

7. What value is the determination of N-*myc* gene copy number in neuroblastoma cases?

Neuroblastoma is among the most heterogeneous of tumors in its morphologic, genetic, and clinical characteristics. Clinical behavior ranges from extremely aggressive and fatal to regression following limited therapy. Amplification of the N-*myc* gene is common in neuroblastoma. In addition to traditional morphologic indicators such as histologic grade, nuclear morphology, and degree of differentiation, the next most significant prognostic indicator is the N-myc gene copy number. Molecular diagnostic techniques can be used to rapidly and accurately determine the N-*myc* copy number. Tumors carrying 10 or more copies have the worst prognosis, with less than 5% long-term survival following conventional therapy.

8. What is microsatellite instability? How is this information useful in cancer diagnosis?

Microsatellite sequences are short, repeated DNA sequences, usually composed of 2–4 nucleotide "units" that are repeated 20 or more times in tandem. These short repeats are abundant in the human genome and do not appear to have any function in most cases. In some instances, when the repeat unit is 3 nucleotides long and it occurs within a protein-coding portion of a gene, the so-called "triplet repeat" is part of the normal protein produced by the gene and does have functional importance. Microsatellite instability (MIN), also called replicative error in repeats (RER), occurs when the number of tandem copies becomes unstable, leading to expansion or contraction in length of the tandem array. In 1993, it was discovered that MIN is a characteristic of some tumor types, particularly colon tumors from families with hereditary nonpolyposis colon cancer (HNPCC), and indicates genetic instability that appears to be common in malignancy. Although MIN occurs sporadically in many nonhereditary tumor types, MIN analysis of tumor tissue has so far proved to be a useful molecular diagnostic tool only in cases where HNPCC is suspected but family history is inconclusive. In such cases, molecular diagnostic MIN analysis of colon tumor tissue (or occasionally other tumors) may be helpful in diagnosing HNPCC.

9. What does T- and B-cell rearrangement reveal about a specific lymphoma case?

Molecular diagnostic methods complement immunologic methods in analysis of tumor specimens for specific rearrangements of the antigen receptor genes of T- and B-lymphoid cells. Tumor cell-specific rearrangements of the V, D, and J segments of the immunoglobulin (B-cells) and the T-cell receptor (TCR) (T-cells) genes can be identified with molecular diagnostic techniques. In general, a tumor-cell-specific rearrangement of the immunoglobulin genes is an indication of B-cell origin, and a clonal TCR rearrangment indicates T-cell origin. A caveat in interpretation is that more than one rearrangement may be found, due to the high sensitivity of molecular diagnostic techniques and the fact that subclones may exist within the sample. Inclusion of significant subpopulations may be a problem in interpretation, and the characteristic genetic instability of tumor cells may lead to a TCR rearrangement occasionally found in a B-cell tumor and vice-versa. Molecular diagnostic information is generally very useful and often definitive for the hematopathologist in this diagnosis. Molecular diagnostic analysis also may be used in determining whether an observation of cellular proliferation (e.g., in a lymph node) is due to clonal growth (signifying malignancy) versus nonclonal inflammatory or reactive cell infiltration.

10. Do all cases of chronic myelogenous leukemia (CML) carry Ph' chromosomal translocations [t(9;22)(q34;q11)]? Are molecular diagnostic techniques preferable to cytogenetics for detecting the Ph' marker?

Greater than 98% of all CML cases have a major *bcr* (M-*bcr*) gene rearrangement (*bcr-abl* translocation), regardless of whether the Ph' chromosome is detected by cytogenetic methods.

The *bcr-abl* translocation also may be present in a subset (about 10%) of acute lymphoblastic leukemia (ALL) and occasionally also acute myelocytic leukemia (AML). Molecular diagnostic characterization of the exact location of the breakpoint in *bcr* indicates that CML is associated with breaks in one part of the *bcr* gene (exons 12 to 16), with breaks characteristic of ALL in a different region (exons 1–2). When CML is suspected, molecular diagnostic techniques can accurately determine *bcr-abl* translocations, including submicroscopic translocations. The absence of a *bcr-abl* translocation detectable with available molecular or cytogenetic technologies may indicate myeloproliferative disease rather than CML, although about 2% of CML cases do not have a *bcr-abl* translocation detectable with available techniques.

The use of fluorescence in-situ hybridization (FISH) to detect the Ph' marker is also common and is based on different technology, including the use of chromosome specific markers (or probes) and fluorescent stains. FISH techniques are an alternative (or complement) to conventional cytogenetic analysis but not a substitute for molecular diagnostic analysis; FISH does not provide the same level of accuracy in determining the exact location of the *bcr* breakpoint as molecular studies can.

11. When is testing for familial breast cancer appropriate? What does it reveal?

Familial breast cancer testing is appropriate when (1) the test result will be useful to the clinician in making decisions about care or surveillance, and (2) when the **patient** decides to undergo testing after a careful discussion with his or her clinician (or genetic counselor) of the risks and benefits of being tested and knowing the result. The family history may include recurrent, early-onset breast cancer, ovarian cancer, and sometimes other forms of cancer as well; multiple independent primary tumors (e.g., a woman affected by both breast and ovarian cancer) should be considered a strong warning sign. Depending on the clinical history, more than one gene may be appropriate for testing. In families with very early-onset breast cancer in addition to sarcomas, brain tumors, and other cancers, the p53 gene may be the first gene to be tested. In families with site-specific breast cancer or breast and ovarian cancer, the BRCA1 and BRCA2 genes are the starting point, but the presence of any breast cancer in males is important to know. Ashkenazi Jewish heritage on either or both sides of the family also will be an important factor in molecular diagnostic testing, because certain specific mutations in BRCA1 and BRCA2 are carried in this population. Finally, in families with a recurrent history of benign breast disease, breast biopsy, thyroid disease, skin tags, and other benign lesions, Cowden disease may be the underlying cause and the PTEN gene (**p**hosphate and **t**ensin analog on chromosome **ten**) may be appropriate for testing.

A positive test result indicates that a person carries a high risk of cancer. In addition to the current literature on that specific gene, the spectrum of cancers that have already occurred in the family—and their ages of diagnosis—provide a starting point as to what cancers may be expected and when they may occur. Surgical or other preventative prophylactic options may be considered, but the value of such interventions is under careful study and a review of the current literature is essential. It is very important to understand that a negative test result for a specific individual is only interpretable if the gene defect carried by other affected members of the family is known. **In lieu of a known family mutation, a "negative DNA test" for a specific individual should not be interpreted as lowering that person's risk.** It also is very important to understand that not all carriers of a cancer-predisposing gene will be affected with cancer. Both sides of the family tree (maternal and paternal) must be examined. A woman is just as likely to have inherited a breast cancer predisposition gene from her father as from her mother!

12. What use is a molecular diagnostic test in a patient already known to have familial adenomatous polyposis (FAP; also called adenomatous polyposis coli [APC])?

Because surveillance is effective in preventing colon cancer, knowledge that a person is at high familial risk for the disease, along with increased and appropriate surveillance involving colonoscopy, allows prevention of the disease or greatly improved chances of successful treatment and long-term survival. However, after a patient with a family history of FAP presents with colonic polyps, a clinical diagnosis can be made without the extra cost of genetic testing. It is still useful to know the specific gene defect carried by that affected person; it may help in care of other members of the family who have not yet presented with symptoms. Patients who do not carry the same defect as their affected family member can be spared the risk, cost, and discomfort of recurrent colonoscopy. In addition, it is now known that variant clinical forms of some familial cancer syndromes with predictable features that are different from the classic syndrome are associated with specific gene defects. Most persons carrying a defect in the APC gene have the classic features of FAP, including hundreds to thousands of colonic polyps presenting early in life. In a subset population with defects in a specific location of the APC gene, the syndrome is different and called attenuated adenomatous polyposis coli (AAPC) or hereditary flat adenoma syndrome (HFAS). Carriers typically have much less obvious colonic manifestations, including so-called flat adenomas rather than pedunculated polyps. They also have different risks of upper gastrointestinal involvement, including fundic gland polyps.

13. What are the risks involved in testing for inherited cancer predisposition syndromes?

Before proceeding with any DNA test for an inherited disease (including cancer predisposition syndromes), it is important to discuss the risks of the test with the patient. Psychological consequences of a positive carrier test in a healthy individual, including anxiety and apprehension about the future, are well documented.

A negative test result may have consequences such as guilt or anxiety if other family members test positive. The potential for loss of insurance coverage may exist, and discrimination or stigma in the workplace also may be a concern. The patient and the clinician should be aware that in some cases, genetic testing often will reveal family secrets such as nonpaternity or undisclosed adoption; although these are not reported by the testing laboratory, they may lead to an "indeterminate" or uninterpretable test result. Depending on the state, laboratory records may be îdiscoverableî in a legal context for paternity determination. Patients often decide to pay for genetic testing out-of-pocket to limit access to the result by their insurance company. The inclusion in the medical record of a genetic test result on an otherwise unaffected person is a subject of much ethical and legal debate.

14. Are molecular diagnostic techniques useful in determining micrometastasis?

Molecular methods have high sensitivity and high specificity in many cases, and may be used to identify extremely small numbers of cancer cells that would not be appreciable on microscopic examination. These cancer cells may represent the earliest phases of metastasis in a natural progression, release into the blood stream during surgery, or the harbinger of residual or recurrent disease post-therapy. These three areas are under very active investigation. Although tumor cells can be detected using molecular diagnostic methods, their significance is almost uniformly unknown and extensive clinical trials are underway to determine how this technology can best support other available means of diagnosis, prognosis, and treatment. For example, pre- or intraoperative hematogenic dissemination of colorectal tumor cells can be detected at the level of 1 cell/ml of blood by molecular analysis of cytokeratin or other markers. Controlled trials to determine the long-term outcome of patients with low levels of micrometastasis will help set thresholds for peri- or postoperative treatment in patients with otherwise localized disease. In almost all cases, the use of molecular diagnosis for determination of micrometastasis is still in clinical trials and not a part of routine care, although it holds great promise for the future.

BIBLIOGRAPHY

1. Arzimanoglou II, Gilbert F, Barber HR: Microsatellite instability in human solid tumors. Cancer 82:1808–1820, 1998.
2. Benz CC, Brandt BH, Zanker KS: Gene diagnostics provide new insights into breast cancer prognosis and therapy. Gene 159:3–7, 1995.
3. Caldas C: Molecular staging of cancer: Is it time? Lancet 350:231, 1997.
4. Crocker J: The importance of molecular pathology in oncology. Clin Oncol (R Coll Radiol) 10:191–193, 1998.
5. Fearon ER, Vogelstein B: A genetic model for colorectal tumorigenesis. Cell 61:759–767, 1990.

6. Glassman AB: Cytogenetics, in situ hybridization and molecular approaches in the diagnosis of cancer. Ann Clin Lab Sci 28:324–329, 1998.
7. Harris CC, Hollstein M: Clinical implications of the p53 tumor-suppressor gene. N Engl J Med 329:1318–1327, 1993.
8. Harrison CJ, Secker-Walker LM: The importance of cytogenetics and associated molecular techniques in the management of patients with leukemia. Clin Oncol (R Coll Radiol) 10:255–261, 1998.
9. Kinzler KW, Nilbert MC, Vogelstein B, et al: Identification of a gene located at chromosome 5q21 that is mutated in colorectal cancers. Science 251:1366–1370, 1991.
10. Lion T, Izraeli,S, Henn T, et al: Monitoring of residual disease in chronic myelogenous leukemia by quantitative polymerase chain reaction. Leukemia 6:495–499, 1992.
11. Nichols KE, Li FP, Haber DA, Diller L: Childhood cancer predisposition: Applications of molecular testing and future implications. J Pediatr 132:389–397, 1998.
12. Ross DW: Molecular markers of cancer. Arch Pathol Lab Med 115:402, 1991.
13. Sidransky D: Nucleic acid-based methods for the detection of cancer. Science 278:1054–1059, 1997.
14. Tsongalis GJ, Coleman WB: Molecular oncology: Diagnostic and prognostic assessment of human cancers in the clinical laboratory. Cancer Invest 16:485–502, 1998.
15. Vogt PK: Cancer genes. West J Med 158:273–278, 1993.
16. Weitz J, Kienle P, Lacroix J, Willeke F, et al: Dissemination of tumor cells in patients undergoing surgery for colorectal cancer. Clin Cancer Res 4:343–348, 1998.
17. Woodhouse E, Emmert-Buck M, Zhuang Z: The Revolution in cancer molecular diagnostics. Cancer J Sci Am 2:197–206, 1996.
18. Yurij Ionov M, Peinado S, Malkhosyan D, et al: Ubiquitous somatic mutations in simple repeated sequences reveal a new mechanism for colonic carcinogenesis. Nature 363:558–561, 1993.

90. COUNSELING FOR CANCER GENETICS

Lisa G. Mullineaux, M.S., C.G.C., and
Amy Strauss Tranin, R.N., M.S., O.C.N.

1. What information is necessary to determine an inherited risk for cancer?

A detailed family medical history is the key to determine inherited risk for cancer. Obtain a patient's personal history of benign and malignant neoplasms as well as any history of neoplasms from biologic relatives on both the maternal and paternal sides. Family members to ask about include parents, siblings, children, aunts, uncles, grandparents, nieces, nephews, and cousins. For each individual with cancer or a tumor, identify the age of diagnosis, the primary site of the neoplasm, if the neoplasm was bilateral or multifocal, and age of death. Record any common environmental exposures (e.g., tobacco).

2. Define inherited predisposition to cancer.

Inherited predisposition to cancer is defined as increased risk of cancer due to a single gene abnormality inherited in a mendelian fashion (autosomal dominant, autosomal recessive, x-linked dominant, x-linked recessive). The gene abnormality does not cause cancer; it increases the risk for cancer.

Indicators and Examples of Inherited Predisposition to Familial Cancer

INDICATOR	EXAMPLE
Onset of primary cancer earlier than expected	Prostate cancer with onset before age 50
Multiple primary neoplasms in the same individual	Female diagnosed with osteogenic sarcoma at age 17 and breast cancer at age 35
Bilateral primary cancers	An individual with bilateral renal cell carcinoma

Table continued on following page.

Indicators and Examples of Inherited Predisposition to Familial Cancer (Continued)

INDICATOR	EXAMPLE
Multifocal centers	An individual diagnosed with colon cancer at age 51 and 65
Two or more relatives within the same genetic lineage diagnosed with the same types of cancer	Ovarian cancer in a mother and her daughter
Two or more relatives within the same genetic lineage with a unique pattern of neoplasms	A mother with clear cell renal carcinoma and her son with cerebellar hemangioblastoma
Rare cell types	Medullary thyroid carcinoma

3. Describe the genetic characteristics of inherited predisposition to cancer.

Most of the identified genetic syndromes that predispose individuals to cancer exhibit an autosomal dominant pattern of inheritance; thus, each offspring of an individual who has a constitutional alteration in a predisposing gene has a 50% probability of inheriting the same alteration. Variable expressivity also may be present in families. Different members of the same family with an identical alteration may have different neoplasms as well as variability in the age of onset of a neoplasm. Reduced penetrance is also observed. Not everyone who has an alteration will get cancer. For example, a woman with a BRCA1 alteration has an 85% lifetime probability of getting breast cancer and a 15% chance of *not* getting breast cancer. Women who have an alteration in a gene that increases the risk for prostate cancer will not get prostate cancer but may pass the alteration on to her sons and/or daughters.

4. How accurate is the family history obtained from a patient?

The closer (in genetic as well as social terms) the relative, the more accurate the report of cancer and its specific primary site. Love et al. reported a decrease in the accuracy of cancer-history reporting the further genetically removed the patient is to the relative with cancer. Accuracy was determined by reviewing pathology reports of the relative in question. The study also showed that patients were accurate about 90% of the time in reporting a history of colon or breast cancer in a first-degree relative (parent, sibling, or child). For all other primary sites the patients were accurate 84% of the time in reporting cancer and the primary site in such first-degree relatives. Accuracy was 71% in second- and third-degree relatives of the patient (grandparents, aunts, uncles, nieces, nephews, cousins). Verification of family history with pathology reports, surgical reports, medical records, and/or death certificates is important for an accurate diagnosis. If records are not available, contact the affected relative or his or her closest living relative after obtaining permission from the patient.

5. Which families are appropriate candidates for genetic testing?

A family that meets clinical criteria (see chapter 92) or appears to have an autosomal dominant pattern of inheritance is a good candidate for genetic testing. The American Society of Clinical Oncology (ASCO) recommends genetic testing when a strong family history or early onset age of cancer is present (probability ≥ 10% that an alteration will be found), when the test results can be interpreted, and when results will affect medical management. The family member affected with the cancer or neoplasm at the earliest stage of onset is the person to test first. If an unaffected person is tested without knowledge of a family's alteration, a negative result may have one of two explanations: either the proper gene was not tested for or the individual does not have an alteration. A negative test result in such a case cannot be used to eliminate inherited risk in the unaffected individual. If an unaffected individual is tested first and an alteration is present, and if an unaffected individual within the family does not have this specific alteration, a true negative result is indicated. A true negative result means that the individual does not have an inherited risk. The risk is not zero, but is assumed to be that of the general population.

6. Who should *not* be offered genetic testing for a cancer-predisposing condition?

Children should not be tested when genetic test results will not alter treatment or medical management. It may not be wise to test an individual who is not mentally competent. Some controversy exists about testing people who may not be psychologically prepared for the consequences. Difficult cases should be presented to a locally available ethics committee.

7. Why is informed consent and respect for autonomy important when considering predisposition genetic testing?

Many clinicians, ethicists, and patients are concerned that genetic test results may be used inappropriately by insurance companies to deny coverage and by employers to discontinue or affect employment of people with a gene alteration predisposing them to a medical condition. Genetic testing also may impact family relationships and an individual's and family's psychological well-being. Coercion should be avoided.

8. Describe some of the benefits of genetic testing for inherited predisposition to cancer.

Genetic testing may assist individuals in making choices about medical care, reproductive planning, and lifestyle. A true negative test result may offer the patient much relief. A positive test result may help individuals who have a need for increased certainty about their genetic status. Medical intervention strategies, such as prophylactic surgery, for genetically identified high-risk patients may reduce their risk of cancer. Genetic testing in some cases also may enhance family communication.

9. Discuss some of the reasons not to perform genetic testing for inherited predisposition to cancer.

A patient may not want to understand his or her genetic status as it relates to cancer risk and may be ill-prepared psychologically to accept genetic risk, especially if he or she has recently been diagnosed with cancer. The test result may not change the medical management of the patient or his or her approach to surveillance. Positive test results may produce feelings of guilt over the potential passing of the deleterious mutation to future generations. The patient may experience genetic discrimination and stigmatization. A negative result may remove an unaffected individual's favored status in a family and also may result in "survivor guilt." Understanding the genetic status of one family member may have overriding family implications; the genetic status of other family members may be inferred. As a result, genetic testing may interfere with family relations and communication.

10. If an alteration is found in one family member, is it assumed that each family member affected with that particular at-risk neoplasm also has the same alteration?

Not necessarily. Because cancer is a common medical condition, individuals affected by a particular type of cancer may carry the same alteration, and others may not. For example, in a family with an alteration in BRCA1, some women in the family diagnosed with breast cancer may not have an alteration in BRCA1; their breast cancer is caused by sporadic genetic mutations. Unless it is from a known homogenous population, it is highly unlikely that a family would have more than one genetic alteration that causes cancer predisposition.

CONTROVERSIES

11. Should prenatal genetic testing be offered for an inherited predisposition to cancer?

Many laboratories do not offer prenatal genetic testing for certain adult-onset genetic conditions. Debate exists about whether or not prenatal testing should be offered.

For:

Offering genetic testing for inherited predisposition to cancer may have substantial benefits for the parents. A true negative test result may give the parents a great deal of relief. Prenatal testing gives the parents autonomy in making reproductive decisions and planning for the future.

Prenatal testing is currently being offered for some childhood-onset inherited neoplasms, such as von Hippel-Landau disease and multiple endocrine neoplasia syndrome type 2.

Against:

Many of the inherited predispositions to cancer syndromes result in adult-onset cancer. Such conditions may be preventable or easily detectable in the future. The fetus with a positive result has some probability of not ever getting the cancer in question because of reduced penetrance. Prenatal testing has the potential to reveal the genetic status of the at-risk parent who may or may not want to know his or her genetic risk. The high degree of uncertainty and potential breach of autonomy of other family members currently makes prenatal genetic testing inadvisable.

12. How important is pre- and post-test genetic counseling for a patient undergoing genetic testing?

ASCO recommends pre- and post-test genetic counseling for patients and their families. Education about risk, options for screening and prevention, informed consent, counseling, and support regarding social, psychological, and ethical issues are essential components of such risk counseling. Some medical professionals suggest a waiting period between the pretest counseling visit and blood draw for genetic testing.

Cancer Risk Counseling Process

PRETEST COUNSELING	POST-TEST COUNSELING
Obtain and verify family and personal medical history.	Determine if the patient wants to receive his/her results.
Determine patient's reasons for risk assessment/testing.	Reveal results.
Provide risk assessment.	Explain implications of test results.
Educate about inheritance, prevention, surveillance strategies, and risk factors.	Review medical management and surveillance options.
Discuss other medical management options and concerns.	Assist in development of coping strategies and family communication.
Present risks and benefits of testing.	Refer to resources as needed.
Explain testing process, sensitivity, and specificity.	Do a follow-up several months after results are received.
Review implications of testing—psychological, genetic discrimination, impact on family.	
Provide supportive counseling.	
Obtain written informed consent.	

13. Where can I find information about local centers and health professionals that offer cancer risk counseling?

The CancerNet web site http://cancernet.nci.gov/wwwprot/genetic/genesrch.html contains a searchable database (The Familial Cancer Risk Counseling and Genetic Testing Directory) of health professionals who take referrals for cancer genetics education and counseling. The Cancer Information Service (1-800-4-CANCER) is another National Cancer Institute source that provides information about cancer risk counseling resources.

BIBLIOGRAPHY

1. Garber JE, Patenaude AF: Ethical, social and counselling issues in hereditary cancer susceptibility. Cancer Surv 25:381–297, 1995.
2. Kash KM: Psychological and ethical implications of defining genetic risk for cancers. Ann N Y Acad Sci 768:41–52, 1995.
3. Lancaster JM, Wiesman RW, Beichauch A: An inheritable dilemma: Prenatal testing for mutations in BRCA1 breast-ovarian cancer gene. Obstet Gynecol 87:306–309, 1996.

4. Lapham EV, Kozma C, Weiss JO: Genetic discrimination: Perspectives of consumers. Science 274: 621–624, 1996.
5. Lerman C, Schwartz MD, Lin TH, et al: The influence of psychological distress on use of genetic testing for cancer risk. J Consult Clin Psychol 65:414–420, 1997.
6. Love RR, Evans AM, Josten DM: The accuracy of patient reports of a family history of cancer. J Chronic Dis 38:289–293, 1985.
7. MacDonald D: The oncology nurse's role in cancer risk: Assessment and counseling. Semin Oncol Nurs 13:123–128, 1997.
8. Peters JA: Familial cancer risk, part I: Impact on today's oncology practice. J Oncol Management 3:18–30, 1994.
9. Schneider KA: Counseling about Cancer: Strategies for Genetic Counselors. Graphic Illusions, 1994, pp 57–102.
10. Scheuner MT, Wang S, Raffel LJ, et al: Family history: A comprehensive genetic risk assessment method for chronic conditions of adulthood. Am J Hum Genet 71:315–324, 1997.
11. Statement of the American Society of Clinical Oncology: Genetic Testing for Cancer Susceptibility. Cancer Surv 25:381–397, 1995.

91. CANCER SCREENING AND PREVENTION STRATEGIES

Mona Bernaiche Bedell R.N., B.S.N., M.S.P.H., O.C.N.

1. Has a high-risk population for ovarian cancer been described?

Three hereditary cancer syndromes have been identified that place women at highest risk for development of ovarian cancer: site-specific ovarian cancer syndrome, breast-ovarian syndrome, and Lynch syndrome II (nonpolyposis colorectal cancer, endometrial cancer, and ovarian cancer). Women with one of these syndromes have a 14–80% lifetime risk of developing ovarian cancer. These syndromes are rare and account for less than 5% of all women diagnosed with ovarian cancer. High-risk screening for ovarian cancer is often recommended, but studies have not yet demonstrated clear benefit.

2. Is there a role for prophylactic oophorectomy in women at high risk for ovarian cancer?

Effectiveness of prophylactic oophorectomy has not been established. It has been offered as an option for women with BRCA1 gene mutations, but the data are insufficient to support a recommendation for or against the procedure as a measure to reduce ovarian cancer risk. Cases of intraabdominal carcinomatosis after prophylactic oophorectomy have been reported. The optimal age for surgery has not been determined, although it has been suggested that women at high risk be offered the option of prophylactic oophorectomy after the completion of childbearing or at age 35 years.

3. What are the screening recommendations for people at increased risk for colorectal cancer?

People at high-risk should be identified for special surveillance. People with intermediate risk should be offered the same screening options as people with average risk, but surveillance should begin 10 years earlier or at age 40. Screening options include:

• Fecal occult blood testing each year
• Flexible sigmoidoscopy every 5 years
• Double-contrast barium enema every 5–10 years or colonoscopy every 10 years

Special surveillance should be considered for high-risk people with first-degree relatives (siblings, parents, or children) who have had colorectal cancer or an adenomatous polyp; people with a family history of familial adenomatous polyposis (FAP) or hereditary nonpolyposis colorectal cancer (HNPCC); and patients with a history of adenomatous polyps, colorectal cancer, or inflammatory bowel disease. (See chapter 66 for further details.)

4. When should special surveillance begin in people with inflammatory bowel disease?

Surveillance colonoscopy to look for colonic dysplasia is commonly performed every 1–2 years after 8 years of disease in patients with pancolitis or after 15 years in patients with colitis involving only the left colon. Prophylactic colectomy eliminates the risk of colon cancer in such patients and should be considered as a preventive strategy.

5. What potential advantages does genetic screening offer over current colorectal screening methods?

High-risk people in families with FAP or HNPCC can be identified at an early age when they may benefit most from intensive surveillance, screening, and possible prophylactic procedures such as colectomy.

6. When is gene testing for hereditary colorectal cancer appropriate?

Genetic counseling and testing are available for two well-described forms of hereditary colorectal cancer, familial adenomatous polyposis (FAP) and hereditary nonpolyposis colorectal cancer (HNPCC). Testing for FAP or HNPCC is mainly useful for confirming the diagnosis of hereditary colorectal cancer in clinically affected patients who meet diagnostic criteria. Secondly, first-degree relatives and other family members of the affected patient also may be at risk and should be offered genetic testing. Gene testing provides the potential to identify most people with HNPCC and FAP before cancer develops. Genetic testing also may be helpful in avoiding intensive screening in potential gene carriers if no mutation is found in a person whose blood relatives are known to carry a specific gene abnormality.

7. How should you explain test results for HNPCC to a person who is related to known carriers of HNPCC gene alterations?

Gene testing distinguishes affected from nonaffected members. Gene penetrance for HNPCC is 70–80%. The remaining 20–30% do not carry the germline mutation and will not develop colorectal cancer or other HNPCC-associated cancers. People with negative test results should be aware that their risk for colorectal cancer remains the same as that for the general population; routine screening and other preventive strategies should be encouraged.

8. Name other cancers for which HNPCC gene carriers may be at risk.

Endometrial, ovarian, small bowel, stomach, and transitional cell carcinoma of the ureters are associated with HNPCC gene mutations. Endometrial cancer is found in almost 50% of families with HNPCC gene defects. Annual screening for endometrial cancer should begin at age 25–35 years. Optimal screening methods have not yet been determined, but endometrial aspirate and transvaginal ultrasound have been studied. Recommendations for screening the other cancers have not been established.

9. What surveillance is required for HNPCC-associated mutation carriers?

Colonoscopy of the entire colon is recommended every 1–2 years, starting between the ages of 20 and 30 years and every year after age 40 for persons known to have HNPCC-associated mutations. HNPCC does not have a predictable onset date; disease may develop at any age from 20–80 years.

10. Does prophylactic colectomy reduce risks for HNPCC in gene carriers?

The efficacy of colonoscopy in decreasing the incidence or reducing mortality from colorectal cancer has not been established by randomized control trials. Subtotal colectomy is recommended for HNPCC-associated mutation carriers who have been diagnosed with colon cancer or adenomas at the time of surveillance. Even if the risk of developing colorectal cancer is reduced by surgery, the risk of extracolonic cancers remains a concern. Prophylactic colectomy remains an option for HNPCC-associated mutation carriers who are not physically able or willing to undergo prescribed surveillance.

11. At what age should screening begin for a potential gene carrier of FAP?

Gene counseling and testing should be offered to people with a family history of FAP but not before puberty. Polyps may develop as early as puberty; the mean age at onset is 16 years. Less than 1% of all colorectal cancers result from a mutation of the APC gene, but nearly 100% of those who test positive will develop colorectal cancer, usually by age 40. False negatives occur in about 20% of patients with FAP. Close surveillance is not helpful because there are too many polyps and it is too difficult to identify early cancers or polyps with more advanced pathology. Colectomy is the only preventive strategy.

12. What other clinical manifestations of FAP may aid in identification of affected patients?

Extracolonic manifestations of FAP include osteomas of the skull and long bones, retinal pigmentation, soft tissue tumors (such as epidermoid cysts, fibroma, and lipomas), and other adenomas of the gastrointestinal tract. Patients with FAP are also more likely to develop other cancers such as thyroid, duodenal, or pancreatic carcinoma or hepatoblastoma and medulloblastoma.

13. What is the significance for men who inherit the altered BRCA1 gene?

Men with the altered BRCA1 gene are not at increased risk for breast cancer, but they can pass the altered gene to their children. Each child of a parent who carries an altered gene has a 50% chance of inheriting the mutation. Men with the altered BRCA1 gene also have a slightly higher risk of colon and prostate cancer than the general population.

14. How should BRCA1 and BRCA2 gene test results be interpreted?

Test results can be positive, negative, or inconclusive. A positive result indicates presence of the altered gene and significant risk of breast, ovarian, and other cancers. The lifetime risk for breast cancer may be as high as 85%; for ovarian cancer, 10–40%. A negative test result for a predisposing gene means that the risk is not as high, but lifetime risk remains the same as for the general population. Continued prevention and surveillance efforts should be emphasized. A negative test result in a family in which an inherited cancer has not been identified also may mean that a mutation has occurred in another predisposing gene not tested. An inconclusive result may be either a polymorphism that has not previously been identified or a mutation of uncertain significance (the function of the mutation is not known). Therefore, an inconclusive result is neither positive nor negative.

15. Should prophylactic mastectomy be recommended for women who carry a gene defect that sharply increases their risk of developing breast cancer?

The issue of prophylactic mastectomy remains highly controversial and presents a clinical dilemma for women at high risk and their physicians. Surgery may reduce but not totally eliminate the risk of breast cancer. Breast cancer has been reported in residual breast tissue after mastectomy. The exact incidence of breast cancer after prophylactic mastectomy is unknown. To date there are no recommendations for or against prophylactic bilateral mastectomy. Women may be more apt to consider this option if they are at very high risk, and less than 50 years old and have dense mammograms that are difficult to interpret. Women with BRCA1 gene mutation who undergo prophylactic mastectomy are still at high risk for ovarian cancer.

16. Should a woman who is a known BRCA 1 mutation carrier and desires a prophylactic mastectomy have reconstruction? If so what type?

This issue is controversial. Some argue against reconstruction so that if a cancer develops, it can be easily identified on the chest wall. Others argue that subpectoral implants are the safest, because any residual breast tissue is easily accessible by physical examination. Most surgeons who do reconstructive procedures believe that if the procedure is done properly, little breast tissue is left behind; therefore, even autologous reconstruction (i.e., transverse rectus abdominis muscle [TRAM] flap) is safe.

17. How efficacious is aspirin as a chemopreventive agent against colorectal cancer?

Evidence from basic science research and several observational studies have demonstrated the beneficial effects of aspirin in reducing the incidence of colorectal cancer by 40% and the mortality rate by 40–50%. Data about other nonsteroidal antiinflammatory drugs (NSAIDs) are more limited but also show great promise. Randomized clinical trials are needed to confirm current findings before recommendations can be made. Future research will determine the optimal drug, dosage, and frequency to minimize gastric irritation and other side effects and to establish optimal duration for chemoprevention.

18. Who should have early prostate cancer screening?

It is estimated that 9% of prostate cancers may be inherited. Men who have early onset of prostate cancer or families with multiple affected members and/or generations are most likely to have inherited forms. African-American men also have an increased risk of prostate cancer. Early screening with yearly digital rectal examination and serum determination of PSA, starting at age 40, is recommended. The efficacy of early screening modalities is unproved.

BIBLIOGRAPHY

1. Burke W, Petersen G, Lynch P, et al: Recommendations for follow-up care of individuals with an inherited predisposition to cancer. I: Hereditary nonpolyposis colon cancer. JAMA 277:915–919, 1997.
2. Burke W, Daly M, Garber J, et al: Recommendations for follow-up care of individuals with an inherited predisposition to cancer. II: BRCA1 and BRCA2. JAMA 277:997–1003, 1997.
3. DuBois RN, Giardiello FM, Smalley WE: Nonsteroidal anti-inflammatory drugs eicosanoids, and colorectal cancer prevention. Gastroenterol Clin North Am 25:773–791, 1996.
4. Giardiello FM. Genetic testing in hereditary colorectal cancer. JAMA 278:15;1278–1281, 1997.
5. Gronberg H, Isaacs SD, Smith JR, et al: Characteristics of prostate cancer in families potentially linked to the hereditary prostate cancer 1 (HPC1) locus. JAMA 278:1251–1255, 1997.
6. Winawer SJ, Fletcher RH, Miller L, et al: Colorectal cancer screening: Clinical guidelines and rationale. Gastroenterology 112:594–642, 1997.

92. BREAST CANCER GENETICS

Wendy C. McKinnon, M.S., and Catherine E. Klein, M.D.

1. What is the difference between familial and hereditary breast cancer?

Familial breast cancer refers to families with at least two cases of breast cancer in close relatives. Approximately 20% of women with breast cancer have at least one relative with breast cancer. The breast cancer in the family may be due to chance coincidence, environmental factors, hormonal factors, a specific inherited genetic abnormality, or some combination of these factors.

Hereditary breast cancer implies mendelian inheritance of breast cancer. Hereditary breast cancer often appears in a familial pattern. However, in small families, with inherited traits of low penetrance, or in cases of paternal transmission, it may be difficult to detect the familial component.

2. What is the frequency of hereditary breast cancer? What clinical features suggest hereditary breast cancer in an individual or family?

One in 9 women develops breast cancer in her lifetime. Current estimates suggest that approximately 5–10% of breast cancers are due to a mutation in an inherited cancer-susceptibility gene. Hereditary breast cancer is suspected in individuals and families with early onset (< age 50), bilateral or multifocal breast cancer, other tumors associated with hereditary breast cancer (e.g., ovarian cancer), and multiple affected relatives in the same lineage with an autosomal dominant pattern of transmission. Several inherited cancer syndromes have breast cancer as a component; these syndromes are due to mutations in a number of different cancer-susceptibility genes.

3. What are the known hereditary cancer syndromes in which breast cancer may appear?
Hereditary breast cancer may run in families with no other apparent cancers (hereditary site-specific breast cancer), in families afflicted with ovarian cancer in addition to breast cancer (breast-ovarian cancer syndrome), or in families with Li-Fraumeni syndrome. Additional tumors in families with Li-Fraumeni syndrome include sarcomas, gliomas, leukemias, and adrenocortical carcinomas. In addition, families with Cowden disease have an increased incidence of breast cancer as well as papillary and follicular thyroid carcinoma and are recognized by multiple facial and oral papules, trichelimmomas, and keratoses. Families with hereditary nonpolyposis colon cancer (HNPCC) or Lynch II syndrome appear to have an increased incidence of breast cancer in addition to colon cancer, endometrial cancer, ovarian cancer, and transitional cell tumors of the ureter. Ataxia-telangiectasia is a disorder inherited in a recessive manner, unlike the other dominantly inherited diseases; heterozygotes appear to be at increased risk for breast cancer, but this theory is currently under debate.

4. What is the genetic basis of inherited cancer syndromes? What are the associated cancer risks?
1. **Hereditary breast/ovarian cancer syndrome.** Mutations in the BRCA1 and BRCA2 breast cancer-susceptibility genes probably account for approximately 80% of inherited breast cancer. BRCA1 (breast cancer gene no. 1) is located on chromosome number 17, and BRCA2 (breast cancer gene no. 2) is located on chromosome number 13. Approximately 45% of families with hereditary breast cancer manifest a BRCA1 gene mutation, and approximately 35% manifest a BRCA2 mutation. Most families with both breast and ovarian cancer have an alteration in BRCA1 rather than BRCA2. Women who inherit mutated copies of these genes have an approximately 85% lifetime risk of developing breast cancer. Female BRCA1 mutation carriers have an approximately 20% risk of developing breast cancer by age 40, 51% risk by age 50, and 87% risk by age 70. The cumulative risk for developing a second primary breast cancer in BRCA1 mutation carriers is estimated to be 65% by age 70. Carriers of a BRCA1 mutation have an approximately 40–50% risk of developing ovarian cancer by age 70. BRCA2 mutation carriers appear to have a later age of onset; 28% of female carriers develop breast cancer by age 50 and 84% by age 70. The corresponding ovarian cancer risks for BRCA2 mutation carriers have been estimated to be approximately 0.4% by age 50 and 27% by age 70. There are other clinical differences between families who harbor mutations in the two genes; male breast cancer and pancreatic cancer are more commonly associated with BRCA2 mutations. In families with BRCA2 mutations, men have an approximate 6% lifetime risk for developing breast cancer (100-fold increase over the general population). Colon cancer rates may be increased in BRCA1 gene carriers (6% lifetime risk), and male BRCA1 mutation carriers appear to have an increased risk for prostate cancer (8% lifetime risk).
2. **Li-Fraumeni syndrome.** Approximately one-half of families that fit the clinical criteria for Li-Fraumeni syndrome have mutations in the P53 gene, located on chromosome number 17. The most commonly associated tumors are early-onset breast cancer, leukemia, osteosarcoma, brain tumors, soft tissue sarcomas, and carcinomas of the adrenal gland. Approximately 30% of tumors occur before age 15. Individuals with germline mutations in P53 have an approximately 50% risk of developing cancer by age 30 and a 90% risk by age 70. Family members are at risk for developing multiple primary cancers and may be susceptible to carcinogenic exposures.
3. **Cowden syndrome.** Mutations in PTEN, also referred to as MMAC, a recently identified gene on chromosome number 10, appear to account for most cases of Cowden disease. Hamartomatous growths of the skin, oral mucosa, breast (often classified as fibrocystic breast disease), thyroid, and colon are hallmarks of the syndrome. Patients with Cowden disease have an approximately

30–50% lifetime risk for developing breast cancer and an approximately 10% risk for developing thyroid cancer.

4. **Hereditary nonpolyposis colon cancer (HNPCC).** HNPCC is a genetically heterogeneous disorder; mutations in several different genes result in a similar clinical presentation. The two most common genes are MSH2 and MLH1; mutations in either confer risks primarily for colon cancer but also for endometrial, breast, ovarian, and transitional cell tumors of the ureter. The lifetime risk for developing colon cancer in people with mutations in one of these two genes appears to be approximately 80–90%. The lifetime risk for endometrial cancer appears to be 30–40%; the risk for other cancers, including breast, appears to be much lower but may depend on the specific mutation segregating in the family.

5. **Ataxia-telangiectasia (AT).** AT is due to mutations in a gene located on chromosome 11. Homozygotes are affected with ataxia and ocular telangiectasias. Patients are also radiation-hypersensitive and at risk for developing cancer. There have been conflicting reports in the literature about whether women who are heterozygous for AT are also radiation-hypersensitive and at increased risk for developing cancer, particularly breast cancer.

5. Describe the BRCA1 and BRCA2 mutations associated with an increased risk for cancer development.

Both BRCA1 and BRCA2 are large tumor suppressor genes, and well over 100 deleterious mutations have been identified in each. Most identified mutations are frameshift and nonsense mutations, which cause premature truncation of the protein. A small proportion of mutations (estimates range from 5–15%) are located in the regulatory part of the gene and usually are not identified with standard mutation detection techniques. Missense mutations comprise a minor proportion of mutations, and their clinical significance is often not clear.

Three specific mutations appear more frequently, particularly in people of Ashkenazi Jewish descent, and are thought to be the result of founder effects. Deletion of adenine and guanine at position 185 in BRCA1 (185delAG) is present in about 1% of Ashkenazi Jews. Two other specific mutations, 5382insC (insertion of cytosine at position 5382 in BRCA1) and 6174delT (deletion of thymine at position 6174 in BRCA2), are found in another 1–2% of Ashkenazi Jews. Some studies suggest that Jewish women with these mutations, although at high risk for breast and ovarian cancer, do not have risks quite as high as described earlier. For example, Jewish women who carry one of the three specific mutations appear to have an approximate 56% lifetime risk for developing breast cancer rather than an 85% risk. The lifetime risk for developing ovarian cancer appears to be approximately 16%. Founder effects for other mutations in other populations also have been identified and described.

6. Are breast cancers due to BRCA mutations pathologically different from other breast cancers?

Several studies have identified histopathologic characteristics in breast tumors of women with germline mutations in BRCA1. In general, such tumors have more adverse pathologic indicators, including more aneuploidy and an increased incidence of high S-phase, than noninherited breast tumors. In addition, inherited tumors are more likely to have negative progesterone and estrogen receptors. Medullary histology is overrepresented, whereas tubular and lobular histology is less common.

7. Do patients harboring a BRCA mutation have a survival advantage?

Despite the more adverse pathologic indicators seen in tumors of BRCA1 mutation carriers, initial studies suggested, paradoxically, that BRCA1 mutation carriers had a better prognosis and a survival advantage compared with women with sporadic breast cancer. Some experts suggest that this advantage may be due to the overrepresentation of medullary breast cancers, which has a favorable outcome. More recent studies do not indicate a survival advantage for BRCA1 mutation carriers but rather a similar and, in some cases, worse prognosis than in women with sporadic, noninherited, breast cancer.

8. When is genetic testing indicated for possible hereditary breast cancer?

Commercial tests are now available to search for deleterious mutations in BRCA1 and BRCA2, P53, and HNPCC, but because of the large size and distribution of mutations in these genes, the testing is technically difficult and costly. When and how to use these tests in clinical practice are controversial issues. They are not screening tests for the general population and should be offered only when the likelihood of a positive test result is high, the test can be adequately interpreted, and the result will influence medical management. It is difficult to make testing recommendations today that will hold true tomorrow. Rather than stating specific criteria for testing, certain principles of genetic testing are listed to help ensure that genetic testing for cancer susceptibility is performed in a reasonable and cost-effective manner.

1. Testing must be initiated by a family member who has had cancer, except under special circumstances (e.g., Ashkenazi Jew with strong family history of breast and/or ovarian cancer in which all affected relatives are deceased). If a specific genetic mutation is identified. genetic testing may be offered to other family members, both affected and unaffected with cancer. In general, a genetic test result from an unaffected family member cannot be interpreted without prior testing of an affected family member.

2. All people having genetic testing for cancer susceptibility should have pretest genetic counseling that includes (1) formal pedigree analysis; (2) documentation of cancer cases in the family; (3) assessment by professionals with expertise in cancer genetics that, based on the family history, a significant probability exists that a genetic mutation will be identified; (4) education and counseling about the risks, benefits, and limitations of genetic testing; and (5) written informed consent before testing.

3. Genetic test results should be disclosed in a face-to-face encounter by a medical professional knowledgeable about implications and limitations. The professional should be someone involved in the testing process who has an established relationship with the person tested.

9. Discuss genetic testing for BRCA1 and BRCA2 in people of Ashkenazi Jewish ancestry.

Ashkenazi background lowers the threshold for testing because the probability of harboring a deleterious mutation is about 4-fold compared with non-Ashkenazi women. Testing in this setting is technically less difficult and less costly, because tests are targeted to look specifically for the three mutations associated with hereditary breast/ovarian cancer and Jewish ancestry. Although these three mutations account for the majority of hereditary breast cancer in the Jewish population, some families that have none of the mutations clearly have hereditary breast cancer by pedigree analysis. They may have mutations in other parts of BRCA1 or BRCA2 or in another gene that has not yet been identified. Again, testing should be undertaken only after pretest genetic counseling and informed consent in a setting that allows anonymous reporting of results and thoughtful support.

10. What health care maintenance recommendations should be offered to a carrier of a BRCA mutation?

When a deleterious mutation is discovered in someone as yet unaffected, options for subsequent care can be tailored to the risk. Increased surveillance can be initiated, and prophylactic removal of the tissue at risk (mastectomy or oophorectomy) may be considered. Cancer prevention intervention, when available, may be offered, and lifestyle modification may be chosen. The Cancer Genetics Consortium has published guidelines for following BRCA gene carriers. These guidelines are based on expert opinion, not proven studies. Mammography should be initiated 10 years earlier than the earliest case of breast cancer documented in the family (or between 25 and 35 years) and continued at yearly intervals. Clinical breast exams every 6 months, beginning at age 25, and monthly breast self-exam are recommended, although no studies have documented the efficacy of such an approach. Patients should be counseled to pursue any abnormality aggressively.

Screening for early detection of ovarian cancer is recommended for BRCA gene carriers, although no good screening techniques have been clearly shown to decrease mortality. Nevertheless, many clinicians recommend transvaginal ultrasound and a blood test called CA-125 in addition to routine pelvic examinations at 6–12-month intervals. Any abnormality must be followed by laparoscopy or laparotomy for definitive diagnosis. These screening tools may increase the ability to detect early ovarian cancer in high-risk women, but their efficacy remains unproven.

Although there appears to be an increased incidence of colon and prostate cancer in BRCA gene carriers, diagnosis does not appear to occur at younger ages than in the general population. Therefore, the consortium recommends that BRCA gene carriers follow the American Cancer Society recommendations for colon and prostate cancer. The colon cancer recommendations entail yearly fecal occult blood testing and flexible sigmoidoscopy every 3–5 years, beginning at age 50. For men, yearly digital rectal exams and prostate-specific antigen testing, beginning at age 50, are recommended.

11. What is the role of prophylactic surgery in BRCA gene carriers?

Women identified as BRCA gene carriers may have as high as an 85% lifetime risk for developing breast cancer and an approximately 50% risk for developing ovarian cancer. It is appropriate to discuss the option of prophylactic mastectomy and oophorectomy as a preventative measure. Affected women must understand that all of the at-risk tissue cannot be removed and that a residual risk for cancer development remains after surgery. Current estimates suggest that less than 5% of breast tissue remains after a prophylactic mastectomy; breast cells remain in the axilla and over the rectus muscle (in the epigastric and supraclavicular areas). A recent study estimated a 92% reduction in breast cancer risk after prophylactic mastectomy. There are no estimates for risk reduction for prophylactic oophorectomy. Several studies have estimated that 2–11% of high-risk women who undergo prophylactic oophorectomy develop abdominal carcinomatosis, which is thought to arise from either residual ovarian cells or tissue similar embryonically to ovarian epithelium. The decision to proceed with prophylactic surgery must be a personal one and should be discussed with at-risk women in a sensitive manner.

12. What is the role of hormonal therapies in BRCA gene carriers?

Hormone replacement and use of oral contraceptives are topics of great concern to patients and health care providers alike, but definitive recommendations are unavailable. Pros and cons of each should be discussed with the patient while we await the results of studies to help predict the actual risk:benefit ratios. In regard to hormone replacement therapy, the risk for breast cancer must be discussed along with the potential benefits of decreased cardiovascular and osteoporosis risks and alternative therapies. Although long-term oral contraceptive use may be associated with an increase in breast cancer risk, it also may help to prevent ovarian cancer.

13. Do epidemiologic factors play a role in cancer development in gene mutation carriers?

From epidemiologic data, breast cancer is associated with obesity, lack of exercise, high-fat diet, smoking, and excessive use of alcohol. Recommendations for healthy lifestyle modifications seem appropriate, although no data support their efficacy in this high-risk population. This is an area of active research interest. Counseling BRCA gene carriers about a healthy lifestyle may help them to gain control in a situation that seems beyond their control.

BIBLIOGRAPHY

1. Burke W, Daly M, Garber J, et al: Recommendations for follow-up care of individuals with an inherited predisposition to cancer. II: BRCA1 and BRCA2. JAMA 277:1003, 1997.
2. Eng C: Cowden syndrome. J Gen Couns 6(2):181–192, 1997.
3. Easton DF, Ford D, Bishop DT, and the Breast Cancer Linkage Consortium: Breast and ovarian cancer incidence in BRCA1 mutation carriers. Am J Hum Gen 56:265–271, 1995.
4. Ford D, Easton DF, Bishop DT, and the Breast Cancer Linkage Consortium: Risk of cancer in BRCA1 carriers. Lancet 343:692–695, 1994.
5. Ford D, Easton DF, Stratton M, et al: Genetic heterogeneity and penetrance analysis of the BRCA1 and BRCA2 genes in breast cancer families. Am J Hum Genet 62:676–689, 1998.
6. Fitzgerald MG, MacDonald DJ, Krainer M, et al: Germ-line BRCA1 mutation in Jewish and non-Jewish women with early-onset breast cancer. N. Engl J Med 334:143–149, 1996.
7. Hoskins KF, Stopfer JE, Calzone KA, et al: Assessment and counseling for women with a family history of breast cancer. JAMA 273:577–585, 1995.

8. Langston AA, Malone KE, Thompson JD, et al: BRCA1 mutation in a population-based sample of young women with breast cancer. N Engl J Med 334:137–142, 1996.

9. Marcus JN, Watson P, Page DL, et al: Hereditary breast cancer: Pathobiology, prognosis, and BRCA1 and BRCA2 gene linkage. Cancer 77:697–709, 1996.

10. Struewing JP, Hartge P, Wacholder S, et al: The risk of cancer associated with specific mutations of BRCA1 and BRCA2 among Ashkenazi Jews. N Engl J Med 336:1401–1408, 1997.

11. Wooster R, Bignell G, Lancaster J, et al: Localization of a breast cancer susceptibility gene, BRCA2, to chromosome 13q12-13. Science 265:2088–2090, 1994.

93. COLON CANCER GENETICS

Steven P. Lawrence, M.D., and Dennis J. Ahnen, M.D.

1. Why is an understanding of the genetic aspects of colorectal cancer clinically relevant?

Colon cancer can be prevented by the application of appropriate screening strategies to average and high-risk groups. Selecting the appropriate screening methods requires a working knowledge of colon cancer genetics to distinguish people at average risk from those at high risk. Risk depends primarily on family history but must take into account the age at diagnosis of affected persons, the number of persons within a family diagnosed with colonic neoplasia, and the presence of any known inherited colorectal cancer syndromes. Recent advances in the understanding of colonic carcinogenesis have significant application to cancer prevention and have made possible genetic testing for inherited syndromes.

2. What is the genetic difference between sporadic and hereditary colon cancer?

Sporadic colorectal carcinoma, the most common form, occurs in 5–6% of the U.S. population over the age of 50. Sporadic cancer is thought to result from a somatic mutation followed by clonal expansion of the mutant clone. Further cycles of mutation and clonal expansion ultimately produce clones of cells with multiple mutations. Environmental factors such as diet and physical activity probably play a major role in the process. This process ultimately gives rise to cancer via the adenoma-carcinoma sequence. The earliest abnormality in this transformation, not detectable by current screening methods, is the aberrant crypt focus, a clonal expansion of neoplastic cells in a single or a few colonic crypts. Unrestricted growth allows these cells to form an adenoma over a period of years. Most colorectal adenomas do not progress to cancer. Progression to malignancy appears to require further somatic mutation(s) within the adenoma, a process which takes an additional 5–10 years.

Hereditary forms of colon cancer arise from predisposing germline mutations that are inherited and already present in all colonocytes at birth. Thus, all colonic mucosal cells are at risk, and fewer steps are necessary for the transition to overt malignancy. Clinically, these hereditary syndromes have the propensity to cause colon cancer at a younger age and at multiple sites.

3. List the hereditary syndromes of colorectal cancer and their variants. How are they inherited?

Syndrome	Variants
1. Adenomatous polyposis coli (APC)	Familial adenomatous polyposis (FAP)
	Gardner's syndrome
	Brain tumor-polyposis syndrome type 2
	(Turcot's syndrome)
	Attenuated adenomatous polyposis coli (AAPC)

Table continued on following page.

Syndrome	*Variants*
2. Hereditary nonpolyposis colorectal cancer (HNPCC)	Hereditary site-specific colon cancer syndrome (Lynch syndrome I)
	Cancer family syndrome (Lynch syndrome II)
	Muir-Torre syndrome
	Hereditary flat adenoma syndrome
	Brain tumor-polyposis syndrome type 1 (Turcot's syndrome)

All of these syndromes are inherited in an autosomal dominant manner with high penetrance.

4. What are the clinical manifestations of familial adenomatous polyposis (FAP)?

FAP is characterized by the development of hundreds or thousands of adenomatous polyps throughout the colon, with an average age of onset at 16 years. These polyps inevitably progress to colon cancer in virtually all FAP patients by age 50. The mean age at cancer diagnosis is 39 years in gene carriers; approximately 7% of malignancies may occur before the age of 21. The site distribution of colon cancer in FAP is more commonly left-sided and typically occurs in the same location as other affected family members.

Upper gastrointestinal tract polyps are also common in patients with FAP. Fundic gland polyps, which occur in the upper stomach, are hyperplastic and pose a minimal risk of malignancy. Duodenal adenomas occur in over 90% of FAP patients and progress to duodenal cancer in approximately 5% of cases.

Congenital hypertrophy of the retinal pigment epithelium, which is detectable by routine ophthalmoscopy, is a phenotypic marker in some FAP families.

5. What genetic mutation causes FAP?

Mutations within the adenomatous polyposis coli (APC) gene, on the long arm of chromosome 5, have been identified as the genetic alteration responsible for FAP and its variants. Almost all of the APC gene mutations identified in families with FAP code for a truncated APC protein. The production of a truncated protein results in abnormal function by mechanisms that have yet to be fully elucidated.

The APC gene mutation occurs in about 1 in 10,000 births, although approximately 20% of new FAP cases appear to arise from spontaneous mutation of the gene. The location of the mutation and hence the length of the abnormally shortened APC protein play a major role in determining the clinical manifestations of the disease. Colon polyp density, the occurrence of retinal lesions, and the risk of variant forms correlate with the locations of point mutations or microdeletions that produce these syndromes.

6. How does attenuated adenomatous polyposis coli (AAPC) differ from classic FAP?

AAPC is a recently described variant of APC characterized by the development of fewer colonic adenomas (< 100), which appear a decade or more later in life than those seen with classic FAP. Unlike the uniform polyp distribution seen in FAP, adenomas in AAPC are predominantly right-sided, occurring above the splenic flexure. The average age of colon cancer diagnosis is similarly delayed by about 10 years compared with FAP, although the long-term risk appears to be equivalent. Of interest, APC gene mutations that give rise to AAPC typically occur at the proximal 5' end of the gene, resulting in a markedly shortened gene product.

7. What is Gardner's syndrome?

Gardner's syndrome is FAP with extraintestinal manifestations. This artificial distinction arose before genetic investigation proved that they represent a spectrum of phenotypic expression of dysfunction of a single gene. The extraluminal abnormalities associated with Gardner's syndrome include:

1. Osteomas of the skull, mandible, and long bones
2. Mandibular cysts, supernumerary teeth
3. Epidermoid and sebaceous cysts
4. Lipomas and fibromas
5. Desmoid tumor

The same mutation in the APC gene can cause FAP without prominent extraintestinal manifestations in some families and the Gardner's syndrome variant in others, suggesting that modifier genes or environmental factors are important in the phenotypic expression of disease.

8. Is genetic testing available for FAP?

When a family member is diagnosed with FAP or a variant syndrome, an in vitro protein synthesis assay may be performed to search for the presence of a truncated APC protein. This commercially available assay, which utilizes leukocyte DNA from a standard blood draw, identifies the truncated APC protein in about 80% of families with FAP. Once the abnormal protein is identified, at-risk family members can be similarly tested. The finding of the same truncated protein in an at-risk family member is diagnostic for FAP. This method is nearly 100% accurate when a known kindred mutation is documented first. Families offered this testing must be provided with pre- and posttesting genetic counseling, preferably with the input of a medical geneticist, to interpret fully the results and their ramifications.

9. What is the treatment for FAP?

At present, total colectomy, usually with an ileoanal anastomosis, is the recommended approach once colonic adenomas arise in an at-risk family member. Sulindac, a nonsteroidal anti-inflammatory drug, has been shown to prevent new adenoma formation and induce polyp regression in FAP in controlled trials. Although this medical therapy remains investigational at present, it may offer hope for alternative treatment strategies in the future. Upper endoscopy is recommended every 1–3 years after colonic polyposis develops to screen for duodenal adenomas.

10. What is hereditary nonpolyposis colorectal cancer (HNPCC)? How does it differ from sporadic colon cancer?

The HNPCC syndromes, also known as the Lynch syndromes, are characterized by the onset of colon cancer at a relatively young age in a predominantly right-sided distribution. As opposed to FAP, HNPCC shows no propensity to develop large numbers of polyps, although adenomas that arise in HNPCC have a much higher risk of malignant transformation. The average age at colon cancer diagnosis in HNPCC is the mid-40s, whereas in sporadic carcinomas risk increases progressively after age 50. Almost 70% of first cancers in HNPCC are seen proximal to the splenic flexure, whereas in sporadic cases slightly over one-half arise above this anatomic region. The exact penetrance of the HNPCC gene mutations are unknown, but studies of large families suggest that as many as 80% of people who carry HNPCC genes will develop colon or one of the other HNPCC-linked cancers. They also have a high risk of synchronous (two or more separate colon cancers diagnosed simultaneously) and metachronous (nonanastomotic new tumors developing at least 6 months after the initial diagnosis) cancers.

11. What are the Amsterdam criteria for HNPCC?

The Amsterdam criteria define a set of clinical criteria that help to identify families at high risk of harboring an HNPCC gene. Although these guidelines do not identify all families with HNPCC, the presence of all three criteria within a kindred warrants genetic testing and counseling. The Amsterdam criteria can be remembered as the rules of 3–2–1:
   • At least 3 relatives with colorectal cancer, two of whom must be first-degree relatives.
   • Involvement of 2 or more generations.
   • At least 1 case diagnosed before age 50.

12. What is the difference between Lynch I and Lynch II syndromes?

Before the evolution of the genetic details of HNPCC, investigators noted that some families had inheritable cancers confined to the large intestine, whereas other families were at risk for both colonic and extracolonic malignancies. The former came to be known as hereditary site-specific colon cancer, or Lynch syndrome I. Families exhibiting both colonic and noncolonic tumors were classified into the cancer family syndrome or Lynch syndrome II. As more families are studied and the genetic basis of HNPCC becomes better understood, the distinction between Lynch syndromes I and II, if real, will be clarified.

13. List the extracolonic malignancies associated with Lynch syndrome II.

1. Endometrial carcinoma—most common; may affect up to 25% of women in some families.
2. Ovarian carcinoma
3. Gastric and small intestine adenocarcinoma
4. Transitional cell carcinoma of the upper urinary tract
5. Hepatobiliary malignancies

14. What is the genetic basis of HNPCC?

Mutations in DNA repair genes, collectively termed the mismatch repair (MMR) system, have been identified as the genetic basis for HNPCC. The MMR proteins repair mismatches in DNA synthesis, which frequently occur during cell division. Mutation in an MMR gene results in a truncated, dysfunctional MMR protein that cannot effectively correct the replication errors. To date, four MMR gene mutations that may lead to HNPCC have been described: hMSH2, hMLH1, hPMS1, and hPMS2. Colonic malignancies that arise from such mutations and hence exhibit many DNA mismatches are termed replication error-positive (RER+) tumors or are said to have microsatellite instability.

Genetic testing methods to detect MMR system defects are under development, using truncated gene product analyses similar to those used for FAP or direct sequencing of the MMR genes. Fulfilling all of the Amsterdam criteria increase the success rate of finding an MMR mutation. When commercially available, genetic testing for HNPCC requires the same caveats recommended for APC gene testing.

15. Describe the clinical management of HNPCC.

Families that meet the Amsterdam criteria or persons at high risk for HNPCC based on genetic testing should undergo screening with colonoscopy. Such screening should begin at age 25 or 10 years younger than the age of the earliest case of colon cancer in the family, whichever comes first. Colonoscopy should be repeated every 2 years. Subtotal colectomy is recommended if a carcinoma or advanced adenoma is found, given the high risk of subsequent cancer. Screening for uterine cancer should be considered, especially in women with a positive family history, although the optimal screening methods have not been determined. Periodic pelvic ultrasonography, endometrial biopsy, or uterine washings have been advocated.

16. How are sebaceous gland tumors associated with colon cancer?

Sebaceous gland tumors, which may occur as adenomas, epitheliomas or carcinomas, are rare neoplasms associated with the Muir-Torre variant of HNPCC. People with single or multiple sebaceous tumors have a significantly increased risk of colon cancer, adenomatous polyps, or a noncolonic malignancy associated with the cancer family syndrome. The occurrence of a sebaceous lesion and a HNPCC-related internal malignancy, even if separated by several years, establishes the diagnosis of Muir-Torre syndrome. In approximately 40% of patients, the cutaneous tumor is found prior to or concurrent with the associated internal cancer. Additional primary malignancies may arise many years after the syndrome is initially diagnosed. Patients with sebaceous gland tumors and family members of patients with Muir-Torre syndrome should undergo the same screening protocols as other HNPCC groups.

17. What is Turcot's syndrome? Why are there two types?

Recent investigations have suggested that Turcot's syndrome, also referred to as brain tumor-polyposis (BTP) syndrome, actually comprises two distinct subtypes—one related genetically and clinically to HNPCC and the other to FAP. Both subtypes are rare, and both appear to result from germline mutations in the MMR system or APC gene that are similar to those identified for HNPCC and FAP, respectively. BTP syndrome type 1 is characterized by the association of glioblastoma multiforme and colorectal carcinoma or adenomas of the HNPCC variety. The predominant brain tumor in BTP syndrome type 2 is medulloblastoma, which occurs in the setting of FAP. The genetic alterations that subsequently lead to primary brain malignancies in some people with inherited colon cancer syndromes are unknown.

18. What percentage of the total colorectal cancer burden is accounted for by the inherited syndromes of colon cancer?

Although important for understanding the molecular basis of colonic malignancy, the inherited colon cancer syndromes account for a relatively small percentage of the total number of cases. Colon carcinoma resulting from FAP represents < 1% of total cases, whereas HNPCC accounts for 2–5%. Sporadic colorectal cancer, therefore, remains the predominant form, and inheritable risk plays a major role in its epidemiology.

19. Describe the importance of family history to the risk of sporadic colorectal cancer.

A positive family history of colon cancer has a significant impact on future risk of developing colorectal carcinoma. Although the exact susceptibility gene or genes that confer this increased risk are not known, it is hypothesized that 20–50% of the total colon cancer risk in the population is due to inherited predisposition. The importance of a positive family history is illustrated by the following:

• A single first-degree relative with colon cancer increases an individual's risk about 1.5- to 2-fold over that of the general population.
• Two first-degree relatives with colon cancer confer a 3- to 4-fold increase in risk.
• One first-degree relative diagnosed with colon cancer between the ages of 45–55 increases risk in that family by approximately 3-fold.
• Persons with one first-degree relative diagnosed with colon cancer at age < 45 have about a 4-fold increased risk.
• Persons with more than two first-degree relatives with colon cancer have approximately a 40–50% risk of the same malignancy.
• Colon cancer risk is increased approximately 2.5-fold if a parent or sibling is diagnosed with an adenomatous polyp of the colon before age 60.

These risk factors have important implications for colorectal cancer screening and thus should be taken as a routine part of a patient's medical history. Screening recommendations, as outlined below, depend on careful assessment of these risk factors.

20. What is the multistep process of colonic carcinogenesis?

The development of a colon carcinoma occurs over several decades and involves a series of stepwise genetic events that transform a normal colonic mucosal cell, through several stages, into a malignancy. The investigations that established this multistep process have had ground-breaking implications in the field of tumor oncogenesis.

At least seven genetic alterations appear to be required to transform a normal colonocyte into a carcinoma. These genetic changes involve varying accumulations of germline and/or spontaneous mutations. A single colonic cell, once genetically altered, undergoes clonal expansion and eventually forms a single, abnormal, and neoplastic crypt—the aberrant crypt focus. Although still benign, this aberrant crypt grows, through further genetic change, to form an early adenoma. As more steps in the process occur, an early adenomatous polyp enlarges and becomes more dysplastic—hence the term "advanced adenoma." Cytologic changes within the adenoma cells evolve from low-grade to high-grade dysplasia. Likewise, the architecture of the polyp may change from a tubular to a villous adenoma, which further increases the risk of malignant transformation. Cancer within a polyp usually arises from a small area and may remain, for a certain period, above the muscularis mucosa, termed a carcinoma-in-situ. At this point, further progression inevitably leads to invasion and a malignant colonic tumor.

21. What role does the multistep process play in colon cancer screening strategies?

The multistep process described above forms the basis of the adenoma-carcinoma sequence. The intermediate step in this process, at which lesions are identifiable, benign, and removable, is the adenomatous polyp. Adenoma removal by colonoscopic polypectomy has been shown to reduce the incidence of colorectal cancer by 76–90%, compared with reference groups. One of the most important goals in colon cancer screening and prevention is the identification and removal of colonic adenomas before malignant transformation occurs.

22. What genetic mutations have been associated with the multistep process and the adenoma-carcinoma sequence?

Obviously the sequence in which genetic mutations occur in the multistep process has a significant impact on the risk of subsequent transformation. Mutations of the tumor suppressor gene *p53* or the oncogene *K-ras*, common in colon carcinomas, have little impact if they are the sole mutation within the colonic cell. Acquired mutations in the APC gene appear to be the dominant initiating factor for aberrant crypt foci and early adenomas. The genetic alterations common to most colon cancers are not uniformly present in all cases. The reason for this heterogeneity and the missing genetic alterations that accompany them have yet to be explained. Similarly, the role which environmental factors such as diet play in triggering these events is unknown. The following table depicts the hypothesized genetic changes most commonly associated with colorectal tumorigenesis.

Clinical Event	Gene Involved	Chromosome	% of Colon Cancers
Normal mucosa	***	***	***
Early adenoma	APC	5q	85
Intermediate adenoma	*K-ras*	12	47
Advanced adenoma	*DCC*	18q	73
Carcinoma	*p53*	17p	85
Metastases	*? DCC, p53*	18q, 17p	***

DCC = deleted in colon cancer gene; APC = adenomatous polyposis coli gene.

23. What are the normal functions of the genes involved in colon cancer?

The APC gene product, the APC protein, modulates the activity of a cytosolic protein, β-catenin, which is important in cellular adhesion and signal transduction pathways. The normal APC protein may target β-catenin for destruction; thus loss of APC protein function may dysregulate these important cell mechanisms. It is theorized that the APC protein also may play a role in apoptosis (programmed cell death) of colonocytes.

K-ras is an oncogene that codes for a small GTP-binding protein (p21). The *ras* protein serves as a signal transduction switch that can stimulate cell growth in response to growth factors. *K-ras* mutations in colon cancer lead to constituitive activation of signal transduction pathways and unregulated cellular growth.

DCC and *p53* are tumor-suppressor genes. The *DCC* protein is thought to be involved in cell adhesion. Loss of *DCC* function may be important in the processes of invasion and metastasis. The *p53* protein has been termed the guardian of the genome, given its role in preventing cells with DNA mutations from replicating. DNA damage causes the formation of *p53* protein, a nuclear phosphoprotein that serves as a transcriptional activator of several genes. This results in cell cycle arrest in the G1 phase. Mutations are then repaired, or the cell undergoes apoptosis. Thus, *p53* mutations abolish this repair mechanism, and cells with significant DNA damage are allowed unrestricted replication.

24. What colorectal screening strategies should be considered based on genetically determined risk stratification for colon cancer?

The following table highlights the currently recommended screening strategies for colorectal cancer based on inheritable risk. Any positive fecal occult blood test or adenoma found on sigmoidoscopy warrants further evaluation, usually by colonoscopy.

Risk Group	Beginning Age	Interval	Method
Average risk = no (+) family history	50	Yearly q 5 yr	Fecal occult blood + Sigmoidoscopy
One (+) FDR	40	Yearly q 5 yr	Fecal occult blood + Sigmoidoscopy
Two or more (+) FDRs	40	q 5 yr	Colonoscopy
(+) FDR < 55 yr old	10 yr < age at diagnosis	q 5 yr	Colonoscopy
FAP	10–12	Yearly until age 40	Sigmoidoscopy*
Attenuated APC	20	q 1–2 yr	Colonoscopy*
HNPCC	25 or 10 yr < age at diagnosis—whichever is first	q 2 yr; yearly after age 40	Colonoscopy

(+) FDR = first-degree relative diagnosed with colorectal cancer; age at diagnosis = age at diagnosis of earliest case of colorectal cancer in family.
* Polyps found on screening examination should prompt consideration of definitive therapy.

BIBLIOGRAPHY

1. Burt RW, DiSario JA, Cannon-Albright L: Genetics of colon cancer: Impact of inheritance on colon cancer risk. Annu Rev Med 46:371–379, 1995.
2. Cannon-Albright LA, Skolnick MH, Bishop T, et al: Common inheritance of susceptibility to colonic adenomatous polyps and associated colorectal cancers. N Engl J Med 319:533–537, 1988.
3. Cohen PR, Kohn SR, Kurzrock R: Association of sebaceous gland tumors and internal malignancy: The Muir-Torre syndrome. Am J Med 90:606–613, 1991.
4. Giardiello FM, Brensinger JD, Petersen GM, et al: The use and interpretation of commercial *APC* gene testing for familial adenomatous polyposis. N Engl J Med 336:823–827, 1997.
5. Kinzler KW, Vogelstein B: Lessons from hereditary colorectal cancer. Cell 87:159–170, 1996.
6. Lynch HT, Smyrk TC, Watson P, et al: Genetics, natural history, tumor spectrum, and pathology of hereditary nonpolyposis colorectal cancer: An updated review. Gastroenterology 104:1535–1549, 1993.
7. Marra G, Boland CR: Hereditary nonpolyposis colorectal cancer: The syndrome, the genes, and historical perspectives. J Natl Cancer Inst 87:1114–1125, 1995.
8. Paraf F, Jothy S, Van Meir EG: Brain tumor-polyposis syndrome: Two genetic diseases? J Clin Oncol 15:2744–2758, 1997.
9. Rustgi AK: Hereditary gastrointestinal polyposis and nonpolyposis syndromes. N Engl J Med 331:1694–1702, 1994.
10. Vogelstein B, Fearon ER, Hamilton SR, et al: Genetic alterations during colorectal-tumor development. N Engl J Med 319:525–532, 1988.
11. Winawer SJ, Fletcher RH, Miller L, et al: Colorectal cancer screening: Clinical guidelines and rationale. Gastroenterology 112:594–642, 1997.
12. Winawer SJ, Zauber AG, Gerdes H, et al: Risk of colorectal cancer in the families of patients with adenomatous polyps. N Engl J Med 334:82–87, 1996.

94. HEREDITARY MALIGNANCIES

Marie E. Wood, M.D., Henry T. Lynch, M.D., and Jane F. Lynch, R.N., B.S.N.

1. What do the terms *hereditary* and *familial* cancer mean?

Hereditary cancer implies a mendelian inheritance pattern. The cancer may involve a specific anatomic site, such as breast cancer, or an association with other cancer types, such as the hereditary breast/ovarian cancer syndrome. The pattern of segregation of the cancer(s) within the family follows the mendelian inheritance pattern of the particular hereditary syndrome: autosomal dominant, autosomal recessive, or X-linked. Recent work has identified abnormalities of specific genes associated with many forms of hereditary cancer.

The term **familial** describes a clustering of cancer within a family. Although no clear pattern of mendelian inheritance is shown, individuals in the family have a somewhat increased risk for cancer and should be monitored closely.

2. How extensively should the physician pursue a family history of cancer?

Ideally, the family history should be compiled through the modified nuclear pedigree, which involves a detailed description of cancer history in first-degree relatives, including mother and father, siblings, and progeny, and second-degree relatives, especially both sets of grandparents, aunts, and uncles. Extending the history to older second-degree relatives includes people who more than likely have passed through the age of highest cancer risk and thus provide more genetic information than siblings and progeny. The history should include cancer of *all* anatomic sites and any premonitory stigmata, such as café au lait spots or neurofibromas in von Recklinghausen's neurofibromatosis (NF-1) and multiple atypical moles in the familial atypical multiple mole melanoma (FAMMM) syndrome. It is important to pursue the history through the paternal as well as maternal lineage, because even in sex-limited tumors, such as breast, ovary, or endometrium, cancer-free males may be obligate gene carriers.

3. What are the cardinal features of hereditary forms of cancer?

1. Early age of cancer onset, although the range in age of onset may be quite variable within and between families

2. Multiple primary cancers with specific combinations, such as colon and endometrium in Lynch Syndrome II or breast and ovary in hereditary breast-ovarian cancer syndrome

3. Premonitory physical stigmata, biomarkers of genotypic susceptibility, or both in certain syndromes (e.g., multiple atypical moles in FAMMM syndrome)

4. Distinctive pathologic features, such as medullary thyroid carcinoma in multiple endocrine neoplasia type II and type III

5. Mendelian patterns of tumor transmission

Not all of these features apply to specific patients or families, because there may be marked variation in expression of any phenotypic feature of the natural history. Nevertheless, these cardinal features are sufficiently pervasive to assist the clinician in identifying hereditary cancer-prone families.

4. How important is the patient's age at cancer diagnosis as a predictor of genetic etiology?

The fraction of cancer that is believed to be genetically induced is substantially greater in patients below age 40. Age at onset of cancer is particularly important in several of the major cancer sites, particularly breast, colon, and ovary. For example, it is estimated that as many as 50% of patients with onset of any of these cancers before age 40 have family histories consonant with a hereditary cancer syndrome. The likelihood of a genetic etiology appears to increase in direct proportion to the decrease in age at onset of cancer. In patients with strikingly early age of cancer onset and a negative family history, a new germline mutation may have occurred in one of the parents. Other explanations for a negative family history in patients with cancer of potential genetic etiology include death of key relatives at early ages from causes other than cancer, lack of accurate data about cause of death, or reduced penetrance of the deleterious gene.

5. What is meant by Knudson's "two-hit" hypothesis for the explanation of cancer etiology? How does it relate to the function of the gene?

In 1971 Knudson proposed what is now known as the "two-hit" or two-mutation model for carcinogenesis. This model was based on studies of patients with retinoblastoma. Knudson proposed that people with the hereditary form of cancer harbored a germline mutation and required a second "hit," which was a postconceptional somatic mutation. Sporadic cases, on the other hand, lack the germline mutation and thereby require two somatic mutations for retinoblastoma to occur. The two-hit model explained the earlier age of onset and the excess of bilaterality in the hereditary form of retinoblastoma compared with its sporadic variant. The sporadic variant required two somatic "hits," a fact that partially explains its later age of onset and the decrease in occurrence of bilateral cancer.

Most genes associated with cancer family syndromes are tumor suppressor genes, the normal function of which is to suppress the malignant (or benign) tumor phenotype. If both copies of the gene are inactivated, suppression is released and the tumor phenotype is expressed.

6. What is the tumor spectrum that characterizes Li-Fraumeni syndrome (LFS)?

The acronym **SBLA** was coined by Lynch et al. to explain the tumor spectrum of LFS:

S = **S**arcoma
B = **B**reast cancer and **b**rain tumors
L = **L**ung and **l**arynx carcinoma, **l**eukemia, and **l**ymphoma
A = **A**drenocortical carcinoma

This exceedingly complex disorder is most likely due to the pleiotropic effects of a p53 germline mutation, which appears to be responsible for the litany of cancer types. Early age of onset and multiple primary cancer are characteristics of LFS and most forms of hereditary cancers. Other tumors that appear to be integral to LFS include neuroblastoma, Wilms' tumor, and pancreatic carcinoma. Undoubtedly, as data about more families are accrued and extended with meticulous attention to cancer of *all* anatomic sites and correlation of molecular genetic studies of newly identified germline (p53) mutations, knowledge about its full tumor complement will increase.

7. Can people be genetically tested for LFS? If so, what is the value of testing?

Germline mutations of the p53 gene are found in 50% of families who meet criteria for LFS. Thus one-half of the families appear to have classic LFS/SBLA but no mutation is found. For the other 50% it is not clear how helpful testing will be. A negative result may be reassuring, but for people who carry a mutation but are not yet affected with cancer the benefits are not clear. There are no good screening protocols for cancers associated with LFS other than breast cancer. We may do nothing more than raise anxiety. Studies are under way to answer this question.

8. Do neuroendocrine tumors have a hereditary etiology?

Various neuroendocrine tumors appear to have a hereditary etiology. Foremost of these is multiple endocrine neoplasia (MEN) type I, which involves parathyroid, pituitary, and pancreatic islet cell tumors. MEN type IIA (or MEN II) involves a predisposition to medullary thyroid carcinoma and pheochromocytoma, which are often bilateral. MEN type IIB (MEN III) is also referred to as the multiple mucosal neuroma syndrome. In addition to the predisposition to medullary thyroid carcinoma and pheochromocytoma, MEN IIB shows multiple mucosal neuromata (dysplasias of neurocristic Schwann cells) and peripheral extensions of neurocristic ganglion cells as well as a marfanoid habitus and abnormalities of intestinal neural plexuses (gangliomatosis of the bowel). The MEN syndromes are inherited in an autosomal dominant pattern.

9. How can pheochromocytoma be inherited?

In addition to its integral association with MEN IIA and IIB, pheochromocytoma also occurs in von Recklinghausen's neurofibromatosis (NF-1 variety) and von Hippel-Lindau disease. Each of these disorders has an autosomal dominant mode of inheritance, as may isolated pheochromocytoma.

10. What is the tumor spectrum in MEN I (Werner's syndrome)? Where is the MEN I locus located?

Tumors of the parathyroid, anterior pituitary, and endocrine pancreas constitute the tumor spectrum in MEN I. Genetic-linkage studies of patients with MEN I and deletion findings in their tumors have enabled the mapping of the MEN I locus to chromosome 11q13. The gene has been identified, and germline mutations have been found in patients with MEN I. The normal function of the gene (named *menin*) is not known, but it is a tumor suppressor gene.

11. Are abnormalities of a single gene responsible for MEN IIA, MEN IIB, and hereditary site-specific medullary thyroid cancer?

Yes. Germline abnormalities of the *RET* protooncogene are found in individual patients and families with all three syndromes. Mutations are found in 95% of patients with MEN IIB, 92% of patients and families with MEN IIA, and 88% of patients with familial medullary thyroid carcinoma (FMTC).

12. Should all patients with medullary thyroid carcinoma be screened for a germline abnormality in the *RET* protooncogene?

The simple answer is yes. Most patients with a positive family history and about 25% of patients with sporadic MTC (and a negative family history) have genetic abnormalities. Family members of patients who are found to have germline abnormalities are candidates for presymptomatic testing. Presymptomatic testing can identify people who have the greatest likelihood of developing MTC and would be candidates for prophylactic thyroidectomy.

13. Does pancreatic cancer show familial aggregation?

Two case-control studies have demonstrated a significant familial aggregation of pancreatic cancer. Studies of extended kindreds have also shown, albeit rarely, pancreatic cancer occurring though multiple generations in a pattern of transmission suggestive of an autosomal dominant inherited factor. Pancreatic cancer has also occasionally been shown to be integrally associated with hereditary pancreatitis, MEN I, Lynch syndrome II, von Hippel-Lindau syndrome, and a subset of the FAMMM syndrome. It also has been seen in excess in BRCA2 families.

14. What is the evidence for hereditary etiology in carcinoma of the stomach?

Gastric carcinoma has been identified in families with familial adenomatous polyposis (FAP), particularly from Japan, as well as in Lynch syndrome II kindreds. Family reports of site-specific gastric cancer appearing through multiple generations are consistent with an autosomal dominant mode of inheritance. Gastric cancer also has been observed at extremely early ages in patients with ataxia-telangiectasia. There also is believed to be an association between pernicious anemia and stomach cancer. Gastric cancer is frequently associated with blood group A. The relationship between gastric cancer and *Helicobacter pylori* may account for some of the familial aggregation.

15. Does intraocular melanoma (IOM) show evidence of a genetic etiology?

There have been rare occurrences of families with IOM occurring on a site-specific basis consonant with an autosomal dominant mode of inheritance. IOM also has been shown to be an integral finding in a subset of families with FAMMM syndrome. In a survey of medical records of 45 patients with histologically diagnosed IOM at the University of Texas M.D. Anderson Hospital and Tumor Institute, one patient with IOM had a similarly affected sibling with histologically verified IOM. A second, unrelated family in which IOM was found through three generations was referred during the course of the study.

16. What is the evidence for the role of genetic factors in Hodgkin's disease (HD) and non-Hodgkin's lymphoma (NHL)?

Knowledge of the role of genetics in the etiology of HD and NHL is limited. There have been occasional families with a remarkably increased occurrence of HD, NHL, or both. In one such family, NHL was histologically verified in a mother and all five of her daughters. One of the NHL-affected daughters had a daughter with HD. It was suggested that these hematogenous malignancies were inherited in an autosomal dominant pattern. There also have been reports of families with only HD, families with only NHL and, more rarely, families with both HD and NHL transmitted in a manner suggestive of the autosomal dominant mode. However, familial occurrences of lymphoma are relatively rare, and familial aggregation of NHL occurs less frequently than familial aggregation of HD.

X-linked lymphoproliferative disease of Purtillo is a special example of NHL occurring at a markedly early age and restricted to males, because the gene is located on the X chromosome. In SBLA syndrome, lymphoma is one of the integral forms of cancer and is transmitted in an autosomal dominant pattern.

Evidence linking genetics, immunology, and environmental factors in the etiology of lymphomas has emerged during the past two decades. For example, immunologic anomalies and/or disorders in lymphomas have been shown to occur in the following mendelian inherited settings:

1. Several sex-linked recessive disorders, including Bruton's agammaglobulinemia, Wiskott-Aldrich syndrome, and X-linked lymphoproliferative disorder of Purtillo

2. Traits inherited in an autosomal recessive mode, including ataxia-telangiectasia, Chédiak-Higashi syndrome, common variable immunodeficiency, Sjögren's syndrome, and familial microcephaly syndrome

Lymphoma also has been described in families prone to systemic lupus erythematosus, which may be a familial disorder in some cases.

17. What are cancer-associated genodermatoses? How many of these syndromes are known?

A diagnosis of cancer-associated genodermatosis implies that the disorder harbors a specific form of benign cutaneous stigmata in association with cancer and is inherited in a mendelian pattern. At least 50 differing hereditary cancer-associated genodermatoses show autosomal dominant, autosomal recessive, and X-linked modes of inheritance. Therefore, one should be aware of the important dermatologic signs, because these stigmata may facilitate diagnosis of a hereditary cancer syndrome. Examples of cancer-associated genodermatoses include the following:

1. **FAMMM syndrome** is characterized by the presence of multiple atypical moles and cutaneous malignant melanoma. Intraocular melanoma and/or pancreatic cancer may occur in a subset of FAMMM kindreds.

2. **Multiple hamartoma syndrome (Cowden's disease)** includes cutaneous lesions such as dome-shaped, flat-topped papules, verrucous lesions, punctate keratoderma of the palms, multiple angiomas and lipomas, and gingival and palatal papules as well as a scrotal tongue. Patients are at high risk for carcinoma of the breast, including bilateral occurrence. Papillary thyroid cancer and uterine cancer occur in excess.

3. **Peutz-Jeghers syndrome** is characterized by multiple pigmented macular spots of the lips, buccal mucosa, conjunctiva, periorbital area, and digits. Patients also have multiple intestinal hamartomatous polyps that may contain adenomatous features and are predisposed, albeit weakly, to adenocarcinoma of the colon and small bowel (duodenum). Granulosa cell tumors of the ovaries also occur.

4. In **xeroderma pigmentosum (XDP)** patients have an exquisite cutaneous photosensitivity to sunlight with excessive freckling in sun-exposed areas of the skin in the first years of life and early degeneration of the skin leading to freckling, telangiectasia, keratosis, papillomas, and eventually to carcinomas and melanomas. The eyes may be affected with photophobia, lacrimation, and keratitis, with resulting opacities. Deficiency of DNA repair with exposure to ultraviolet light has shown heterogeneity with at least eight complementation groups based on DNA repair phenotypes.

18. Has a gene for Cowden's disease been identified? What cancer risk is associated with this disease?

The *PTEN* gene on chromosome 10 has been found to contain germline mutations in patients with Cowden's disease. The disease carries a 30–50% lifetime risk of breast cancer and a 10% risk of nonmedullary thyroid cancer. Uterine cancer is seen at an increased rate in patients with Cowden's disease.

19. Where is the retinoblastoma gene located? Has it been cloned?

The retinoblastoma gene, the first tumor suppressor gene identified, is found on the long arm of chromosome 13. It has been localized and cloned.

20. Do other cancers occur in patients with retinoblastoma?

Various cancers, especially osteogenic sarcoma and soft tissue sarcoma, occur in the radiation field of patients treated for the hereditary form of retinoblastoma. There appears to be a dose-response relationship between radiation and sarcoma development. Other cancers seen in patients with hereditary retinoblastoma include brain tumors, melanoma, pineoblastoma, breast cancer, and sometimes Hodgkin's disease.

21. At least two distinct forms of neurofibromatosis exist—NF-1 and NF-2. What is the difference between the two?

NF-1 is an autosomal dominant disorder that affects about 1 in 5000 people. It was previously called von Recklinghausen's disease or peripheral neurofibromatosis. The term NF-1 was adopted in 1987 to make a clear distinction between the two definite categories of neurofibromatosis. NF-1 is characterized by the presence of multiple hyperpigmented macules known as café au lait spots; dermal, subcutaneous, and plexiform neurofibromas; iris (Lisch) nodules; axillary freckling; and optic nerve gliomas. The gene for NF-1 is on the proximal long arm of chromosome 17 (17q11.2).

NF-2 was previously called central neurofibromatosis, bilateral acoustic neurofibromatosis, and hereditary bilateral vestibular schwannoma syndrome. This autosomal dominant disorder affects about 1 in 50,000 people. It is characterized by bilateral acoustic neuromas, posterior subcapsular cataracts, meningiomas, trigeminal nerve tumors, schwannomas, spinal cord ependymomas, and dermal, subcutaneous, and plexiform neurofibromas. The gene for NF-2 is located on the distal long arm of chromosome 22.

22. What is the tumor spectrum in von Hippel-Lindau (VHL) disease?

VHL is a hereditary cancer syndrome with autosomal dominant inheritance characterized by a predisposition to the development of retinal, cerebellar, and spinal hemangioblastomas. In addition, patients have a markedly increased susceptibility to renal cell carcinoma and pheochromocytoma. Two types can be distinguished: VHL type I (without pheochromocytoma) and VHL type II (with pheochromocytoma).

23. Has VHL been linked to a gene?

The gene for VHL has been mapped to chromosome 3p25–p26. The gene has been cloned and sequenced. Seventy-five percent of patients with VHL have a mutation in the VHL gene, which is another tumor suppressor gene. The seven different missense mutations in exons I and III vary in their biologic consequence from a minimal VHL II phenotype with pheochromocytoma only to a full VHL phenotype with renal cell carcinoma and pancreatic lesions.

24. How can genetic testing for VHL be helpful?

Recommended screening for unaffected members of VHL families begins at age 5, with yearly ophthalmologic examination. Additional screening for brain tumors, renal cancer, and pheochromocytoma is also recommended at later ages. For members of a family with a known mutation who test negative, avoidance of extensive life-long screening can be an emotional and economic savings.

25. Is there an excessive risk of cancer among heterozygous carriers of the ataxia-telangiectasia gene?

Ataxia-telangiectasia (A-T) is an autosomal recessive disorder in which cancers develop in affected homozygous individuals at an enormous rate (approximately 100 times higher than in unaffected age-matched controls). Because A-T is inherited as an autosomal recessive disorder, there are many heterozygous people in the general population; indeed, they constitute about 1% of the general population.

Several studies have examined the relationship between breast cancer and A-T. It was previously thought that A-T heterozygotes had an increased risk of breast cancer. Newer studies performed after the gene for A-T (the *ATM* gene) had been identified and sequenced, demonstrate no increased risk for carriers of one abnormal *ATM* gene (heterozygotes).

26. Is prostate cancer genetic?

Some families clearly demonstrate autosomal dominant transmission of prostate cancer, and it is thought that about 5% of prostate cancer is inherited. Recently a gene on chromosome 1 (*HPC1*) has been linked to hereditary prostate cancer. Characteristics of prostate cancer in families linked to this genetic locus include early age of onset, higher-grade tumors, and advanced stage at diagnosis. Men with a family history of prostate cancer should begin prostate cancer screening early (at age 40 or 5–10 years before the earliest diagnosis).

BIBLIOGRAPHY

1. Anderson RJ, Lynch HT: Familial risk for neuroendocrine tumors. Curr Opin Oncol 5:75–84, 1993.
2. Chandrasekharappa SC, Guru SC, Manickam P, et al: Positional cloning of the gene for multiple endocrine neoplasia-type 1. Science 276:404–407, 1997.
3. Gronberg H, Isaacs S, Smith J, et al: Characteristics of prostate cancer in families potentially linked to the hereditary prostate cancer 1 (*HPC1*) locus. JAMA 278:1251–1255, 1997.
4. Liaw D, Marsh D, Li J, et al: Germline mutations of the *PTEN* gene in Cowden disease, an inherited breast and thyroid cancer syndrome. Nat Gen 16:64–67, 1997.
5. Lynch HT, Anderson DE, Krush AJ, et al: Hereditary and intraocular malignant melanoma. Cancer 21:119–125, 1968.
6. Lynch HT, Mulcahy GM, Harris RE, et al: Genetic and pathologic findings in a kindred with hereditary sarcoma, breast cancer, brain tumors, leukemia, lung, laryngeal, and adrenal cortical carcinoma. Cancer 41:2055–2064, 1978.
7. Lynch HT, Marcus JN, Weisenberger D, et al: Genetic and immunopathologic findings in a lymphoma family. Br J Cancer 59:622–626, 1989.
8. Malkin D, Li FP, Strong LC, et al: Germ line p53 mutations in a familial syndrome of breast cancer, sarcomas, and other neoplasms. Science 250:1233, 1990.
9. Roos KL, Dunn DW: Neurofibromatosis. Cancer 42:241–254, 1992.
10. Swift M, Morrell D, Massey R, et al: Incidence of cancer in 161 families affected by ataxia-telangiectasia. N Engl J Med 325:1831–1836, 1991.
11. Wong F, Boice J, Abramson D, et al: Cancer incidence after Retinoblastoma: Radiation dose and sarcoma risk. JAMA 278: 1262–1267, 1997.

95. GENE THERAPY

Austin L. Spitzer, B.A., and William E. Lee, M.D.

1. What is gene therapy?

Gene therapy is the transfer of foreign genetic material into an individual's cells to alter the course of disease. The process involves the replacement of absent or defective genes, the introduction of toxin genes to induce cellular death, or the insertion of genes to stimulate or enhance the immune response.

2. Name and describe the two routes of gene delivery.

1. The ex vivo approach removes cells from the individual, genetically modifies them, and then reinfuses the altered cells into the patient.

2. The in vivo approach directly places the genetic material into the affected tissue (in situ) or systemically introduces the genetic material into the individual.

3. What are the mechanisms for delivering the genetic material?

Early laboratory methods relied on cell engulfment of DNA precipitates or altered cellular membranes with the use of electrical current to facilitate DNA transfer. Although successful, the method was not highly efficient and is not applicable for use in vivo. Subsequently, techniques to increase the efficiency of gene delivery, integration, and expression were developed. Mechanical methods include direct nucleic acid injection or particle-mediated bombardment of target tissue. More recent strategies have focused on enveloping nucleic acids within lipids to form liposomes or using viral particles as vehicles for transfer of genetic material.

4. What are the common nonviral strategies of gene delivery?

The nonviral approaches are direct naked DNA injections, liposomes (nucleic acids conjugated with polycationic lipids that facilitate cell entry), and particle-mediated gene transfer. Particle-mediated transfer is the firing of DNA-covered gold or tungsten particles with a "gene gun" into target tissue. Nonviral methods are not limited by the size of the genetic material to be transferred and are less immunogenic because of their lack of protein. However, they deliver and express the genetic material poorly in vivo.

5. Why are viruses the most common gene therapy delivery vehicles (vectors)?

Viruses are considered ideal vectors because they have evolved to transfer genetic material into a host's cell. The engineered viruses are not pathogenic because they are void of the necessary components for replication. The vectors are produced from packaging cell lines that provide all the essential elements for synthesis of viral particles that contain the therapeutic gene. Based on the clinical trials to date, concerns of production of recombinant wild-type virus and insertional mutagenesis appear to be unfounded.

6. List the advantages and disadvantages of the common viral vectors for gene transfer.

Advantages and Disadvantages of the Common Viral Vectors for Gene Transfer

VECTOR	ADVANTAGES	DISADVANTAGES
Adenovirus	High-efficiency gene transfer. Targets minority of cells, dividing and nondividing. High titers.	Nonspecific gene transfer. Sometimes elicits inflammatory response result. Immunity from prior exposures may limit clinical usefulness.
Adeno-associated virus	Targets dividing and many nondividing cells. Long duration of action in vivo.	Smaller genome limits size of gene transfer.
Lentivirus	Gene transfer to both dividing and nondividing cells. Integration into host DNA.	Concern that recombination may produce pathogenic virus. Random integration.
Retrovirus	Capable of producing long-term gene transfer. Integration into host DNA	Requires target cells that are dividing. Random integration. Low titers.

7. Which candidate genes are currently used in cancer gene therapy protocols?

1. Immunotherapy genes that express HLA-B7 or interleukins can augment immune responses against the transduced cancer cells.

2. Toxin genes that induce cell death when expressed.

3. Wild-type tumor suppressor genes can restore the normal function of the mutated gene in the cancer cells, leading to cell death.

4. Chemoprotection genes, such as the multidrug resistance gene, may protect hematopoietic cells against chemotherapy-induced myelosuppression.

5. Antisense genes and ribozymes are used to neutralize the expression of oncogenes.

8. Explain the bystander effect.

The bystander effect is cell toxicity within the direct vicinity of cells expressing an introduced toxin gene. Herpes simplex virus thymidine kinase (HSVtk) can render a cancer cell susceptible to killing by the antiviral agent ganciclovir. HSVtk in eukaryotic cells phosphorylates ganciclovir, which disrupts the cell's normal DNA synthesis and results in cell death. Furthermore, in some tissues neighboring cells that have not been transduced with HSVtk also are susceptible to the effects of ganciclovir. The bystander effect is speculated to occur through intercellular communications.

9. What challenges are common to all gene therapy protocols?

Gene transfer and expression, regulation, and safety concerns are pertinent to all current strategies.

10. When did the first clinical gene therapy trials occur and what did they demonstrate?

In 1989, a gene-marking study was initiated in which the *Escherichia coli* gene for neomycin resistance was successfully transferred into extracted tumor-infiltrating lymphocytes of patients with advanced cancer. The study demonstrated the safety of foreign gene transfer and the ability to identify cells that had been reintroduced with marker genes.

In 1990, a therapeutic trial was initiated involving retroviral-mediated transfer of the adenosine deaminase (ADA) gene into the autologous T lymphocytes of two girls with ADA deficiency. The transfer apparently improved their clinical condition, but interpretation was complicated because PEG (polyethylene glycol)-ADA therapy also had to be continued.

11. What contribution to bone marrow transplantation did marker gene transfer studies make?

In one study, bone marrow grafts from cancer patients were marked with the *E. coli* neomycin-resistance gene and reinfused. The marker gene was found in the recurrent tumors, which demonstrated that unpurged autologous bone marrow contained tumor cells that contribute to relapse.

12. To what medical problem are most gene therapy protocols directed?

The majority of clinical protocols are directed at the treatment of cancer. Currently, retroviral vectors are used in most strategies based on their efficiency of transfer and level of expression. Immunotherapy and toxin genes are being used in a variety of tumor types, including brain, melanoma, and ovarian.

BIBLIOGRAPHY

1. Anderson WF: Human gene therapy. Nature 392(supp):25–30, 1998.
2. Blaese RM, Culver KW, Miller AD, et al: T Lymphocyte-directed gene therapy for ADA-SCID: Initial trial results after 4 years. Science 270:475–480, 1995.
3. Brenner MK, Rill DR, Moen RC, et al: Gene-marking to trace origin of relapse after autologous bone-marrow transplantation. Lancet 341:85–86, 1993.
4. Culver KW, Ram Z, Walbridge S, et al: In vivo gene transfer with retroviral vector producer cells for treatment of experimental brain tumors. Science 256:1550–1552, 1992.
5. Kay MA, Liu D, Hoogerbrugge PM: Gene therapy. Proc Natl Acad Sci USA 94:12744–12746, 1997.
6. Ross G, Erickson R, Knorr D, et al: Gene therapy in the United States: A five-year status report. Hum Gen Ther 7:1781–1790, 1996.
7. Verma IM, Somia N: Gene therapy—Promises, problems and prospects. Nature 389:239–242, 1997.

INDEX

Page numbers in **boldface type** indicate complete chapters.